D1810626

OSTERGARD'S
Urogynecology
and Pelvic Floor
Dysfunction
SIXTH EDITION

SIXTH EDITION

OSTERGARD'S Urogynecology and Pelvic Floor Dysfunction

Editors

Alfred E. Bent, MD
Professor
Department of Obstetrics and Gynaecology
Dalhousie University School of Medicine
Head, Division of Gynaecology
Izaak Walton Killam Health Centre
Halifax, Nova Scotia, Canada

Geoffrey W. Cundiff, MD
Professor
Department of Obstetrics and Gynaecology
University of British Columbia
Vancouver, British Columbia
Head,
Department of Obstetrics and Gynaecology
Providence Health Care
Vancouver, British Columbia, Canada

Steven E. Swift, MD
Professor
Department of Obstetrics and Gynecology
Medical University of South Carolina
Charleston, South Carolina

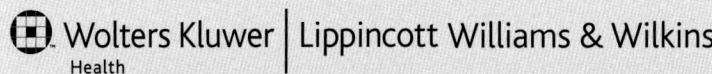

Wolters Kluwer | Lippincott Williams & Wilkins
Health

Philadelphia · Baltimore · New York · London
Buenos Aires · Hong Kong · Sydney · Tokyo

Acquisitions Editor: Sonya Seigafuse
Managing Editor: Ryan Shaw
Marketing Manager: Kimberly Schonberger
Senior Manufacturing Manager: Ben Rivera
Project Manager: Nicole Walz
Art Director: Risa Clow
Cover Designer: Melissa Walter
Production Services: Maryland Composition

Copyright © 2008 by Lippincott Williams & Wilkins, a Wolters Kluwer business

Copyright © 2003 by Lippincott Williams & Wilkins. Copyright © 1996, 1991, 1985, and 1980 by Williams & Wilkins, under the title *Urogynecology and Urodynamics: Theory and Practice*.

530 Walnut Street
Philadelphia, PA 19106

All rights reserved. This book is protected by copyright. No part of this book may be reproduced in any form or by any means, including photocopying, or utilizing by any information storage and retrieval system without written permission from the copyright owner, except for brief quotations embodied in critical articles and reviews. To request permission, please contact Lippincott Williams & Wilkins at 530 Walnut Street, Philadelphia, PA 19016, via email at permissions@lww.com or via our website at lww.com (products and services).

Printed in the United States of America

Library of Congress Cataloging-in-Publication Data
Ostergard's urogynecology and pelvic floor dysfunction. — 6th ed. / editors, Alfred E. Bent, Geoffrey W. Cundiff, Steven E. Swift.
p. ; cm.
Includes bibliographical references and index.
ISBN-13: 978-0-7817-7095-8
ISBN-10: 0-7817-7095-5
1. Urogynecology. 2. Urodynamics. 3. Pelvic floor—Pathophysiology. I. Ostergard, Donald R., 1938- II. Bent, Alfred E. III. Cundiff, Geoffrey W. IV. Swift, Steven E. V. Title: Urogynecology and pelvic floor dysfunction.
[DNLM: 1. Female Urogenital Diseases. 2. Genital Diseases, Female. 3. Pelvic Floor—physiopathology. 4. Prolapse. 5. Urinary Incontinence. WJ 190 O85 2007]
RG484.U76 2007
616.6—dc22   2007012309

Care has been taken to confirm the accuracy of the information presented and to describe generally accepted practices. However, the authors, editors, and publisher are not responsible for errors or omissions or for any consequences from application of the information in this book and make no warranty, expressed or implied, with respect to the currency, completeness, or accuracy of the contents of the publication. Application of this information in a particular situation remains the professional responsibility of the practitioner; the clinical treatments described and recommended may not be considered absolute and universal recommendations.

The authors, editors, and publisher have exerted every effort to ensure that drug selection and dosage set forth in this text are in accordance with current recommendations and practice at the time of publication. However, in view of ongoing research, changes in government regulations, and the constant flow of information relating to drug therapy and drug reactions, the reader is urged to check the package insert for each drug for any change in indications and dosage and for added warnings and precautions. This is particularly important when the recommended agent is a new or infrequently employed drug.

Some drugs and medical devices presented in this publication have Food and Drug Administration (FDA) clearance for limited use in restricted research settings. It is the responsibility of health care providers to ascertain the FDA status of each drug or device planned for use in their clinical practice.

The publishers have made every effort to trace copyright holders for borrowed material. If they have inadvertently overlooked any, they will be pleased to make the necessary arrangements at the first opportunity.

To purchase additional copies of this book, call our customer service department at (800) 638-3030 or fax orders to 1-301-223-2400. Lippincott Williams & Wilkins customer service representatives are available from 8:30 am to 6:00 pm, EST, Monday through Friday, for telephone access. Visit Lippincott Williams & Wilkins on the Internet: http://www.lww.com.

10 9 8 7 6 5 4 3 2 1

I wish to dedicate this edition to our son, Nathaniel Jon Bent, better known as Nate. He has always provided that joy to parents that we wish for, and we proudly reflect on times from infancy through childhood, adolescence, college youth, and now young adult. His kindness, understanding, and interpersonal skills fit well with his chosen profession in dentistry. I acknowledge the continued support from my wife, Callie, and her dedication to the men in her life.

-Alfred E. Bent

I have benefited from so many mentors in my life, but wish to dedicate this edition to my first mentors, my parents, Edward and Margaret Cundiff. My interest in academics undoubtedly sprang from growing up in a home with two professors. I will miss their optimism, their joy for life, and their endless pursuit of truth, but will continue to benefit from their influence for all of my life to come.

-Geoffrey W. Cundiff

I would like to dedicate this edition to those who are most important to me: my God, my wife Alisa, and my children Dylan, Brooks, and Taylor. In addition, I would like to thank my mentors, Robert Kirk, MD, and Donald Ostergard, MD, who took my interest in urogynecology and helped me turn it into a career.

-Steven E. Swift

Contents

SECTION I:
Normal Pelvic Floor and Outcome Assessment

SECTION II:
Disorders of Lower Urinary Tract

SECTION III:
Disorders of Anus and Rectum

SECTION IV:
Disorders of Pelvic Support

SECTION V:
Appendices

Contributing Authors

Karen Abraham, PT, PhD, OCS
Associate Professor
Division of Physical Therapy
Shenandoah University
Winchester Rehabilitation Center
Winchester, Virginia

Olugbenga A. Adekanmi, MRCOG
Department of Obstetrics and Gynecology
York Hospital
York, United Kingdom

Matthew D. Barber, MD, MHS
Associate Professor of Surgery
Department of Obstetrics and Gynecology
Glickman Urologic Institute
Section of Urogynecology and Pelvic
    Reconstructive Surgery
Cleveland Clinic
Cleveland, Ohio

Alfred E. Bent, MD
Professor of Obstetrics and Gynecology
Dalhousie University
Head, Division of Gynecology
IWK Health Centre
Halifax, Nova Scotia, Canada

Joan L. Blomquist, MD
Clinical Instructor
Johns Hopkins University
Fellowship Director
Division of Female Pelvic Surgery and
    Reconstructive Pelvic Surgery
Greater Baltimore Medical Center
Baltimore, Maryland

Toby C. Chai, MD, FACS
Associate Professor of Surgery
Division of Urology
University of Maryland School of Medicine
Baltimore, Maryland

Ralph R. Chesson, Jr., MD
Jack A. Andonie Professor of Gynecologic
    Surgery
Professor of Obstetrics and Gynecology
Section of Female Pelvic Medicine and
    Reconstructive Surgery
Louisiana State University Health Sciences
    Center
New Orleans, Louisiana

Geoffrey W. Cundiff, MD, FACOG, FACS
Professor of Obstetrics and Gynecology
University of British Columbia
Head, Department of Obstetrics and
    Gynecology
Providence Health Care
Vancouver, British Columbia, Canada

G. Willy Davila, MD
Chairman, Department of Gynecology
Head, Section of Urogynecology and
    Reconstructive Pelvic Surgery
Cleveland Clinic Florida
Weston, Florida

R. Mark Ellerkmann, MD
Department of Gynecology and Obstetrics
Johns Hopkins Medicine
Division of Urogynecology, Department of
    Gynecology
Greater Baltimore Medical Center
Baltimore, Maryland

Matthew Fagan, MD
Urogynecology Associates of Philadelphia
Philadelphia, Pennsylvania

Melissa C. Fischer, MD
Fellow in Female Pelvic Medicine and
    Reconstructive Surgery
New York University School of Medicine
New York, New York

Robert M. Freeman, MD, FRCOG
Directorate of Obstetrics and Gynecology
Urogynecology Unit
Derriford Hospital
Plymouth, Devon, United Kingdom

Robert E. Gutman, MD
Johns Hopkins Hospital
Baltimore, Maryland

Gopal N. Gupta, MD
University of Maryland School of
    Medicine
Baltimore, Maryland

Victoria L. Handa, MD
Johns Hopkins University
Johns Hopkins Bayview Medical Campus
Baltimore, Maryland

Okechukwu A. Ibeanu, MD
Urogynecology Fellow
Division of Urogynecology and Female Pelvic
   Reconstructive Surgery
Department of Obstetrics and Gynecology
Louisiana State University School of Medicine
New Orleans, Louisiana

Marjorie Jean-Michel, MD
Clinical Fellow
Urogynecology and Reconstructive Pelvic
   Surgery
Cleveland Clinic Florida
Weston, Florida

Scott M. Kambiss, DO, FACOG
Assistant Professor of Obstetrics and Gynecology
Uniformed Services University of Health
Fellow, Female Pelvic Reconstructive Surgery
University of Massachusetts Memorial
Worcester, Massachusetts

Mickey M. Karram, MD
MD Good Samaritan Hospital Seton Center
Cincinnati, Ohio

Kathleen C. Kobashi, MD
Clinical Associate Professor
University of Washington
Co-Director, Continence Center
Section of Urology and Renal Transplantation
Virginia Mason Medical Center
Seattle, Washington

Richard P. Marvel, MD
Assistant Professor of Obstetrics and Gynecology
Johns Hopkins School of Medicine
Medical Staff
Greater Baltimore Medical Center
Johns Hopkins Medical Institutes
Board of Directors, International Pelvic Pain
   Society
Towson, Maryland

Mary T. McLennan, MD, FACOG
Associate Professor of Obstetrics, Gynecology,
   and Women's Health
St. Louis University
St. Louis, Missouri

Jennifer Mile-Thomas, MD
James Buchanan Brady Urological Institute
Johns Hopkins Medicine
Baltimore, Maryland

Joseph M. Montella, MD
Associate Professor of Obstetrics and
   Gynecology
Jefferson Medical College
Director, Division of Urogynecology
Jefferson University Hospital
Philadelphia, Pennsylvania

Mikio A. Nihira, MD, MPH
Associate Professor of Obstetrics and
   Gynecology
Division of Female Pelvic Medicine and
   Reconstructive Surgery
University of Oklahoma Health Sciences Center
Fellow, American College of Obstetrics and
   Gynecology
Fellow, American College of Surgeons
Oklahoma City, Oklahoma

Victor W. Nitti, MD, FACS
Professor and Vice Chairman
Department of Urology
New York University School of Medicine
New York, New York

David D. Rahn, MD
University of Texas Southwestern Medical Center
Dallas, Texas

Holly E. Richter, PhD, MD
Professor and Division Director
Department of Obstetrics and Gynecology
Women's Pelvic Medicine and Reconstructive
   Surgery
University of Alabama at Birmingham
Birmingham, Alabama

Joseph Schaffer, MD
Professor of Obstetrics and Gynecology
Chief of Gynecology and Urogynecology
University of Texas Southwestern Medical Center
Dallas, Texas

Laura Scheufele, BScPT, BCIA-PMDB
Johns Hopkins Bayview Medical Center
Baltimore, Maryland

Sam Siddighi, MD
Department of Obstetrics and Gynecology
University of Cincinnati
Division of Urogynecology, Reconstructive
   Pelvic Surgery
Good Samaritan Hospital
Cincinnati, Ohio

Steven E. Swift, MD
Associate Professor of Obstetrics and
  Gynecology
Medical University of South Carolina
Charleston, South Carolina

Marc R. Toglia, MD
Assistant Professor of Obstetrics and Gynecology
Thomas Jefferson School of Medicine
Director, Division of Urogynecology
Mainline Hospital System
Philadelphia, Pennsylvania

Thomas L. Wheeler, II, MD
Instructor/Fellow in Obstetrics and Gynecology
Women's Pelvic Medicine and Reconstructive
  Surgery
University of Alabama at Birmingham
Birmingham, Alabama

Cecilia K. Wieslander, MD
Department of Obstetrics and Gynecology
Division of Urogynecology and Reconstructive
  Surgery
University of Texas Southwestern Medical Center
Parkland Memorial Hospital
St. Paul University Hospital
Dallas, Texas

Patrick J. Woodman, DO, FACOOG, FACS
Assistant Clinical Professor Obstetrics and
  Gynecology
Indiana University School of Medicine
Methodist Hospital/Clarian Health Partners
Indianapolis, Indiana

E. James Wright, MD
Assistant Professor
Johns Hopkins Medical Institutions
Director of Neurology
Chief of Urology
Johns Hopkins Bayview Medical Center
Baltimore, Maryland

Brian S. Yamada, MD
Virginia Mason Medical Center
Seattle, Washington

Stephen B. Young, MD
Professor of Obstetrics and Gynecology
University of Massachusetts Medical School
Chief, Division of Urogynecology and
  Reconstructive Pelvic Surgery
University of Massachusetts Memorial Medical
  Center
Worcester, Massachusetts

Foreword

by Donald R. Ostergard, MD, FACOG

The first edition of *Ostergard's Urogynecology and Pelvic Floor Dysfunction* was the product of a series of postgraduate courses in urogynecology with speakers who were leaders in the fledgling field at that time. Up to that point, there was no formality of any kind in this discipline. These lectures were taped and transcribed. After translation of the spoken word into printed word, the chapter was returned to the authors who further edited the chapters and supplied the illustrations. At that time, the clinician felt that the anterior vaginal repair was the best way to treat stress incontinence and a chapter was devoted to a comparison of that technique with the retropubic approach. There was no mention of paravaginal defects or grafts and meshes for augmentation of prolapse and incontinence repairs. The anatomy of the bladder and urethra was poorly understood and urodynamics was just coming into being. The measurements of pressures within the bladder and urethra initially utilized a spinal manometer with an open ended catheter which was gradually replaced by microtransducer recording devices and physiological recorders. Data collection from the tracings was labor-intensive, requiring calipers to measure distances that were then translated to closure pressure or functional length. Subtracted channels facilitated the search for detrusor instability now known as detrusor overactivity. Computers for automatic computations did not exist.

In the mid-1960s, Dr. Jack Robertson did his early work with the urethroscope utilizing carbon dioxide for visualization and for cystometry and, through his publications, called attention to this scientifically neglected component of gynecology and urology (1). An Incontinence Clinic was established at Harbor/UCLA Medical Center where I was a resident at the time and we put this new objective approach to the incontinent patient to work in caring for our patients with good success. Prior to this time the clinical history of stress incontinence was the only preoperative evaluation required and was an automatic ticket to the operating room for an anterior repair. At this time the scientific literature was sparse and consisted of isolated bits of information scattered in a plethora of medical journals with only a few people who would be considered experts existing throughout the world and only about five academic centers pursuing research. The field was in need of organization, collation, and research collaboration and dissemination of what was known at the time. The International Continence Society was founded in 1971 in Europe primarily by urologists, physiologists, and medical engineers with very few gynecologists participating and represented the only group that met to exchange information.

The premier sites in female incontinence research included academic centers in Oslo, Norway, with Drs. Torkel Rud and Mogens Asmussen; Uppsala, Sweden, with Drs. Ulf Ulmsten and Axel Ingleman-Sundberg; London, England, with Mr. Stuart Stanton; and San Francisco, California, with Dr. Emil Tanagho. Each of them was developing urodynamic techniques in different ways. In Scandinavia, the microtransducer catheter was being used for the first time; in England, videocystourethrography was in development; and, in California, urodynamics were performed with fluid-charged double balloon catheters and the use of a Beckman physiological recorder. In 1976, our Incontinence Clinic was enhanced with urodynamics utilizing the Beckman physiological recorder and microtransducer catheters. Micro calipers and other instruments were used to manually measure all cystometric events, urethral pressure profiles (functional length, closure pressure, and area under the curve), and electromyographic activity. We were fortunate that this recorder could subtract pressures to give closure pressure curves and, more importantly, detrusor pressures. It soon became evident that urodynamic study had application to the routine care of incontinent patients and that dissemination of this information, along with formation of an academic research base in this new field, was very important, so I started the first Fellowship Program in Urogynecology in 1977. My first fellow soon left to practice general obstetrics and gynecology. In 1978, Dr. Tom McCarthy became the first full-time fellow in the field. He currently practices in Santa Maria, California.

In 1976 about 25 of us, at the direction of Dr. Axel Ingleman-Sundberg from Sweden, formed the International Urogynecological Association at the FIGO meeting in Mexico City. Due to the interest in physicians attending our postgraduate courses in the United States, five of us founded the American Urogynecologic Society in 1979: President, Dr. Jack Robertson; Secretary-Treasurer, myself; Drs. Finis Wiggins and Fred Jansen; and Dr. Earl Fuller who was the editor of the first newsletter with his wife, an attorney, drawing up the formal papers. The first meeting in 1980 had about 60 physicians from all over the world in attendance with no exhibits. This was the year the first edition of this textbook was published.

Tremendous change in this field has occurred in the interim—not only with dedicated computers to analyze and record urodynamic data, but with digitization of urodynamic and radiological studies which have greatly enhanced our abilities to gather and store data and also to care for our patients now having evidence-based medicine to back up our clinical practice.

It is somewhat disturbing, however, to see that in spite of the efforts of many investigators, evidence-based medicine is being neglected when new surgical procedures and diagnostic techniques are introduced by industry. Prior to the early 1990s, new surgical procedures carried the names of the physicians who studied them and published their results. Now new procedures carry names adopted by industry and one is being billed as "revolutionary." There are intensive medical marketing campaigns with no controlled clinical trials to back up these claims. New meshes and grafts are being introduced at a blinding rate, mostly in response to the complications that develop in response to the utilization of these untested products. Most unfortunately, patient safety in the performance of the procedures as described by industry is often neglected. For example, Pereyra taught us in the 1970s to protect the bladder and bowel during the performance of a needle procedure for incontinence by placing a finger into the retropubic space up to the undersurface of the rectus muscle to minimize the possibility of placing the needle transperitoneally or into the bladder (2). Stamey emphasized cystoscopy to further evaluate for bladder penetration (3). None of the procedures currently marketed include Pereyra's teachings and newer procedures are minimizing the need to perform cystoscopy. Many patients have died as a result of bowel injury after the performance of newer procedures (4).

The United States Food and Drug Administration (FDA) has not approved these new surgical procedures, only the mesh or graft and the instruments to perform the procedure that are included in the kit for sale carry this level of approval. For example, the FDA approves the mesh based on the claim that this material is substantially equivalent to something that the FDA has previously approved. As a case in point, when pressure injected bovine collagen was approved by the FDA as ProteGen® its predicate was accepted. No papers were ever published regarding the efficacy or level of adverse events associated with this product that accompanied the first surgical procedure for incontinence for sale by industry. When the high level of adverse events was recognized, which included urethrovaginal fistulae (5), it was withdrawn from the market and the FDA then said that obviously the product was adulterated and misbranded and agreed with the recall. Of interest is the fact the mesh used in the transvaginal tape procedure used ProteGen® as its predicate and most of the subsequently approved polypropylene meshes follow forming the lower parts of a pyramid with a withdrawn product at the apex.

Only the transvaginal tape procedure currently sold for incontinence has been subjected to a controlled clinical trial against the Burch procedure, albeit with a different mesh configuration than is used in the United States today (6). If the physician who utilizes these meshes today does not have sufficient information on efficacy for the specific procedure in comparison to a gold standard, how can that physician obtain informed consent from the patient for the performance of the procedure? In a controlled clinical trial one graft was shown to deteriorate rather than enhance the efficacy of standard posterior vaginal repair and another sling material to result in an unacceptably low success rate (7). Neither had a prior publication on efficacy. The American College of Obstetricians and Gynecologists has published on this issue and other editorials or clinical commentaries have appeared questioning the wisdom of using new techniques without the backing of evidence-based medicine (8-13). There are potential ethical, financial, and legal concerns for physicians in this regard. Companies marketing new products and procedures should volunteer controlled clinical trials to back up their marketing claims prior to their use in routine clinical practice. The chapters in this textbook discuss these clinical procedures and graft choices.

We are all very grateful for those individuals who shared in the organized development of this field on a sound scientific basis, conducted research to expand the knowledge base, and who continue to lead in the field. My special thanks go to those who have contributed to all the editions of this textbook to make it what it has become today and especially to Dr. Alfred Bent who has taken the lead for this edition and to his very capable co-editors, Drs. Geoffrey Cundiff and Steven Swift. The bottom line is that as a subspecialty we have made a positive difference in the health care of women and should not succumb to using procedures for sale by industry for which evidence-based medicine does not exist. First, do no harm!

REFERENCES

1. Robertson, JR. Gynecologic urethroscopy. *Am J Obstet Gynec* 1973;115:986.
2. Pereyra AJ, Lebherz TB. Combined urethrovesical suspension and vaginourethroplasty for correction of urinary stress incontinence. *Obstet Gynec* 1967;30:537–546.
3. Stamey TA. Endoscopic suspension of the vesical neck for urinary incontinence in females. Report on 203 consecutive patients. *Ann Surg* 1980;192:465–471.
4. Deng DY, Rutman M, Raz S, et al. Presentation and management of major complications of midurethral slings: Are complications under-reported? *Neurourol Urodyn* 2007;26:46–52.
5. Kobashi KC, Dmochowski R, Mee SL, et al. Erosion of woven polyester pubovaginal sling. *J Urol* 1999;162:2070–2072
6. Ward KL, Hilton P. A prospective multicenter randomized trial of tension-free vaginal tape and colposuspension for primary urodynamic stress incontinence: Two year follow up. *Am J Obstet Gynec* 2004;190:324–331.
7. Owens DC, Winters JC. Pubovaginal sling using DuradermTM graft: Intermediate follow-up and patient satisfaction. *Neurourol Urodyn* 2004;23:115–118.
8. Paraiso MFR, Barber MD, Muir TW, et al. Rectocele repair: A randomized trial of three surgical techniques including graft augmentation. *Am J Obstet Gynec* 2006;108:1589–1596.
9. American College of Obstetricians and Gynecologists, Committee Opinion, Committee on Ethics. Innovative Practice: Ethical Guidelines. *Obstet Gynec* 2006;108:1762–1771.
10. American College of Obstetricians and Gynecologists, Practice Bulletin, Pelvic Organ Prolapse. *Obstet Gynec* 2007; 109:461–473.
11. 2005 IUGA Grafts Roundtable. *Int Urogynecol J* 2006;17:Suppl1.
12 Hilton P. Of porcupines and poodles—A joint challenge to industry and the profession. *Int Urogynecol J* 2007;18:3–11
13. Norton P. New technology in gynecologic surgery: Is new necessarily better? *Obstet Gynec* 2004;190:324–331.
14. Ostergard DR. Lessons from the past: Directions for the future. Do new marketed surgical procedures and grafts produce ethical, personal liability and legal concerns for physicians? *Int Urogyn J* 2007;18: Epub ahead of print.

Preface

A great challenge in any medical field is to maintain skills and current knowledge. Textbook preparation only attempts to fill the gaps in the second challenge, and unfortunately, by the time all is prepared, the material is already partly out of date. While the last edition was only published in 2003, the publishers have determined the need to close the window of decreasing educational value and bring this edition to fruition. I would like the authors of these various chapters to know how much I appreciate their dedication and work in supplying information in a timely fashion, and with a great amount of effort in preparation. It is also of importance to acknowledge the work of prior authors who have paved the way for updated information to be added or substituted for their chapters. Author contributions are what make this book so valuable to all of us, and by introducing new authors for their input on material presented previously, we all benefit from another perspective to understanding the subspecialty and provision of medical care.

New topics in the Sixth Edition include pelvic pain, voiding dysfunction, pathophysiology of pelvic floor disorders as relates to childbirth and aging, and graft materials and sutures. The presentation has been changed considerably in the section on pelvic organ prolapse, with more detailed material including an overview, emphasis on specific compartmental defects in anterior, posterior, and apical support, as well as a section on obliterative procedures. Authors directly involved in providing this kind of treatment have prepared the nonsurgical management. Outcome assessment has provided a good source for various questionnaires and their use.

Medical student, resident, private practitioner, faculty, and even the trained subspecialist in female pelvic medicine should find value in reading this text. We encourage critique and appraisal with appropriate feedback on areas for discussion and improvement.

Normal Pelvic Floor and Outcome Assessment

CHAPTER 1

Anatomy of the Pelvic Viscera

Geoffrey W. Cundiff

BACKGROUND

Value of Surgical Anatomy

As in all surgical specialties, the reconstructive pelvic surgeon is frequently faced with situations that are best addressed by applying a clear understanding of the pertinent anatomy. Ideally, the art of surgery should involve the application of a repertoire of surgical techniques to the given pathology. However, given the phenotypic and pathophysiologic variations that exist in nature, a firm understanding of anatomical variation is paramount to good surgical outcomes. Often, when faced with a challenging case, what separates a great surgeon from an average surgeon is a confidence in the given anatomy that allows for informed actions. In short, anatomical understanding is the foundation of sound surgical technique.

Many of you who read this book are more than reconstructive surgeons. As investigators, the mastery of three-dimensional anatomy provides a framework for understanding the complex pathophysiology of pelvic floor dysfunction. This in turn provides insight that allows us to teach female pelvic medicine and surgery in a meaningful way.

General Considerations

There are a number of factors that make the study of pelvic anatomy particularly challenging. These include gender differences, physical constraints due to a surrounding bony pelvis, and challenging three-dimensional relationships. In this context it is wise to begin our tour of the pelvic anatomy by reviewing some underlying principles. First, all of the pelvic viscera, including the uterus, function primarily as storage units with a secondary role of the timely release of the stored material. The function of the pelvic organs places certain constraints on their physical form. Towards achieving these constraints, the pelvic viscera uniformly comprise a hollow viscus capable of significant distention, as well as a sophisticated closure mechanism. Moreover, the mouth or opening of the viscus is generally well anchored with a three-dimensional tether, while the distensible body of the viscus is relatively mobile to facilitate the increased volume of distention.

ANATOMY OF SUPPORT

Bony Pelvis

In considering the functions of the bony pelvis, the skeletal roles, provision of a supportive base for the osseous framework surrounding the viscera of the thorax, and a stable point of articulation for the lower extremities, should not overshadow the important functions that the bony pelvis provides for the pelvic viscera. These roles become apparent when considering experiments of nature, and phenotypic variation that can have a negative impact on pelvic floor function.

The skeletal anomalies associated with bladder exstrophy offer a dramatic example. Affected women have a wide transverse inlet, shortened anterior posterior pelvic diameter, and absent symphysis pubis. These variations have such an impact on support that nearly 100% of affected women develop pelvic organ prolapse (1). Less severe versions of the skeletal anomalies found in bladder exstrophy are associated with the development of pelvic floor disorders in women without congenital anomalies. Two matched case–control studies showed that women with prolapse and other pelvic floor disorders, when compared to controls, have wider transverse inlets and narrower anterior–posterior diameters (2,3). Even subtle variations in the orientation of the bony pelvis appear to affect function. Loss of lumbar lordosis that results in a less vertically oriented pelvic inlet, for example, is also associated with pelvic organ prolapse (4,5). These morphologic variations may provide a larger hiatus for abdominal pressure transmission. Alternatively, these skeletal variations may predispose women to maternal soft-tissue injury during parturition (2). Recognizing the impact of these morphological variations highlights the central function of the bony pelvis in pelvic support, namely serving as points of attachment for the pelvic floor musculature and connective tissue supports.

The coxal or innominate bones, commonly known as the hip bones, articulate posteriorly with the sacrum at the sacroiliac joints and anteriorly with each other at the pubic symphysis. Developmentally, the coxal bone forms as a fusion of three constituent bones: the ilium superiorly, the ischium inferiorly and posteriorly, and the pubic bone inferiorly and anteriorly. These smaller bones fuse to create the acetabulum and articulate with the paired coxal bone at the pubic symphysis.

Taken together, the coxal bones and sacrum create an angulated cylinder, or stove pipe cavity.

The superior portion is the inlet to the true pelvis, circumscribed by the linea terminalis. It is described by the posterior pubic symphysis, the inner aspects of the superior pubic rami, also known as the arcuate line of the ilium, as well as the alar portions and promontory of the sacrum. In the standing female, this inlet lies in a plane 60 to 65 degrees from the horizontal plane. This pelvic orientation places the anterior iliac spines and pubic tubercule (the anterior edge of the symphysis pubis) in the same vertical plane. Similarly, the anterior border of the greater sciatic foramen is almost vertical in this orientation (Fig. 1.1).

The pelvic outlet is diamond-shaped, with the apices defined by bony landmarks—the symphysis pubis anteriorly, the ischial tuberosities laterally, and the tip of the coccyx posteriorly. The diamond can be further dissected into two triangles, with the anterior triangle defined by the symphysis and two tuberosities and the posterior triangle defined by the coccyx and two tuberosities (Fig. 1.2).

These triangles lie in different planes. In the standing position, the anterior triangle is horizontal, while the posterior triangle is angled posteriorly at approximately 130 degrees. The anterior triangle provides the exit point for the bladder and

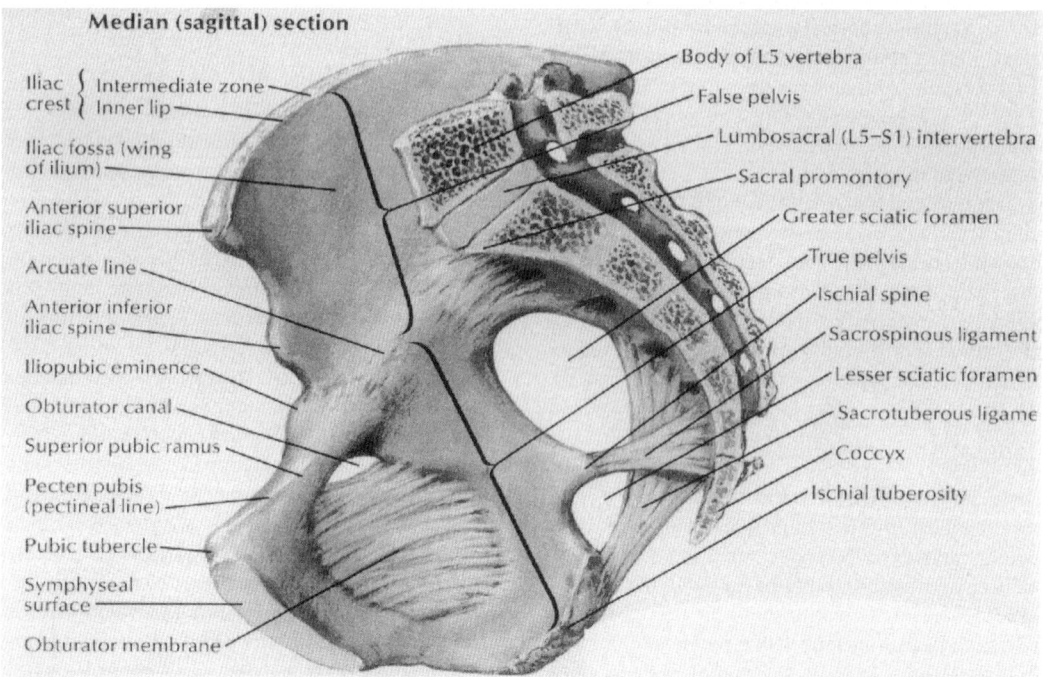

FIGURE 1.1 ●   The bony pelvis and ligaments in sagittal cross-section oriented in anatomical standing position. The anterior iliac spines and pubic tubercle are in the same vertical plane. (From Netter FH. *Atlas of human anatomy*. East Hanover, NJ: Novartis, 1997, Plate 330. Copyright © 1997 Icon Learning Systems, LLC. A subsidiary of MediMedia, USA, Inc. All rights reserved.)

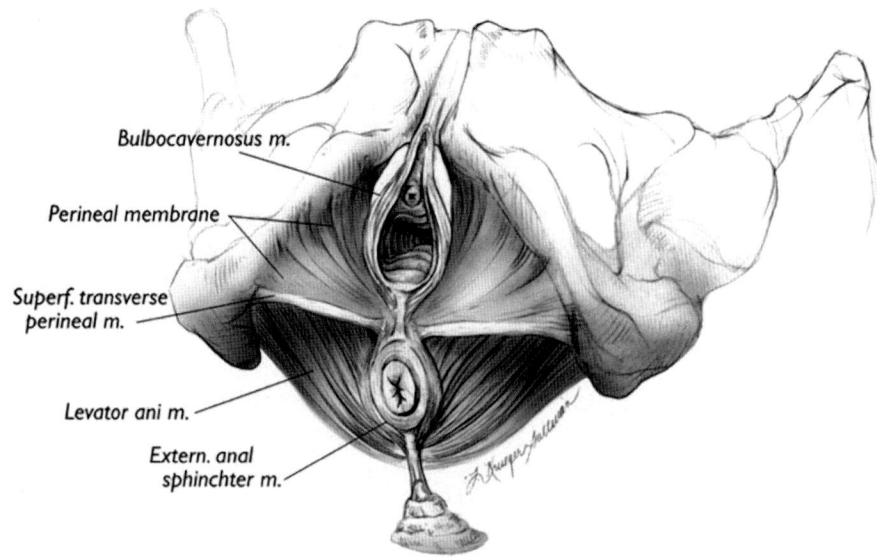

Bulbocavernosus m.

Perineal membrane

Superf. transverse
perineal m.

Levator ani m.

Extern. anal
sphinchter m.

FIGURE 1.2 ● Oblique view of the perineum. Note the diamond shape of the pelvic outlet defined by the symphysis pubis anteriorly, the ischial tuberosities laterally, and the tip of the coccyx posteriorly. The anterior triangle and the posterior triangle that make the diamond lie in different planes. (Reproduced with permission of the artist, Lianne Krueger-Sullivan.)

urethra and is called the urogenital triangle. Similarly, the posterior triangle is the exit point for the anus and is called the anal triangle. The lateral edges of the anteior triangle are the ischiopubic rami, while the lateral edges of the posterior triangle are the sacrotuberous ligaments (see Fig. 1.1). The sacrotuberous ligaments travel medially and superiorly from the ischial tuberosities to the lateral and posterior aspects of the lower half of the sacrum. These ligaments form the posterior border of the pelvic outlet and perineum.

Ischial Spine

The anterior border of the greater sciatic foramen ends in a blunt projection pointing medially, called the ischial spine. In thc standing pelvis, thc ischial spine is about 2 to 3 cm above the level of the pubic crest. This orientation provides an almost horizontal relationship between the posterior aspect of the pubic bone and ischial spine. The sacrospinous ligament travels medially and posteriorly from the ischial spine to the lateral and anterior aspects of the lower portion of the sacrum and the coccyx. Lying superior to the sacrotuberous ligament, this ligament transects the greater sciatic notch, creating the greater and lesser sciatic foramen (see Fig. 1.1).

The greater and lesser sciatic foramen, as well as the obturator foramen, serve as conduits for muscles, vasculature, and nerves that enter and exit the true pelvis. Knowledge of these structures'

spatial relationships helps to avoid surgical injuries. Because the ischial spine is easily palpated, it serves as an excellent surgical reference point, and consequently, a surgeon is well served by a three-dimensional understanding of the anatomy surrounding the ischial spine (Fig. 1.3). This invaluable landmark indicates the normal axis of the vagina, as the arcus tendineus fascia pelvis ends at the spine. The pelvic ureter leaves the sidewall 1 to 2 cm from the spine to pass medially on the pubocervical fascia before entering the inferior bladder wall. The pudendal nerve and vessels exit the pelvis through the greater sciatic foramen only to course beneath the ischial spine and sacrospinous ligament before re-entering the lesser sciatic foramen. The ischial spine is consistently found beneath the intermediate portion of the uterosacral ligament, although its location with respect to the anterior and posterior edges is variable (6).

Obturator Foramen

Recent surgical advances have utilized the obturator membrane and surrounding muscles to anchor implanted grafts. For many pelvic surgeons, this surgical approach is unfamiliar, necessitating the acquisition of new anatomical knowledge of the obturator compartment.

The obturator foramen is a large oval window bounded by the pubic ramus and ischium. The obturator membrane covers this opening. The obtura-

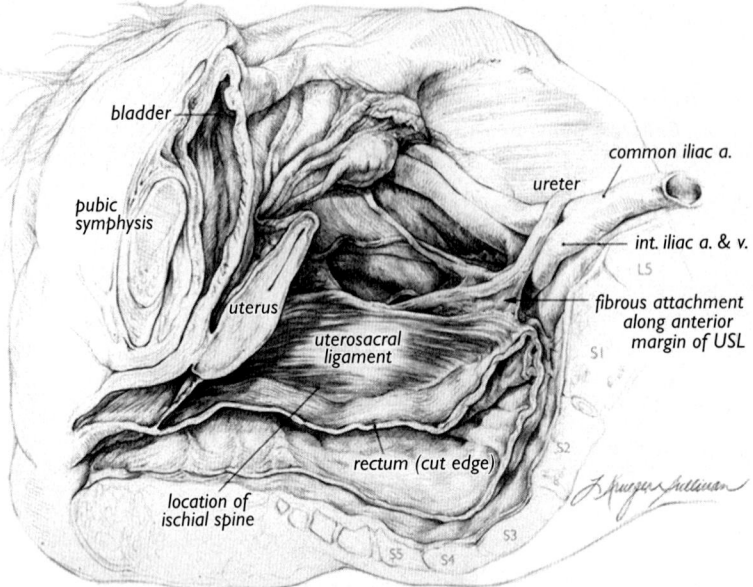

A

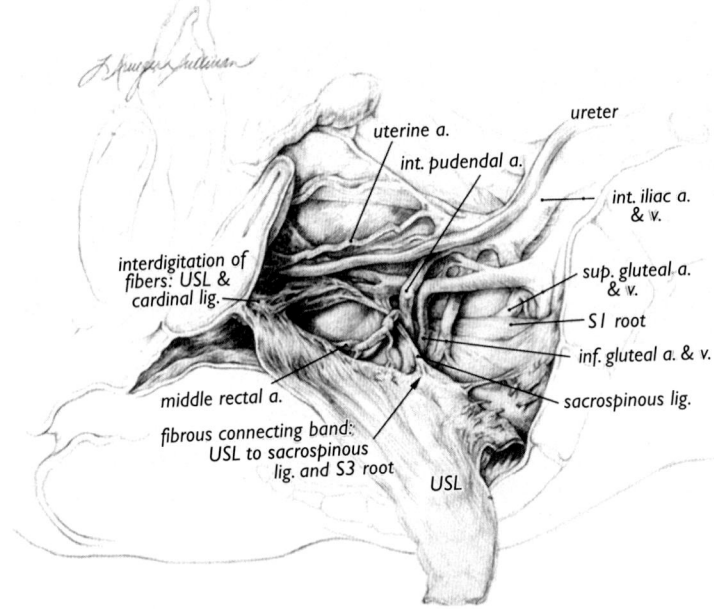

B

FIGURE 1.3 ● **(A)** Sagittal view of the pelvic sidewall illustrating the relationships of the surface anatomy to the ischial spine. **(B)** The uterosacral ligament has been dissected medially to reveal the underlying structures. The ischial spine lies at the end of the visible sacrospinous ligament. (Reproduced with permission of the artist, Lianne Krueger-Sullivan.)

tor internus muscle originates from the entire bony margin of the obturator foramen on the pelvic side of the obturator membrane. This broad origin allows the muscle to compose most of the lateral pelvic sidewall. The tendon of the obturator inter-

nus muscle exits the lesser sciatic foramen on its way to insert onto the greater trochanter, providing for external rotation of the femur. Anteriorly and lateral to the edge of the obturator foramen is a groove in the body of the pubic bone. The obturator membrane's attachment here creates the obturator canal, through which pass the obturator vessels and nerve as they course anteriorly from the posterior aspect of the pelvic sidewall.

The obturator compartment lies on the outside of the obturator membrane. The adductor muscles of the lower extremity find their origin in this region. With the patient in the lithotomy position the adductor muscles originate on the ischiopubic ramus and course along the inner aspect of the thigh. Most superficial, from anterior to posterior, are the adductor longus, gracilis, and adductor magnus. Deep to these muscles are the adductor brevis anteriorly and the obturator externus posteriorly (Fig. 1.4). The adductor muscles are innervated by the obturator nerve, which emerges from the obturator canal between the adductor longus and adductor brevis, and beneath the gracilis. The nerve then bifurcates into anterior and posterior divisions. Some authors have described a similar course for the branches of the obturator artery, although recent cadaver work from Whiteside suggests variable courses for these branches (7). Regardless, the medial aspect of the obturator foramen is relatively safe between the level of the clitoris anteriorly and the anus posteriorly.

Pelvic Floor Musculature

Within the bony pelvis is a basin open at the pelvic inlet but closed beneath, except for the levator hiatus, by a muscular lining composed of the pelvic musculature. Anteriorly, this group of skeletal muscles includes the obturator internus muscles, which originate on the pubic ramus lateral to the symphysis pubis and cross over the inner aspect of the obturator membrane. Posteriorly, the piriformis muscles originate from the anterior and lateral aspects of the sacrum in its middle to upper portion. They then course laterally through the greater sciatic foramen to insert on the greater trochanter beside the obturator internus tendon. Inferiorly, the pelvic diaphragm, a group of paired muscles that include the levator ani and coccygeus muscles, creates the pelvic floor (Fig. 1.5).

The levator ani muscles are subdivided, from medial to lateral, into the puborectalis, pubococcygeus, and iliococcygeus muscles. The puborectalis and pubococcygeus muscles originate from the inner aspect of the pubic rami on either side of the midline at the level of the pubic symphysis. The muscle fibers pass laterally to the vagina and rectum, creating a U-shaped sling surrounding the genital hiatus medially. The muscle fibers of the il-

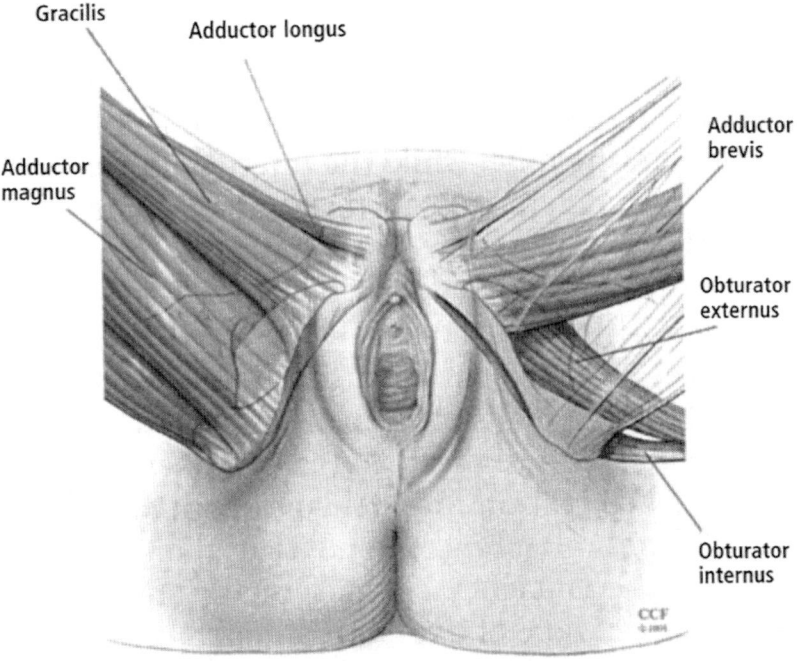

FIGURE 1.4 ● Muscles of the obturator compartment. The superficial muscles are illustrated on the left. On the right, the superficial muscles have been made transparent to allow depiction of the deeper muscles. (From Barber MD. Contemporary views on female pelvic anatomy. *Cleveland Clin J Med* 2005;72:S3–11, with permission.)

iococcygeus muscles pass laterally to the pubococcygeus muscles, fanning out to create the pelvic floor posteriorly and laterally.

The iliococcygeus muscles are unique in their origin from a curvilinear thickening of the parietal fascia overlying the obturator internus muscle known as the arcus tendineus levator ani or muscle white line (see Fig. 1.5). This tendinous muscle origin runs on top of the parietal surface of the obturator internus muscle, from the posterior symphysis pubis to the ischial spines. The iliococcygeus muscles insert on the lower aspect of the lateral sacrum.

The muscles of the pelvic diaphragm are composed of a unique type of striated muscle that contains a majority of type I (slow twitch) muscle fibers that maintain a constant resting tone over time. Each muscle group also contains a smaller proportion of type II (fast twitch) fibers, permitting them to respond quickly during sudden increases in intra-abdominal pressures (8). Contraction of the pelvic diaphragm closes the genital hiatus and provides a horizontal levator plate on which the pelvic viscera lie.

Orientation of the Pelvic Viscera

The urethra, lower vagina, and anus all exit the pelvic outlet via the levator hiatus. The puborectalis and pubococcygeus muscles bound this muscular opening in the pelvic floor. The constant resting tone of the puborectalis and pubococcygeus not only closes the genital hiatus but also pulls the distal vagina and anorectal junction toward the pubic symphysis, creating a near-right angle between the anal and rectal canals. This angle is referred to as the anorectal angle. The posterior deflection is also present in the urethra and vagina. The acuity of the angle results from the opposing forces of the baseline contraction of the pelvic diaphragm, actively pulling anteriorly, countered by the passive force of the posterior connective tissue attachments, which maintain the upper portion of the pelvic viscera deflected posteriorly. This results in consistent anatomical relationships between the vaginal apex, the ischial spines, and the sacrum in women with normal support. A recent study defined these relationships based on magnetic resonance imaging of the pelvis in nulliparous adult females who had a normal gynecologic examination. In the standing female patient, the bladder, the upper two thirds of the vagina, and the rectum lie in a horizontal axis over the muscular levator plate (9). As the vaginal canal courses past the ischial spines toward the sacrum, the posterior fornix or vaginal apex normally lies anterior to S2, about 4 to 5 cm medial, 1 to 2 cm anterior, and 1 to 2 cm superior (cranial) to the ischial spines (10) (Fig. 1.6).

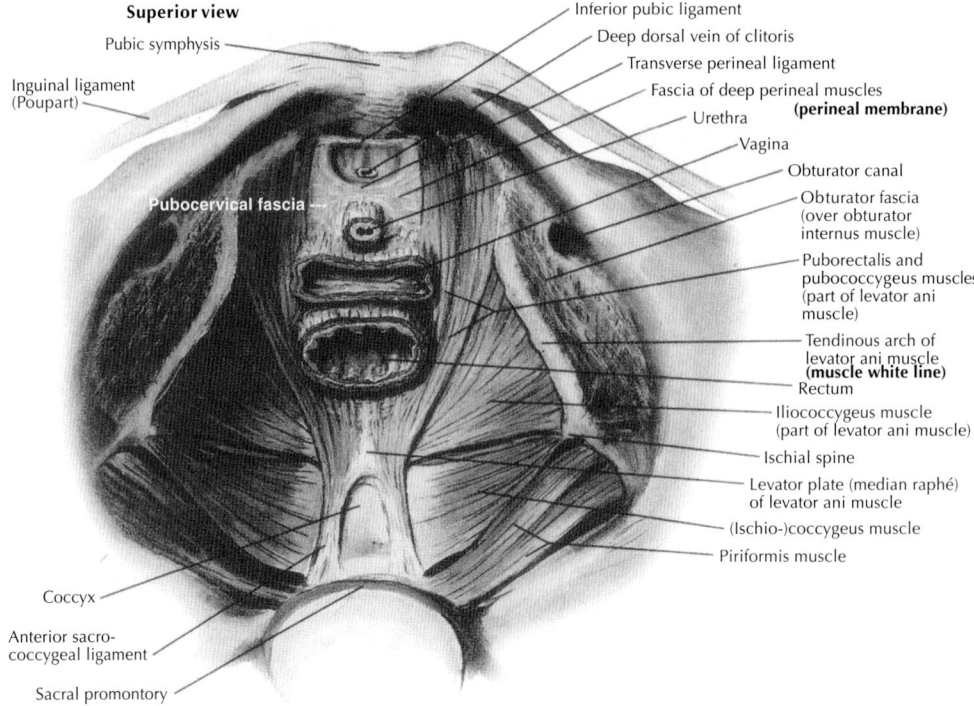

FIGURE 1.5 ● Muscles of the pelvic floor. (From Netter FH. *Atlas of human anatomy.* East Hanover, NJ: Novartis, 1997, Plate 333. Copyright © 1997 Icon Learning Systems, LLC. A subsidiary of MediMedia, USA, Inc. All rights reserved.)

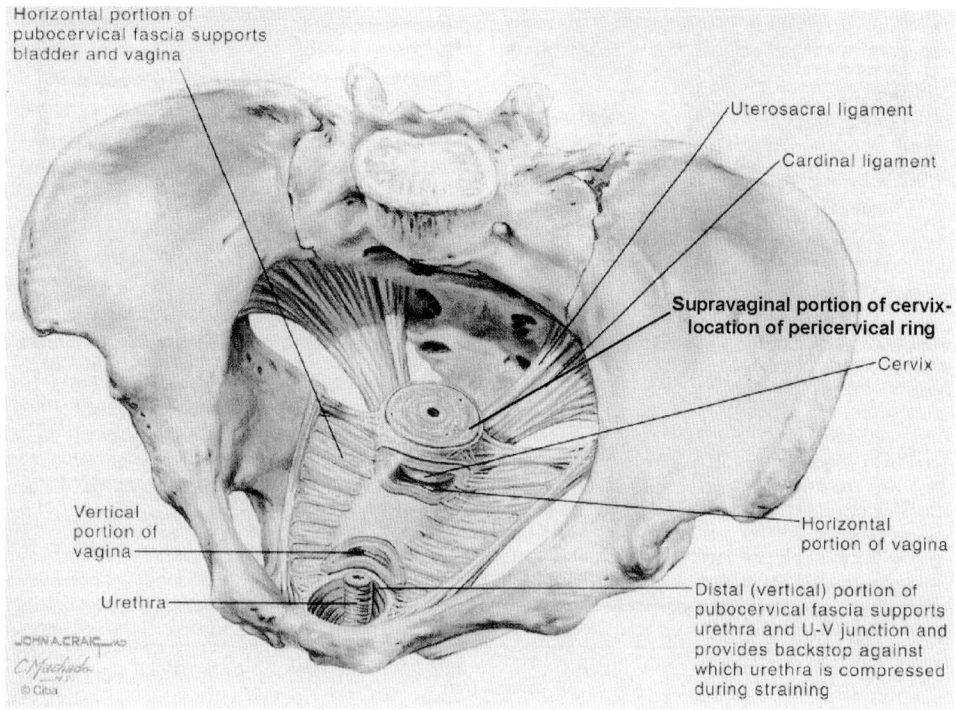

Horizontal portion of pubocervical fascia supports bladder and vagina

Uterosacral ligament

Cardinal ligament

Supravaginal portion of cervix-location of pericervical ring

Cervix

Vertical portion of vagina

Horizontal portion of vagina

Urethra

Distal (vertical) portion of pubocervical fascia supports urethra and U-V junction and provides backstop against which urethra is compressed during straining

FIGURE 1.6 ● Orientation and connective tissue support of the vagina. (From Retzky SS, Rogers RM. Urinary incontinence in women. In: *Clinical symposia*. Summit, NJ: Ciba-Geigy Corp, 1995;47(3), adapted from Plate 3, p. 7. Copyright © 1995 Icon Learning Systems, LLC. A subsidiary of MediMedia, USA, Inc. All rights reserved.)

Connective Tissue Support

The connective tissue support of the pelvis arises from both the parietal fascia covering the pelvic musculature and the visceral fascia investing the pelvic viscera. The visceral fascia surrounds and mechanically supports the pelvic viscera as well as enveloping the supplying vasculature, nerves, and lymph channels. This visceral web runs from the pelvic brim along the upper sidewalls and back wall of the pelvis to the anatomic level of the ischial spine, where the network then proceeds horizontally (in the standing patient) to the obturator internus muscles laterally, and the pubic bones and perineal body inferiorly. This support network is continuous and interdependent within the three-dimensional muscular pelvic basin. Importantly, these visceral connective tissues vary in composition, thickness, strength, and elasticity, depending on the mechanical and physiologic support requirements in each particular location within the network.

The parietal fascia covering the pelvic musculature is a mechanically dense matrix of connective tissue consisting predominantly of collagen fibers coalescing into thick bundles that are then interwoven into a strong, three-dimensional sheet (11). The vascular supply is limited, and active fibroblasts are few in number within this dense connective tissue. In contrast, visceral fascia, also referred to as the endopelvic fascia, is a loose, three-dimensional meshwork of collagen, elastin, and smooth muscle with a richer vascular supply. The term *fascia* is ambiguous as this fibromuscular tissue layer lacks the dense collagen usually associated with the term, but it includes a soft ground substance with different connective tissue cells, including fibroblasts, smooth muscle cells, and elastin in addition to type III collagen, all loosely arrayed to create an elastic fibromuscular layer (11). This meshwork surrounds and peripherally supports the viscera in both the abdominal and pelvic cavities. It is flexible and elastic within limits, as this visceral connective tissue mechanically stretches within limits, but beyond these limits, it breaks.

The endopelvic fascia serves two important roles. The first is the provision of flexible conduits and physical supports for the vasculature, visceral nerves, and lymph tissue that service the viscera. The visceral fascial capsules envelop the bladder, urethra, cervix, vagina, rectum, and anal canal (12). They are intimately attached to the surrounding smooth muscle coat of each viscus. Within these capsules are the vasculature, visceral nerves, lymph nodes and channels, and adipose tissue (areolar tissue). The fascial covering of each hollow viscus provides support during storage, distention, and evacuation.

The second role of the visceral fascia is to suspend the viscera mechanically over the pelvic floor. The horizontal orientation of the pelvic viscera over the pelvic diaphragm creates a flap-valve mechanism that prevents prolapse of the pelvic viscera through the genital hiatus. Increased intra-abdominal pressure, such as with Valsalva straining, generates force perpendicular to the longitudinal axis of the vagina and pelvic viscera, compressing these organs against the simultaneously contracting levator plate.

While the connective tissue support of the pelvis provides a seamless system of meshwork support for the pelvic viscera, the system is more easily comprehended when broken up into constituent parts. DeLancey introduced the concept of dividing the connective tissue support in the pelvis into three levels, with levels I, II, and III representing apical, middle, and distal vaginal support, respectively (13) (Fig. 1.7). Level I support of the paracolpium and parametrium is provided by the cardinal and uterosacral ligaments, which suspend the vaginal vault. Level II is the support of the midvagina, produced by the lateral attachments of the anterior and posterior endopelvic fascia to the pelvic sidewalls. Level III support results from the fusion of these same sheets with the pubic symphysis anteriorly and perineal body posteriorly. Although assigning these levels artificially divides what is actually a continuum of connective tissue in the pelvis, the levels can provide a useful anatomical tool to understand normal support and loss of support at different levels.

The origin of the uterosacral ligament is fanlike at the sacrum, narrowing to its smallest width just proximal to the cervix. Although some texts report the uterosacral ligament to have its origin only from S2-4, anatomical investigations show the uterosacral ligament to be attached broadly to S1, S2, and S3 and variably to S4, with additional attachments to the sacral periosteum and sacrospinous ligament (6,14). This broader attachment disperses the suspensory forces acting on the uterosacral ligament (see Fig. 1.3A).

Campbell identified three distinct histological regions of the uterosacral ligament (14). The superior third, which attaches to the sacrum, is composed of loose strands of connective tissue and intermingled fat, with few vessels, nerves, or lymphatics. The intermediate portion has denser connective tissue with a few scattered smooth muscle fibers, nerve elements, and blood vessels. At the cervical attachment, the uterosacral ligament coalesces into closely packed bundles of smooth muscle with abundant medium-sized and small blood vessels and nerve bundles. The

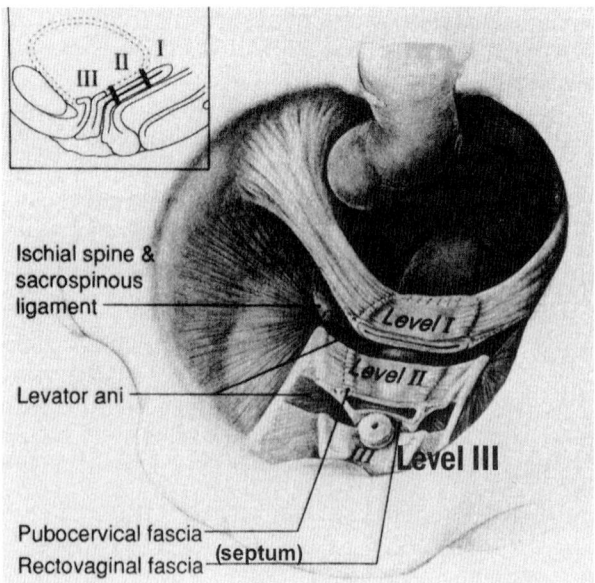

FIGURE 1.7 ● Levels of pelvic support. (From DeLancey JOL. Anatomic aspects of vaginal eversion after hysterectomy. _Am J Obstet Gynecol_ 1992;166:1719, with permission.)

Ischial spine & sacrospinous ligament

Levator ani

Pubocervical fascia

Rectovaginal fascia (septum)

Level I

Level II

Level III

uterosacral ligament is, therefore, densest where it inserts into the paracervical ring. However, the distal uterosacral ligament attachments to the cervix also extend down the posterior lateral aspects of the vagina (6,14). Together these attachments draw the cervix posteriorly towards the hollow of the sacrum (10) (see Fig. 1.6).

This direction is balanced by the lateral tension of the cardinal ligaments. The fan-shaped cardinal ligament creates a sheath that envelops the uterine artery and vein, fusing with the paracervical ring medially. The internal iliac artery courses along this border and helps to establish the cardinal ligament sheath. The fibers of the uterosacral and cardinal ligaments intermingle at the cervical portion to create a smaller, fanlike insertion with fibers extending anteriorly above the internal cervical os and posteriorly down onto the proximal third of the vagina. Together the cardinal and uterosacral ligaments create the paracervical ring of connective tissue surrounding the cervix at the vaginal apex. This is also the attachment for the endopelvic fascia of the anterior and posterior vaginal walls. The cervix, with its surrounding paracervical ring, therefore, acts like the hub of a wheel for the connective tissue support of the vagina (see Fig. 1.6).

There are two prominent lateral connective tissue structures that play a key role in both muscular and connective tissue support of the pelvis: the arcus tendineus levator ani and the arcus tendineus fascia pelvis. Arising as condensations of the parietal fascia of the obturator internus and levator ani muscles, these dense aggregations of connective tissue contain more organized fibrous collagen than the visceral or endopelvic fascia (15). As previously discussed, the arcus tendineus levator ani provides the anchorage for the origin of the levator ani muscles, the iliococcygeus and pubococcygeus muscles. Anteriorly, the arcus tendineus levator ani inserts at the pubic rami and then crosses over the obturator internus muscle to insert posteriorly at the ischial spine (Fig. 1.8).

The arcus tendineus fascia pelvis is a condensation of the parietal fascia of the obturator internus muscle and the visceral fascia enveloping the anterior and posterior vagina. The arcus tendineus fascia pelvis is medial to and runs nearly parallel to the arcus tendineus levator ani. It inserts at the anterior pubic rami, adjacent to the pubic symphysis and slightly anterior to the arcus tendineus levator ani. Posteriorly, the arcus tendineus fascia pelvis joins with the arcus tendineus levator ani to insert at or just above the ischial spine (see Fig. 1.8). The arcus tendineus fascia pelvis provides the lateral anchoring sites for the anterior vaginal wall and posterior vaginal wall.

Anteriorly, the fibromuscular layer of the anterior vaginal wall, known as the pubocervical fascia, bridges the two arcus tendineus fascia pelvi, providing support for the bladder and urethra. The fibromuscular layer of the posterior vaginal wall is also known as Denonvilliers' fascia or the rectovaginal septum. It arises from fusion of the two walls of the embryological peritoneal cul-de-sac (16). This creates a fibromuscular sheet that spans the posterior vaginal wall and coalesces with surrounding structures. Recent histological work demonstrates that this layer is synonymous with the vaginal muscularis of the posterior vaginal wall (17). Superiorly it thins out centrally and attaches to the cervix and the cardinal uterosacral support of the vaginal apex. Laterally the rectovaginal fascia attaches to the pelvic sidewall (18). In the upper vagina the lateral attachment coalesces with the lateral support of the anterior vaginal wall at the arcus tendineus fascia pelvis. The lower half of the rectovaginal fascia fuses with the aponeurosis of the levator ani muscle along a line referred to as the arcus tendineus fascia rectovaginalis (18) (Fig. 1.9). It converges with the arcus tendineus fasciae pelvis at a point approximately midway between the pubic symphysis and the ischial spine to form a Y configuration on the sidewall of the pelvis. The point of convergence of the two lines is at the point along the tube of the vagina where the pelvic floor becomes wider than the vagina. Superior to this point the fascia endopelvina bridges the gap between the vaginal tube and the pelvic sidewall (12) (Fig. 1.10). This web of connective tissue coalesces with the fascia of the obturator internus muscle to create the arcus tendineus fascia pelvis, as well as with extensions of the uterosacral ligaments. The fascia endopelvina in the upper vagina, and separate attachments of the pubocervical fascia and rectovaginal septum posteriorly, result in different cross-sections of the vagina at different levels. The anatomical attachments are reflected on coronal magnetic resonance imaging (MRI) images that show a characteristic H shape to the vaginal lumen distally, as compared with an oval shape superiorly.

Urethral Support

Distally, the pubocervical fascia has fascial and muscular attachments that provide passive and active support of the distal third of the urethra. This is the only portion of the urethra that is fixed to the pubic bone. The passive support sometimes referred to as a hammock of support (19) results from a connective tissue bridging of the pubocervical fascia and its distal lateral attachments, often termed pubourethral ligaments (Fig. 1.11). The

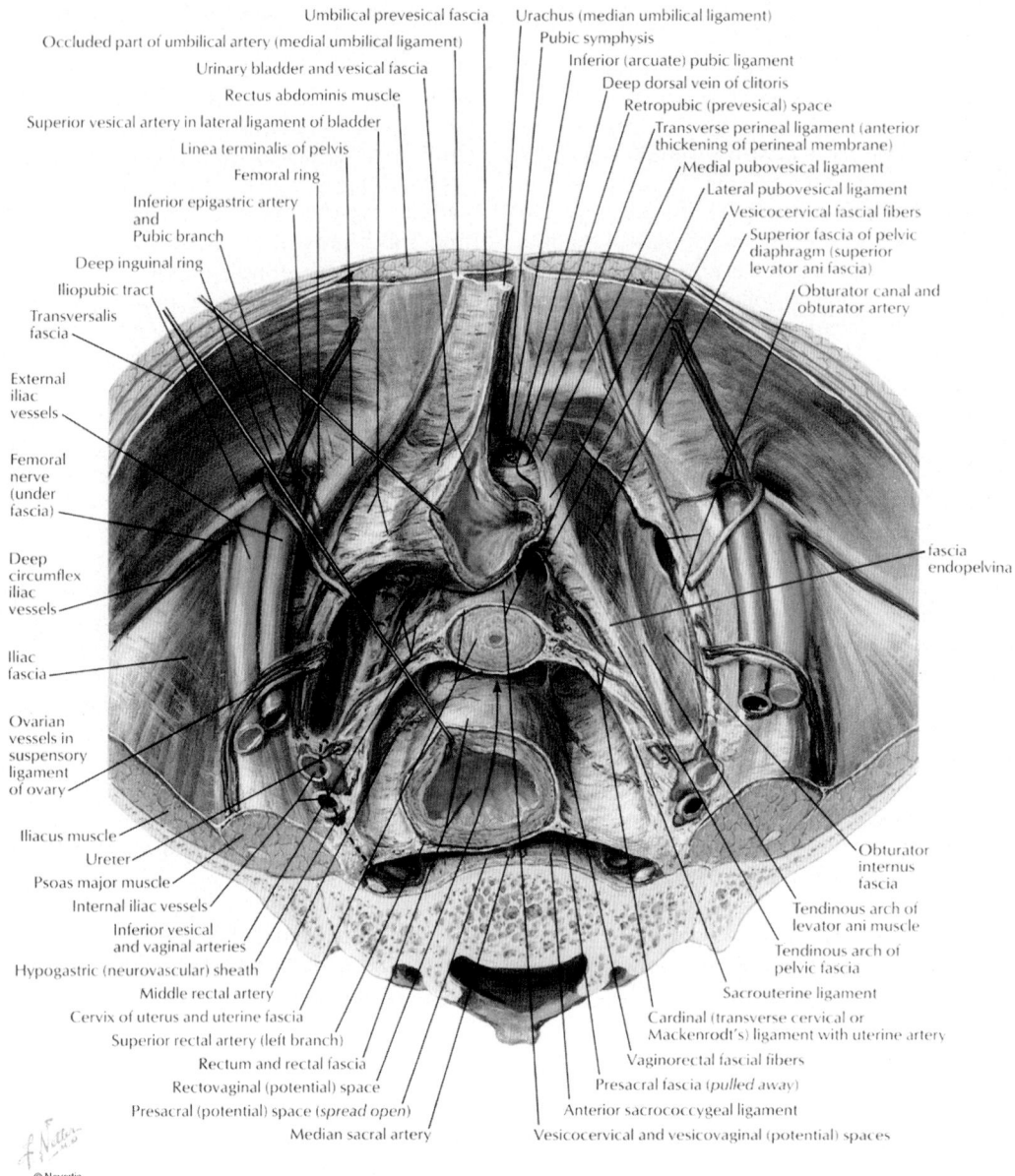

Umbilical prevesical fascia
Occluded part of umbilical artery (medial umbilical ligament)
Urinary bladder and vesical fascia
Rectus abdominis muscle
Superior vesical artery in lateral ligament of bladder
Linea terminalis of pelvis
Femoral ring
Inferior epigastric artery and Pubic branch
Deep inguinal ring
Iliopubic tract
Transversalis fascia
External iliac vessels
Femoral nerve (under fascia)
Deep circumflex iliac vessels
Iliac fascia
Ovarian vessels in suspensory ligament of ovary
Iliacus muscle
Ureter
Psoas major muscle
Internal iliac vessels
Inferior vesical and vaginal arteries
Hypogastric (neurovascular) sheath
Middle rectal artery
Cervix of uterus and uterine fascia
Superior rectal artery (left branch)
Rectum and rectal fascia
Rectovaginal (potential) space
Presacral (potential) space (spread open)
Median sacral artery

Urachus (median umbilical ligament)
Pubic symphysis
Inferior (arcuate) pubic ligament
Deep dorsal vein of clitoris
Retropubic (prevesical) space
Transverse perineal ligament (anterior thickening of perineal membrane)
Medial pubovesical ligament
Lateral pubovesical ligament
Vesicocervical fascial fibers
Superior fascia of pelvic diaphragm (superior levator ani fascia)
Obturator canal and obturator artery
fascia endopelvina
Obturator internus fascia
Tendinous arch of levator ani muscle
Tendinous arch of pelvic fascia
Sacrouterine ligament
Cardinal (transverse cervical or Mackenrodt's) ligament with uterine artery
Vaginorectal fascial fibers
Presacral fascia (pulled away)
Anterior sacrococcygeal ligament
Vesicocervical and vesicovaginal (potential) spaces

© Novartis

FIGURE 1.8 ● Endopelvic fascial sheaths and pelvic musculature. Note the *arcus tendineus levaotor ani* or tendinous arch of the levator ani muscle and the *arcus tendineus fascia pelvis* or tendinous arch of the pelvic fascia. (From Netter FH. *Atlas of human anatomy.* East Hanover, NJ: Novartis, 1997, Plate 341. Copyright © 1997 Icon Learning Systems, LLC. A subsidiary of MediMedia, USA, Inc. All rights reserved.)

active support results from the attachment to the arcus tendineus levator ani. A separate structure, the pubovesical "ligament" or muscle, composed of smooth muscle, extends from the detrusor muscle to the arcus tendineus fascia pelvis and pubic bone (Fig. 1.12). The pubovesical ligament is distinct from the urethral supports and is an extension of the smooth muscle of the detrusor of the blad-

der. It may assist in opening the bladder neck during micturition (20).

Perineum

At its most inferior portion, the rectovaginal septum fuses with the perineal body. The perineal body is a pyramidal structure located between the

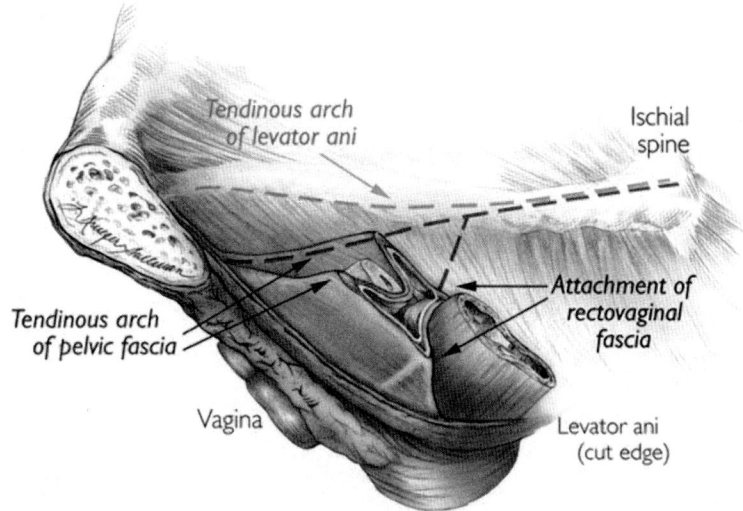

FIGURE 1.9 ● Lateral attachments of the endopelvic fascia to the pelvic sidewall, demonstrating the arcus tendineus fascia rectovaginalis. (Reproduced with permission of the artist, Lianne Krueger-Sullivan.)

vaginal introitus and anus with the base of the pyramid on the perineum (see Fig. 1.2). Much like the hub of a wheel, it is a confluence of the perineal membrane (composed of the bulbocavernosus muscles, superficial transverse perineal muscles, and investing fascia), a portion of the levator ani muscles, the external anal sphincter, and the rectovaginal fascia. Through its attachment to

the cardinal and uterosacral ligaments the rectovaginal septum stabilizes the perineal body, which is essentially suspended from the sacrum. The perineal body is further stabilized through the lateral attachments of the perineal membrane to the ischiopubic rami (21).

The perineal membrane is a sheet of connective tissue consisting primarily of fibrous connective

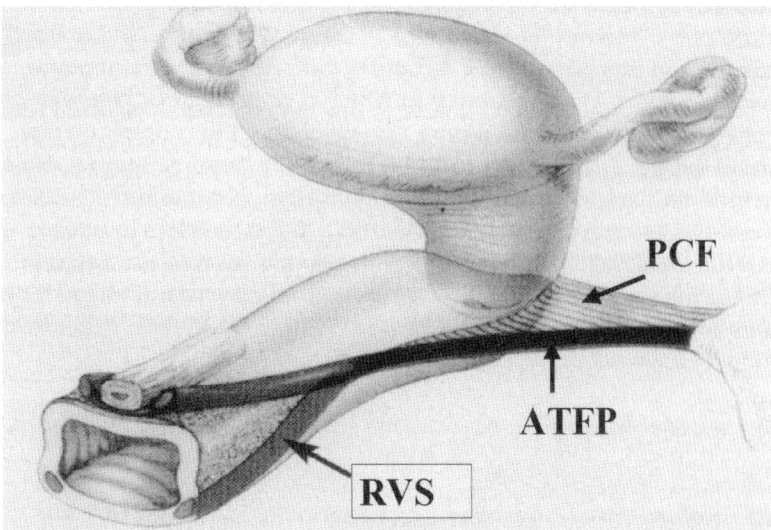

FIGURE 1.10 ● Attachment of rectovaginal septum and arcus tendineus fascia pelvis to pelvic sidewall, demonstrating the intervening web of tissue in the upper vagina, the fascia endopelvina. RVS, rectovaginal septum; ATFP, arcus tendineus fascia pelvis; PCF, pubocervical fascia. (From Leffler KS, Thompson JR, Cundiff GW, et al. Attachment of the rectovaginal septum to the pelvic sidewall. *Am J Obstet Gynecol* 2001;185:43, with permission.)

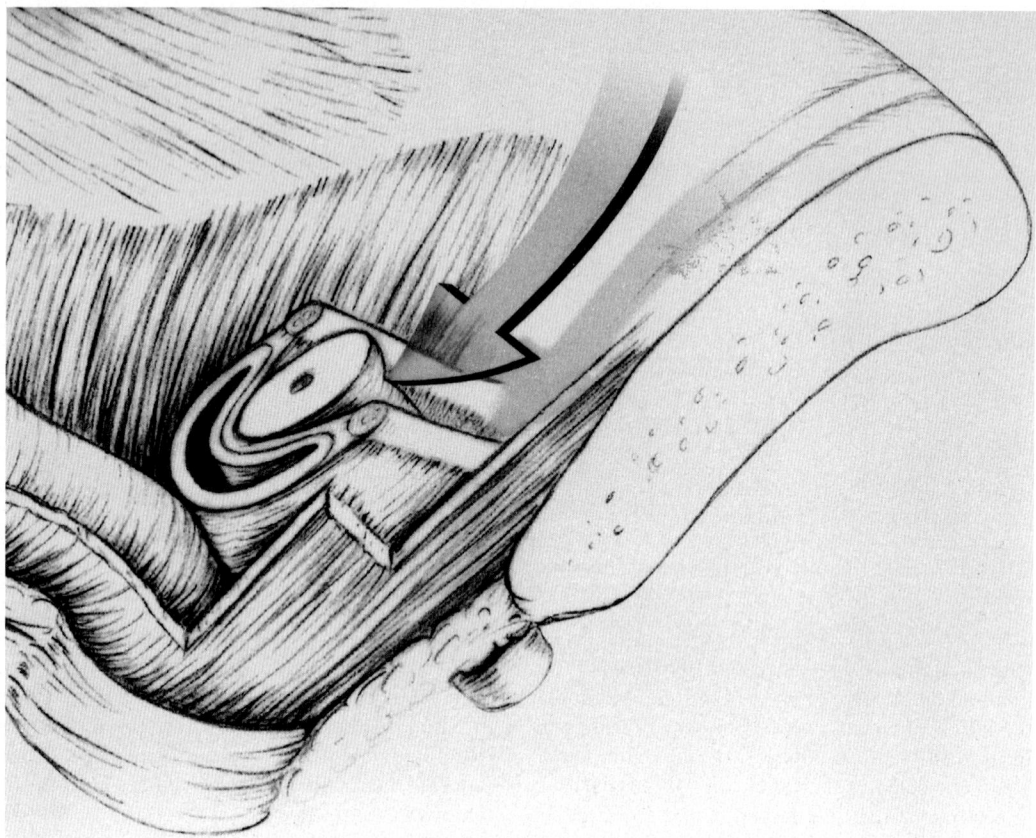

FIGURE 1.11 ● The urethral support system seen after the urethra and vagina have been transected just below the vesical neck. The *arrow* represents the force generated by increased abdominal pressure. (From DeLancey JOL. Structural support of the urethra as it relates to stress urinary incontinence: the hammock hypothesis. *Am J Obstet Gynecol* 1994;170:1713–1720, with permission.)

tissue that spans the region between the ischiopubic rami. The perineal membrane was previously described as the urogenital diaphragm, and has been erroneously depicted as two fascial layers sandwiching a transverse layer of muscle. In fact, this muscle is an important part of the distal urethral sphincter discussed later, but does not have a cranial fascial covering (22). Between the lateral and superior support, there is limited downward mobility of the perineal body, which normally lies within 2 cm of an imaginary line between the ischial tuberosities (23).

Importantly, detachments of the rectovaginal fascia from the perineal body can compromise the support of the perineum, resulting in perineal descent. Excessive perineal descent was first described in the colorectal literature by Parks and Hardcastle in 1966 (24). Since that time multiple studies have associated perineal descent with a variety of defecatory disorders, including constipation, solitary rectal ulcer syndrome, rectal pain, and fecal incontinence (25–28). Neurophysiologic

studies have demonstrated that one mechanism for fecal incontinence is pudendal neuropathy, due to stretching of the pudendal nerve associated with perineal descent (29,30).

Interactions Between Muscular and Connective Tissue Support

It is essential to understand that vaginal support arises from interactions between the pelvic musculature and connective tissue. DeLancey's analysis of the posterior vaginal wall provides excellent evidence of this interrelationship (31). Through its attachments to the lateral rectovaginal fascia and the perineal body, the resting tone of the pelvic diaphragm augments the support of the posterior vaginal wall and perineal body. Moreover, under normal conditions the anterior displacement provided by the resting tone of the puborectalis muscles brings the posterior vaginal wall into direct contact with the anterior vaginal wall. With this arrangement, pressure applied to the anterior and posterior vagi-

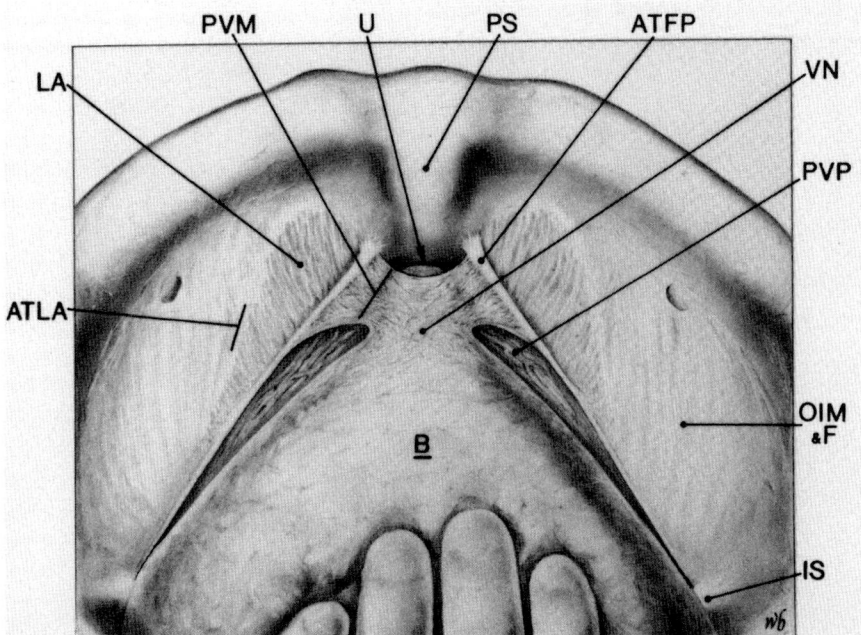

FIGURE 1.12 ● Space of Retzius. Pubovesical muscle (PVM) can be seen going from vesical neck (VN) to arcus tendineus fasciae pelvis (ATFP) and running over the paraurethral vascular plexus (PVP). ATLA, arcus tendineus levator ani; B, bladder; IS, ischial spine; LA, levator ani muscles; OIM&F, obturator internus muscle and fascia; PS, pubic symphysis; U, urethra. (From DeLancey JOL. Pubovesical ligament: a separate structure from the urethral supports [pubo-urethral ligaments]. *Neurourol Urodynam* 1989;8:53–61. Copyright © 1989 John Wiley & Sons, Inc. Reprinted with permission of Wiley-Liss, Inc., a division of John Wiley & Sons, Inc.)

nal walls is balanced, and the force is carried to the levator ani muscles and perineal body. Denervation of the pelvic diaphragm results in opening of the genital hiatus and separation of the anterior and posterior vaginal walls. In this circumstance, pressures applied to the anterior and posterior vaginal walls must be borne by the connective tissue alone. Due to its lateral attachments to the levator ani muscles, the loss of muscular tone also produces laxity in the rectovaginal fascia (see Fig. 1.9)

Innervation and Vasculature

Innervation of the levator ani and coccygeus muscles derives directly from the third and fourth sacral motor nerve roots on the superior surface of the muscles (32–34). The innervation of the puborectalis portion of the levator ani muscle is controversial. While postmortem dissections suggest that the puborectalis muscle innervation is via the pudendal nerve from the caudal side of the muscle, in vivo nerve conduction studies demonstrate direct innervation via the third and fourth sacral nerve roots, from the cephalad side of the muscle (35,36). The rest of the pelvic floor musculature receives innervation from the ventral roots of the

second, third, and fourth sacral nerve roots via the pudendal nerve. For example, the inferior rectal (hemorrhoidal) branches of the pudendal nerve innervate the external anal sphincter and the perineal branches innervate the striated urogenital sphincter muscle. Autonomic innervation of the pelvic viscera is complex. The internal anal sphincter receives parasympathetic innervation from the first, second, and third sacral nerve roots via the pelvic plexus (37). Sympathetic innervation is carried via the hypogastric nerves, derived from L5 (Fig. 1.13). The hypogastric nerves split at variable distances to the left of the sacral promontory. The inferior hypogastric plexus lies in the cardinal ligament inferior to the point where the uterine branch of the iliac artery crosses the distal ureter (Fig. 1.14). By blocking the external anal sphincter innervation with a bilateral pudendal block, Frenckner and Euler found that 85% of the resting tone of the anus is due to internal anal sphincter tone (38). Burleigh provides an excellent summary of conflicting information that exists regarding the sympathetic and parasympathetic innervation of the internal anal sphincter (39). Excitation of the sympathetic nervous system usually inhibits the smooth muscle along the gastrointestinal tract,

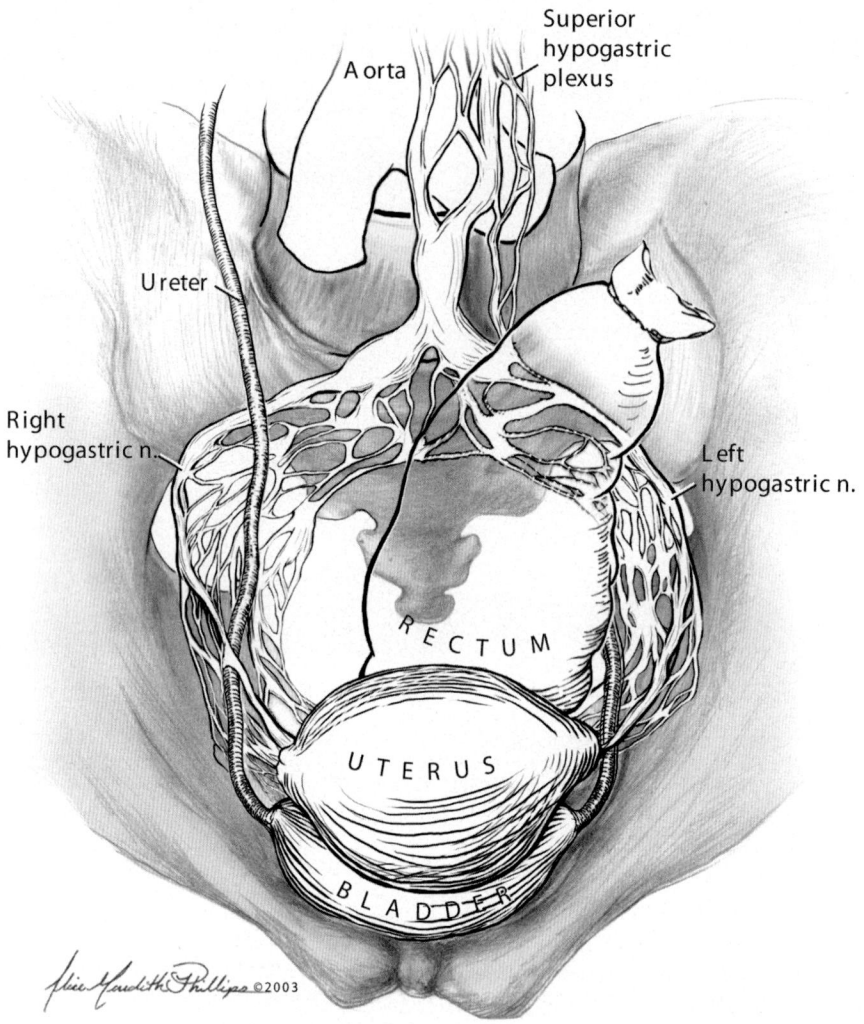

FIGURE 1.13 ● Superior hypogastric plexus with the peritoneum, endopelvic fascia, and veins removed. The relationship of the right and left hypogastric nerves to the uterus, bladder, and rectum is shown. The uterosacral ligament. (Reproduced with permission of the artist, Alice Meridith Phillips.)

whereas parasympathetic stimulation usually increases activity. At the gastrointestinal sphincters, however, sympathetic excitation results in contraction of smooth muscle and increased tone. Increased sphincter tone has been documented by stimulation of cut presacral nerves derived from the thoracolumbar region of anesthetized women, while 50% loss of resting sphincter tone occurs with blockade of the sympathetic nervous system with a high spinal anesthesia (40,41). In addition, sympatholytic agents such as the alpha-receptor blocker phentolamine result in decreased tone and alpha agonists result in increased tone (39).

Coordination of urine storage and appropriately timed micturition requires an intact and mature central nervous system (42). The innervation to the urethra and bladder combines sensory, motor, and autonomic input to coordinate the detrusor muscle, urethral sphincter muscles, and levator ani muscles. The perineal branch of the pudendal nerve provides innervation to the striated urogenital sphincter muscle. Like the internal anal sphincter, the autonomic innervation to the bladder and urethra is carried via the pelvic plexus and the hypogastric nerve. The second, third, and fourth sacral roots provide parasympathetic innervation via the pelvic plexus, mediating detrusor muscle contraction through acetylcholine receptors. The hypogastric nerve carries sympathetic nerve roots from the thoracic levels 10 through 12 and lumbar segments 1 and 2. Beta receptors predominate in the bladder detrusor muscle and alpha receptors at

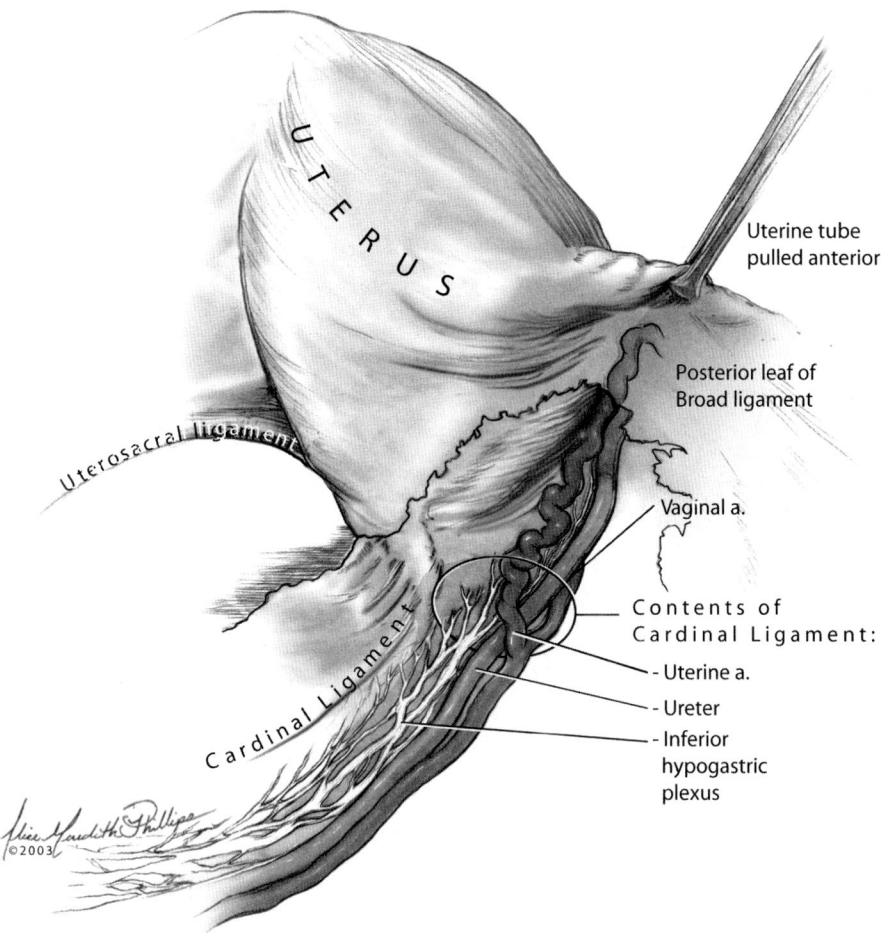

UTERUS

Uterine tube
pulled anterior

Posterior leaf of
Broad ligament

Uterosacral ligament

Vaginal a.

Contents of
Cardinal Ligament:

- - Uterine a.

- - Ureter

- - Inferior
hypogastric
plexus

Cardinal Ligament

©2003

FIGURE 1.14 ● Oblique view of the inferior hypogastric plexus of the right hypogastric nerve showing its relationship to the uterine artery and ureter. (Reproduced with permission of the artist, Alice Meridith Phillips.)

the urethral sphincter (43). Sympathetic stimulation via the hypogastric nerve assists in storage of urine, with central nervous system modulation and learned inhibition of detrusor contraction. Storage of urine is facilitated by beta receptor–mediated smooth muscle relaxation at the bladder neck and alpha receptor–mediated contraction of the urethral smooth muscle.

The majority of the pelvic viscera receive their primary blood supply from the branches of the internal iliac artery. There is an extensive collateral blood flow within the pelvis and much of this arises from the ovarian vessels. The ovarian arteries originate from the anterior abdominal aorta just beneath the renal arteries and cephalic to the inferior mesenteric artery. As they pass inferiorly toward the pelvis, they course from a medial to lateral location, crossing the ureter at the level of the pelvic brim. At this level they provide branches

that serve the ureter and fallopian tube. They then cross the proximal aspect of the external iliac vessels lateral to medial, and run medially in the infundibulopelvic ligament. The left ovarian vein drains into the left renal vein, whereas the right ovarian vein drains directly into the inferior vena cava.

The common iliac arteries are the terminal branches of the aorta. The bifurcation of the aorta occurs at approximately the level of L4. After 3 to 4 cm, the common iliac similarly bifurcates into the external and internal iliac arteries. The internal iliac artery provides much of the blood supply to the pelvic viscera and pelvic floor (Fig. 1.15). Although there is some variance in the branching pattern, the internal iliac artery generally splits into the anterior and posterior divisions. The branches of the anterior division include the obturator, umbilical, uterine, vaginal, inferior and su-

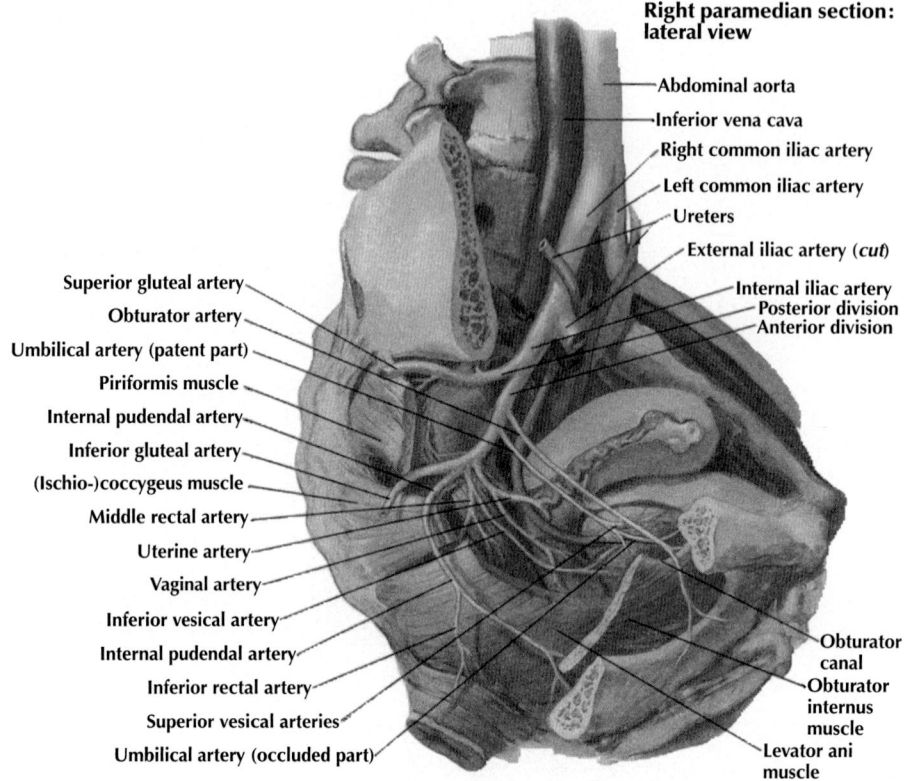

Right paramedian section: lateral view

- Abdominal aorta
- Inferior vena cava
- Right common iliac artery
- Left common iliac artery
- Ureters
- External iliac artery (*cut*)
- Internal iliac artery
  - Posterior division
  - Anterior division

- Superior gluteal artery
- Obturator artery
- Umbilical artery (patent part)
- Piriformis muscle
- Internal pudendal artery
- Inferior gluteal artery
- (Ischio-)coccygeus muscle
- Middle rectal artery
- Uterine artery
- Vaginal artery
- Inferior vesical artery
- Internal pudendal artery
- Inferior rectal artery
- Superior vesical arteries
- Umbilical artery (occluded part)

- Obturator canal
- Obturator internus muscle
- Levator ani muscle

FIGURE 1.15 ● Sagittal view of the branches of the internal iliac artery with the ischium removed. (From Netter FH. *Atlas of human anatomy.* East Hanover, NJ: Novartis, 1997, Plate 373. Copyright © 1997 Icon Learning Systems, LLC. A subsidiary of MediMedia, USA, Inc. All rights reserved.)

perior vesical, middle rectal, internal pudendal, and inferior gluteal arteries. The posterior division branches include the iliolumbar, lateral sacral, and superior gluteal arteries. The external iliac artery is the principal blood supply to the lower extremities but also provides important collateral flow to the pelvis. The deep epigastric and deep circumflex iliac arteries branch from the external iliac artery before it travels under the inguinal ligament and into the femoral canal. After passing beneath the inguinal ligament, the external iliac artery becomes the femoral artery.

VISCERAL ANATOMY

Lower Urinary Tract

Within the pelvis, the urinary tract includes the pelvic ureters, bladder, vesical neck, and urethra. Functionally, the lower urinary tract provides storage and appropriate evacuation. These are the functions of the bladder, consisting of the detrusor musculature and underlining mucosa, and urethra, with a specialized mucosal and vascular lining.

The vesical neck represents that region of the bladder base where the urethral lumen traverses the wall of the bladder. Although the ureters are functionally part of the upper urinary tract, a firm understanding of their course is fundamental to pelvic surgery and is, therefore, included.

Ureters

The ureters are expansile muscular tubes that transmit urine from the kidneys to the bladder. The transitional cell epithelium is supported by smooth muscle in a circular orientation. The ureters are retroperitoneal in location and are enveloped in their own endopelvic fascial covering that is closely adherent to the peritoneum. Small arterioles that travel in this adventitial layer provide the ureter with its blood supply.

The ureter exits the medial aspect of the renal pelvis, coursing inferiorly and medially over the psoas muscles in the retroperitoneal space of the upper abdomen. The pelvic ureter is easily identified as it traverses the common iliac artery at the posterior pelvic brim. From here it follows the branches of the internal iliac artery through the pararectal space, and can frequently be seen peristalsing just beneath the peritoneal lining of the pelvic sidewall. In the lateral pelvic sidewall, the intrapelvic ureter is in close proximity to the insertion of the uterosacral ligament at the cervix (6,14). At the level of the sacrum, the ureter is approximately 4 cm from the anterior margin of the uterosacral ligament but converges on its course so that it lies less than 1 cm from the anterior margin of the uterosacral ligament at the level of the cervix (see Fig. 1.3A). Anatomical studies have shown a variable fibrous attachment of the ureter to the distal uterosacral ligament (6). Understanding this close association between the ureter and the uterosacral ligament can prevent injury to the ureter during both routine gynecologic and urogynecologic surgery. Distal to the uterosacral ligament, the ureter passes beneath the uterine artery and changes course medially, coursing over the pubocervical fascia towards the bladder trigone (see Fig. 1.15).

Bladder

The bladder is a hollow viscus with the bladder wall composed of coarse bundles of smooth muscle called the detrusor muscle. The mucosal lining is a transitional epithelium that rests on a loose submucosa. Functionally, the bladder can be further subdivided into the dome and the bladder base roughly at the level of the ureteral orifices. The bladder wall of the dome is relatively thinnner, providing for its easy distensibility, whereas the bladder wall of the base has a thicker musculature that undergoes less distention during filling.

The detrusor musculature is a complex matrix of coordinated smooth muscle. Separate layers are described and are more distinct in the bladder base, but are not nearly as well defined as the layers of smooth muscle in the gut. The outermost layer is primarily longitudinal in orientation. Within this outer longitudinal layer is an intermediate layer of oblique and circular fibers, although the fiber directions in this portion of the dome are less well defined than those in the outer layer. The innermost layer is plexiform, creating the pattern of trabeculations seen at cystoscopy.

Within the region of the vesical neck are two oppositely oriented U-shaped bands of detrusor fibers. The more prominent Heiss's loop (detrusor loop) passes anterior to the internal meatus, with the U opening posteriorly. The second loop provides the intermediate circular layer of the detrusor under the trigone, and opens anteriorly. The urethral lumen passes through these opposed muscular loops, which may provide a sphincteric action to close the urethral lumen when the two straps of

muscle pull in opposite directions (44). There is some evidence of a different autonomic innervation of this part of the detrusor musculature that would permit reciprocal activity of the dome and base (45). Together with the urinary trigone, these fibers form the thickened musculature described as the bladder base.

Embryologically, the trigone arises separately from the bladder dome. The trigonal primordium leads to a specialized body of smooth muscle comprising the base of the bladder and extending down the vesical neck and into the urethra. There are three definable portions: the urinary trigone, the trigonal ring, and the trigonal plate (46,47). The urinary trigone is a triangular body of smooth muscle with its apices at the internal urinary meatus and ureteral orifices. At cystoscopy, it appears slightly elevated above the rest of the detrusor musculature due to its intimate attachment to the upper third of the anterior vaginal wall. Inferior to the urinary trigone and at the level of the internal urinary meatus, the trigonal musculature spreads out to encircle the proximal urethra, forming the trigonal ring. This ring surrounds the urethral lumen of the vesical neck. Given the location of the trigonal ring within the α-adrenergically innervated aspect of the vesical neck, it conceivably plays a role in the closure of the proximal urethra. Extending below the level of the trigonal ring is the trigonal plate, a column of trigonal tissue extending along the dorsal aspect of the urethra, between the ends of the striated urogenital sphincter.

Urethra

The urethra's archictecture reflects its dual functions as barrier and conduit, as well as its intimate yet independent relationship to the function of bladder. Although only 3 to 4 cm in length, this muscular lumen has a complex layered structure. The proximal 15% of its longitudinal length lies within the muscular wall of the bladder base, whereas the distal 20% passes through the perineal membrane (48). Between these two ends is the sphincteric mechanism.

The sphincteric mechanism has three components that each provide approximately one third of the resting urethral pressure. The striated urogenital sphincter is the outermost layer. Different authors refer to it as the striated circular muscle, striated sphincter, or rhabdosphincter. This striated muscle surrounds the smooth muscle sphincter, a thin circular layer of smooth muscle and inner longitudinal layer of smooth muscle. Lastly is the vascular cushions, lying between the smooth muscle and the mucosa of the urethra. This submucosa is unusually rich in its vascular supply and produces a hermetic seal (49–51).

The striated urogenital sphincter is really two muscle groups with different but coordinated functions (Fig. 1.16). The upper sphincteric portion or *sphincter urethrae* has muscle fibers in a circular orientation surrounding the upper 40% of the lumen just distal to the intramural urethra. This corresponds to what previous authors called the rhabdosphincter (52). The fibers of the sphincter ure-

thrae do not completely encircle the urethral lumen, but insert on the lateral aspects of the trigonal plate of the dorsal urethral wall. Fibers in this region do not form a complete circle, and the gap between its two ends is bridged by the trigonal plate, which completes the circle. This does not impair contraction as the trigonal plate functions as a tendon, bridging the gap between the two muscle ends.

The second portion of the striated urogenital sphincter occupies the distal one third of the ure-

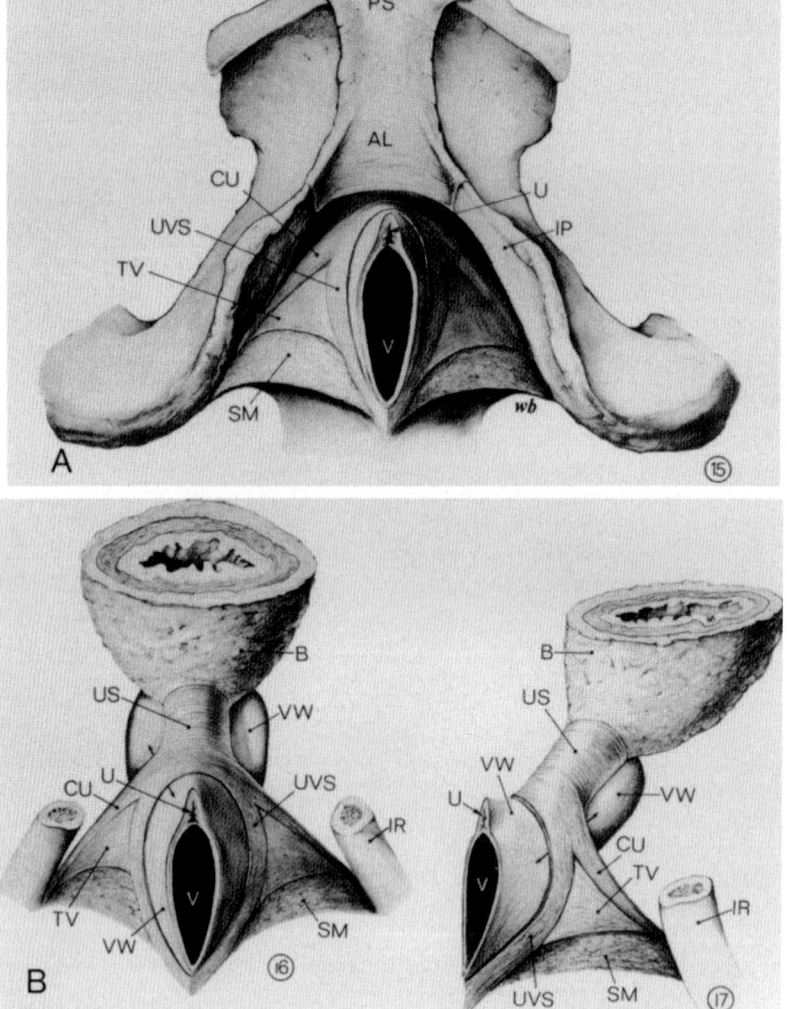

FIGURE 1.16 ● The striated urogenital sphincter muscle after removal of the perineal membrane. **(A)** Pubic bones intact. **(B)** Pubic bones removed. AL, arcuate pubic ligament; B, bladder; CU, compressor urethrae; IP, ischiopubic ramus; IR, ischial ramus; PS, pubic symphysis; SM, smooth muscle; TV, transverse vaginae muscle; U, urethra; US, urethral sphincter; UVS, urethrovaginal sphincter; V, vaginal orifice; VW, vaginal wall. (From Oelrich TM. The striated urogenital sphincter muscle in the female. *Anat Rec* 1983;205:223–232. Copyright © 1983 John Wiley & Sons, Inc. Reprinted with permission.)

thra (see Fig. 1.16). It consists of two bands of striated muscle that arch over the ventral urethra. One of these bands interdigitates with the muscular wall of the vagina and is called the urethrovaginal sphincter muscle. The other band of muscle, called the compressor urethrae, originates near the ischiopubic ramus. These two bands differ primarily in their lateral projections as both drape over the distal ventral urethra. Although their innervation is complex, all three portions of the striated urogenital sphincter muscle function as a single unit. The fibers within this muscle are primarily slow twitch muscle, ideal for maintaining constant tone while retaining the ability to contract when additional occlusive force is needed (8). Contraction of the striated urogenital sphincter muscle constricts the lumen of the upper portion of the urethra and compresses its ventral wall in the lower one third. Given their common derivation from the urogenital sinus, the urethra and vagina are intimately related structures (50). In fact, they are fused along the distal two thirds of the urethra. This connection to the endopelvic fascia of the anterior vaginal wall means that the support of the urethra depends not only on the attachments of the urethra to adjacent structures but also on the connection of the vagina and its connection to the muscles and fasciae of the pelvic wall.

There are two distinct smooth muscle layers within the urethra: the outer layer with a circular orientation and the inner with a longitudinal orientation. The circular muscle of the urethra is less developed, but is adjacent to and distal to the trigonal ring. While contiguous with the detrusor muscle, it is not a downward extension of the bladder muscle and actually has a different embryological derivation. The longitudinal muscle that lies inside the circular layer is more distinct, with considerable bulk. It is not continuous with the detrusor musculature but does extend to the level of the trigonal ring (49). It probably serves to shorten the urethra during micturition.

The vascular cushions provide a watertight seal resulting from the coaptation of urothelium due to the vascular plexus in the underlying submucosa. While the urothelium of the urethra is a downward extension of the transitional epithelium of the bladder, it is uniquely hormonally sensitive, specifically to estrogens (49,53). Moreover, the distal urethra has a stratified squamous epithelium. The line of demarcation between these two epithelia varies depending, in part, on the hormonal status of the individual. It can occur in the midurethra, as it does postmenopausally, or may extend well up into the bladder during the reproductive years.

Within the submucosa are a series of glands that empty into the dorsal surface of the urethra (54). These glands, while variable in number, are concentrated mainly in the lower and middle thirds. Cystic dilation of these glands can result in a urethral diverticulum.

The submucosal urethral vasculature is a highly organized arteriovenous complex capable of specific filling and emptying (49,55,56). Filling of the venous plexus has a direct impact on resting urethral pressure and is responsible for up to one third of the resting pressure of the urethra (56). At the same time, constriction of the urethral lumen during increased activity of the muscular sphincter tends to empty the vascular plexus, as during times of increased muscular activity the vasculature would be of less importance.

Continence Mechanism

While the concept of a "continence mechanism" is intellectually satisfying, it can be misleading if it creates a simplistic view of the complex interactions between the muscular and nonmuscular components of the urethral sphincter, and the passive and active support provided by the anterior vagina wall, which all contribute to urinary continence. Reviewing the contributions of the sphincteric mechanism and support mechanism will demonstrate the coordinated role both play in continence.

As noted previously, the sphincteric mechanism arises from an intricate interplay of striated muscle, the smooth muscle of the urethra and bladder, and the urothelium and submucosal vascular plexus. The proximal intramural urethra is affected by the opposing U-shaped bands of detrusor muscle and the trigonal ring. Below this intramural region lies the midportion of the urethra that extends from 20% to 60% of the total urethral length. Here the striated urogenital sphincter muscle and the circular and longitudinal smooth muscle act on the urethral lumen, providing a near-circumferential closure. More distal to this area but above the perineal membrane (from 60% to 80%), the compressor urethrae and urethrovaginal sphincter portions of the striated urogenital sphincter function by compressing the urethral lumen against the anterior vaginal wall (see Fig. 1.16). The importance of the compressor urethrae to continence is demonstrated by the occurrence of stress urinary incontinence after radical vulvectomy, when the distal urethra containing the compressor urethrae and urethrovaginal sphincter is excised. The compressor urethrae and urethrovaginal sphincter also provide the backup continence mechanism in 50% of continent women with an incompetent vesical neck (57). The distal urethra includes the distal one fifth of the total urethral length, ending at the external urinary meatus. It is primarily fibrous and functions to aim the urine stream almost like a nozzle rather than as part of the continence mechanism.

The intimate relationship between the urethra and anterior vaginal wall highlights the importance of normal vaginal wall function and support to normal urethral function. The muscular and connective tissue components of pelvic floor support create an environment in which the urethra, vesical neck, and bladder can function effectively. Loss of urethral support has been implicated in the pathophysiology of stress urinary incontinence, although there is not a one-to-one relationship between urethral support and stress continence (see Fig. 1.11) (58). In addition, stress incontinence also occurs with a poorly functioning vesical neck despite normal urethral support (59). Clearly, urethral support is one but not the only factor involved in continence.

The distal two thirds of the dorsal urethra is fused to the anterior vaginal wall by the endopelvic connective tissue so that the support of the urethra depends not only on the attachments of the urethra to adjacent structures but also on the connection of the vagina and periurethral tissues to the muscles and fasciae of the pelvic side wall. The lateral attachments of the pubocervical fascia provide a stable backboard or hammock of support for the urethra. The integrity of the attachment includes the connective tissue attachment to the arcus tendineus fascia pelvis as well as muscular attachments to the medial border of the levator ani muscle (20). Also embedded within the endopelvic connective tissue in this region are the pubovesical muscles, which are extensions of the detrusor muscle (20,60,61). In this configuration, an increase in the intra-abdominal pressure compresses the urethra against the passive support of the pubocervical fascia. An insult to the lateral stabilization of the pubocervical fascia, therefore, compromises the compression of the urethra and can be seen clinically as a compromise of the urethral support.

In addition to the passive support of the urethra provided by the pubocervical fasica and its lateral attachments, there is evidence of a dynamic support as well. In fact, while the distal urethra is fixed, fluoroscopic studies suggest that the proximal urethra is relatively mobile (62). The fixation of the distal portion of the urethra results from attachments to the pubocervical fascia as well as direct attachment to the pubic bones via the perineal membrane and the lower portions of the striated urogenital sphincter. The point of inflection be-

tween the mobile and immobile portions of the urethra has been called the "knee" of the urethra, and lies at approximately 50% of urethral length (22,48). The mobility of the proximal urethra is demonstrated at the onset of micturition, when women allow the vesical neck to descend by relaxing the levator ani muscles (63). This voluntary muscle action opens the posterior urethrovesical angle that is created by the normal resting tone of the levator ani muscles (45). This connection of the levator ani muscles to the endopelvic fascia surrounding the vagina and urethra allows the normal resting tone of the levators to maintain the retropubic position of the vesical neck (64). When the muscle relaxes at the onset of micturition, this allows the vesical neck to rotate downward to the limit of the elasticity of the fascial attachments. Contraction at the end of urination allows the vesical neck to resume its normal position.

The constituent parts of the pelvic floor that invest the urethra and attach it to its surrounding bony and muscular supports are the active contracting floor that provides a dynamic component of the continence mechanism. If the passive transmission of intra-abdominal pressure to the urethra were the only factor involved in continence, pressures during a cough would be maximal in the proximal urethra. Instead, studies reveal that the distal urethra, in the region of the compressor urethrae and urethrovesical sphincter, has the highest pressure elevations (65,66). This suggests that contraction of these muscles during a cough augments urethral pressure in this region. These pressures frequently exceed intra-abdominal pressure, indicating that factors other than abdominal pressure play a role (67). Moreover, the pressure rise precedes the rise in cough pressure, suggesting that the pelvic floor muscles are contracting in preparation for the cough (67). Kinesthesiologic electromyogram recordings of pelvic floor muscles show a similar reflexive contraction of the levator ani muscles during a cough. This contraction elevates the urethral supports, not only stabilizing the supportive hammock against abdominal pressure but also adding to the forces favoring urethral closure during times of increased abdominal pressure.

In summary, the continence mechanism is a complex interplay of both dynamic and passive support and sphincteric function. This suggests that the symptom of stress incontinence could result from different and at times multiple pathophysiologic insults. As a result, stress incontinence likely does not result from a single anatomical defect.

Lower Alimentary Tract

Rectum

The rectum serves both as a conduit between the sigmoid colon and anus and a reservoir for stool prior to defecation. Approximately 12 cm in length, it is contiguous with the sigmoid colon at the level of S3 and gives way to the anus at the levator hiatus. The caliber of the rectum is narrowest cranially but then widens to form the distensible rectal ampulla just above the pelvic floor.

While a retroperitoneal organ, the distal third of the rectum is beneath the level of the peritoneal cavity and therefore has no other peritoneal covering. The peritoneum does cover the anterior and lateral surfaces of the upper third of the rectum and the anterior surface of the middle third of the rectum. The rectum is surrounded by a fascial sheath and is loosely attached to the anterior surface of the sacrum via lateral and posterior stalks known as the lamina propria. This causes the rectum to follow the curve of the sacrum and coccyx, curving posteriorly in the sagittal plane. Inferiorly it passes through a fibrous sheet called Waldeyer's fascia. In the coronal plane, the rectum has a serpentine morphology, characterized by three concavities indicated by three flexures that result from the transverse rectal folds (see Fig. 1.16). The superior and inferior transverse rectal folds are on the left, while the middle transverse rectal fold is on the right. These folds arise from mucous membrane covering thickened circular smooth muscle summarizes prolongations of the taeniae coli, and serve to partially close the rectum.

There are five rectal arteries providing blood supply to the rectum (see Fig. 1.15). The superior rectal artery is a continuation of the inferior mesenteric artery. It crosses the left common iliac artery and descends into the pelvis within the sigmoid mass colon but then divides into two branches that descend on either side of the rectum. The more distal blood supply arises from the middle rectal arteries, branches of the internal iliac arteries, and the inferior rectal arteries, which are branches of the internal pudendal arteries.

Anal Canal

The anal canal is the terminal portion of the large intestine. The canal itself is 2.5 to 6 cm in length, running from where the rectal ampulla narrows, due to the anterior displacement of the puborectalis muscle, to the anal verge. The canal is surrounded by the puborectalis muscles superiorly and the internal and external anal sphincters below this (Fig. 1.17).

The internal anal sphincter is a continuation of the circular smooth muscle layer of the rectum (see Fig. 1.17). Anal manometric data during pudendal nerve block confirm that the internal anal sphincter contributes up to 85% of the maximal anal resting pressure (68,69). The internal anal sphincter is surrounded by the striated external anal sphincter muscle, which provides voluntary squeeze tone to the sphincter complex. In a study of 17 cadavers, DeLancey found the external anal sphincter to overlap the internal anal sphincter by an average of 17 mm, while the external sphincter extended only 3.7 cm caudal to the internal sphincter (70).

Classically, the external anal sphincter is described with three components—the deep, superficial, and subcutaneous portions—although these are not reflected by functional studies of the sphincter (71) (see Fig. 1.17). The external anal sphincter may contribute up to 60% of the anal canal pressure if there is sudden distention of the rectum, but it cannot maintain sustained tone (72). Haadem and Enck both found that resting and squeeze anal pressures decline with aging (73,74). Similarly, previous studies of the anatomy of the anal sphincter complex have described a narrow anterior wall in comparison to the thick posterior diameter, including both internal and external components (71,75). Recent studies with MRI depict the sphincter complex as cylindrical, with an anterior length almost equaling the posterior length (76,77). The internal anal sphincter contributes 54% of the anterior width of the anal sphincter complex (77). Fenner et al confirmed the cylindrical shape of the internal anal sphincter by imaging 10 nulliparous women with MRI (76). They found that the anterior and posterior thicknesses of the internal anal sphincter were similar. They also identified that the manometric high-pressure zone corresponds to the posterior anal sphincter length and that the external anal sphincter has a thicker posterior wall, especially in the cephalad portion.

The internal anal sphincter receives its sympathetic supply from L5, which passes through the pelvic plexus via the hypogastric plexus. The parasympathetic supply from S2-4 synapses at the pelvic plexus, where it joins the sympathetic nerves. The internal anal sphincter acts through reflex arcs at the spinal cord without voluntary control. The puborectalis (levator ani) is innervated by branches of the S2-4 sacral roots and does not receive direct innervation from the pudendal nerve. The external anal sphincter is innervated bilaterally by the pudendal nerve (S2-4) via Alcock's canal (see Fig. 1.15). The pudendal nerve fibers cross over at the level of the spinal cord, allowing

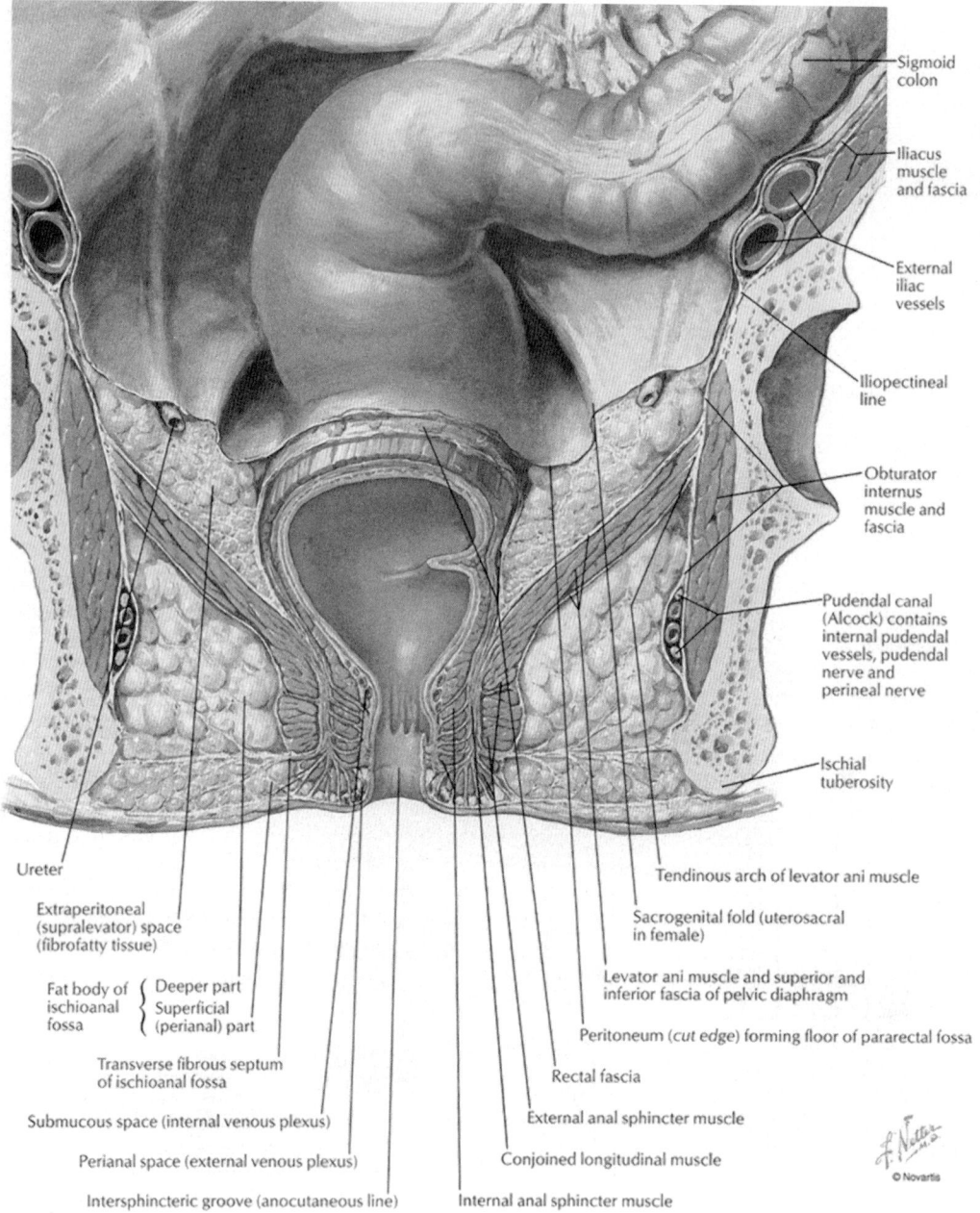

Sigmoid colon

Iliacus muscle and fascia

External iliac vessels

Iliopectineal line

Obturator internus muscle and fascia

Pudendal canal (Alcock) contains internal pudendal vessels, pudendal nerve and perineal nerve

Ischial tuberosity

Ureter

Extraperitoneal (supralevator) space (fibrofatty tissue)

Fat body of ischioanal fossa { Deeper part / Superficial (perianal) part

Transverse fibrous septum of ischioanal fossa

Submucous space (internal venous plexus)

Perianal space (external venous plexus)

Intersphincteric groove (anocutaneous line)

Tendinous arch of levator ani muscle

Sacrogenital fold (uterosacral in female)

Levator ani muscle and superior and inferior fascia of pelvic diaphragm

Peritoneum (*cut edge*) forming floor of pararectal fossa

Rectal fascia

External anal sphincter muscle

Conjoined longitudinal muscle

Internal anal sphincter muscle

FIGURE 1.17   ●   Coronal section of the lower rectum and anal sphincters. (From Netter FH. *Atlas of human anatomy*. East Hanover, NJ: Novartis, 1997, Plate 364. Copyright © 1997 Icon Learning Systems, LLC. A subsidiary of MediMedia, USA, Inc. All rights reserved.)

preservation of external anal sphincter function in the event of unilateral damage. The rich sensory supply from the anal canal travels along the inferior rectal branch of the pudendal nerve.

Continence Mechanism

The key muscles of the continence mechanism are the puborectalis, internal anal sphincter, and exter-

nal anal sphincter. Contraction of the puborectalis muscle narrows the genital hiatus, developing the nearly 90-degree anorectal angle. The resting tone of the puborectalis muscle serves as the primary continence mechanism for solid stool, whereas the internal anal sphincter and external anal sphincter are essential for continence of flatus and liquid stool. The internal sphincter maintains the majority of resting tone for the sphincter complex through autonomic reflex arcs and is essential for passive continence. Although the external sphincter also maintains constant resting tone, it is ultimately responsible for preventing fecal urgency and stress incontinence associated with sudden increases in intra-abdominal pressure. This function is under both voluntary and involuntary control. The anal cushions act as the final anatomic barrier. They fill with blood, causing occlusion of the anal canal.

CONCLUSIONS

Form follows function, and the anatomy of the pelvic viscera reflects their function in storage and evacuation. As a corollary, injury to the normal anatomical arrangements can have a negative impact on pelvic floor function. A clear understanding of the normal visceral anatomy and the supporting structures of the pelvic viscera not only helps to prevent surgical misadventures but also helps the surgeon restore normal pelvic floor function.

REFERENCES

1. Muir TW, Aspera AM, Rackley RR, et al. Recurrent pelvic organ prolapse in a woman with bladder exstrophy: a case report of surgical management and review of the literature. *Int Urogynecol J Pelvic Floor Dysfunct* 2004;15:436–438.
2. Handa VL, Pannu HK, Siddique S, et al. Architectural differences in the bony pelvis of women with and without pelvic floor disorders. *Obstet Gynecol* 2003;102: 1283–1290.
3. Sze EH, Kohli N, Miklos JR, et al. Computed tomography comparison of bony pelvis dimensions between women with and without genital prolapse. *Obstet Gynecol* 1999;93:229–232.
4. Mattox TF, Lucente V, McIntyre P, et al. Abdominal spinal curvature and its relationship to pelvic organ prolapse. *Am J Obstet Gynecol* 2000;183:1381–1384.
5. Nguyen TT, Lind LR, Choe JY, et al. Lumbosacral spine and pelvic inlet changes associated with pelvic organ prolapse. *Obstet Gynecol* 2000;95:332–336.
6. Buller JL, Thompson JR, Cundiff GW, et al. Uterosacral ligament: Description of anatomic relationships to optimize surgical safety. *Obstet Gynecol* 2001;97:873–879.
7. Whiteside JL, Walters MD. Anatomy of the obturator region: relations to a transobturator sling. *Int Urogynecol J Pelvic Floor Dysfunct* 2004;15:223–226.
8. Gosling JA, Dixson JS, Critchey HOD, et al. A comparative study of the human external sphincter and periurethral levator ani muscles. *Br J Urol* 1983;53:35–41.
9. DeLancey JOL. Standing anatomy of the pelvic floor. *J Pelvic Surg* 1996;2:260–263.
10. Gutman RE, Pannu HK, Cundiff GW, et al. Anatomical relationship between the vaginal apex and the bony architecture of the pelvis: a magnetic resonance imaging evaluation. *Am J Obstet Gynecol* 2005;192:1544–1548.
11. Strohbehn K. Normal pelvic floor anatomy. *Obstet Gynecol Clin North Am* 1998;25:683–705.
12. Uhlenhuth ER, Day E, Smith R, et al. The visceral endopelvic fascia and the hypogastric sheath. *Surg Gynecol Obstet* 1948;86:9–15.
13. DeLancey JOL. Anatomic aspects of vaginal eversion after hysterectomy. *Am J Obstet Gynecol* 1992;166: 1717–1728.
14. Campbell R. The anatomy and histology of the sacrouterine ligaments. *Am J Obstet Gynecol* 1950;59:1–12.
15. Norton PA. Pelvic floor disorders: The role of fascia and ligaments. *Clin Obstet Gynecol* 1993;36:926–938.
16. Van Ophoven A, Roth S. The anatomy and embryological origins of the fascia of Denonvilliers: a medico-historical debate. *J Urol* 1997;157:3–9.
17. Kleeman SD, Westermann C, Karram MM. Rectoceles and the anatomy of the posterior vaginal wall; revisited. *Am J Obstet Gynecol* 2005;193:2050–2055.
18. Leffler KS, Thompson JR, Cundiff GW, et al. Attachment of the rectovaginal septum to the pelvic sidewall. *Am J Obstet Gynecol* 2001;185:41–43.
19. DeLancey JOL. Structural support of the urethra as it relates to stress urinary incontinence: The hammock hypothesis. *Am J Obstet Gynecol* 1994;170:1713–1723.
20. Delancey JOL. Pubovesical ligament: A separate structure from the urethral supports (pubourethal ligaments). *Neurourol Urodynam* 1989;8:53–61.
21. DeLancey JOL. Structural anatomy of the posterior pelvic compartment as it relates to rectocele. *Am J Obstet Gynecol* 1999;180:815–823.
22. Oelrich TM. The striated urogenital sphincter muscle in the female. *Anat Rec* 1983;205:223–232.
23. Skomorowska E, Hegedus V, Christiansen J. Evaluation of perineal descent by defecography. *Int J Colorectal Dis* 1988;3:191–194.
24. Parks AG, Hardcastle J. The syndrome of the descending perineum. *Proc R Soc Med* 1966;59:477–482.
25. Henry MM, Parks AG, Swash M. The pelvic floor musculature in the descending perineum syndrome. *Br J Surg* 1982;69:470–472.
26. Bartolo DC, Read NW, Jarett JA, et al. Differences in anal sphincter function and clinical presentation in patients with pelvic floor descent. *Gastroenterology* 1982; 85:68–75.
27. Snooks SJ, Nicholls RJ, Henry MM, et al. Electrophysiological and manometric assessment of the pelvic floor in solitary rectal ulcer syndrome. *Br J Surg* 1985;2: 131–133.
28. Hudson CN. Female genital prolapse and pelvic floor deficiency. *Int J Colorect Dis* 1988;3:181–185.
29. Ho YH, Goh HS. The neurophysiological significance of perineal descent. *Int J Colorect Dis* 1995;10: 107–111.
30. Henry MM, Parks AG, Swash M. The anal reflex in idiopathic fecal incontinence: an electrophysiological study. *Br J Surg* 1980;67:781–783.
31. DeLancey JOL. Structural anatomy of the posterior pelvic compartment as it relates to rectocele. *Am J Obstet Gynecol* 1999;180:815–823.
32. Lawson JON. Pelvic anatomy I: Pelvic floor muscles. *Ann R Coll Surg Engl* 1974;54:244–252.
33. Snooks SJ, Swash M. Innervation of the muscles of continence. *Ann R Coll Surg Engl* 1986;68:45–49.
34. Wall LL. The muscles of the pelvic floor. *Clin Obstet Gynecol* 1993;36:910–925.
35. Percy JP, Neill ME, Swash M, et al. Electrophysiological study of motor nerve supply of the pelvic floor. *Lancet* 1981;1:16–17.
36. Wood BA, Kelly AJ. Anatomy of the anal sphincters and pelvic floor. In: Henry MM, Swash M, eds. *Colo-*

proctology and the pelvic floor, 2nd ed. London: Butterworth-Heineman, 1992:3–19.

37. Burleigh DE. Pharmacology of the internal anal sphincter. In: Henry MM, Swash M, eds. *Coloproctology and the pelvic floor*, 2nd ed. London: Butterworth-Heineman, 1992:37–53.

38. Frenckner B, von Euler C. Influence of pudendal block on the function of the anal sphincters. *Gut* 1975;16: 482–489.

39. Burleigh DE. Pharmacology of the internal anal sphincter. In: Henry MM, Swash M, eds. *Coloproctology and the pelvic floor*, 2nd ed. London: Butterworth-Heineman, 1992:37–53.

40. Frenckner B, Ihre T. Influence of autonomic nerves on the internal anal sphincter in man. *Gut* 1976;17: 306–312.

41. Rankin FW, Learmonth JR. Section of the sympathetic nerves of the distal portion of the colon and rectum in the treatment of Hirschsprung's disease and certain types of constipation. *Ann Surg* 1930;92:710–720.

42. Chai TC, Steers WD. Neurophysiology of micturition and continence in women. *Int Urogynecol J Pelv Floor Dysfunct* 1997;8:85–97.

43. Ek A. Innervation and receptor functions of the human urethra. *Scand J Urol Nephrol Suppl* 1977;45:1–50.

44. Jeffcoate TNA, Roberts H. Observations on stress incontinence of urine. *Am J Obstet Gynecol* 1952;64: 721–738.

45. Elbadawi A. Neuromuscular mechanisms of continence. In: Yalla SV, McGuire EJ, Elbadawi A, et al, eds. *Neurourology and urodynamics*. New York: Macmillan, 1989:3–35.

46. Droes JT. Observations on the musculature of the urinary bladder and urethra in the human fetus. *Br J Urol* 1974;46:179–185.

47. Huisman AB. Aspects on the anatomy of the female urethra with special relation to urinary continence. *Contrib Gynecol Obstet* 1983;10:1–31.

48. DeLancey JOL. Correlative study of paraurethral anatomy. *Obstet Gynecol* 1986;68:91–97.

49. Huisman AB. Aspects on the anatomy of the female urethra with special relation to urinary continence. *Contrib Gynecol Obstet* 1983;10:1–31.

50. Krantz KE. The anatomy of the urethra and anterior vaginal wall. *Am J Obstet Gynecol* 1951;62:374–386.

51. Ricci J, Lisa JR, Thom CH. The female urethra: a histologic study as an aid in urethral surgery. *Am J Surg* 1950;79:499–505.

52. Gosling JA. The structure of the female lower urinary tract and pelvic floor. *Urol Clin North Am* 1985;12:207–214.

53. Smith P. Age changes in the female urethra. *Br J Urol* 1972;44:667–676.

54. Huffman J. Detailed anatomy of the paraurethral ducts in the adult human female. *Am J Obstet Gynecol* 1948; 55:86–101.

55. Berkow SG. The corpus spongiosum of the urethra: its possible role in urinary control and stress incontinence in women. *Am J Obstet Gynecol* 1953;65:346–351.

56. Rud T, Anderson KE, Asmussen M, et al. Factors maintaining the intraurethral pressure in women. *Invest Urol* 1980;17:343–347.

57. Versi E, Cardozo LD, Studd JWW, et al. Internal urinary sphincter in maintenance of female continence. *Br Med J* 1986;292:166–167.

58. Fantl AJ, Hurt WG, Bump RC, et al. Urethral axis and sphincteric function. *Am J Obstet Gynecol* 1986;155: 554–558.

59. McGuire EJ. Urodynamic findings in patients after failure of stress incontinence operations. *Prog Clin Biol Res* 1981;78:351–360.

60. Gil Vernet S. *Morphology and function of the vesico-prostato-urethral musculature*. Treviso: Edizioni Canova, 1968.

61. Woodburne RT. Anatomy of the bladder and bladder outlet. *J Urol* 1968;100:474–487.

62. Westby M, Asmussen M, Ulmsten U. Location of maximum intraurethral pressure related to urogenital diaphragm in the female subject as studied by simultaneous urethrocystometry and voiding urethrocystography. *Am J Obstet Gynecol* 1982;144:408–412.

63. Muellner SR. Physiology of micturition. *J Urol* 1951; 65:805–810.

64. Parks AG, Porter NH, Melzak J. Experimental study of the reflex mechanism controlling muscles of the pelvic floor. *Dis Colon Rectum* 1962;5:407–414.

65. Constantinou CE. Resting and stress urethral pressures as a clinical guide to the mechanism of continence in the female patient. *Urol Clin North Am* 1985;12:247–258.

66. Hilton P, Stanton SL. Urethral pressure measurement by microtransducer: the results in symptom-free women and in those with genuine stress incontinence. *Br J Obstet Gynaecol* 1983;90:919–933.

67. Constantinou CE, Govan DE. Spatial distribution and timing of transmitted and reflexly generated urethral pressures in healthy women. *J Urol* 1982;127:964–969.

68. Frenckner B, von Euler C. Influence of pudendal block on the function of the anal sphincters. *Gut* 1975;16: 482–489.

69. Wunderlich M, Parks AG. Physiology and pathophysiology of the anal sphincters. *Int Surg* 1982;67:291–298.

70. DeLancey JOL, Toglia MR, Perucchini D. Internal and external anal sphincter anatomy as it relates to midline obstetric lacerations. *Obstet Gynecol* 1997;90:924–927.

71. Dalley AF. The riddle of the sphincters: The morphophysiology of the anorectal mechanism revisited. *Am Surgeon* 1987;53:298–306.

72. Frenckner B, Ihre T. Influence of autonomic nerves on the internal anal sphincter in man. *Gut* 1976;17:306–312.

73. Haadem K, Dahlström JA, Ling L. Anal sphincter competence in healthy women: Clinical implications of age and other factors. *Obstet Gynecol* 1991;78:823–827.

74. Enck P, Kuhlbusch MTA, Lübke H, et al. Age and sex and anorectal manometry in incontinence. *Dis Colon Rectum* 1989;32:1026–1030.

75. Oh C, Kark AE. Anatomy of the external anal sphincter. *Br J Surg* 1972;59:717–723.

76. Fenner DE, Kriegshauser JS, Lee HH, et al. Anatomic and physiologic measurements of the internal and external anal sphincters in normal females. *Obstet Gynecol* 1998;91:369–374.

77. Aronson MP, Lee RA, Berquist TH. Anatomy of anal sphincters and related structures in continent women studied with magnetic resonance imaging. *Obstet Gynecol* 1990;76:846–851.

CHAPTER 2

Epidemiology of Pelvic Organ Prolapse and Urinary Incontinence

Steven E. Swift

INTRODUCTION

The epidemiology of urinary incontinence and pelvic organ prolapse are often included together in the literature; however, these two diseases are distinct and separate entities that have only superficial similarities in their epidemiology. They are both common diseases, occurring in 5% to 30% of the population, and both can be managed surgically, often simultaneously. It has been reported that there is an incidence of 2.04 to 2.63 surgical procedures to correct prolapse or genuine stress incontinence per 1,000 women-years, with an increasing incidence as women age, and a lifetime risk of undergoing surgery for prolapse or incontinence of 5% to 11.1% (1,2). One reason these two conditions are often lumped together involves the role of pelvic floor muscle relaxation in the development of both stress urinary incontinence and pelvic organ prolapse. While this is true, it should be remembered that only about half of the urinary incontinence cases encountered are stress-related, and the remaining types of incontinence have little to do with pelvic floor muscle relaxation, while all of prolapse is related to pelvic floor muscle relaxation and attenuation of ligamentous structures.

DEFINITIONS

Another similarity between these two entities involves the use of condition-specific definitions in the literature. Most of the older literature concerning the epidemiology of pelvic organ prolapse used a nonspecific definition that was unique to that paper (3). Recent efforts by international organizations to standardize a definition of pelvic organ prolapse have provided some guidance but have not cleared up the situation. The American College of Obstetrics and Gynecology (ACOG) technical bulletin defines pelvic organ prolapse as the protrusion of the pelvic organs into or out of the vaginal canal (4). The International Continence Society (ICS) defines the absence of prolapse as any subject with pelvic organ prolapse quantification system (POPQ) stage 0 support (5). Finally, the National Institutes of Health (NIH) defines pelvic organ prolapse as (POPQ) stage II, III, and IV exams (6). These definitions range from the very loose ACOG definition to the very specific but different ICS and NIH definitions. Currently there is no clinical definition of pelvic organ prolapse; however, several investigators are suggesting that prolapse of any vaginal segment beyond the hymenal remnants may be the best working definition (this includes some POPQ stage II and all stage III and IV exams).

There is less controversy regarding the definition of urinary incontinence, but here as well the epidemiologic literature is fraught with confusion. In this body of literature, while the definitions are standard and recognized, they are seldom used when querying subjects, and therefore the studies reported in the literature often have disparate findings not due to true population differences but secondary to differences in how incontinence is defined. The ICS has taken the lead in defining incontinence through their Standardization of Terminology Committee, which publishes a series of documents setting the international standards for defining lower urinary tract disorders. This committee has recently changed the definition of urinary incontinence in a subtle manner that will likely influence future studies. The older ICS definition of urinary incontinence (in place since 1982) is involuntary loss of urine which is objectively demonstrable and is a social or hygienic problem (7). The new ICS definition of urinary incontinence (as of 2002) is the complaint of any involuntary leakage of urine (8). While these changes are subtle, any studies that were based on responses using a questionnaire employing the older definition may vary from responses using a questionnaire using the newer definition.

Another problem in studying urinary incontinence is that there are various forms or types of urinary incontinence that probably have very different etiologies. Stress urinary incontinence is generally thought to be due to a defective urethral sphincter mechanism arising from damage to the pudendal nerve and fascia of the pelvis as a result of childbirth. Urge urinary incontinence is due to uninhibited detrusor contractions that may have a subtle or overt neurologic etiology. Mixed incontinence is a combination of both and may be due to multiple factors. These types of incontinence, along with rarer forms such as overflow incontinence and fistulas, cannot be easily distinguished based on history and physical examination and may require complex urodynamic testing (9). Therefore, any epidemiologic study findings based solely on responses to a questionnaire would be suspect in identifying specific etiologies for the various types of incontinence.

Despite these limitations, the literature in this area is growing and we are beginning to understand and appreciate the epidemiology of these disorders. This will eventually allow us to recommend prevention strategies. A corollary to this developing body of epidemiologic literature is the development of questionnaires specifically designed to identify these conditions in large general populations (10). These will allow us to perform population-based studies and will help settle some old controversies based on conflicting reports.

EPIDEMIOLOGY OF PELVIC ORGAN PROLAPSE

Incidence of Pelvic Organ Support Defects

Determining the difference between normal and abnormal pelvic organ prolapse is complicated, not only because we lack a validated definition, but also because there is a lack of knowledge regarding the distribution of pelvic organ support in the normal female population. It can be difficult to define something as pathologic without some understanding of normal, particularly in the patient

who is asymptomatic. Therefore, prior to describing the etiology of pelvic organ prolapse, a discussion on the state of our current understanding regarding the distribution of pelvic organ support in the female population is in order.

Several reports have described the distribution of pelvic organ support in female populations employing the POPQ exam to define the degree of pelvic organ support in their subjects (11–14). The POPQ is a classification system for documenting the degree of pelvic organ support that describes five stages (0 through IV), with stage 0 representing excellent support and stage IV representing complete vaginal vault eversion or complete uterine procidentia. This classification system has been found to be a reliable and reproducible tool for quantifying pelvic organ support (15,16). Three of the four large studies to date had similar findings, with the majority of subjects examined having POPQ stage I or II exams and only 3% to 9% having stage III and IV exams. The distribution of POPQ stages demonstrates a bell curve distribution (Fig. 2.1). Two of these studies (11,13) represent patients presenting to outpatient gynecology clinics for annual Pap smears and pelvic exams. The other (12) was a true population-based study of women living in a Danish city. The one outlying study was done on a group of perimenopausal women presenting for a study on soy supplements to treat menopausal symptoms (14). The drawback to all of these reports is that the populations studied may not necessarily be reflective of the general female population. However, despite being different populations, three of the four studies have strikingly similar results, suggesting that most women will have stage I or II exams and that only 3% to 11% will have advanced degrees of prolapse.

Etiology of Pelvic Organ Prolapse

Increasing parity and advancing age are consistently identified as risk factors for the development of pelvic organ prolapse. Several other factors have also been implicated: vaginal versus abdominal delivery of a term infant, antecedent surgery to correct prolapse, hysterectomy, congenital defects, race, lifestyle, and chronic disease states that increase intra-abdominal pressure (i.e., chronic constipation, pulmonary disease, obesity). However, here the literature is not as consistent, and the role that these factors play is still not fully understood.

Childbirth

Vaginal delivery of a term infant has been postulated to be the most significant contributor to the

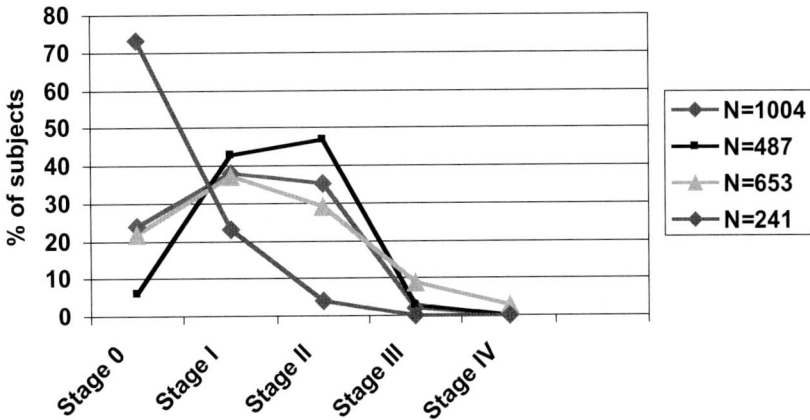

FIGURE 2.1 ● Percent of subjects in each POPQ stage from four population-based studies. (N, the number of subjects examined in each study.)

subsequent development of pelvic organ prolapse (1,2,11–13,17,18). It is postulated that as the fetal vertex passes through the vaginal canal, it stretches the levator ani muscles and the pudendal nerve, leading to damage with permanent neuropathy and muscle weakness. This damage is felt to be ultimately responsible for pelvic organ prolapse noted later in life.

If stretching of the pelvic floor plays a significant role in the development of pelvic organ prolapse, then larger infants should exacerbate this damage, and this should be reflected in the etiology of prolapse. When this was specifically addressed, it was reported that there is a 10% increase in the association of pelvic organ prolapse with each 10- to 16-ounce increase in the birthweight of a vaginally delivered infant (13,18).

Also, it would be expected that the birth route would play a role in the subsequent development of prolapse. It has been demonstrated that the pudendal nerve damage caused by vaginal delivery can be avoided by cesarean section (19–21). However, several recent articles have demonstrated conflicting results when evaluating the risk of a vaginal over cesarean delivery on the eventual development of pelvic organ prolapse (13,22). Therefore, it remains unclear whether it is the pregnancy or the delivery route that places an individual at risk for prolapse.

Age

Another area where the literature is in agreement involves the increasing prevalence of pelvic organ prolapse in a population as it ages (2,11,12, 13,17,18,22,23). This is intuitive to the clinician, as there are very few patients in their twenties and thirties with significant pelvic organ prolapse. Figure

2.2 demonstrates the distribution of pelvic organ support as women age. The peak or median POPQ stage of support shifts to the right as the population described increases in age. It has been shown that there is roughly a 30% to 50% increase in the incidence of pelvic organ prolapse with each 10 years of advancing age (13,17,18). This confirms data on the incidence of surgically managed pelvic organ prolapse from several studies that showed a 50% to 100% increase per decade in the incidence of surgery to correct pelvic organ prolapse up until age 70, where it appears to plateau (2,23).

Menopause

The literature is consistent that the risk of pelvic organ prolapse increases with advancing age, but what role menopause and hormone replacement therapy have on pelvic organ prolapse is unknown. One study has identified menopausal status as a risk factor to develop prolapse (17). However, they did not determine which patients were taking hormone replacement therapy and which were not. In other studies, menopausal status and whether or not a subject was taking hormone replacement therapy were not identified as risk factors for developing pelvic organ prolapse (13,18). Therefore, it may be that advancing age is more responsible for the increased risk of developing pelvic organ prolapse than is menopausal status. Currently, the role of estrogen in the area of pelvic organ support is unclear, but while it may not prevent the development of prolapse it probably does not promote its development, and its use in subjects with significant pelvic organ support defects should be viewed as neutral. Whether or not it can prevent or delay the onset of pelvic organ prolapse remains to be determined.

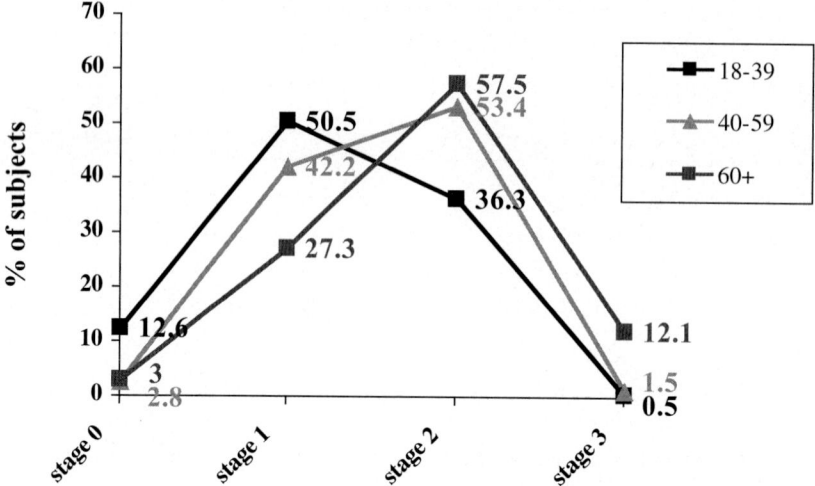

FIGURE 2.2 ● Percent of subjects with POPQ stage exams by age group. Note how the peak shifts to the right with advancing age.

Previous Surgery to Correct Pelvic Organ Support Defects

This may not be a fair addition to the etiologies of pelvic organ prolapse, as these subjects already have manifested pelvic organ support defects and have the underlying pathologic processes that lead to this disease. Recurrence rates for surgical correction of pelvic organ prolapse are in the 10% to 30% range (2,24,25). Therefore, it is not surprising that when subjects identified with previous surgery to correct prolapse are included in studies, this is consistently identified as a risk factor. When the various risk factors for developing severe (POPQ stage 3 and 4) pelvic organ prolapse were analyzed, it was determined that previous surgery to correct prolapse was the single greatest risk factor for the subsequent development of severe prolapse (18). This appears to be a statement on the inadequacies of our current surgical procedures for correcting significant pelvic organ prolapse.

Hysterectomy

The role of hysterectomy as a cause of subsequent development of pelvic organ prolapse is controversial, with no current consensus. The overall incidence of severe pelvic organ prolapse following hysterectomy has been estimated to be 2 to 3.6 per 1,000 women-years (26,27). This is similar to the rates of surgically corrected pelvic organ prolapse and incontinence noted for the general population (2.04 to 2.63 per 1,000 women-years) and would suggest that there is no excess of pelvic organ prolapse in subjects with a prior hysterectomy (1,2). When the role of hysterectomy was specifically

addressed, the results are mixed, with some studies identifying it as a risk factor for prolapse and others suggesting it is not (1,13,18). The next question regarding hysterectomy is whether the route of surgery influences the subsequent development of pelvic support defects. The general opinion is that the incidence of pelvic support defects is greater following a vaginal hysterectomy than an abdominal hysterectomy (11,13,26,28). However, the rates and degree of prolapse appear similar regardless of the type of antecedent hysterectomy (1,26). While the route of hysterectomy may not predict subsequent development of pelvic organ prolapse, there is a correlation between subsequent prolapse and the initial indication for the hysterectomy. Pelvic organ prolapse rates as high as 15 per 1,000 women-years have been noted in patients whose indication for hysterectomy was uterine prolapse (2). This confirms the above findings of an increased risk of pelvic organ prolapse following surgery to correct pelvic support defects and may explain some of the data suggesting vaginal hysterectomy as a cause of pelvic organ prolapse.

The disruption of the attachments of the uterosacral cardinal ligament complex to the cuff is felt to be the cause of posthysterectomy vaginal vault prolapse. Most authors feel that paying particular attention to reattaching these ligaments to the cuff and obliterating the cul-de-sac can reduce the incidence of prolapse. There are a few uncontrolled reports that the incidence of enterocele following a hysterectomy can be reduced by greater than 50% if cul-de-sac obliteration is performed at the time of hysterectomy (28,29). It would seem that if disruption of the attachments of the uterosacral and cardinal ligaments were the main reason for subsequent prolapse, then supracervical hysterectomies would provide some degree of protection. In one case series, an investigator reported that in his practice there were 31 cases of eversion of the vagina and cervical stump and only 7 cases of vaginal eversion of the cuff. This was despite the mention that more total abdominal than supracervical hysterectomies were performed in that practice (30). This suggests that preservation of the uterosacral and cardinal ligamentous attachment to the cervix does not prevent subsequent prolapse.

Prolapse following hysterectomy is controversial and apparently unrelated to the route of surgery. It may be related to the indication, with vaginal vault prolapse occurring most commonly following a hysterectomy for prolapse.

Congenital Defects

One of the biggest questions concerning the etiology of pelvic organ prolapse is the question of which patients are at risk. From the above discussion, it appears that pudendal neuropathy and pelvic floor damage occur with almost all vaginal deliveries, yet severe pelvic organ prolapse occurs in only about 3% to 11% of the population. Therefore, do those patients destined to develop prolapse have an underlying congenital defect that prevents recovery of their pelvic support mechanism from the trauma of vaginal delivery, and might this also account for prolapse that is occasionally seen in the nulliparous patient?

One obvious congenital anomaly that could be involved in pelvic support defects is collagen vascular disease. There is evidence that women with pelvic organ prolapse have less total collagen in their pubocervical fascia when compared to controls and that the collagen present is of a weaker type than noted in controls with normal support (31,32). There is also the observation that subjects with pelvic organ prolapse have a greater degree of joint hypermobility, suggesting a collagen defect (33). Therefore, if pelvic organ prolapse is related to collagen defects, then women with congenital connective tissue diseases should have a greater incidence of prolapse. However, when women with Ehlers-Danlos syndrome were evaluated, there was no relationship between greater degrees of joint mobility and more prominent pelvic organ prolapse (34).

Another congenital defect that is felt to play a role in pelvic organ prolapse is spina bifida. While this is often quoted as a cause of prolapse, particularly in the young nulliparous patient, there are only a few case reports describing its relationship to prolapse, and most of these were in the newborn (35,36). In the report by Torpin there was mention of a group of adult women with prolapse who had a 28% incidence of spina bifida occulta compared with a 10% incidence in their control population without prolapse (35). While the relationship may not be straightforward, in the young nulliparous woman with severe prolapse an evaluation to identify spina bifida occulta is warranted.

Is there a congenital predilection for pelvic support dysfunction in some subjects that may be responsible for the more severe degrees of pelvic organ prolapse? Currently this question remains unanswered, and no recommendations regarding screening or prevention can be made.

Racial Differences

One factor that may predict those subjects likely to develop pelvic organ prolapse is their genetic make-up as reflected in their race. There are a few anecdotal reports that certain populations (Asians) have a lower incidence of pelvic organ prolapse then other racial groups, but these tend to be more opinion than fact (37). These reports showed a greater collagen content in the fascial supports of Asians compared to Caucasian women. The populations compared and contrasted were not adequately described to determine what other influences may have explained the results. Also, a recent study on the incidence of urinary incontinence (a condition commonly associated with pelvic organ prolapse) in Asian women demonstrated similar rates to those published for predominately Caucasian populations (38). When race was specifically addressed in one large population-based study, Hispanic race seemed to have the greatest risk of developing prolapse (13). While this study had adequate representation of Caucasian, Blacks, and Hispanics, there were very few Asians. The other large studies have not had enough racial diversity to comment on this factor.

There is some evidence that Hispanic females are at greater risk of developing prolapse than either Black or Caucasian women. While there may be differences in collagen and pelvic anatomy between races, how this translates into risk of developing pelvic organ prolapse remains speculative.

Lifestyle

It is widely believed that women who participate in high-impact activities, whether at work or play, will have more complications with prolapse and associated symptoms than their sedentary counterparts. Heavy lifting at work appears to be related to pelvic organ prolapse. In one study, the number of prolapse surgeries performed on over 28,000 nursing assistants demonstrated a 60% increase over the general population (39). It was felt this was secondary to their work-related duties. In several studies women who reported their occupation as laborer or housewife demonstrated a greater risk of pelvic organ prolapse, suggesting that work-related physical stressors may indeed be an etiology for pelvic organ prolapse (13,40,41).

Chronic Disease

Chronic illnesses that result in constant stress and strain on the pelvic floor are often quoted as a significant predisposing condition for pelvic organ prolapse (1,42). Conditions such as chronic obstructive pulmonary disease or chronic cough, chronic constipation, and obesity are the diseases most often implicated, but there is little data in the literature to substantiate these statements.

There are two studies that describe an association between chronic constipation and pelvic organ prolapse (43,44). In one study 61% of subjects with uterovaginal prolapse reported straining with stool as young adults prior to the onset of the prolapse. In a control group only 4% reported straining with stool as young women (43). In the other study there was an association between straining at stool and anterior vaginal wall prolapse (36).

It is felt that increasing weight places greater pressure on the abdominal cavity, displacing the pelvic organs out through the urogenital hiatus. Increasing BMI has demonstrated increased risk for prolapse, with a 2.5-fold increase for subjects with a BMI greater than 25 when compared to subjects with a BMI less than 25 (13). However, this finding is not consistent, and another study found no association between increasing weight and prolapse (23).

Diabetes mellitus is a disease that is associated with poor wound healing and therefore has been mentioned as a factor in the development of pelvic organ prolapse. It is felt that diabetics may not be able to fully recover following the damage that occurs to the pelvic floor with childbirth, and this puts them at increased risk to develop pelvic organ prolapse later in life. However, when studied, there is no apparent association between the two (13,18). Other chronic illnesses such as pulmonary disease and hypertension have been evaluated as risk factors for developing severe pelvic organ prolapse, and again no relationship was found between these chronic illnesses and prolapse (13,18).

Increasing physical stressors at work and chronic constipation appear to be related to the development of pelvic organ prolapse. What role other illnesses play in the development of pelvic organ prolapse has not been defined. Conditions such as chronic obstructive pulmonary disease that result in ongoing continuous insults to the pelvic floor also probably play a role in the etiology of this condition but have not been sufficiently investigated.

Summary

The role of childbirth and aging in the development of pelvic organ prolapse has been firmly established, but whether there are congenital conditions that place the individual at risk remains controversial. Also, are there conditions that can be identified and corrected to reduce the individual's risk of subsequently developing pelvic organ prolapse? From a limited amount of literature it would appear that chronic constipation and physical stressors at work are two areas that deserve attention. However, these are important considerations that need more investigation before conclusive recommendations can be made.

EPIDEMIOLOGY OF URINARY INCONTINENCE

Prevalence of Urinary Incontinence

It is estimated that between 23% and 35% of adult women have urinary incontinence (45–48). Trying to identify what percent have stress urinary incontinence versus urge incontinence versus mixed is impossible from the large epidemiologic studies. As mentioned above, responses to specific questions regarding symptoms of incontinence cannot adequately discriminate between the various forms of incontinence, and therefore any large symptom-based study can only guess at the relative contribution of each. One study that correlated types of incontinence as reported on a validated questionnaire and urodynamically determined diagnosis found poor correlation (49). A good rule of thumb is that roughly one half will have stress urinary incontinence, one quarter will have urge incontinence, and one quarter will have mixed incontinence. The prevalence of urinary incontinence is not evenly distributed throughout the population. Instead, much like pelvic organ prolapse, it is a disease that disproportionately affects the elderly. In one large epidemiologic study the prevalence increased steadily from a low of 8% to 9% in women age 20 to 24 years to 30% in women aged 50 to 54, where it plateaued and remained between 30% and 35% (45) (Fig. 2.3).

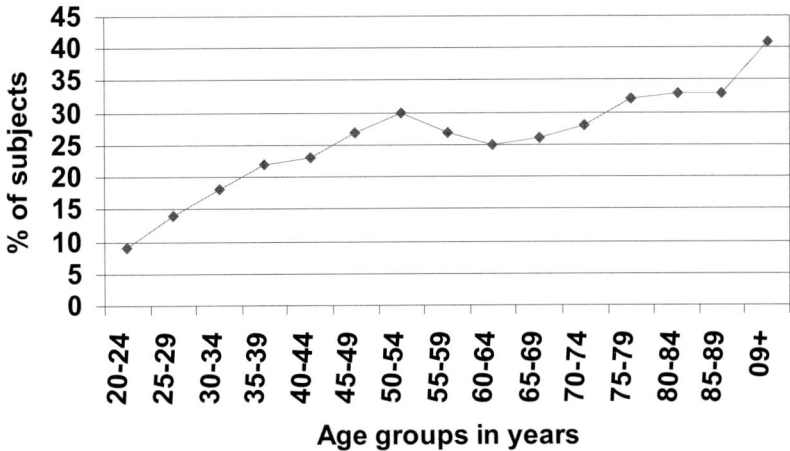

FIGURE 2.3 ● Percent of subjects with urinary incontinence by age in a Norwegian study of more than 27,000 subjects. (From Hannestad YS, Rotveit G, Sandvik H, et al. A community-based epidemiologic survey of female urinary incontinence: The Norwegian EPINCOT study. *J Clin Epidemiol* 2000;53:1150–1160.)

Natural History of Urinary Incontinence

Several studies published in the past decade have shed light on the incidence of urinary incontinence over 3- to 5-year periods (50–54). The annual incidence of new incontinence is between 5% and 8%, but what is surprising is that the annual remission rates (the development of continence without intervention in a previously incontinent subject) are between 10% and 38%. It was long held that once an individual began to experience incontinence, she would remain symptomatic until undergoing corrective therapy, but this thought may no longer be valid.

It can be said that urinary incontinence is a common disease, affecting between 15% and 30% of adults at any given time. The prevalence increases with age until age 50, where it plateaus, and importantly the remission rate of incontinence is as high as 38% per year. While the data on who is likely to have a spontaneous remission versus continued complaints is unknown, it should be kept in mind that subjects with minimal symptoms do not always require intervention, as many of them will become continent with time. This does not mean that therapy to correct incontinence should be withheld (while awaiting a spontaneous resolution) but rather that subjects with minimal incontinence may decide to watch and wait before proceeding on an invasive course of therapy.

Etiology of Urinary Incontinence

Age

As mentioned above, age plays a very significant role in the development of urinary incontinence.

The relationship is linear, with a steady rise in the prevalence of urinary incontinence from age 20 to 50, after which there is a plateau until women reach their seventies, where we see another slight rise (45). It is felt that several changes in the pelvic floor musculature and overall health that occur with aging are responsible for the increasing incontinence that occurs as women age.

Another observation is that the relative contribution of each type of incontinence changes with age. Younger women tend to report more stress incontinence symptoms, whereas older women tend to report more urge symptoms. This may be due to the effect of urogenital atrophy on lower urinary tract symptoms. This leads to another proposed etiologic risk factor for urinary incontinence, menopause, which is also age-related. It is felt that estrogen is beneficial in promoting continence and that its absence can eventually lead to urinary incontinence. While this simplistic view of the relationship between estrogen and menopause is probably invalid, it is well known that women with urogenital atrophy are at increased risk for urinary tract infections and have more irritative voiding symptoms (55,56), both of which are corrected with the application of estrogen therapy. Therefore, it may be that hypoestrogenic women have more severe symptoms, which has fed the supposition that menopause leads to incontinence. In addition, while estrogen therapy may improve irritative lower urinary tract symptoms, it has proved ineffective in treating incontinence (57). Finally, the rise in the prevalence of urinary incontinence plateaus at age 50. If menopause were a significant risk factor, one would expect a sharp rise within a few years of menopause (roughly age 51) as estrogen levels fall and menopause begins to exert its effect on the lower urinary tract.

Aging is one of the greatest risk factors for developing pelvic organ prolapse, but this appears to be unrelated to hormonal changes that women pass through during the aging process.

Pregnancy/Childbirth

The relationship between pregnancy and urinary incontinence goes back to Howard Kelly's landmark 1914 article on the surgical correction of incontinence, in which he wrote, "There is a type of urinary incontinence in women, without manifest injury to the bladder and having no relationship to fistula, which most frequently comes on following childbirth" (58). Since then most of the epidemiologic literature has identified pregnancy as a cause of urinary incontinence. However, the debate continues as to whether it is the pregnancy or the mode of delivery that has the greatest impact on future development of urinary incontinence.

It is well known that urinary incontinence is very common during pregnancy, with prevalence rates of between 30% and 60%, but the majority of these subjects will have resolution of their incontinence in the first 6 to 12 months postpartum (59–62). Which patients go on to develop long-term problems with urinary incontinence and which will obtain resolution has not been established. It is felt that the mechanism by which pregnancy causes urinary incontinence is similar to that proposed for pelvic organ prolapse discussed previously in this chapter. However, if the main insult of pregnancy involves stretching and damage to the pelvic fascia, levator musculature, and nerves innervating the pelvic viscera, then it would be expected that vaginal delivery would have the greatest impact. This may not be the case. The literature on the relationship between mode of delivery and subsequent development of urinary incontinence is mixed. Several recent large epidemiologic studies specifically addressed the question regarding effects of pregnancy and mode of delivery on subsequent urinary incontinence. Two studies found that women who delivered by cesarean section had a similar risk of urinary incontinence as women with any vaginal delivery (to include women who had delivered by cesarean delivery and vaginal delivery and women who delivered by vaginal delivery only) (45,47). One other study evaluated women who delivered by cesarean section only compared with women who only delivered vaginally and demonstrated that vaginal delivery increased the risk of incontinence (63). All three of these studies noted that any pregnancy increased the risk of sub-

sequent incontinence over nulliparity. However, a recent study of more than 4,000 women participating in one insurance plan found that cesarean delivery had a protective effect equal to nulliparity against the development of pelvic floor disorders (48). Finally, there is a unique study looking at the effect of cesarean only versus vaginal delivery in identical twins (64). Among 271 identical twin pairs, cesarean delivery–only twins had 50% less urinary incontinence over their identical twin who delivered vaginally. Therefore, it may be that delivering by cesarean only does provide some degree of protection.

However, before we can state with any degree of accuracy what effect vaginal delivery has on pelvic floor function, a large long-term prospective randomized trial should be carried out, but the chances of this are slim owing to the logistics involved. To date, there is only one prospective randomized trial comparing planned cesarean to vaginal delivery that was performed in subjects with breech presentation (65). The outcome of urinary incontinence was measured at 3 months postdelivery, and these investigators found only a small but statistically significant difference in urinary incontinence between the two groups, with cesarean delivery being protective.

Another area of concern involves instrumented vaginal delivery. When compared to a normal spontaneous vaginal delivery or vacuum-assisted vaginal delivery, a forceps-assisted delivery increased the risk of incontinence at 1 year by fivefold (62).

It can be said that pregnancy increases the risk of developing urinary incontinence. That risk can be lessened slightly with cesarean section and is probably increased with forceps.

Hysterectomy

The effects of hysterectomy on urinary incontinence continue to be debated. It has been suggested that disrupting the musculofascial attachment of the cervix to the cardinal uterosacral ligament complex will lead to relaxation and subsequent development of stress incontinence. In addition, the disruption of the autonomic nervous innervation of the bladder during dissection of the cardinal uterosacral ligament complex can lead to urge incontinence. However, again the evidence linking any type of urinary incontinence to hysterectomy is poor and contradictory. If this disruption played a significant role, then it could be surmised that a supracervical hysterectomy would provide protection. A recent large prospective randomized study comparing supracervical hysterectomy to a total abdominal hysterectomy failed to show any difference in lower urinary tract complaints at 1 year of follow-up (66). A recent review of the literature involving the effects of hysterectomy on urinary incontinence demonstrated no increased incontinence rates for 2 years following a hysterectomy (67).

Racial Differences

There have been anecdotal suggestions that Caucasian women have more incontinence than Black women. Most of the literature supporting this supposition comes from referral practices or in populations with a very small subset of minorities (51,68). In the few large population-based studies there is the suggestion that there is more severe incontinence among Caucasians than Blacks, but other minorities are underrepresented (69,70).

Obesity

The relationship between obesity and urinary incontinence has been consistently confirmed in several large epidemiologic studies (47,51,69–72). Even women who are modestly overweight, with a BMI between 26 and 30, have up to a 50% increase in their incontinence compared to women with a BMI below 25 (47). Obese women with a BMI above 30 have a twofold increase in urinary incontinence compared to women with BMIs below 25 (47). Further, in morbidly obese women (with BMIs between 40 and 81), the prevalence of urinary incontinence is as high as 66% (73). It is felt that the increasing abdominal girth increases the intra-abdominal pressure, which causes increased stress and strain on the viscera, nerves, and muscles of the pelvic floor, much like pregnancy. In addition, there is evidence that weight loss, either surgically induced or attained through diet and exercise, can relieve or at least reduce the incontinence symptoms (74–76).

Chronic Illnesses/Lifestyle

A recent large observational study of more than 5,000 women participating in a health maintenance organization demonstrated an increased risk of incontinence among its participants who carried diagnoses of Parkinson's disease, dementia, stroke, depression, and congestive heart failure (77). There is very little data on how other chronic illnesses affect urinary incontinence, but it is well established that hypertensive subjects on diuretics have more severe symptoms.

Another chronic illness/lifestyle choice, cigarette smoking, appears to promote urinary incontinence. Smokers have demonstrated a 2.5-fold increase in the risk of developing genuine stress incontinence over nonsmokers independent of other risk factors (78). In a large epidemiologic study, only those smoking greater than 20 cigarettes per day had an increased risk of incontinence (79). It is felt that the forceful coughing associated with cigarette smoking is responsible for the increased incidence of stress incontinence in smokers. What effect COPD and other pulmonary diseases with increased coughing have is less certain.

There are reports on the incidence of urinary incontinence during high-impact activities, particularly sports, with up to 25% of young physically fit women reporting some urinary incontinence (80). However, when elite athletes are followed over time, the incidence of incontinence developing later in life is similar to age-matched controls (81).

Family History

Whether urinary incontinence is an inherited disease is a question that has been asked repeatedly, but to date there are only a few reports. In a large epidemiologic study from Norway on urinary incontinence, the authors reported that daughters of incontinent women had a 30% increased risk of having incontinence, and younger sisters of women with incontinence had a 60% increased risk of incontinence (82). In a study of postmenopausal sister pairs (one being nulliparous and the other parous), it was determined that the prevalence of incontinence was similar between sisters regardless of parity, suggesting that it was genetics and not parity that played the greater role in determining who would have urinary incontinence (83).

Summary

Urinary incontinence is a common disease and its prevalence increases with age. Pregnancy appears to place one at risk for incontinence, but how much effect is from the pregnancy itself versus the delivery route remains debatable. Lifestyle choices like smoking and obesity also place one at risk, while weight loss improves incontinence. Whether or not smoking cessation will lessen the risk of incontinence remains speculative. Finally, from the few studies available, it would appear that genetics predisposes some individuals to urinary incontinence. It is the genetics of incontinence that need to be fully explored before we can make recommendations on prevention strategies.

REFERENCES

1. Mant J, Painter R, Vessey M. Epidemiology of genital prolapse: observations from the Oxford Family Planning Association study. *Br J Obstet Gynecol* 1997;104: 579–585.

2. Olsen AL, Smith VJ, Bergstrom JO, et al. Epidemiology of surgically managed pelvic organ prolapse and urinary incontinence. *Obstet Gynecol* 1997;89:501–506.

3. Brubaker L, Norton P. Current clinical nomenclature for description of pelvic organ prolapse. *J Pelvic Surg* 1996;2:257–259.

4. American College of Obstetricians and Gynecologists. *Pelvic organ prolapse.* ACOG Technical Bulletin 214. Washington, DC: ACOG, 1995.

5. Bump RC, Mattiasson A, Brubaker LP, et al. The standardization of terminology of female pelvic floor dysfunction. *Am J Obstet Gynecol* 1996;175:10–17.

6. Weber AM, Abrams P, Brubaker L, et al. The Standardization of terminology for researchers in female pelvic floor disorders. *Int Urogynecol J* 2001;12:178–186.

7. Abrams P, Blaivas JG, Stanton S, et al. The standardisation of terminology of lower urinary tract function. *Neurourol Urodyn* 1988;7:403–426.

8. Abrams P, Cardozo L, Fall M, et al. The standardization of terminology in lower urinary tract function: Report from the Standardization Subcommittee of the International Continence Society. *Neurourol Urodyn* 2002; 21:167–178.

9. Jensen JK, Nielsen FR, Ostergard DR. The role of patient history in the diagnosis of urinary incontinence. *Obstet Gynecol* 1994;83:904–910.

10. Lukacz ES, Lawrence JM, Buckwalter JG, et al. Epidemiology of prolapse and incontinence questionnaire: validation of a new epidemiologic survey. *Int Urogynecol J* 2005;16:272–284.

11. Swift SE. The distribution of pelvic organ support in a population of female subjects seen for routine gynecologic health care. *Am J Obstet Gynecol* 2000;183: 277–285.

12. Slieker-ten H, Vierhout M, Bloembergen H, et al. *Distribution of pelvic organ prolapse in a general population: Prevalence, severity, etiology, and relation with the function of pelvic floor muscles.* Abstract presented at the Joint Meeting of the ICS and IUGA, August 25–27, 2004, Paris, France.

13. Swift SE, Woodman P, O'Boyle A, et al. Pelvic Organ Support Study (POSST); the distribution, clinical definition, and epidemiology of pelvic organ support defects. *Am J Obstet Gynecol* 2005;192:795–806.

14. Bland DR, Earle BB, Vitolins MZ, et al. Use of the pelvic organ prolapse staging system of the International Continence Society, American Urogynecologic Society, and the Society of Gynecologic Surgeons in perimenopausal women. *Am J Obstet Gynecol* 1999;181: 1324–1328.

15. Hall AF, Theofrastous JP, Cundiff GC, et al. Interobserver and intraobserver reliability of the proposed International Continence Society, Society of Gynecologic Surgeons, and American Urogynecologic Society pelvic organ prolapse classification system. *Am J Obstet Gynecol* 1996;175:1467–1471.

16. Kobak WH, Rosenberger K, Walters MD. Interobserver variation in the assessment of pelvic organ prolapse. *Int J Urogynecol Pelvic Floor Dysfunct* 1996; 7:121–124.

17. Gurel H, Gurel SA. Pelvic relaxation and associated risk factors: the results of logistic regression analysis. *Acta Obstet Gynecol Scand* 1999;78:290–293.

18. Swift SE, Pound T, Dias JK. Case-control study of the etiologic factors in the development of severe pelvic organ prolapse. *Int Urogynecol J* 2001;12:187–192.

19. Snooks SJ, Swash M, Henry MM, et al. Risk factors in childbirth causing damage to the pelvic floor innervation. *Int J Colorectal Dis* 1986;1:20–24.

20. Smith ARB, Hosker GL, Warrell DW. The role of partial denervation of the pelvic floor in the aetiology of genital prolapse and stress incontinence of urine. A neurophysiological approach. *Br J Obstet Gynecol* 1989; 96:24–28.

21. Allen RE, Hosker GL, Smith ARB, et al. Pelvic floor damage and childbirth: a neurophysiological study. *Br J Obstet Gynecol* 1990;97:770–779.

22. MacLennan AH, Taylor AW, Wilson DH, et al. The prevalence of pelvic floor disorders and their relationship to gender, age, and mode of delivery. *Br J Obstet Gynecol* 2000;107:1460–1470.

23. Samuelsson EU, Victor FTA, Tibblin G, et al. Signs of genital prolapse in a Swedish population of women 20 to 59 years of age and possible related factors. *Am J Obstet Gynecol* 1999;180:299–305.

24. Brown JS, Waetjen LE, Subak LL, et al. Pelvic organ prolapse surgery in the United States, 1997. *Am J Obstet Gynecol* 2002;186:712–716.

25. Benson JT, Lucente V, McClellan E. Vaginal versus abdominal reconstructive surgery for the treatment of pelvic support defects: a prospective, randomized study with long-term outcome evaluation. *Am J Obstet Gynecol* 1996;175:1418–1422.

26. Symmonds RE, Williams TJ, Lee RA, et al. Posthysterectomy enterocele and vaginal vault prolapse. *Am J Obstet Gynecol* 1981;140:852–859.

27. Richter K. Massive eversion of the vagina: pathogenesis, diagnosis, and therapy of the "true" prolapse of the vaginal stump. *Clin Obstet Gynecol* 1982;25:897–899.

28. Virtanen HS, Makinen JI. Retrospective analysis of 711 patients operated on for pelvic relaxation in 1983 to 1989. *Int J Obstet Gynecol* 1993;42:109–115.

29. Waters EG. Vaginal prolapse: technique for prevention and correction at hysterectomy. *Obstet Gynecol* 1956;8: 432–436.

30. Phaneuf LE. Inversion of the vagina and prolapse of the cervix following supracervical hysterectomy and inversion of the vagina following total hysterectomy. *Am J Obstet Gynecol* 1952;64:739–743.

31. Jackson SR, Avery NC, Tarlton JF, et al. Changes in metabolism of collagen in genitourinary prolapse. *Lancet* 1996;347:1658–1661.

32. Makinen J, Soderstrom KO, Kiilhoma P, et al. Histological changes in the vaginal connective tissue of patients with and without uterine prolapse. *Arch Gynecol* 1986;239:17–20.

33. Norton P, Baker J, Sharp H, et al. Genitourinary prolapse: relationship with joint mobility. *Neurourol Urodynam* 1990;9:321–322.

34. McIntosh LJ, Stanitski DF, Mallett VT, et al. Ehlers-Danlos syndrome: relationship between joint hypermobility, urinary incontinence, and pelvic floor prolapse. *Gynecol Obstet Invest* 1996;41:135–139.

35. Torpin R. Prolapse uteri associated with spina bifida and clubfeet in newborn infants. *Am J Obstet Gynecol* 1942;43:892–894.

36. Ajbor LN, Okojie SE. Genital prolapse in the newborn. *Int Surg* 1976;61:496–497.

37. Zacharin RF. "A Chinese anatomy"—the pelvic supporting tissues of the Chinese and Occidental female compared and contrasted. *Aust NZ J Obstet Gynecol* 1977;17:1–11.

38. Brieger GM, Yip SK, Hin LY, et al. The prevalence of urinary dysfunction in Hong Kong Chinese women. *Obstet Gynecol* 1996;88:1041–1044.

39. Jorgensen S, Hein HO, Gyntelberg F. Heavy lifting at work and risk of genital prolapse and herniated disc in assistant nurses. *Occup Med* 1994;44:47–49.

40. Chiaffarino F, Chatenoud L, Dindelli M, et al. Reproductive factors, family history, occupation, and risk of urogenital prolapse. *Eur J Obstet Gynecol* 1999; 82:63–67.

41. Woodman PJ, Swift SE, O'Boyle AL, et al. Prevalence of severe pelvic organ prolapse in relation to job description and socioeconomic status: a multicenter cross-sectional study. *Int Urogynecol J* 2006 [on-line].

42. DeLancey JOL. Pelvic floor dysfunction: causes and prevention. *Contemp Obstet Gynecol* 1993 (Jan):68–80.

43. Spence-Jones C, Kamm MA, Henery MM, et al. Bowel dysfunction: a pathogenic factor in uterovaginal prolapse and urinary stress incontinence. *Br J Obstet Gynecol* 1994;101:147–152.

44. Kahn MA, Breitkopf CR, Valley M, et al. Pelvic organ support study (POSST) and bowel symptoms: Straining is associated with perineal and anterior vaginal defects in a general gynecologic population. *Am J Obstet Gynecol* 2005;192:1516–1522.

45. Hannestad YS, Rotveit G, Sandvik H, et al. A community-based epidemiologic survey of female urinary incontinence: the Norwegian EPINCOT study. *J Clin Epidemiol* 2000;53:1150–1160.

46. MacLennan AH, Taylor AW, Wilson DH, et al. The prevalence of pelvic floor disorders and their relationship to gender, age, parity, and mode of delivery. *Br J Obstet Gynecol* 2000;107:1460–1470.

47. McKinnie V, Swift S, Wang W, et al. The effect of pregnancy and mode of delivery on the prevalence of urinary and anal incontinence. *Am J Obstet Gynecol* 2005;193:512–518.

48. Kukacz ES, Lawrence JM, Contreras R, et al. *Parity, mode of delivery, and pelvic floor dysfunction.* Abstract presented at the American Urogynecology Society 26th annual meeting, Atlanta, GA, September 15–17, 2005.

49. Sandvik H, Hunskaar S, Vanvik A, et al. Diagnostic classification of female urinary incontinence: an epidemiologic survey corrected for validity. *J Clin Epidemiol* 1995;48:339–345.

50. Herzog AR, Diokno AC, Brown MB, et al. Two-year incidence, remission, and change patterns of urinary incontinence in noninstitutional older adults. *J Gerontol* 1990;45:M67.

51. Burgio KL, Matthews KA, Engel BT. Prevalence, incidence, and correlates of urinary incontinence in healthy, middle-aged women. *J Urol* 1991;146:1255–1260.

52. Sammuelson E, Victor A, Tibblin G. A population study of urinary incontinence and nocturia among women aged 20 to 59 years. Prevalence, well-being, and wish for treatment. *Acta Obstet Gynecol Scand* 1997; 76:74–79.

53. Moller LA, Lose G, Jorgensen T. Prevalence and bothersomeness of lower urinary tract symptoms in women 40 to 60 years of age. *Acta Obstet Gynecol Scand* 2000; 79:298–303.

54. Sammeulson EC, Victor FT, Svardsudd KF. Five-year incidence and remission rates of female urinary incontinence in a Swedish population less than 65 years old. *Am J Obstet Gynecol* 2000;183:568–572.

55. Cardozo L, Lose G, McClish D, et al. A systematic review of estrogens for recurrent urinary tract infections: Third Report of the Hormones and Urogenital Therapy (HUT) Committee. *Int Urogynecol J* 2001;12:15–20.

56. Cardozo L, Bachman G, McClish D, et al. Meta-analysis of estrogen therapy in the management of urogenital atrophy in post menopausal women: second report of the Hormones and Urogenital Therapy Committee. *Obstet Gynecol* 1998;92:722–727.

57. Fantl JA, Cardozo L, McClish D. Estrogen therapy in the management of urinary incontinence in post-menopausal women: a meta-analysis. First report of the Hormones and Urogenital Therapy Committee. *Obstet Gynecol* 1994;83:12–18.

58. Kelly HA, Dunn WM. Urinary incontinence in women, without manifest injury to the bladder. *Surg Gynecol Obstet* 1914;18:444–450.

59. Burgio KL, Locher JL, Zcyzynski H, et al. Urinary incontinence during pregnancy in a racially mixed sample: characteristics and predisposing factors. *Int Urogynecol J* 1996;7:69–73.

60. Iosif S. Stress incontinence during pregnancy and in the puerperium. *Int J Obstet Gynecol* 1981;19:13–20.

61. Viktrup L, Lose G, Rolff M, et al. The symptom of stress urinary incontinence caused by pregnancy or delivery in the primiparas. *Obstet Gynecol* 1992;79:945–949.

62. Arya LL, Jackson ND, Meyers DL, et al. Risk of new-onset urinary incontinence after forceps and vacuum delivery in primiparous women. *Am J Obstet Gynecol* 2001;185:1318–1324.

63. Rotveit G, Daltveit AK, Hannestad YS, et al. Urinary incontinence after vaginal delivery or cesarean section. *N Engl J Med* 2003;348:900–907.

64. Goldgerg RP, Abramov Y, Botros S, et al. *Delivery mode is the major environmental determinant of SUI: results of the Evanston Identical Twin Sisters Study.* Presented at the 30th annual meeting of the International Urogynecological Association, Copenhagen, Denmark, August 9–12, 2005.

65. Hannah ME, Hannah WJ, Hodnett ED, et al. Outcomes at three months after planned cesarean versus planned vaginal delivery for breech presentation at term. *JAMA* 2002;287:1822–1831.

66. Gimbel H, Zobbe V, Andersen BM, et al. Lower urinary tract symptoms after total and subtotal hysterectomy: results of a randomized controlled trial. *Int Urogynecol J* 2005;16:257–262.

67. Thom DH, Brown JS. Reproductive and hormonal risk factors for urinary incontinence in later life: a review of the clinical and epidemiological literature. *J Am Geriatr Soc* 1998;46:1411–1420.

68. Bump RC. Racial comparisons and contrasts in urinary incontinence and urogenital prolapse in a black inner city population. *Am J Obstet Gynecol* 1993;81: 421–424.

69. Brown JS, Gady D, Ouslander JG, et al. Prevalence of urinary incontinence and associated risk factors in post-menopausal women. *Obstet Gynecol* 1999;94:66–71.

70. Thom DH, Van Den Eeden SK, Brown JS. Evaluation of parturition and other reproductive variables as risk factors for urinary incontinence in later life. *Obstet Gynecol* 1997;90:983–987.

71. Wingate L, Wingate MB, Hassanein R. The relationship between overweight and urinary incontinence in post-menopausal women: a case control study. *Menopause* 1994;1:199–203.

72. Dwyer PL, Lee ET, Hay DM. Obesity and urinary incontinence in women. *Br J Obstet Gynecol* 1988;95: 91–96.

73. Richter HE, Burgio KL, Clements RH, et al. Urinary and anal incontinence in morbidly obese women considering weight loss surgery. *Obstet Gynecol* 2005;106: 1272–1277.

74. Bump RC, Sugarman HJ, Fantl JA, et al. Obesity and lower urinary tract function in women: Effect of surgically induced weight loss. *Am J Obstet Gynecol* 1992; 167:392–399.

75. Subak LL, Johnson C, Whitcomb E, et al. Does weight loss improve incontinence in moderately obese women? *Int Urogynecol J* 2002;13:40–43.

76. Auwad W, Bomberi L, Freeman R. *The effects of weight reduction on obese women with urinary incontinence.* Abstract presented at the 30th annual International Urogynecology Association meeting, Copenhagen, Denmark, August 9–12, 2005.

77. Thom DH, Hann MN, Van Den Eeden S. Medically recognized urinary incontinence and risks of hospitalization, nursing home admission, and mortality. *Age Aging* 1997;26:267–272.

78. Bump RC, McClish DK. Cigarette smoking and urinary incontinence in women. *Am J Obstet Gynecol* 1992; 167:1213–1218.

79. Hannestad YS, Rortveit G, Daltveit AK, et al. Are smoking and other lifestyle factors associated with female urinary incontinence? The Norwegian EPINCOT study. *Br J Obstet Gynecol* 2003;110:247–254.

80. Nygaard IE, Thompson FL, Svengalis SL, et al. Urinary incontinence in elite nulliparous athletes. *Obstet Gynecol* 1994;84:183–187.

81. Nygaard IE. Does prolonged high-impact activity contribute to later urinary incontinence? A retrospective cohort study of female Olympians. *Obstet Gynecol* 1997; 90:718–722.

82. Hannestad YS, Rolv T, Rortveit G, et al. Familial risk of urinary incontinence in women: population-based cross-sectional study. *Br Med J* 2004;329:889–891.

83. Buschbaum GH, Duecy EE, Kerr LA, et al. Urinary incontinence in nulliparous women and their parous sisters. *Obstet Gynecol* 2005;106:1253–1258.

CHAPTER 3

Outcomes Assessment

Brian S. Yamada and Kathleen C. Kobashi

INTRODUCTION

Pelvic floor disorders include a wide range of interrelated clinical conditions, such as urinary incontinence, voiding dysfunction, pelvic organ prolapse, defecatory dysfunction, and sexual dysfunction. While pelvic floor disorders seldom lead to severe morbidity or mortality, their primary impact is on quality of life. Consequently, quality of life assessment is critical when evaluating treatments for urinary incontinence and pelvic prolapse (1). Traditional means of assessing efficacy of treatments for pelvic floor disorders include objective measures such as urodynamic studies, pad tests, clinical examinations, and voiding diaries. While objective measures are typically a part of the treatment assessment, clinical and research questionnaire tools are now playing a more prominent role in outcomes assessment.

When reviewing the literature for urinary incontinence and pelvic floor disorders, it is apparent that the overall quality of the body of literature is suboptimal. Even today, many practice guidelines are based on studies using objective measures alone. More recent literature suggests that objective measures are often poorly correlated to patient goals and quality of life (2). This is further complicated by the fact that much of the literature has inadequate follow-up, lack of standard definitions for the success or failure of treatments, lack of sufficient power, and a paucity or underreporting of complications.

Multiple questionnaires have been developed over the past decade and are beginning to encompass the various components associated with pelvic floor disorders. Currently, no standard questionnaire for pelvic floor disorders exists. The goal of this chapter is to give an overview of the tools currently available to the clinical and research urologist and urogynecologist. Most of the available instruments focus on only one component of the multifaceted pelvic floor, but recently questionnaires have begun to include symptoms reflective of the multiple compartments, with specific items designed to address quality of life.

QUESTIONNAIRE DEVELOPMENT

Although a detailed discussion is beyond the scope of this chapter, a brief summary of the steps necessary for developing a questionnaire is provided. The initial focus in questionnaire development is the compilation of pertinent items via evaluation of existing scales and the addition of questions based on input from "experts" in the field and discussion with patients. A new questionnaire is assessed for *content validity* to see whether it appears to cover all the relevant or important domains. The questions are then assessed for *face validity*, which determines that the items actually measure what they are intended to measure. Validity testing also involves testing the criteria against a gold standard, if one exists (3).

Next, *reliability testing* is performed to ensure that the items in a questionnaire are measured in a reproducible fashion. Reliability is usually quoted as a ratio of the variability between individuals to the total variability in the scores. It is expressed as a number between 0 and 1, with 0 indicating no reliability and 1 indicating perfect reliability (3). Reliability testing includes intraobserver reliability, interobserver reliability, and test–retest reliability. *Intraobserver reliability* assesses the consistency between observations made by the same rater on two different occasions. *Interobserver reliability* assesses the degree of agreement between different observers. *Test–retest reliability* assesses the consistency of responses on a given item separated by an interval of time to evaluate whether the item would be interpreted and answered the same way twice by the same individual (3).

Internal consistency further confirms reliability and refers to the degree of correlation between the questionnaire items. Items forming a domain should moderately correlate with each other but also contribute independently to the overall domain score (4). These correlations are calculated using Cronbach's alpha and should exceed a value of 0.8. *Responsiveness* is the ability of an instrument to detect a small but clinically important change. This psychometric property is often neglected in the literature (5,6).

Finally, the questionnaire must have adequate interpretability, meaning that ambiguous or incomprehensible items should be eliminated. The method of questionnaire administration may also affect participant responses. For example, a better correlation to urodynamic findings was found in patients who were administered the Bristol Female Lower Urinary Tract Symptoms questionnaire in the mailed self-administered form versus interview-assisted administration (7).

This chapter contains descriptions of numerous questionnaires available for evaluation of symptoms and quality of life pertaining to urinary incontinence, pelvic organ prolapse, and sexual dysfunction. Each of the questionnaires to be discussed underwent a thorough validation process. Some of the described instruments have been updated with short-form versions. Short-form questionnaires are potentially useful when an instrument is frequently used or the assessment time is limited. Long questionnaires are time-consuming and may increase the number of unanswered items (8).

TRADITIONAL OUTCOMES MEASURES: URODYNAMICS, PAD TESTS, BADEN-WALKER, PELVIC ORGAN PROLAPSE QUANTIFICATION (POP-Q)

Two traditional outcomes measures used to measure success of therapy for stress urinary incontinence include urodynamics and the 1-hour pad test. These tests, however, do not necessarily correlate well to questionnaire results. For example, urodynamics has not been proven to be accurate in detecting the presence or severity of incontinence unless the bladder volume is fixed at 200 to 300 cc or 50% to 75% of bladder capacity. These measures do not assess quality of life and therefore provide an incomplete picture of patient status.

Pelvic organ prolapse is assessed in part by physical examination. Physical examination has also traditionally been used to determine the success of prolapse repair. The two standard systems for assessing prolapse are the Baden-Walker system and the Pelvic Organ Prolapse Quantification (POP-Q) system. The International Continence Society recognizes the POP-Q as the standard measurement system. While useful as part of patient assessment, it is controversial whether these measures correlate to clinical symptoms and quality of life. Further description of the POP-Q exam as it pertains to symptoms is presented later in this chapter.

CURRENT INSTRUMENTS: URINARY INCONTINENCE AND PELVIC PROLAPSE

Urogenital Distress Inventory (UDI) and Incontinence Impact Questionnaire (IIQ)

The Urogenital Distress Inventory (UDI) was developed by Shumaker in 1994 with the goal of assessing the degree to which symptoms associated with urinary incontinence are bothersome. The original UDI has 19 questions and encompasses three domains (symptoms related to stress urinary incontinence, detrusor overactivity, and bladder outlet obstruction). The Incontinence Impact Questionnaire (IIQ) was developed at the same time and assesses the impact of urinary incontinence on activities, social roles, and emotional states in women (9). It consists of 30 questions and covers four domains (physical activity, social relationships, travel, and emotional health). Each question has a 4-point response scale (0 = not at all, 1 = slightly, 2 = moderately, 3 = greatly). Both the UDI and IIQ were developed for simple self-administration. Both questionnaires are strong psychometrically and numerous authors have supported their validity (10,11). Neither questionnaire specifically addresses pelvic prolapse or its associated symptoms.

In 1995, short-form versions of the UDI and IIQ were created (Figs. 3.1 and 3.2). The 19-item UDI was condensed into a 6-item questionnaire and named the UDI-6. The 30-item IIQ was condensed into the 7-item IIQ-7. Regression analysis of each short form suggested that they would accurately predict the results of the long form. Both questionnaires were validated and are considered to be more useful than their long forms in many clinical and research applications (12). The UDI-6 has been shown to correspond to findings on urodynamics. Lemack et al demonstrated that most patients reporting moderately or greatly bothersome stress incontinence on the UDI-6 were found to have stress leakage on urodynamics, which differed significantly from those who reported no bother. Valsalva leak point pressure did not correlate to symptom severity on the scale. Urgency symptoms described as moderately or greatly bothersome were found to have a significantly

Do you experience, and, if so, how much are you bothered by

		Not at all	A little bit	Moderately	Greatly
1	Frequent urination	0	1	2	3
2	Urine leakage related to urgency	0	1	2	3
3	Urine leakage related to physical activity	0	1	2	3
4	Small amounts of urine leakage (drops)	0	1	2	3
5	Difficulty emptying your bladder	0	1	2	3
6	Pain or discomfort in the lower abdomen/genitalia	0	1	2	3

FIGURE 3.1 ● Urogenital Distress Inventory–Short Form (UDI-6).

greater incidence of detrusor overactivity on urodynamics compared to women who did not have this complaint (13).

Other authors have suggested certain limitations of the IIQ and UDI. Handa found that most items in the IIQ were useful for discriminating incontinence among women with mild-to-moderate urinary incontinence but tended to underestimate the magnitude of changes of incontinence severity in women with severe urinary incontinence (11). Harvey found that the IIQ and UDI appeared to be valid in women with a urodynamic diagnosis of incontinence but were of questionable validity as markers of incontinence severity in women without a urodynamic diagnosis (14).

International Consultation on Incontinence (ICIQ) Modular Questionnaire

Sponsored by the World Health Organization and organized by the International Continence Society and the International Consultation on Urological Diseases, the first International Consultation on Incontinence (ICI) was held in 1998. This committee supported the idea that a universally applicable questionnaire should be developed for urinary incontinence (15). The goal was that such a questionnaire could be widely applied both in clinical practice and research, used in different settings and studies, and allow for cross-comparisons. For example, the questionnaire could cross-compare a drug treatment to an operation used for the same condition, in the same way that that the International Prostate Symptoms Score (IPSS) has been used (15). The end result was the development of the ICIQ Modular Questionnaire.

The first module developed was the ICIQ-UI Short Form for urinary incontinence, which has been validated and published (16). Other modules have been added to the ICIQ Modular Questionnaire by the adoption and renaming of several pre-existing, validated scales (17–22). The adopted questionnaires pertaining to female pelvic floor disorders are listed in Figure 3.3. Additional modules are being developed for urinary tract, vaginal, and lower bowel symptoms. Each of these modules deal with quality of life and sexual function in a

Has the urine leakage and/or prolapse affected your

		Not at all	A little bit	Moderately	Greatly
1	Ability to do household chores (cooking, house-cleaning, laundry)?	0	1	2	3
2	Physical recreation such as walking, swimming, or other exercise?	0	1	2	3
3	Entertainment activities (movies, concerts, etc.)?	0	1	2	3
4	Ability to travel by car or bus more than 30 minutes from home?	0	1	2	3
5	Participation in social activities outside your home?	0	1	2	3
6	Emotional health (nervousness, depression, etc.)?	0	1	2	3
7	Feeling frustrated?	0	1	2	3

FIGURE 3.2 ● Incontinence Impact Questionnaire–Short Form (IIQ-7).

dicted long-form scores (Fig. 3.7). The short form was also correlated to the IIQ-7, SHF-12, and Symptom Score (25).

Female Sexual Function Index (FSFI)

The Female Sexual Function Index (FSFI) is a 19-item, validated self-report measure of female sexual function (Fig. 3.8). It is geared toward a wide range of women, including postmenopausal women. It encompasses four domains of potential dysfunction: desire disorders, arousal disorder, orgasmic disorder, and sexual pain disorders. The questionnaire is designed and validated for assessment of female sexual function and quality of life in clinical trials or epidemiological studies (26).

PATIENT GOALS

Patient goals are an important but often overlooked component of outcomes assessment for women seeking care for pelvic floor disorders and medical care in general. Two studies have specifically addressed this topic. Hullfish compared preoperative patient goals and postoperative perceived achievement of goals in women undergoing pelvic surgery. Of 194 goals listed by participants, 40.2% had to do with resuming previous activities or lifestyle, 38.1% with symptom relief, 9.3% with improving self-image and social relationships, 7.7% with improving general health, and 4.6%

with improving physical appearance (27). In this study, 72% of goals were attained at short-term follow-up and 68% were attained at long-term follow-up. Long-term goal achievement correlated to UDI-6 and IIQ-7 scores and was inversely associated with surgical complications. Goal achievement was not associated with other clinical or demographic variables (27).

In another study, 78 women undergoing pelvic reconstructive surgery were asked to state their goals for surgery. Most commonly, goals involved improvement of urinary incontinence (58%), pelvic organ prolapse (53%), general health lifestyle (50%), and activity (44%). Less commonly reported goals were related to urgency/frequency (12%), sexual function (11%), and relief of urinary retention (6%) (2). Seventy-five percent of patients indicated they met all or most of their goals. Twelve percent met less than half and 9% met none of their goals. Patient satisfaction was moderately correlated to goal achievement. Objective cure, defined as no urodynamic stress incontinence and stage 0 or 1 prolapse, was not related to satisfaction. Lifestyle factors seemed to play a large role: many women focused on return to missed activities, whereas others focused on resolution of the particular problem (i.e., "I want the bulge gone," "I don't want to leak when I cough") (2). Understanding what the patient wants to achieve with surgery can help with presurgical counseling. However, the authors observed that

1	How frequently do you feel sexual desire? This may include wanting to have sex, planning to have sex, feeling frustrated due to lack of sex, etc.
2	Do you climax (have an orgasm) when having sexual intercourse with your partner?
3	Do you feel sexually excited (turned on) when having sexual activity with your partner?
4	How satisfied are you with the variety of sexual activities in your current sex life?
5	Do you feel pain during sexual intercourse?
6	Are you incontinent of urine (leak urine) with sexual activity?
7	Does fear of incontinence (either stool or urine) restrict your sexual activity?
8	Do you avoid sexual intercourse because of bulging in the vagina (either the bladder, rectum, or vagina falling out?
9	When you have sex with your partner, do you have negative emotional reactions such as fear, disgust, shame, or guilt?
10	Does your partner have a problem with erections that affects your sexual activity?
11	Does your partner have a problem with premature ejaculation that affects your sexual activity?
12	Compared to orgasms you have had in the past, how intense are the orgasms you have had in the past six months?

☐ Always   ☐ Usually   ☐ Sometimes   ☐ Seldom   ☐ Never

FIGURE 3.7 ● Pelvic Organ Prolapse/Urinary Incontinence Sexual Function Questionnaire–Short Form (PISQ-12).

1. Over the past 4 weeks, how often did you feel sexual desire or interest?	5 = Almost always or always 4 = Most times (more than half the time) 3 = Sometimes (about half the time) 2 = A few times (less than half the time) 1 = Almost never or never
2. Over the past 4 weeks, how would you rate your level (degree) of sexual desire or interest?	5 = Very high 4 = High 3 = Moderate 2 = Low 1 = Very low or none at all
3. Over the past 4 weeks, how often did you feel sexually aroused ("turned on") during sexual activity or intercourse?	0 = No sexual activity 5 = Almost always or always 4 = Most times (more than half the time) 3 = Sometimes (about half the time) 2 = A few times (less than half the time) 1 = Almost never or never
4. Over the past 4 weeks, how would you rate your level of sexual arousal ("turn on") during sexual activity or intercourse?	0 = No sexual activity 5 = Very high 4 = High 3 = Moderate 2 = Low 1 = Very low or none at all
5. Over the past 4 weeks, how confident were you about becoming sexually aroused during sexual activity or intercourse?	0 = No sexual activity 5 = Very high confidence 4 = High confidence 3 = Moderate confidence 2 = Low confidence 1 = Very low or no confidence
6. Over the past 4 weeks, how often have you been satisfied with your arousal (excitement) during sexual activity or intercourse?	0 = No sexual activity 5 = Almost always or always 4 = Most times (more than half the time) 3 = Sometimes (about half the time) 2 = A few times (less than half the time) 1 = Almost never or never
7. Over the past 4 weeks, how often did you become lubricated ("wet") during sexual activity or intercourse?	0 = No sexual activity 5 = Almost always or always 4 = Most times (more than half the time) 3 = Sometimes (about half the time) 2 = A few times (less than half the time) 1 = Almost never or never
8. Over the past 4 weeks, how difficult was it to become lubricated ("wet") during sexual activity or intercourse?	0 = No sexual activity 5 = Extremely difficult or impossible 4 = Very difficult 3 = Difficult 2 = Slightly difficult 1 = Not difficult
9. Over the past 4 weeks, how often did you maintain your lubrication ("wetness") until completion of sexual activity or intercourse?	0 = No sexual activity 5 = Almost always or always 4 = Most times (more than half the time) 3 = Sometimes (about half the time) 2 = A few times (less than half the time) 1 = Almost never or never
10. Over the past 4 weeks, how difficult was it to maintain your lubrication ("wetness") until completion of sexual activity or intercourse?	0 = No sexual activity 5 = Extremely difficult or impossible 4 = Very difficult 3 = Difficult 2 = Slightly difficult 1 = Not difficult

FIGURE 3.8 ● Pelvic Organ Prolapse/Urinary Incontinence Sexual Function Questionnaire–Short Form (PISQ-12). *(continued)*

11. Over the past 4 weeks, when you had sexual stimulation or intercourse, how often did you reach orgasm (climax)?	0 = No sexual activity 5 = Almost always or always 4 = Most times (more than half the time) 3 = Sometimes (about half the time) 2 = A few times (less than half the time) 1 = Almost never or never
12. Over the past 4 weeks, when you had sexual stimulation or intercourse, how difficult was it for you to reach orgasm (climax)?	0 = No sexual activity 5 = Extremely difficult or impossible 4 = Very difficult 3 = Difficult 2 = Slightly difficult 1 = Not difficult
13. Over the past 4 weeks, how satisfied were you with your ability to reach orgasm (climax) during sexual activity or intercourse?	0 = No sexual activity 5 = Very satisfied 4 = Moderately satisfied 3 = About equally satisfied and dissatisfied 2 = Moderately dissatisfied 1 = Very dissatisfied
14. Over the past 4 weeks, how satisfied have you been with the amount of emotional closeness during sexual activity between you and your partner?	0 = No sexual activity 5 = Very satisfied 4 = Moderately satisfied 3 = About equally satisfied and dissatisfied 2 = Moderately dissatisfied 1 = Very dissatisfied
15. Over the past 4 weeks, how satisfied have you been with your sexual relationship with your partner?	5 = Very satisfied 4 = Moderately satisfied 3 = About equally satisfied and dissatisfied 2 = Moderately dissatisfied 1 = Very dissatisfied
16. Over the past 4 weeks, how satisfied have you been with your overall sexual life?	5 = Very satisfied 4 = Moderately satisfied 3 = About equally satisfied and dissatisfied 2 = Moderately dissatisfied 1 = Very dissatisfied
17. Over the past 4 weeks, how often did you experience discomfort or pain during vaginal penetration	0 = Did not attempt intercourse 5 = Almost always or always 4 = Most times (more than half the time) 3 = Sometimes (about half the time) 2 = A few times (less than half the time) 1 = Almost never or never
18. Over the past 4 weeks, how often did you experience discomfort or pain following vaginal penetration?	0 = Did not attempt intercourse 5 = Almost always or always 4 = Most times (more than half the time) 3 = Sometimes (about half the time) 2 = A few times (less than half the time) 1 = Almost never or never
19. Over the past 4 weeks, how would you rate your level (degree) of discomfort or pain during or following vaginal penetration?	0 = Did not attempt intercourse 5 = Very high 4 = High 3 = Moderate 2 = Low 1 = Very low or none at all

For the questionnaire instructions and scoring algorithm, please see www.FSFIquestionnaire.com

FIGURE 3.8 ● *(Continued)*

extensive presurgical counseling did not necessarily eliminate unrealistic hopes (such as relief of urinary frequency and urgency) from the personal goals list, nor did it dissuade these women from having surgery (2).

ANATOMIC MEASURES

The POP-Q system is recognized by the International Continence Society as the standard physical examination tool for measurement of pelvic organ prolapse. Currently, the significance of findings using this examination system is unclear. Several authors have attempted to quantify correlations between POP-Q measurements and pelvic prolapse and urinary symptoms.

Ghetti et al assessed women by both POP-Q exam and two questionnaires: the UDI-6 with three questions from the original UDI about bulge symptoms and an Oregon Health Sciences University questionnaire (OHSU). The authors determined that frequency of bother increases when the leading edge descends from point –3 to 0, and at measurements between +1 and +5, 90% of women report bother. A sensation of "bulging" correlated most strongly to prolapse both on the UDI-6 and OHSU questionnaires (28). However, 30% of subjects with no prolapse reported being bothered by the sensation of vaginal bulge (although half of these subjects reported being only slightly bothered). Many symptoms of bowel and bladder dysfunction showed negligible correlations with overall prolapse severity. Anterior compartment prolapse did not correlate to urinary incontinence, frequency, and difficulty voiding in this study (28).

Bradley et al compared findings from the POP-Q exam to the PFDI in non–care-seeking women with an intact uterus. This study determined that obstructive urinary symptoms increased as anterior descensus and maximal vaginal descensus increased. Urinary incontinence (including stress urinary and urge urinary incontinence) and bowel symptoms were not associated with descensus of any vaginal component. Prolapse symptom scores from the PFDI increased as anterior wall prolapse increased on the POP-Q. However, these symptoms did not correlate to posterior wall and apical prolapse on the POP-Q. Patient report of "seeing or feeling a bulge" was associated with increasing descensus in all compartments. Bradley et al and other authors have not been able to determine the point at which vaginal descensus clearly became symptomatic (29,30).

Digesu et al compared findings from the POP-Q exam to questionnaire responses on the P-QOL questionnaire in a study assessing 233 symptomatic and 122 asymptomatic women. Overall, the symptomatic women had greater symptom severity by questionnaire and significantly greater prolapse on exam compared to the asymptomatic population. Similar to Bradley's findings, urinary symptoms were not correlated to uterovaginal prolapse (including the anterior component), with the exception of the "feeling of incomplete bladder emptying" and the "need of straining during voiding" (31). Interestingly, the need to strain during voiding also correlated to posterior vaginal wall prolapse and uterine descent. In contrast to Bradley's findings, bowel symptoms were strongly associated with posterior vaginal wall prolapse. Sexual dysfunction was assessed and was specifically associated only with cervical descent (measure C on POP-Q) (31).

Ellerkmann observed a weak inverse relationship between worsening anterior compartment prolapse and stress incontinence. This association may be a result of mechanical obstruction or urethral kinking (30). No correlation was identified between worsening anterior compartment prolapse and urge incontinence (30). Worsening prolapse in all compartments was associated with increasing symptoms of pelvic discomfort and visualization of a bulge. Only weak correlations were shown between posterior prolapse and the "sensation of incomplete evacuation and digital manipulation" (30). Romanzi found a significant association between voiding dysfunction and detrusor instability and pelvic organ prolapse (32).

CONCLUSION

Clear and precise outcomes assessment and consideration of the proper outcomes measures to evaluate are becoming more important as the discipline of pelvic floor medicine advances. The use of available questionnaires continues, while the development of newer and more sophisticated instruments is in progress. Researchers are challenged not only with designing proper all-inclusive instruments, but also with defining those outcomes that are most important to assess. Although objective parameters will always maintain their importance, assessment of patient goals, quality of life, and subjective measures are rightfully beginning to gain proper attention.

REFERENCES

1. Barber MD, Kuchibhatla MN, Pieper CF, et al. Psychometric evaluation of 2 comprehensive condition-specific quality of life instruments for women with pelvic floor disorders. *Am J Obstet Gynecol* 2001;185:1388.

2. Elkadry EA, Kenton KS, FitzGerald MP, et al. Patient-selected goals: a new perspective on surgical outcome. *Am J Obstet Gynecol* 2003;189:1551.

3. Streiner DL. *Health measurement scales: A practical guide to their development and use*: Oxford Medical Publications, 1995.

4. Digesu GA, Khullar V, Cardozo L, et al. P-QOL: a validated questionnaire to assess the symptoms and quality of life of women with urogenital prolapse. *Int Urogynecol J Pelvic Floor Dysfunct* 2005;16:176.

5. Crosby RD, Kolotkin RL, Williams GR. Defining clinically meaningful change in health-related quality of life. *J Clin Epidemiol* 2003;56:395.

6. Wiebe S, Guyatt G, Weaver B, et al. Comparative responsiveness of generic and specific quality-of-life instruments. *J Clin Epidemiol* 2003;56:52.

7. Khan MS, Chaliha C, Leskova L, et al. The relationship between urinary symptom questionnaires and urodynamic diagnoses: an analysis of two methods of questionnaire administration. *Br J Obstet Gynaecol* 2004;111:468.

8. Homma Y, Uemura S. Use of the short form of King's Health Questionnaire to measure quality of life in patients with an overactive bladder. *BJU Int* 2004;93:1009.

9. Shumaker SA, Wyman JF, Uebersax JS, et al. Health-related quality of life measures for women with urinary incontinence: the Incontinence Impact Questionnaire and the Urogenital Distress Inventory. Continence Program in Women (CPW) Research Group. *Qual Life Res* 1994;3:291.

10. Hagen S, Hanley J, Capewell A. Test–retest reliability, validity, and sensitivity to change of the urogenital distress inventory and the incontinence impact questionnaire. *Neurourol Urodyn* 2002;21:534.

11. Handa VL, Massof RW. Measuring the severity of stress urinary incontinence using the Incontinence Impact Questionnaire. *Neurourol Urodyn* 2004;23:27.

12. Uebersax JS, Wyman JF, Shumaker SA, et al. Short forms to assess life quality and symptom distress for urinary incontinence in women: the Incontinence Impact Questionnaire and the Urogenital Distress Inventory. Continence Program for Women Research Group. *Neurourol Urodyn* 1995;14:131.

13. Lemack GE, Zimmern PE. Predictability of urodynamic findings based on the Urogenital Distress Inventory-6 questionnaire. *Urology* 1999;54:461.

14. Harvey MA, Kristjansson B, Griffith D, et al. The Incontinence Impact Questionnaire and the Urogenital Distress Inventory: a revisit of their validity in women without a urodynamic diagnosis. *Am J Obstet Gynecol* 2001;185:25.

15. Abrams P, Avery K, Gardener N, et al. The International Consultation on Incontinence Modular Questionnaire: www.iciq.net. *J Urol* 2006;175:1063.

16. Avery K, Donovan J, Peters TJ, et al. ICIQ: a brief and robust measure for evaluating the symptoms and impact of urinary incontinence. *Neurourol Urodyn* 2004;23:322.

17. Jackson S, Donovan J, Brookes S, et al. The Bristol Female Lower Urinary Tract Symptoms questionnaire: development and psychometric testing. *Br J Urol* 1996;77:805.

18. Brookes ST, Donovan JL, Wright M, et al. A scored form of the Bristol Female Lower Urinary Tract Symptoms questionnaire: data from a randomized controlled trial of surgery for women with stress incontinence. *Am J Obstet Gynecol* 2004;191:73.

19. Kelleher CJ, Cardozo LD, Khullar V, et al. A new questionnaire to assess the quality of life of urinary incontinent women. *Br J Obstet Gynaecol* 1997;104:1374.

20. Wagner TH, Patrick DL, Bavendam TG, et al. Quality of life of persons with urinary incontinence: development of a new measure. *Urology* 1996;47:67.

21. Coyne K, Revicki D, Hunt T, et al. Psychometric validation of an overactive bladder symptom and health-related quality of life questionnaire: the OAB-q. *Qual Life Res* 2002;11:563.

22. Donovan JL, Abrams P, Peters TJ, et al. The ICS-"BPH" Study: the psychometric validity and reliability of the ICSmale questionnaire. *Br J Urol* 1996;77:554.

23. Barber MD, Walters MD, Bump RC. Short forms of two condition-specific quality-of-life questionnaires for women with pelvic floor disorders (PFDI-20 and PFIQ-7). *Am J Obstet Gynecol* 2005;193:103.

24. Rogers RG, Kammerer-Doak D, Villarreal A, et al. A new instrument to measure sexual function in women with urinary incontinence or pelvic organ prolapse. *Am J Obstet Gynecol* 2001;184:552.

25. Rogers RG, Coates KW, Kammerer-Doak D, et al. A short form of the Pelvic Organ Prolapse/Urinary Incontinence Sexual Questionnaire (PISQ-12). *Int Urogynecol J Pelvic Floor Dysfunct* 2003;14:164.

26. Rosen R, Brown C, Heiman J, et al. The Female Sexual Function Index (FSFI): a multidimensional self-report instrument for the assessment of female sexual function. *J Sex Marital Ther* 2000;26:191.

27. Hullfish KL, Bovbjerg VE, Steers WD. Patient-centered goals for pelvic floor dysfunction surgery: long-term follow-up. *Am J Obstet Gynecol* 2004;191:201.

28. Ghetti C, Gregory WT, Edwards SR, et al. Pelvic organ descent and symptoms of pelvic floor disorders. *Am J Obstet Gynecol* 2005;193:53.

29. Bradley CS, Nygaard IE. Vaginal wall descensus and pelvic floor symptoms in older women. *Obstet Gynecol* 2005;106:759.

30. Ellerkmann RM, Cundiff GW, Melick CF, et al. Correlation of symptoms with location and severity of pelvic organ prolapse. *Am J Obstet Gynecol* 2001;185:1332.

31. Digesu GA, Chaliha C, Salvatore S, et al. The relationship of vaginal prolapse severity to symptoms and quality of life. *Br J Obstet Gynaecol* 2005;112:971.

32. Romanzi LJ, Chaikin DC, Blaivas JG. The effect of genital prolapse on voiding. *J Urol* 1999;161:581.

Disorders of Lower Urinary Tract

CHAPTER 4

Physiology of Lower Urinary Tract—Bladder and Urethra

Toby C. Chai and Gopal N. Gupta

INTRODUCTION

Normal bladder function is typified by the storage of an adequate volume of urine at low pressure without leakage and unwanted bladder sensations (urgency) interspersed with periods of efficient unimpeded expulsion of urine. The bladder and bladder outlet (internal and external urethral sphincters) are under tightly regulated neural control. This allows for normal urinary storage and expulsion. The bladder and internal urethral sphincter are composed of smooth muscle fibers, while the external urethral sphincter is composed of skeletal striated muscle fibers. While we have learned much of bladder neurophysiology from studying animal models, the actual pathologic defects in bladder dysfunction frequently encountered clinically, such as urinary incontinence (both stress and urge), nonneurogenic detrusor overactivity, hypersensitive bladder syndromes (e.g., overactive bladder and interstitial cystitis), and nonobstructive urinary retention remain elusive. Animal models have helped test etiologic theories and define treatment modalities for disorders of micturition and urinary continence. This chapter will focus on data obtained from experiments performed with human tissues if available.

There is less published literature about neurophysiologic control of the urethra compared with that of the bladder. Additionally, the functional framework of the urethra is opposite to that of the bladder: during urine storage, the urethra is contracted while the bladder is relaxed, and during expulsion, the urethra is relaxed while the bladder is contracted. Therefore, treatments designed to reverse bladder dysfunction would mandate opposite effects on the urethra.

The bladder is unique among autonomically innervated organs due to the high degree of conscious or voluntary control that can be exerted on its function. This means that well-established neural connections from higher neural centers (e.g., cerebral cortex) to the bladder exist. Therefore, the neural control of bladder function is quite complex and a neurophysiologic defect anywhere from the cerebral cortex to the bladder can result in bladder dysfunction. This complexity in part explains our limited understanding of the pathophysiology of bladder dysfunction and also explains the limited treatments available for these bladder problems. The intent of this chapter is not to provide an exhaustive review of the basic science literature, but rather to present neurophysiological facts that have clinical relevance. Literature from experimental studies utilizing humans and/or human bladder tissues will be emphasized for maximal clinical relevance.

BLADDER EFFERENT PATHWAY

Peripheral Efferent Neural Pathways

The motor pathway to the bladder is autonomic. The bladder efferent neuronal bodies originate from the S2–S4 spinal cord within the sacral parasympathetic nucleus, which is situated between the ventral and dorsal horn gray matter. The preganglionic axons exit the spinal cord in the ventral roots and merge into the periphery in the pelvic nerves. These pelvic nerves synapse at ganglia within the periphery at the pelvic plexus or even within the bladder wall (intravesical ganglia) (1,2). The postganglionic nerves then synapse onto the bladder smooth muscle cells (Fig. 4.1). The

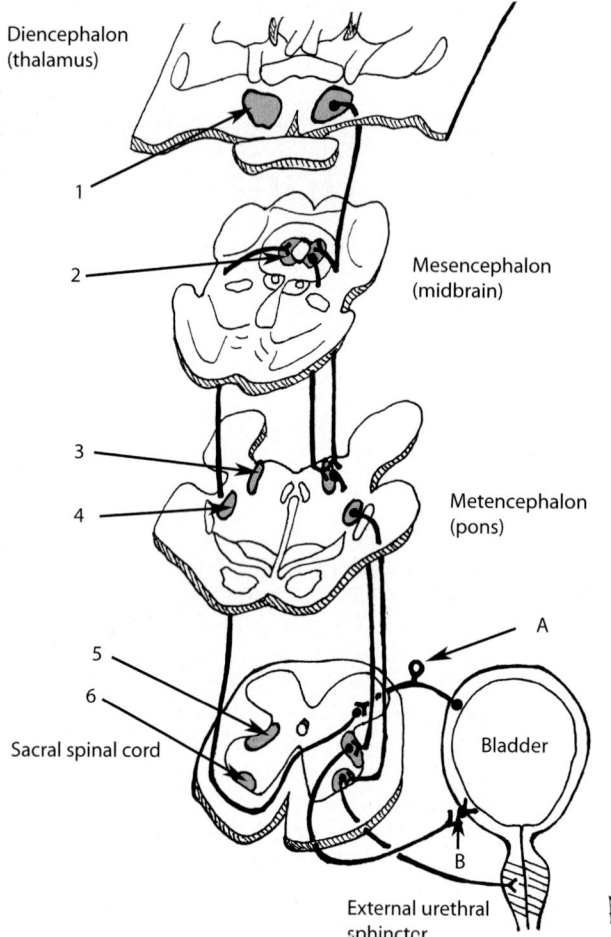

Diencephalon
(thalamus)

Mesencephalon
(midbrain)

Metencephalon
(pons)

Sacral spinal cord

Bladder

External urethral
sphincter

FIGURE 4.1 ● *(1)* Medial preoptic (MPO) area; *(2)* periaqueductal gray (PAG) area; *(3)* pontine micturition center (PMC), M-region, or Barrington's nucleus; *(4)* L-region; *(5)* sacral parasympathetic nucleus; *(6)* Onuf's nucleus; *(A)* dorsal root ganglia; *(B)* intramural ganglia.

end effect of activation of the efferent pathway is a coordinated, efficient bladder contraction that results in bladder emptying.

The sympathetic motor neuronal bodies reside in the thoracolumbar spinal cord. The preganglionic motor fibers also exit the spinal cord within the ventral nerve roots. The preganglionic fibers synapse on the postganglionic nerve at the paravertebral ganglia, which lie close to the spinal cord. The postganglionic nerve becomes the hypogastric nerve following closely to the hypogastric artery to innervate the bladder.

The role of sympathetic motor innervation in normal bladder function is not totally clear in the human. Studies in the cat suggest that it has a role in maintenance of urinary continence. Activation of sympathetic outflow to the bladder via stimulation of bladder afferents in anesthetized cats caused the bladder to relax and the urethra to contract (3,4). This pathway may have importance in maintaining continence in humans. The human bladder smooth muscle has been found to have β3-

adrenergic receptor (β3-AR), which may mediate its relaxation (5). The relaxation of the bladder may be through inhibition of the parasympathetic intravesical ganglia or through activation of β3-AR on the bladder. Therefore, the concept of using a β3-AR agonist for detrusor overactivity is actively being investigated.

The motor pathway to the bladder does not have to be thought of as "isolated" from the afferent pathway (detailed later). Recent data has shown that "micromotions" of the bladder can be detected in humans with sensory urgency (overactive bladder syndrome) (6). These micromotions are presumed to be small localized contractions of the detrusor muscle that cannot be detected with conventional water-filled cystometrography. It is presumed that these bladder micromotions within the smooth muscle can disturb nearby sensory fibers, giving rise to a sense of urinary urgency. Patients with overactive bladder syndrome had much higher frequencies of these detrusor micromotions (6). Therefore, there can be a relationship between detrusor overactivity (in this case micro-motions) and increased sensory awareness of the bladder. It remains to be seen how clinically useful micromotion detection will become and whether this is truly related to overactive bladder syndrome.

Detrusor Smooth Muscle Signaling

The neurotransmitter released by the preganglionic and postganglionic parasympathetic nerves is acetylcholine. Acetylcholine released by the postganglionic cells binds to muscarinic receptors (M2 and M3) on the bladder smooth muscle cells to initiate the excitation–contraction event. Bladder smooth muscle contraction mechanisms have been extensively studied because it is easy to obtain smooth muscle from animal models, both in normal and experimentally induced diseased states (e.g., bladder outlet obstruction, diabetes, inflammation models). One must remember that these are in vitro studies in which the bladder has been typically stripped of the urothelium and neural input; thus, the findings from organ baths do not necessarily reflect the complete in vivo picture.

The normal human bladder is composed of 70% M2 receptors and 30% M3 receptors. It is actually the M3 receptors that are responsible for organ bath–measured contractions (7,8). However, M2 receptors mediate organ bath contractions in spinal cord–injured humans (9). It was also shown that mRNA for M3 receptor decreased as a function of aging in the human bladder (10). This could possibly explain the decreased contractility of the bladder in the elderly. Another study suggested that unique variations in expression of M2 and M3 receptors could explain variable responses to antimuscarinics (11).

Most treatments for patients with urinary urgency, frequency, and urge incontinence (overactive bladder) are aimed at blockade of presumed "uninhibited" bladder smooth muscle contractions mediated by either M2 or M3 receptors. This is based on the supposed mechanism of action of antimuscarinic agents. Whether these presumed pathologic detrusor smooth muscle contractions are pathophysiologic, whether there is an alteration in muscarinic receptor phenotype distribution (M2:M3 ratio), and whether the primary pathology in overactive bladder is in the motor efferent pathway are currently unknown. It is unclear whether the physiologic defect in overactive bladder lies completely in the bladder motor pathway or may involve the sensory pathway. Urinary urgency would seem to involve a component of sensory-initiated phenomenon. Nevertheless, the

efficacy of antimuscarinics for treatment of overactive bladder symptoms has been shown in multiple large clinical trials (12).

The trigger for smooth muscle contraction is the increase in intracellular cytosolic calcium. Muscarinic receptor activation initiates this through cascades of secondary messenger events. The prototypical smooth muscle contraction signaling by increased cytosolic calcium is best explained by M3-receptor activation. M3 activation results in activation of phospholipase C, which hydrolyzes phosphoinositide-4,5-biphosphate, with subsequent release of inositol triphosphate (IP3) and diacylgycerol (13). Diacylgycerol activates protein kinase C, which can increase cytosolic calcium through release of intracellular stores, while IP3 activates the release of calcium from the sarcoplasmic reticulum. These events ultimately result in increased cytosolic calcium. Surprisingly, this prototypical sequence of events of phospholipase C activation and IP3 and diacylgycerol release was not critical to M3-mediated human detrusor smooth muscle contraction (14). This demonstrates that there are species-specific differences in secondary messenger events even if M3-receptor activation is the upstream event. The contractions in human detrusor smooth muscle were largely mediated by calcium influx through L-type, voltage-dependent channels (nifedipine-sensitive channels). These mechanisms are depicted in Figure 4.2.

Although increased cytosolic calcium is still the ultimate event (15,16), the mechanism by which activated M2 receptors mediate detrusor smooth muscle contraction is less direct than the mechanism occurring with activated M3 receptors. Because human bladders obtained from spinal cord–injured patients have M2-mediated contractions (9), it is critical to understand the downstream events after M2-receptor activation. The activated M2 receptor interacts with the Gi protein, which then inhibits adenylyl cyclase, resulting in decreased cytosolic cAMP. cAMP ultimately regulates intracellular calcium. If cAMP is decreased by M2-receptor activation, cytosolic calcium will be increased, leading to contraction. In addition, adenylyl cyclase is the prototypical enzyme that is activated by activation of the β-adrenergic receptor, with resultant increased cAMP and smooth muscle relaxation. In this way, M2-receptor activation could induce smooth muscle contraction by counteracting sympathetic effects on detrusor smooth muscle. These mechanisms are depicted in Figure 4.2.

Receptors other than M3 may also mediate bladder contractions. This was based on findings

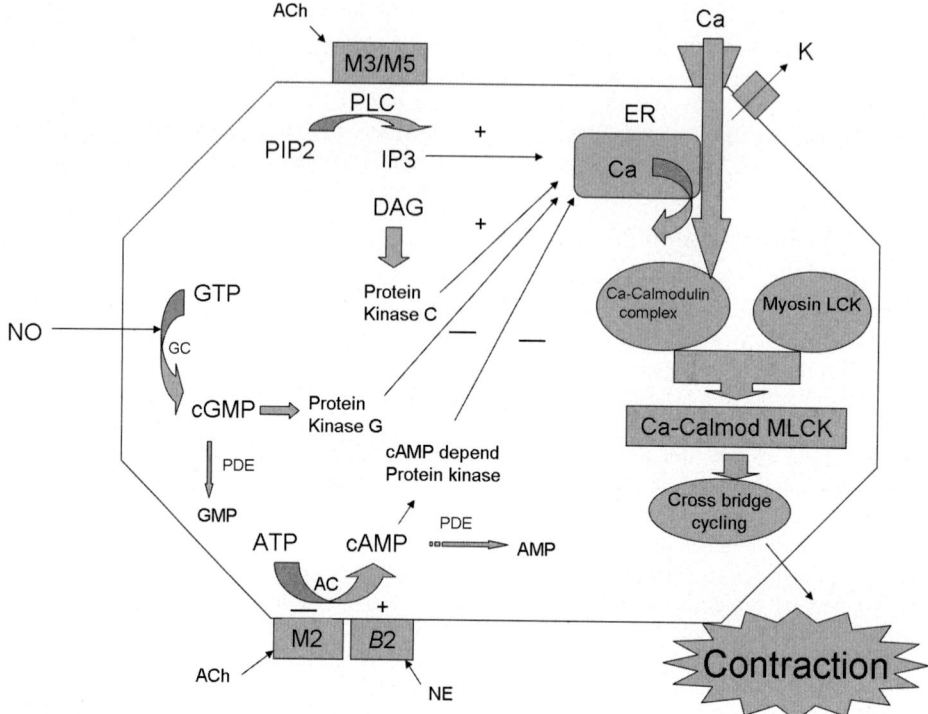

FIGURE 4.2 ● Representative of a detrusor smooth muscle cell.

that bladder contractions in animals were resistant to both cholinergic and adrenergic blockade (termed "nonadrenergic, noncholinergic" [NANC]–mediated bladder contractions) (17). For example, in humans it was shown that the purinergic agent adenosine triphosphate (ATP) can cause bladder smooth muscle contractions (18). These ATP-mediated contractions occur through the P2X1 receptors on the bladder smooth muscle (19). It is possible that in disease states bladder contractions could shift from muscarinic- to purinergic-mediated mechanisms. In humans, it has been shown that bladder smooth muscle strips obtained from patients with interstitial cystitis are much more responsive to ATP compared to control human bladder strips (20). Also, in aging, the human detrusor has an increased purinergic trigger as the basis for its contractions (21).

Detrusor smooth muscle contraction is triggered by increased cytosolic calcium. Calcium binds to calmodulin and causes a conformal change in calmodulin, exposing sites that interact with myosin light-chain kinase (MLCK). MLCK activation phosphorylates MLC protein, which results in cycling of myosin crossbridges (heads) along actin filaments and the development of tension. Furthermore, phosphorylation of MLC also activates myosin ATPase, which hydrolyzes ATP

to provide energy for detrusor smooth muscle contraction. A secondary mechanism that is calcium independent can also occur via the rho-rho-kinase pathway. This pathway is dependent on inhibition of MLC dephosphorylation (via inhibition of myosin phosphatase) (22). The rho-rho-kinase pathway has been shown to mediate human detrusor smooth muscle contractions (14,23). The rho-rho-kinase pathway may represent another therapeutic target, assuming it either is pathologically altered in disease or can be harnessed to compensate for defects in the calcium-dependent excitation–coupling pathway.

A clinical condition that seems to be directly related to the efferent system is that of idiopathic nonobstructive urinary retention. Patients present in urinary retention without an identifiable bladder outlet obstruction. The etiology of the retention is presumed to be the inability of the detrusor smooth muscle to generate a contraction. However, treatment with oral urecholine, a muscarinic agonist, has not proven to be uniformly clinically useful, even though the first description of its use was over half a century ago (24). The failure of the smooth muscle to contract may be caused by a variety of reasons related to the neurophysiology discussed above, including failure of the efferent nerves to release acetylcholine, failure of urethra or bladder outlet to relax, and/or failure of excitation–contraction coupling at any point along the pathway from muscarinic receptor activation to force generation. A synopsis of the complexities of smooth muscle function in the lower urinary tract has been published (25).

Descending Efferent Neural Pathways

Descending neurons from the medullary pons (pontine micturition center [PMC], Barrington's nucleus, or M-region) synapse on the sacral parasympathetic nucleus to modulate efferent outflow to the bladder. In cats this pathway has been demonstrated (26), and stimulation of this area caused the bladder to contract and the urethra to relax (27). Since the PMC is under volitional cortical control, the micturitional reflexes can be consciously suppressed (see Fig. 4.1). These descending pathways respond to adrenergic receptor agonists/antagonists (28,29) in modulating the micturition reflex. Intrathecal adrenergic agonists augment the micturition reflex (promote bladder emptying), whereas adrenergic antagonists inhibit the micturition reflex (promote bladder storage).

In the context of alpha-blocker use in treatment of benign prostatic hyperplasia (BPH) and lower urinary tract symptoms (LUTS) such as urinary frequency and urgency, these findings are relevant and interesting. Traditionally, the mechanism of action of alpha-blockers in the treatment of BPH has been thought to be relaxation of prostatic smooth muscle, with subsequent decreased "dynamic" tone of the prostatic urethra (30). Another effect on the prostate may be apoptosis of prostatic glandular cells (31). However, the therapeutic effect of alpha-blockers in decreasing urinary frequency and urgency may also target the central descending efferent pathways onto the sacral spinal cord and thereby inhibit the micturition reflex. Furthermore, elevated catecholamine states such as hypertension have been shown to be associated with increased LUTS in both animals and humans (32,33). These findings suggest that the beneficial actions of alpha-blockers in LUTS may be more complex than previously thought.

Clinical Measures of Bladder Efferent Pathway

The cystometrogram is the clinical tool used to measure detrusor contraction. During a detrusor contraction an increase in intravesical pressure is measured. A pressure-flow study (PFS) is created when simultaneous uroflowmetry is obtained during the voiding phase of the cystometrogram. The primary goal of analyzing components of the PFS data (e.g., maximum detrusor pressure, maximum urinary flow rate) is to determine whether there is an element of bladder outlet obstruction (BOO). BOO should result in a higher detrusor contraction pressure with decreased maximal flow rate. Various mathematical constructs derived from the PFS data have been proposed to help stratify patients into the obstructed versus nonobstructed category (34,35).

While the goal of the PFS is to determine presence of BOO, measurement of the isovolumetric bladder contraction pressure has been advocated to measure detrusor contractile strength (36) using an outlet occlusive urethral catheter. It has been demonstrated that impaired detrusor contractility has been underrecognized (37), especially if isovolumetric bladder contraction pressures are not determined. Currently, the primary and most effective treatment of detrusor failure remains intermittent clean catheterization.

BLADDER AFFERENT PATHWAY

Afferent Neural Pathways

The bladder wall has been shown to have sensory nerve endings that are responsive or triggered by stretch (38). These afferent fibers were traditionally thought to terminate in the lamina propria; however, recently, sensory afferent fibers were seen to extend into the rat bladder urothelium, intermingling with urothelial cells (39). In humans, substance P–containing nerve terminals (a marker for sensory fibers) have been found to be in close approximation to the urothelium (40). These fibers are part of the bipolar sensory nerve. The neural soma (bodies) reside in the dorsal root ganglia and the other end of the sensory nerve fiber terminates in the dorsal horn of the gray matter in the spinal cord. Here, descending pathways can modulate afferent input (41). In addition, afferent fibers can synapse onto the sacral parasympathetic nuclei to modulate the efferent outflow to the bladder (42).

The bladder sensory nerves travel in the periphery within the pelvic nerve, hypogastric nerve, and pudendal nerve and are composed of A-δ myelinated fibers and unmyelinated c-fibers. The c-fibers are normally silent, but in animal models with experimentally injured states such as inflammation and spinal cord injury, these fibers are activated (43,44). The A-δ fibers respond to pressure and stretch and initiate the micturition reflex (45). Patients with bladder outlet obstruction (males and females) have been shown to have a positive bladder ice-water test, which correlates with activation of the c-fibers (46). These fibers also respond to capsaicin, a neurotoxin isolated from hot peppers. Capsaicin and its derivatives such as resinifera-toxin have been proposed to be used to block acti-vated c-fibers in disease states. It has been hypoth-esized that interstitial cystitis results from activation of c-fibers, which then transmit signals of pain and burning. However, a recent large mul-ticenter placebo-controlled clinical trial of intrav-esical resiniferatoxin for interstitial cystitis symp-toms showed no clinical benefit (47), arguing against c-fiber activation as the cause of interstitial cystitis symptoms.

The lack of appropriate sensory measurement tools and inability to obtain dorsal root ganglia where sensory nerve cells reside have made the study of the human bladder sensory pathway diffi-cult. Most studies have traditionally focused on the efferent pathway, primarily because of the abun-dant resources to study bladder smooth muscle. Much of this research has been borrowed and adapted from other areas such as vascular smooth muscle. Advances in treatment for bladder symp-toms such as urinary frequency, urinary urgency, and bladder pain will require a better understand-ing of how bladder sensory signals are processed. A review of bladder sensory processing has been recently published (48).

The neurotransmitters responsible for sensation in the human bladder are not precisely known. Putative sensory neurotransmitters derived from animal studies include substance P, calcitonin-gene related peptide, and corticotrophin-releasing factor (CRF) (49,50). The importance of P2X3/P2X2 purinergic receptors to the bladder sensory processing has been shown with knockout animal models. P2X3 and P2X2 knockout mice have been shown to have increased bladder capac-ity and decreased voiding frequency. This is con-sistent with decreased afferent signaling into the micturition reflex (51).

Urothelial Afferent Signaling

The bladder urothelium has traditionally been thought to function as a barrier, protecting the un-derlying stroma from urinary irritants. However, recently, the bladder urothelial cell has been shown to have neuronal-like properties (52). Urothelial cells have demonstrated release of neu-rotransmitters such as ATP (53–55), nitric oxide (56), and acetylcholine (21). The urothelial cell also expresses receptors that are typical signal transduction receptors found on neurons. These in-clude muscarinic receptors (57), TRPV1 or "hot" receptors (39,58), TRPM8 or "cool" receptors

(58), and purinergic receptors (P2X3 and P2X2) (59,60). Urothelial sensory ability was first sug-gested by work from Ferguson demonstrating that rabbit bladder urothelium releases ATP in re-sponse to stretch (53). This finding has been repro-duced in human bladder urothelium using different experimental techniques to stretch the urothelium (54,55).

Bladder urothelial sensory signaling has been shown to be important in the human disease state of interstitial cystitis. Increased ATP release in re-sponse to stretch has been demonstrated in human bladder cells from interstitial cystitis patients (54). A common pathologic symptom in interstitial cys-titis is the hypersensation of bladder filling. The increased ATP release could bind to P2X3 recep-tors on sensory nerve endings within the urothe-lium to cause an increased sensation during blad-der filling. Furthermore, interstitial cystitis cells express more P2X3 and P2X3 receptors, which suggests that the augmented ATP release by the in-terstitial cystitis urothelial cells could serve an au-tocrine role (59,60). The pathways in urothelial signaling are depicted in Figure 4.3.

Clinical Measures of Bladder Afferent Activity

Three sensory thresholds—first sensation of fill-ing, first desire to void, and strong desire to void (61)—have been used to assess the clinical meas-urement of bladder sensory signals. These sensa-tions are easily distinguishable from each other and other sensations. These thresholds have clini-cal utility, for example, in interstitial cystitis, in which the bladder capacity is significantly dimin-ished due to pain with bladder filling (62). This study also suggested that central processing of pain was altered in interstitial cystitis patients.

The intent of an ice-water test is to induce a re-flex bladder contraction through rapid infusion of ice water into the bladder and activating the c-fiber afferents, which ultimately trigger a bladder con-traction. The clinical utility of this method of sen-sory testing in routine practice has not been estab-lished. The high incidence of a positive ice-water test in a population of bladder-obstructed patients has been suggested to reflect bladder neuroplastic-ity in these patients (46). The ice-water test is neg-ative in control individuals without voiding symp-toms. A recently described process in which a constant current electrical stimulus was applied to the bladder urothelium via an intravesical elec-trode to determine sensory thresholds was de-scribed (63). This methodology is purported to provide reliable measures of spinal sensory and

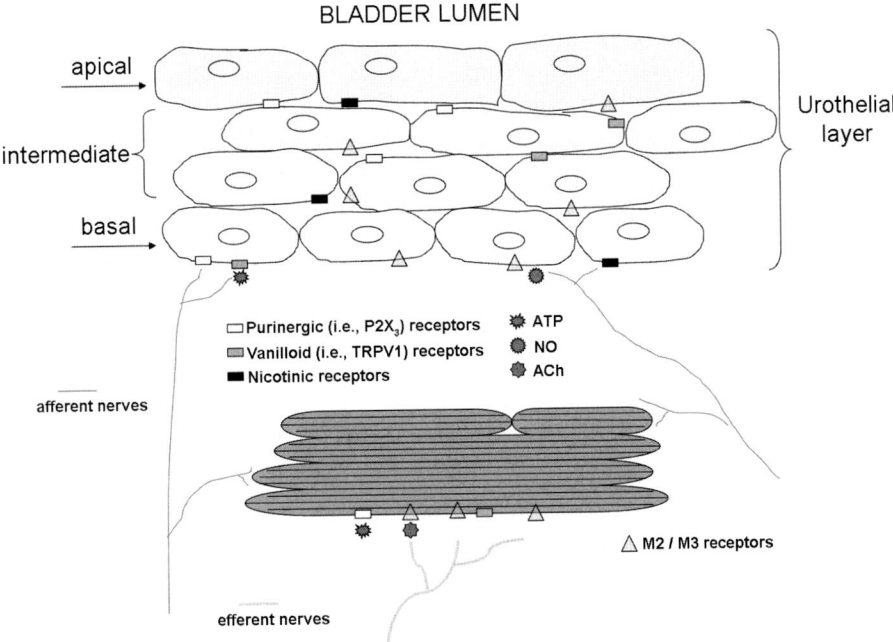

FIGURE 4.3 ● Urothelial cells can function as both sensory and transducer cells by receiving and sending signals to neighboring urothelial cells, nerves, or detrusor smooth muscle.

peripheral sensory nerve function from the large and small myelinated and unmyelinated nerve fibers.

HIGHER-LEVEL CENTRAL NERVOUS SYSTEM PROCESSING OF BLADDER AFFERENT SIGNALS

The bladder is unique among visceral organs in that it is under a high level of volitional control. Investigators studying the brain using either positron emission tomography or functional magnetic resonance imaging (fMRI) during bladder storage and emptying have found similar areas of activation in humans as compared to those found in the cat and rat (64–66). Recent fMRI studies were performed on subjects without neurologic disease but with "poor bladder control" on urodynamics and were compared to control patients with normal bladder parameters on urodynamics (67). Patients with poor bladder control had less activation of the orbitofrontal cortex during bladder filling, suggesting that activity in the orbitofrontal cortex suppresses promicturition signals.

Investigators have found a high association between depression and idiopathic urinary incontinence (e.g., urge incontinence) (68,69). This association further highlights the complexity of bladder control at supraspinal levels. In the rat model, reduction of central nervous system sero-

tonin by clomipramine-induced bladder overactivity (70). Furthermore, the bladder overactivity in serotonin-depleted animals could be reversed by treating the animals with the serotonin reuptake inhibitor fluoxetine.

CRF has been implicated as a neurotransmitter/neuromodulator in a variety of nonhypophyseal neuronal systems, including the neural control of bladder function. The importance of CRF on bladder function was reviewed (71). Barrington's nucleus, or the PMC, which has a central role in coordinating bladder function, is richly innervated with CRF-containing neurons (72). CRF-containing neurons have also been detected in areas such as the dorsal raphe nucleus (associated with depression), amygdala (relay center for emotional stress and visceral pain), and hippocampus (associated with memory). These related findings help support an association between stress responses, depression, visceral pain, and micturitional disturbances. However, it has not been determined whether a primary bladder condition (such as interstitial cystitis or overactive bladder) leads to depression or whether depression may cause bladder symptoms.

URETHRAL EFFERENT PATHWAY

The urethra is composed of both smooth and striated muscle. The smooth muscle component is autonomically innervated, while the striated portion is somatically innervated. The striated portion of the urethra in both males and females is called the rhabdosphincter or the external urethral sphincter. The human rhabdosphincter is composed of both slow and fast fatigue fibers. This may explain the sphincter's ability to maintain tone over a long period of time (73). Innervation of the rhabdosphincter is via a motor neuron arising from the S2–S4 spinal cord at Onuf's nucleus and exits along with the parasympathetic motor nerves. In contrast, somatic motor innervation to the rhabdosphincter is via the pudendal nerve.

The internal urethral sphincter is located proximal to the rhabdosphincter in close proximity to the bladder neck and is primarily sympathetically innervated (74). During ejaculation, the internal sphincter allows closure of the bladder neck, thus preventing retrograde semen flow. Traditionally, alpha-blocking agents were thought to relax the internal sphincter in the face of benign prostatic hyperplasia. However, as mentioned in the section on bladder efferent pathways, alpha-blockers may also work at the level of the spinal cord, modulating (inhibiting) descending influences on micturition pathways.

Descending pathways from higher centers promote urine storage (bladder relaxation and urethral contraction) and synapse on Onuf's nucleus motor neurons. Norepinephrine and serotonin are the neurotransmitters involved at these synapses. The proposed mechanism of action of duloxetine is augmentation of this urine storage reflex. A recent review on the use of duloxetine, a serotonin–norepinephrine reuptake inhibitor, to modulate the contractility of the external urethral sphincter and bladder capacity was published (75). Blockade of reuptake of these neurotransmitters augments activity of motor neurons in Onuf's nucleus, with resultant increased tone of the external urethral sphincter. The effectiveness of duloxetine in decreasing stress urinary incontinence in females has been shown in a placebo-controlled clinical trial (76).

Young males have been reported to have internal urethral dysfunction (77–79). The bladder outlet obstruction is proposed to be due to inappropriately high internal urethral sphincter tone. Treatment with alpha-blockers and incision of the internal urethral sphincter and bladder neck has been described as clinically effective.

URETHRAL AFFERENT PATHWAY

Urethral sensory innervation is similar to the representation of sensory innervation of the bladder.

Sensory nerves can travel along the pudendal, pelvic, and hypogastric nerves (80). These fibers synapse within the dorsal horn of the S2 to S4 spinal cord (those that travel in pudendal and pelvic nerves) and the thoracolumbar spinal cord (hypogastric nerve).

The presence of fluid traversing the urethra activates the afferent pathway. These afferent fibers in turn reinforce the bladder to contract more efficiently, probably through facilitatory descending input. This urethrovesical reflex has been shown in humans (81,82). Alternatively, an urethrovesical reflex that promotes urinary storage is present. Voluntary contraction of the external urethral sphincter can induce inhibition of bladder contractions (83). This reflex may be the basis for how Kegel exercises may induce bladder relaxation and prevent urge incontinent episodes.

REFERENCES

1. Gilpin CJ, Dixon JS, Gilpin SA, et al. The fine structure of autonomic neurons in the wall of the human urinary bladder. *J Anat* 1983;137(Pt 4):705–713.
2. Crowe R, Haven AJ, Burnstock G. Intramural neurons of the guinea-pig urinary bladder: histochemical localization of putative neurotransmitters in cultures and newborn animals. *J Auton Nerv Syst* 1986;15(4):319–339.
3. de Groat WC, Theobald RJ. Reflex activation of sympathetic pathways to vesical smooth muscle and parasympathetic ganglia by electrical stimulation of vesical afferents. *J Physiol* 1976;259(1):223–237.
4. de Groat WC, Lalley PM. Reflex firing in the lumbar sympathetic outflow to activation of vesical afferent fibres. *J Physiol* 1972;226(2):289–309.
5. Takeda M, Obara K, Mizusawa T, et al. Evidence for beta3-adrenoceptor subtypes in relaxation of the human urinary bladder detrusor: analysis by molecular biological and pharmacological methods. *J Pharmacol Exp Ther* 1999;288(3):1367–1373.
6. Drake MJ, Harvey IJ, Gillespie JI, et al. Localized contractions in the normal human bladder and in urinary urgency. *BJU Int* 2005;95(7):1002–1005.
7. Chess-Williams R, Chapple CR, Yamanishi T, et al. The minor population of M3-receptors mediate contraction of human detrusor muscle in vitro. *J Auton Pharmacol* 2001;21(5–6):243–248.
8. Fetscher C, Fleichman M, Schmidt M, et al. M(3) muscarinic receptors mediate contraction of human urinary bladder. *Br J Pharmacol* 2002;136(5):641–643.
9. Pontari MA, Braverman AS, Ruggieri MR Sr. The M2 muscarinic receptor mediates in vitro bladder contractions from patients with neurogenic bladder dysfunction. *Am J Physiol Regul Integr Comp Physiol* 2004; 286(5):R874–880.
10. Mansfield KJ, Liu L, Mitchelson FJ, et al. Muscarinic receptor subtypes in human bladder detrusor and mucosa, studied by radioligand binding and quantitative competitive RT-PCR: changes in ageing. *Br J Pharmacol* 2005;144(8):1089–1099.
11. Sigala S, Mirabella G, Peroni A, et al. Differential gene expression of cholinergic muscarinic receptor subtypes in male and female normal human urinary bladder. *Urology* 2002;60(4):719–725.

12. Chapple C, Khullar V, Gabriel Z, et al. The effects of antimuscarinic treatments in overactive bladder: a systematic review and meta-analysis. *Eur Urol* 2005;48(1): 5–26.

13. Caulfield MP, Birdsall NJM, International Union of Pharmacology. XVII. Classification of muscarinic acetylcholine receptors. *Pharmacol Rev* 1998;50:279–290.

14. Schneider T, Fetscher C, Krege S, et al. Signal transduction underlying carbachol-induced contraction of human urinary bladder. *J Pharmacol Exp Ther* 2004; 309(3):1148–1153.

15. Braverman AS, Ruggieri MR. Selective alkylation of rat urinary bladder muscarinic receptors with 4-DAMP mustard reveals a contractile function for the M2 muscarinic receptor. *J Recept Signal Transduct Res* 1999; 19(5):819–833.

16. Hegde SS, Choppin A, Bonhaus D, et al. Functional role of M2 and M3 muscarinic receptors in the urinary bladder of rats in vitro and in vivo. *Br J Pharmacol* 1997;120(8):1409–1418.

17. de Groat WC, Saum WR. Synaptic transmission in parasympathetic ganglia in the urinary bladder of the cat. *J Physiol* 1976;256(1):137–158.

18. Hoyle CH, Chapple C, Burnstock G. Isolated human bladder: evidence for an adenine dinucleotide acting on P2X-purinoceptors and for purinergic transmission. *Eur J Pharmacol* 1989;174(1):115–118.

19. Hardy LA, Harvey IJ, Chambers P, et al. A putative alternatively spliced variant of the P2X(1) purinoreceptor in human bladder. *Exp Physiol* 2000;85(4):461–463.

20. Palea S, Artibani W, Ostardo E, et al. Evidence for purinergic neurotransmission in human urinary bladder affected by interstitial cystitis. *J Urol* 1993;150(6): 2007–2012.

21. Yoshida M, Miyamae K, Iwashita H, et al. Management of detrusor dysfunction in the elderly: changes in acetylcholine and adenosine triphosphate release during aging. *Urology* 2004;63(3 Suppl 1):17–23.

22. Kitazawa T, Masuo M, Somlyo AP. G protein-mediated inhibition of myosin light-chain phosphatase in vascular smooth muscle. *Proc Natl Acad Sci USA* 1991; 88(20):9307–9310.

23. Takahashi R, Nishimura J, Hirano K, et al. Ca2+ sensitization in contraction of human bladder smooth muscle. *J Urol* 2004;172(2):748–752.

24. Lee LW. The use of urecholine in the management of chronic urinary retention. *J Urol* 1950;64(2):408–412.

25. Christ GJ, Liebert M. Proceedings of the Baltimore smooth muscle meeting: identifying research frontiers and priorities for the lower urinary tract. *J Urol* 2005; 173:1406–1409.

26. Holstege G, Kuypers HG, Boer RC. Anatomical evidence for direct brain stem projections to the somatic motoneuronal cell groups and autonomic preganglionic cell groups in cat spinal cord. *Brain Res* 1979;171(2): 329–333.

27. Holstege G, Griffiths D, de Wall H, et al. Anatomical and physiological observations on supraspinal control of bladder and urethral sphincter muscles in the cat. *J Comp Neurol* 1986;250(4):449–461.

28. Sugaya K, Nishijima S, Miyazato M, et al. Effects of intrathecal injection of tamsulosin and naftopidil, alpha-1A and -1D adrenergic receptor antagonists, on bladder activity in rats. *Neurosci Lett* 2002; 328(1):74–76.

29. Yoshiyama M, De Groat WC. Role of spinal alpha1-adrenoceptor subtypes in the bladder reflex in anesthetized rats. *Am J Physiol Regul Integr Comp Physiol* 2001;280(5):R1414–1419.

30. Lepor H. Alpha adrenergic antagonists for the treatment of symptomatic BPH. *Int J Clin Pharmacol Ther Toxicol* 1989;27(4):151–155.

31. Chon JK, Borkowski A, Partin AW, et al. Alpha 1-adrenoceptor antagonists terazosin and doxazosin induce prostate apoptosis without affecting cell proliferation in patients with benign prostatic hyperplasia. *J Urol* 1999;161(6):2002–2008.

32. Sugaya K, Kadekawa K, Ikehara A, et al. Influence of hypertension on lower urinary tract symptoms in benign prostatic hyperplasia. *Int J Urol* 2003;10(11):569–574.

33. Persson K, Pandita RK, Spitsbergen JM, et al. Spinal and peripheral mechanisms contributing to hyperactive voiding in spontaneously hypertensive rats. *Am J Physiol* 1998;275(4 Pt 2):R1366–1373.

34. Abrams PH, Griffiths DJ. The assessment of prostatic obstruction from urodynamic measurements and from residual urine. *Br J Urol* 1979;51(2):129–134.

35. Schafer W. Analysis of bladder-outlet function with the linearized passive urethral resistance relation, linPURR, and a disease-specific approach for grading obstruction: from complex to simple. *World J Urol* 1995;13(1):47–58.

36. Griffiths DJ. Assessment of detrusor contractility strength or contractility. *Neurourol Urodynam* 1991;10:1.

37. Griffiths DJ. Editorial: bladder failure—a condition to reckon with. *J Urol* 2003;169(3):1011–1012.

38. Bahns E, Halsband U, Janig W. Responses of sacral visceral afferents from the lower urinary tract, colon and anus to mechanical stimulation. *Pflugers Arch* 1987; 410(3):296–303.

39. Birder LA, Kanai AJ, de Groat WC, et al. Vanilloid receptor expression suggests a sensory role for urinary bladder epithelial cells. *Proc Natl Acad Sci USA* 2001; 98(23):13396–13401.

40. Wakabayashi Y, Tomoyoshi T, Fujimiya M, et al. Substance P–containing axon terminals in the mucosa of the human urinary bladder: pre-embedding immunohistochemistry using cryostat sections for electron microscopy. *Histochemistry* 1993;100(6):401–407.

41. de Groat WC, Nadelhaft I, Milne RJ, et al. Organization of the sacral parasympathetic reflex pathways to the urinary bladder and large intestine. *J Auton Nerv Syst* 1981;3(2–4):135–160.

42. Morgan C, Nadelhaft I, de Groat WC. The distribution of visceral primary afferents from the pelvic nerve to Lissauer's tract and the spinal gray matter and its relationship to the sacral parasympathetic nucleus. *J Comp Neurol* 1981;201(3):415–440.

43. Cheng CL, Liu JC, Chang SY, et al. Effect of capsaicin on the micturition reflex in normal and chronic spinal cord–injured cats. *Am J Physiol* 1999;277(3 Pt 2):R786–794.

44. Habler HJ, Janig W, Koltzenburg M. Activation of unmyelinated afferent fibres by mechanical stimuli and inflammation of the urinary bladder in the cat. *J Physiol* 1990;425:545–562.

45. Habler HJ, Janig W, Koltzenburg M. Myelinated primary afferents of the sacral spinal cord responding to slow filling and distension of the cat urinary bladder. *J Physiol* 1993;463:449–460.

46. Chai TC, Gray ML, Steers WD. The incidence of a positive ice water test in bladder outlet obstructed patients: evidence for bladder neural plasticity. *J Urol* 1998;160(1): 34–38.

47. Payne CK, Mosbaugh PG, Forrest JB, et al; ICOS RTX Study Group (Resiniferatoxin Treatment for Interstitial Cystitis). Intravesical resiniferatoxin for the treatment of interstitial cystitis: a randomized, double-blind, placebo-controlled trial. *J Urol* 2005;173(5):1590–1594.

48. Wyndaele JJ, De Wachter S. The basics behind bladder pain: a review of data on lower urinary tract sensations. *Int J Urol* 2003;10 Suppl:S49–55.

49. de Groat WC. Neuropeptides in pelvic afferent pathways. *Experientia* 1987;43(7):801–813.

50. Kawatani M, Suzuki T, de Groat WC. Corticotropin releasing factor-like immunoreactivity in afferent projections to the sacral spinal cord of the cat. *J Auton Nerv Syst* 1996;61(3):218–226.

51. Cockayne DA, Dunn PM, Zhong Y, et al. P2X2 knockout mice and P2X2/P2X3 double knockout mice reveal a role for the P2X2 receptor subunit in mediating multiple sensory effects of ATP. *J Physiol* 2005 [Epub ahead of print].

52. Birder L. Role of the urothelium in bladder function. *Scand J Urol Nephrol Suppl* 2004;(215):48–53.

53. Ferguson DR, Kennedy I, Burton TJ. ATP is released from rabbit urinary bladder epithelial cells by hydrostatic pressure changes—a possible sensory mechanism? *J Physiol* 1997;505(Pt 2):503–511.

54. Sun Y, Keay S, De Deyne PG, et al. Augmented stretch activated adenosine triphosphate release from bladder uroepithelial cells in patients with interstitial cystitis. *J Urol* 2001;166(5):1951–1956.

55. Sun Y, MaLossi J, Jacobs SC, et al. Effect of doxazosin on stretch-activated adenosine triphosphate release in bladder urothelial cells from patients with benign prostatic hyperplasia. *Urology* 2002;60(2):351–356.

56. Birder LA, Apodaca G, De Groat WC, et al. Adrenergic- and capsaicin-evoked nitric oxide release from urothelium and afferent nerves in urinary bladder. *Am J Physiol* 1998;275(2 Pt 2):F226–229.

57. Chess-Williams R. Muscarinic receptors of the urinary bladder: detrusor, urothelial, and prejunctional. *Auton Autacoid Pharmacol* 2002;22(3):133–145.

58. Stein RJ, Santos S, Nagatomi J, et al. Cool (TRPM8) and hot (TRPV1) receptors in the bladder and male genital tract. *J Urol* 2004;172(3):1175–1178.

59. Sun Y, Chai TC. Up-regulation of P2X3 receptor during stretch of bladder urothelial cells from patients with interstitial cystitis. *J Urol* 2004;171(1):448–452.

60. Tempest HV, Dixon AK, Turner WH, et al. P2X and P2X receptor expression in human bladder urothelium and changes in interstitial cystitis. *BJU Int* 2004;93(9):1344–1348.

61. Wyndaele JJ. The normal pattern of perception of bladder filling during cystometry studied in 38 young healthy volunteers. *J Urol* 1998;160(2):479–481.

62. Ness TJ, Powell-Boone T, Cannon R, et al. Psychophysical evidence of hypersensitivity in subjects with interstitial cystitis. *J Urol* 2005;173(6):1983–1987.

63. Ukimura O, Ushijima S, Honjo H, et al. Neuroselective current perception threshold evaluation of bladder mucosal sensory function. *Eur Urol* 2004;45(1):70–76.

64. Blok BF, Willemsen AT, Holstege G. A PET study on brain control of micturition in humans. *Brain* 1997;120(Pt 1):111–121.

65. Blok BF, Sturms LM, Holstege G. Brain activation during micturition in women. *Brain* 1998;121(Pt 11):2033–2042.

66. Zhang H, Reitz A, Kollias S, et al. An fMRI study of the role of suprapontine brain structures in the voluntary voiding control induced by pelvic floor contraction. *Neuroimage* 2005;24(1):174–180.

67. Griffiths D, Derbyshire S, Stenger A, et al. Brain control of normal and overactive bladder. *J Urol* 2005;174(5):1862–1867.

68. Zorn BH, Montgomery H, Pieper K, et al. Urinary incontinence and depression. *J Urol* 1999;162(1):82–84.

69. Nygaard I, Turvey C, Burns TL, et al. Urinary incontinence and depression in middle-aged United States women. *Obstet Gynecol* 2003;101(1):149–156.

70. Lee KS, Na YG, Dean-McKinney T, et al. Alterations in voiding frequency and cystometry in the clomipramine-induced model of endogenous depression and reversal with fluoxetine. *J Urol* 2003;170(5):2067–2071.

71. Klausner AP, Steers WD. Corticotropin-releasing factor: a mediator of emotional influences on bladder function. *J Urol* 2004;172(6 Pt 2):2570–2573.

72. Valentino RJ, Page ME, Luppi PH, et al. Evidence for widespread afferents to Barrington's nucleus, a brainstem region rich in corticotropin-releasing hormone neurons. *Neuroscience* 1994;62(1):125–143.

73. Gosling JA, Dixon JS, Critchley HO, et al. A comparative study of the human external sphincter and periurethral levator ani muscles. *Br J Urol* 1981;53(1):35–41.

74. Tulloch AG. Sympathetic activity of internal urethral sphincter in empty and partially filled bladder. *Urology* 1975;5(3):353–355.

75. Thor KB, Donatucci C. Central nervous system control of the lower urinary tract: new pharmacological approaches to stress urinary incontinence in women. *J Urol* 2004;172(1):27–33.

76. Dmochowski RR, Miklos JR, Norton PA, et al; Duloxetine Urinary Incontinence Study Group. Duloxetine versus placebo for the treatment of North American women with stress urinary incontinence. *J Urol* 2003;170(4 Pt 1):1259–1263.

77. Trockman BA, Gerspach J, Dmochowski R, et al. Primary bladder neck obstruction: urodynamic findings and treatment results in 36 men. *J Urol* 1996;156(4):1418–1420.

78. Nitti VW, Lefkowitz G, Ficazzola M, et al. Lower urinary tract symptoms in young men: videourodynamic findings and correlation with noninvasive measures. *J Urol* 2002;168(1):135–138.

79. Woodside JR. Urodynamic evaluation of dysfunctional bladder neck obstruction in men. *J Urol* 1980;124(5):673–677.

80. Russo A, Conte B. Afferent and efferent branching axons from the rat lumbo-sacral spinal cord project both to the urinary bladder and the urethra as demonstrated by double retrograde neuronal labeling. *Neurosci Lett* 1996;219(3):155–158.

81. Shafik A, Shafik AA, El-Sibai O, et al. Role of positive urethrovesical feedback in vesical evacuation. The concept of a second micturition reflex: the urethrovesical reflex. *World J Urol* 2003;21(3):167–170.

82. Gustafson KJ, Creasey GH, Grill WM. A urethral afferent mediated excitatory bladder reflex exists in humans. *Neurosci Lett* 2004;360(1–2):9–12.

83. Shafik A. A study of the continence mechanism of the external urethral sphincter with identification of the voluntary urinary inhibition reflex. *J Urol* 1999;162(6):1967–1971.

Basic Evaluation of the Incontinent Female Patient

Steven E. Swift and Alfred E. Bent

T here remains considerable debate over what constitutes the minimal or basic evaluation of the incontinent female. Although there are a few published guidelines, no studies to date have determined the effectiveness of these recommendations or their relationship to therapeutic outcomes. Therefore, we are left with conflicting expert opinion regarding which, if any, testing should be done before initiating therapy for incontinence in the female patient.

However, with these limitations in mind, any basic evaluation of the incontinent female should be able to distinguish reliably among stress urinary incontinence and urge urinary incontinence. This is a particularly important point because the therapeutic interventions for the various types of incontinence are dramatically different. While surgery plays a large role in treating stress urinary incontinence, it often makes urge incontinence worse. Mixed urinary incontinence (a combination of stress and urge incontinence) cannot be diagnosed with any degree of certainty without the use of urodynamic testing. If a patient is having detrusor contractions during evaluation, multichannel urodynamic testing is required to ensure that any loss seen with cough or Valsalva is due to a weak urethral sphincter mechanism and not a detrusor contraction. In addition, the evaluation should be able to detect those uncommon forms of incontinence that require referral to a specialist.

BACKGROUND

The Agency for Health Care Policy and Research (AHCPR) first published consensus guidelines for evaluation and management of urinary incontinence in 1992 (updated in 1996) (1). These guidelines were drawn up by a panel of experts who based their recommendations on a critical review of the literature and on expert opinion. They recommended that a basic evaluation should include the following: a thorough history (including a voiding diary), physical examination, postvoid residual urine determination, and urinalysis. The evaluation criteria were subsequently applied retrospectively to a referral-based practice and were found to correctly diagnose only 70% of subjects with the complaint of stress urinary incontinence (2). However, it must be remembered that these guidelines were developed for a primary care practice, but in the study mentioned, they were applied to a tertiary referral population. Therefore, it remains to be determined how effective they are for patients in a primary clinical practice. However, the study did point out some of the shortcomings of the AHCPR guidelines and demonstrated that these recommendations should be constantly tested and updated to reflect changes in our knowledge base.

Since the AHCPR's introduction of guidelines, two other organizations have published guidelines for evaluation of the incontinent female. The American College of Obstetrics and Gynecology (ACOG) has published criteria for evaluating patients prior to surgery for stress incontinence (3) (Table 5.1). These guidelines are more specific to preoperative findings or criteria that should be met prior to embarking on invasive therapy. The International Consultation on Incontinence (ICI) has published an extensive algorithm (that can be viewed on line at www.continent.org open documents) on the evaluation and treatment of the

TABLE 5.1

ACOG Guidelines for Primary Surgery for SUI

Confirmation of Indication	Actions Prior to the Procedure
Documentation of stress incontinence	Document normal voiding habits
Identify and manage transient causes of stress incontinence	Document normal neurological examination
Demonstrate stress loss and confirm low residual urine	Document absence of prior incontinence or radical surgery
	Document absence of pregnancy
	Counsel patient regarding alternative therapy

incontinent female (4). The portion that covers the basic evaluation is complete and furthers that published by the AHCPR and should serve as a thorough clinically practical model (Table 5.2). However, neither of these criteria sets has been evaluated in clinical practice, so while they seem complete, until tested they may prove less then reliable.

This chapter focuses on simple testing techniques for evaluating the incontinent female that

TABLE 5.2

ICI Guidelines for the Initial Evaluation of the Incontinent Female

History and general assessment	Nature and duration of symptoms
	Previous surgical procedures
	Environmental issues
	Patient mobility
	Mental status
	Disease status
	Patient medications
	Patient goals
	Patient expectations
	Fitness for surgery
Urinary diary and symptom score	3- or 7-day diary
	Quality-of-life tool specific for incontinence
Physical examination	Abdominal examination
	Sacral neurologic examination
	Pelvic examination
	Assess estrogen status
Cough stress test	Preferably with a full bladder
Urinalysis +/− urine culture	Dip in office urinalysis may be adequate.
	Culture only for patients suspected of having a UTI by urinalysis
Postvoid residual determination by abdominal examination	I&O catheterization
	Ultrasound Postvoid residual optional

are available to most practitioners and points out some of the situations that require more specialized testing or referral.

HISTORY

All too often the patient's history is used to diagnose the type of incontinence. The following statement is as true today as it was in 1972 and sums up the role of history in diagnosing the type of urinary incontinence in females: "urinary symptoms in the female can be extremely misleading and do not form a scientific basis for treatment . . . . Without some form of objective investigation, the gynecologist who relies on clinical impression is likely to submit some of his (or her) patients to ineffective surgery, and others to needless surgery" (5). History alone is a poor predictor of the type of incontinence, and there is no question or set of questions that can adequately distinguish between the various forms of incontinence (6–9).

Severity of Incontinence

Although history is a poor predictor for the type of incontinence, it does play a major role in evaluation and treatment. A comprehensive urogynecologic history should include duration and characteristics of the incontinent episodes, frequency of incontinent episodes, use of protective devices, previous therapy, and any conditions that may predispose the patient to incontinence. Determining the nature and severity of the patient's incontinence will help direct future therapies, with more severe symptoms suggesting more aggressive therapeutic choices and milder symptoms suggesting less invasive interventions. Although this may seem obvious, it can be overlooked. All too often a patient who has two or three incontinence episodes a year is referred to a specialist. There she undergoes an extensive evaluation with expensive testing and is offered invasive surgery or placed on daily medication simply for responding "yes" to a question about incontinence at an annual exam. Therefore, documenting the degree and severity of the problem is important before offering therapy. There are no validated or recognized severity scales to use in documenting the degree of incontinence, and there is no severity measure or cut-off for determining who will benefit from more or less invasive therapies. Instead, there exists a continuum of patients. Those with symptoms at either extreme represent obvious examples of minimal or severe incontinence for whom the decision to intervene or not is readily apparent. It is the patient with mild-to-moderate symptoms who represents the greatest challenge in determining the extent of

evaluation and treatment. Therefore, documenting the degree of her problem and desire for therapeutic interventions will aid greatly in treatment planning.

Transient Causes of Incontinence

Reversible and transient causes of incontinence should be identified. These are summarized with the mnemonic DIAPPERS (Table 5.3).

Delirium

Delirium is a state of confusion or altered consciousness characterized by acute or subacute onset. Delirium may result from many drugs or medical illnesses, and these should be considered in patients who are very poor historians or whose caretakers demonstrate concern over their change in behavior. The underlying causes of delirium may present atypically and, if unrecognized, may be associated with significant morbidity and mortality (10). Incontinence is a symptom that may abate when the cause of the patient's confusion is identified and treated.

Infection (Recurrent Urinary Tract Infections)

Urogenital atrophy predisposes postmenopausal women to develop urinary tract infections (UTIs). The prevalence of recurrent UTI (defined as greater then three per year) is as high as 8% to 10% in women over the age of 60 years, and it is present in 50% of female nursing home residents (11). Symptoms of UTI in elderly patients may differ from those in younger patients. Dysuria is often absent, and incontinence may be the patient's only symptom.

TABLE 5.3

Transient Causes of Urinary Incontinence

Delirium
Infection
Atrophic vaginitis
Pharmacologic
Psychological
Endocrine
Restricted mobility
Stool impaction

Atrophic Urethritis

Postmenopausal estrogen deficiency and atrophy of the urogenital tissues can lead to increased genitourinary tract sensitivity and irritative symptoms, including frequency, urgency, and nocturia. While atrophy does not cause incontinence per se, it does worsen symptoms, and its treatment with estrogen will resolve many of the irritative urinary symptoms (12,13).

Pharmacologic Causes

Virtually any medication that affects the autonomic nervous system also influences lower urinary tract function. Commonly prescribed antihypertensives, antidepressants, and sedative-hypnotics may exacerbate incontinence. Many over-the-counter multicomponent cold medications, decongestants, and antihistamines can affect the lower urinary tract. Incontinent patients should be asked about both prescription and nonprescription medication use.

One area that deserves special attention is the use of antihypertensive agents, which are commonly prescribed for older females. It has been demonstrated that patients attending hypertension clinics have a relative risk for urinary incontinence of 3.3, with alpha-adrenergic blockers (i.e., prazosin, terazosin, or doxazosin) being the primary culprits (14). A simple change in medication from an alpha-adrenergic blocker can often provide significant clinical improvement. Diuretics, although often implicated in incontinence, may aggravate symptoms but have not been shown to have a causal relationship (15).

Psychological Causes

Incontinence may occasionally be used to gain attention or to manipulate others. Patients may be so profoundly depressed that they do not care about continence.

Endocrine Causes

Diabetes mellitus, diabetes insipidus, and hypercalcemia may induce an osmotic diuresis that exacerbates other causes of incontinence. While this does not lead to incontinence per se, it can lead to frequency, urgency, and nocturia.

Restricted Mobility

Arthritis, hip deformity, or gait instability may impair the elderly patient's ability to reach the bathroom. If mobility cannot be improved, a nearby commode may improve the incontinence. This is often referred to as functional incontinence.

Stool Impaction

Fecal impaction is a common cause of urinary incontinence in bedridden or immobile patients. As the sigmoid and rectum enlarge, they act as a pelvic mass, compressing the bladder and exacerbating other forms of incontinence. It should be suspected in the patient who develops fecal oozing and urinary incontinence with a palpable bladder (16).

VOIDING DIARY

The voiding diary is a helpful evaluation tool for documenting and measuring the severity of incontinence. There are several different techniques for performing a voiding diary. The frequency of urinary episodes can be collected over 3 to 7 days and/or the amount of liquid intake and urine production can be recorded over 1 to 2 days. A 1-week record of leak episodes and voiding is highly reliable for demonstrating urinary frequency, nocturia, and number of incontinent episodes; however, it cannot diagnose the type of incontinence (17). A 3-day voiding diary has demonstrated equivalence to a 1-week diary for documenting frequency and nocturia (18). A 24-hour record of fluid intake and voided volumes has a weak correlation with frequency of voids and incontinent episodes, but it does measure the fluid intake and voided bladder volumes (19). A fluid intake of greater than 4 L/day mandates consideration of diabetes insipidus, and frequent small voids can point to a diagnosis of interstitial cystitis.

PHYSICAL EXAMINATION

The physical examination should include a general physical examination, local neurologic testing, pelvic examination, cotton swab test, postvoid residual, and cough stress test.

General Physical Exam

An overall assessment of the patient is important. This includes a comment about her general state of health, mobility, and cognitive status. Subjects in poor health with limited mobility will require a different set of goals and therapeutic options than a more active, healthy patient. In addition, there are a few other aspects of the general physical that should be noted. An abdominal examination revealing a large abdominopelvic mass or significant ascites will need to be evaluated and addressed prior to embarking on therapy for incontinence. Attempting to treat urinary frequency and urgency with a large mass filling the pelvis or abdomen and compressing the bladder will be met with frustration and poor treatment outcomes. Significant peripheral edema in conjunction with a 24-hour voiding diary that demonstrates nocturia or nocturnal urge incontinence suggests that the patient is mobilizing fluid in the recumbent position. Mobilizing this fluid before bed may aid in the treatment of her symptoms. The individual with limited mobility requires special consideration in any treatment plan. Use of bedside commodes and teaching better transfer techniques are often all that is necessary to treat incontinence.

Neurologic Examination

A brief focused neurologic examination is recommended to screen for neurologic disease but has a low detection rate in the patient with no history of neurologic diseases. If the history or general assessment of the patient suggests a neurologic disorder, then a thorough neurologic examination is required. If the patient appears neurologically intact during the history and there is no past medical history of a significant neurologic insult, then a brief neurologic examination as outlined below is satisfactory.

A brief neurologic examination consists of deep tendon reflex testing of the lower extremities and simple assessment of perineal sensation and clitoral or anal sphincter reflex.

The reflexes to be tested include the knee, ankle, and plantar responses. Any asymmetry of the reflexes may closely reflect the nature of bladder dysfunction. In supranuclear lesions, there is hyperreflexia of the deep tendon reflexes. This is often associated with uninhibited detrusor contractions as demonstrated by cystometry.

Spinal cord segments S2 to S4 contain important neurons involved with micturition. In addition to the autonomic innervation, the periurethral striated muscle is also innervated by the pudendal nerve, originating in the S2 to S4 segments. Stimulation of this nerve causes contraction of the distal periurethral striated muscle. Reflexes, including the anal sphincter, clitoral–anal reflex, and cough reflexes, can produce contraction of the pelvic floor. Stroking the skin lateral to the anus elicits the anal reflex. Contraction of the anus should be observed. When the contraction is not visible, often a contraction can be palpated with an examining finger. The clitoral–anal reflex involves contraction of the bulbocavernosus, ischiocavernosus, and anal sphincter in response to tapping or squeezing of the clitoris (Fig. 5.1).

The absence of reflexes is not always abnormal. Hyperreflexia or asymmetry is more suspicious of an underlying neurologic cause and should warrant a more thorough investigation.

Accurate assessment of sensory function is challenging because of the subjective nature of the response and the need for patient cooperation. Despite these limitations, the examiner can usually determine whether the patient can perceive a stimulus and whether the response is symmetric. The sensation over the S2 to S4 dermatomes can determine if there are specific abnormalities at the level of the nerve root. This would suggest specific nerve or nerve root injuries. Dermatome charts (Fig. 5.2) are useful when a deficit is noted on ex-

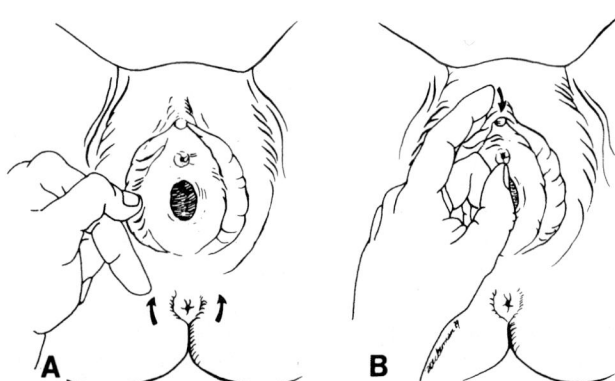

FIGURE 5.1 ● Tests of sacral cord integrity. **(A)** The anal reflex. The skin lateral to the anus is stroked. Contraction of the anus is observed or palpated with an examining finger. **(B)** The clitoral–anal reflex. Contraction of the bulbocavernosus and ischiocavernosus muscles is observed in response to tapping or squeezing the clitoris.

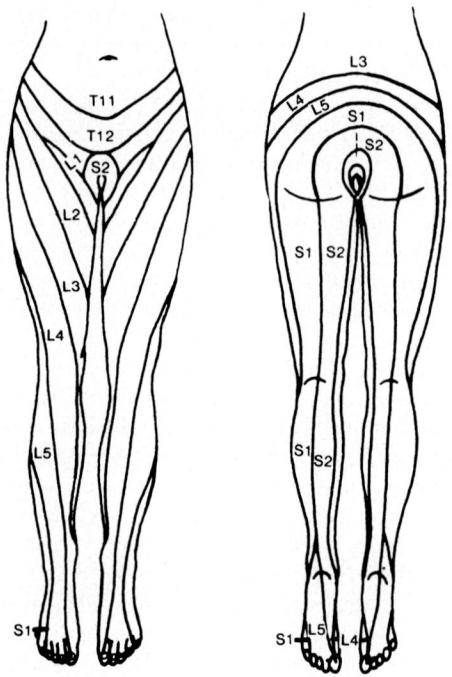

FIGURE 5.2 ● An exemplary dermatome map for use with sensory testing.

amination. Dermatomes overlap, and levels can vary considerably. Sensory testing of the perineum involves gently touching the skin of the perineum with a Q-tip or blunt needle and asking the patient to distinguish between the two. If sensation is absent or the patient cannot distinguish between the two stimuli, this suggests an abnormality that should be evaluated.

If this evaluation reveals any suspicious findings, then referral to a specialist for a more thorough evaluation is indicated.

Thorough Neurologic Examination

The thorough neurologic examination always begins with a detailed history. Attention to the speech and manner of patient responses to questions is necessary. The mode of onset, evolution, and course of each symptom are of paramount importance. It is tempting to shorten the time spent on history taking when the patient is a poor historian. The presence of poor speech or disorganized thoughts may be the first clue to a central nervous system lesion that is related to the urologic complaints. The elicited history should include sequentially the same categories to be explored in the neurologic examination: mental status, strength and sensory changes of the upper and lower extremities, and gait and station.

Mental Status

Mental status testing is performed by determining accuracy in the following areas: recent and past memory; orientation to date, place, and person; calculations; comprehension of simple directions; and reading and writing abilities. The Mini Mental Status Examination is available as a structured, well-tested tool for brief assessment of a patient's mental status (20). It is important to define the severity of any mental deficit because the patient's cognitive and physical abilities will affect treatment options.

Muscle Strength

Skeletal muscles should be inspected for muscle atrophy and fasciculations, spasticity, rigidity, and strength. Muscle strength is assessed by having the patient either resist movement or actively move against resistance. Strength is graded on a scale of 0 to 5: 0, no movement; 1, trace of contraction; 2, active movement when gravity eliminated; 3, active movement against gravity only; 4, active movement against resistance but less than normal; and 5, normal strength.

The maneuvers required to test sacral spinal cord integrity focus on the lower extremities. The basic maneuvers are extension and flexion of the hip, knee, and ankle and inversion or eversion of the foot (Fig. 5.3).

Deep Tendon Reflexes

Evaluation of the deep tendon reflexes provides information regarding segmental and suprasegmental spinal cord function.

An upper motor neuron lesion may also be detected with the plantar toe reflex. The plantar toe reflex is elicited by stroking the handle of a reflex hammer along the lateral aspect of the foot, from the heel to the ball of the foot, and then curving it medially. A normal response produces plantarflexion of the toes. An abnormal (Babinski) response produces fanning of the toes and dorsiflexion of the big toe and indicates interruption of the corticospinal tracts, an upper motor neuron lesion.

Although the absence of a patellar reflex is always abnormal, the ankle reflex diminishes with age; its absence in elderly patients, therefore, may be of no clinical significance (21). In patients with cauda equina lesions or with peripheral neuropathy (lower motor neurons), the deep tendon reflexes may be diminished or absent. Clinically, patients demonstrate detrusor areflexia or varying degrees of decreased bladder contractility. The presence of peripheral nerve impairment, autonomic neuropathy, or spinal cord disease below T12 may be suggested by absent or diminished re-

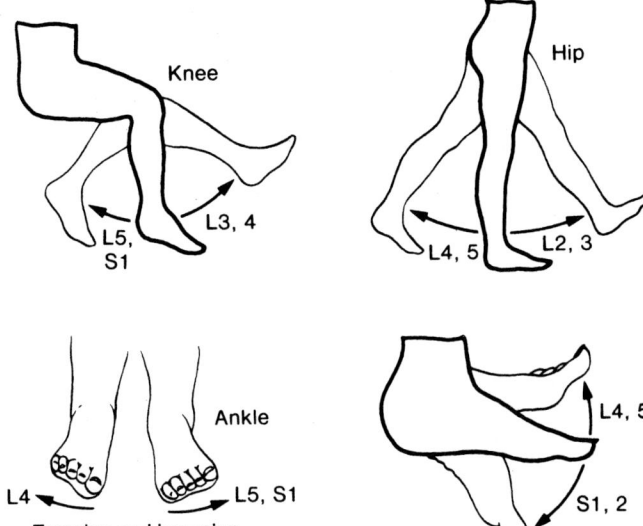

FIGURE 5.3 ● Testing of motor strength. Lower extremity movements and the corresponding spinal cord segments are indicated.

flexes and clinically correlated with symptoms of urinary retention or voiding difficulties.

Cerebellum

The cerebellum has four major functions in the control of micturition: maintenance of the tone of the periurethral striated muscle and the pelvic floor, suppression of the detrusor reflex by modulation of the brain stem detrusor centers, coordination of bladder contraction with urethral relaxation, and regulation of the strength of detrusor and periurethral muscle contractions. Truncal ataxia and the ataxic gait, characteristic of midline cerebellar dysfunction, are frequently observed in patients with multiple sclerosis. Additional cerebellar testing consists of evaluation of finger–nose and heel–shin coordination and examination of the patient's gait, including tandem gait.

Cerebellar disease characteristically produces spontaneous high-amplitude detrusor reflex contractions as observed during cystometry. Poor hand coordination in these patients can impede the use of intermittent self-catheterization.

If a neurologic cause for incontinence is suspected, then appropriate referral is indicated prior to embarking on a treatment course. Once the neurologic abnormality is evaluated and appropriately treated, the patient will often still require therapy for her incontinence, and follow-up should be arranged.

Pelvic Examination

A pelvic examination is central to evaluating the incontinent female, and the presence of uncommon forms of incontinence can be suggested from a careful inspection. The presence of a large pool of urine in the vagina should suggest a vesicovaginal, ureterovaginal, or urethrovaginal fistula. On bimanual examination, a large tender mass palpated along the anterior vaginal wall suggests a suburethral diverticulum. In addition, a large pelvic mass may contribute to urinary frequency and urgency as it presses down on the bladder, although it is unlikely to be the cause of the incontinence. If the examination suggests any of these findings, further evaluation should be directed toward making the proper diagnosis.

During the examination, attention should be paid to pelvic organ support. The pelvic organ prolapse quantification system (POPQ) is a standardized system for measuring and reporting changes in vaginal support (22). The POPQ technique for describing pelvic organ support is covered in detail in Chapter 25. The assessment of pelvic organ support should be conducted during a Valsalva maneuver or cough, and the degree of movement of the various components of the vagina should be noted. A Sims or disarticulated Graves speculum can be used to retract the posterior vaginal wall, allowing for visualization of the entire anterior vaginal wall during straining. A similar technique is employed to visualize the posterior vaginal wall by retracting the anterior vagina. The cervix and apex or cuff can be either visualized directly with a speculum or palpated during straining to determine the degree of support.

There is some controversy regarding whether the patient should be examined in the supine dorsal lithotomy position or standing. In one study, there did not appear to be any difference between examining the subject supine or standing (23). However, other studies have suggested more pronounced prolapse with the subject in a more upright position (24). If a patient complains of a greater degree of prolapse than is visualized supine, then the examination should be performed in an upright position.

Q-tip Test

The mobility of the urethrovesical junction (UVJ) should be assessed by the Q-tip or cotton swab test or by imaging techniques such as ultrasound or cystography (25). The Q-tip test is performed by first cleaning the external urethral meatus with an appropriate antibacterial solution. Next, a sterile Q-tip that has been lubricated with an anesthetic ointment is gently inserted into the urethra until the tip has reached the bladder. Generally, there is a slight decrease in resistance as the tip passes the bladder neck. The Q-tip is then drawn back until a slight resistance is felt, which ensures that the tip is at the UVJ. The resting angle is measured with a simple goniometer, with the reference being parallel to the floor. The subject is then asked to perform the Valsalva maneuver or cough, and the excursion is measured. By the Q-tip test, hypermobility is defined as an excursion with straining of more than 30 degrees from the resting angle or more than 30 degrees from the horizontal (26,27) (Fig. 5.4). The Q-tip test has been a mainstay of the basic evaluation since its introduction in 1971 and has demonstrated good interobserver reliability (28–30). It has never demonstrated clinical utility in diagnosing the type of incontinence but can only determine whether there is UVJ hypermobility or good support. It has

been suggested that mobility of the UVJ can be assessed by simply visualizing the degree of descent of the anterior vaginal wall with Valsalva. However, when direct visual assessment was compared with the Q-tip test, it was deemed inadequate (31). For a full discussion of ultrasound and cystourethrographic definitions of hypermobility, refer to Chapter 26. If surgery is not being contemplated, the Q-tip test can be omitted from a basic evaluation. Its main role is to determine which subjects would benefit from a surgical elevation of the bladder neck and which subjects already have adequate UVJ support and may be better suited to injectable therapy.

Postvoid Residual Urine Determination

A postvoid residual (PVR) urine determination should be made immediately after spontaneous voiding to rule out overflow incontinence in most patients. It has been suggested that PVR can be estimated on bimanual examination by feeling for an enlarged distended bladder. However, this technique had a 14% sensitivity rate for detecting PVR of greater than 50 mL. A more accurate technique is performed by a simple in-and-out catheterization, bladder scan, or ultrasound, if available (32). Consensus seems to exist that a PVR of less than 50 to 100 mL is normal, a PVR of more than 200 mL is abnormal, and any values in between require clinical correlation (1). Abnormal tests should be repeated because the reliability of a single determination is poor (33). There are currently few if any data available to determine what constitutes a clinically significant elevated PVR that results in morbidity (i.e., increased UTIs, overflow incontinence, sensation of bladder pressure or urgency, or reflux with upper tract damage). Therefore, most

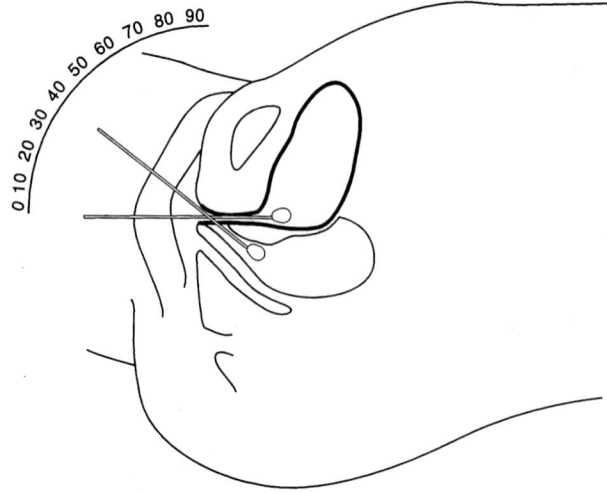

FIGURE 5.4 ● The Q-tip test demonstrating a resting angle of 0 degrees (bladder outlined in bold line) and the Q-tip angle with strain of about 40 degrees.

patients should have a PVR determined, and values of less than 50 mL should reassure the clinician. Values of greater than 50 mL but less than 200 mL should be repeated and correlated clinically. If the patient is asymptomatic with clean urinalysis and no history of UTIs, no therapy is indicated. The patient should be referred for a voiding study to determine whether she has any other pathology (e.g., detrusor–sphincter dyssynergia) if the PVR is greater than 200 mL.

Urinalysis

A test to evaluate for an occult bladder infection should be performed. A dipstick urinalysis has poor sensitivity but high specificity and negative predictive values of 97% to 99% in a urogynecology clinic population (34,35). Therefore, a negative dipstick urinalysis reliably predicts the absence of infection. A positive dipstick urinalysis (meaning the presence of heme, leukocytes, or nitrates) mandates a clean-catch or catheterized microscopic urinalysis with culture and sensitivity to determine whether an infection is present. Alternatively, if a microscope is available, a sample of unspun urine can be inspected for the presence of leukocytes, red blood cells, and bacteria.

There is controversy regarding the need for all patients with incontinence to have a urine culture and sensitivity as part of their initial evaluation. From the previously mentioned data, a good policy would be to screen all patients with either a dipstick or office microscopic urinalysis. In high-risk patients and in subjects undergoing invasive testing, a stronger case can be made to ensure sterile urine by culture and sensitivity.

The physical examination makes up an important part of the basic examination of the incontinent female but does not always lead to the diagnosis. However, empiric conservative treatment can often be initiated after the history and physical examination are completed, with complex testing reserved for treatment failures.

Urodynamic Testing

The diagnosis of urinary incontinence often rests with the urodynamic studies that are performed as part of the evaluation. Although they can be very sophisticated, there are simple means of performing these tests that are readily available to most practitioners in the office setting.

Cystometrogram

Routine office cystometry, which was left out of the AHCPR, ACOG, and ICI recommendations,

should be considered an essential part of the basic evaluation of the incontinent patient because it plays a central role in the diagnosis of both stress urinary incontinence and urge urinary incontinence. It has demonstrated a limited ability to diagnose detrusor overactivity, and even sophisticated multichannel studies detect uninhibited detrusor contractions in only 60% of subjects noted to have detrusor overactivity on ambulatory urodynamics (36). In view of this, the sophistication of the technique employed to perform cystometry may be of limited importance, and simple eyeball cystometry may suffice in the majority of patients.

The technique for performing eyeball cystometry uses 500 mL of sterile saline, a Foley catheter, and a 60-mL Foley-tipped syringe (Fig. 5.5). The urethral meatus is prepared with an antiseptic solution. The catheter is placed, and the bladder is emptied. If the subject has just voided, this can be recorded as the PVR. The subject is then asked to stand, if possible. The plunger of the 60-mL Foley-tipped syringe is removed, and the barrel is attached to the catheter. The barrel is held about 10 to 15 cm above the pubic symphysis. The sterile saline is then poured into the open barrel of the Foley-tipped syringe, filling the bladder in 60-mL increments until the patient states she cannot tolerate more fluid in the bladder. The meniscus of the saline in the syringe barrel is noted throughout the filling process, and if it begins to rise, this should be described as a detrusor contraction. The results

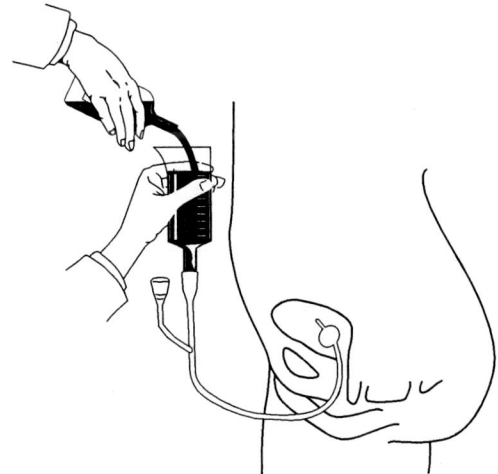

FIGURE 5.5 ● Eyeball cystometry is done in the standing position if possible. The barrel of the Foley-tipped syringe is held roughly 10 cm above the upper extent of the pubic symphysis.

TABLE 5.4

Findings During the Basic Evaluation of the Incontinent Patient That Require Further Evaluation

Findings Suggesting Further Evaluation	Suggested Evaluation
History	
1. Recurrent UTI*	1. Cystoscopy and possibly IVP versus renal ultrasound
2. Continuous incontinence/nonepisodic	2. Rule out fistula with methylene blue testing, cystoscopy, or cystometrogram.
3. Previous failed incontinence surgery*	3. Comprehensive evaluation to include complete urodynamic evaluation
4. Painful frequent voids/urge incontinence	4. Cystoscopy and cystometrogram
5. Greater than 4,000 mL voided volume	5. Evaluation of diabetes insipidus on 24-hour voiding diary
6. Neurologic disease suspected of contributing to the patient's symptoms*	6. Referral to a local expert on female urinary incontinence and/or neurologist
Physical Examination	
1. Vagina with obvious urine	1. Rule out fistula
2. Suburethral tender mass	2. Cystoscopy/radiographic study to rule out diverticula
3. Large pelvic mass	3. Age-appropriate workup
4. Pelvic organ prolapse extending beyond the hymen (POPQ stages 3 and 4)*	4. Evaluation of severe pelvic organ prolapse
Urodynamics	
1. Postvoid residual >200 mL*	1. Referral for urodynamic evaluation of obstructive voiding or underactive detrusor
2. Persistent microscopic hematuria on dip urinalysis in the absence of infection*	2. Cystoscopy and IVP
3. Small-volume bladder on cystometrogram (<300 cc)	3. Cystoscopy with sedation to rule out interstitial cystitis
4. Mixed incontinence on cystometrogram and cough stress test	4. Multichannel urodynamics
5. Positive supine empty stress test	5. Multichannel urodynamics
Overall Impression of Results	
1. Confusion regarding the results of testing*	1. Referral to a local expert on female urinary incontinence
2. Patients failing treatment based on your evaluation*	2. Referral to a local expert on female urinary incontinence

*Correspond to AHCPR guidelines for further evaluation after a basic workup of the incontinent female (1).

IVP, intravenous pyelogram; POPQ, pelvic organ prolapse quantification system of eyeball cystometry were found to be comparable to more sophisticated urodynamics (37).

The other piece of information that a cystometrogram can provide is bladder capacity. Normal bladder capacity is at least 350 to 400 mL. If the bladder volume by cystometry is very small (less than 300 mL), interstitial cystitis should be considered; conversely, if the capacity is more than 350 mL, interstitial cystitis is effectively ruled out (38). Various techniques for performing simple cystometry have been described employing the intrauterine pressure channel of a fetal monitor and an old-fashioned manometer (39,40). Regardless of the technique employed, the results of cystometry should always be interpreted with an open mind, remembering that a negative cystometrogram does not rule out the presence of urinary urge incontinence.

Cough Stress Test

A cystometrogram is not always effective at documenting uninhibited detrusor contractions, but it allows for bladder filling so that the cough stress test can be performed with a known bladder volume. The cough stress test involves filling a patient's bladder to at least 300 mL or symptomatic fullness. Then, while standing (or supine if she is unable to stand), the patient coughs while the physician directly visualizes the urethral meatus. If urine is noted to leak from the external urethral meatus, the result is a positive cough stress test. It has been demonstrated that performing a cough stress test before filling the bladder is extremely unreliable and may miss 80% of cases of stress incontinence, but when performed at a bladder volume of 300 mL or symptomatic fullness, this test becomes highly reliable (41–45). A negative cough stress test effectively rules out most cases of stress incontinence (46).

Some patients do not cough forcibly in the laboratory setting, and they may consciously hold in (contract the muscles of the pelvic floor) during the test. A positive cough stress test correlates highly with the presence of stress incontinence; however, if uninhibited detrusor contractions are noted during a cystometrogram preceding the cough stress test, the results become suspect (45,46).

One other caveat regarding the cough stress test is the supine empty stress test. This refers to subjects who are noted to leak urine from the urethral meatus during a cough or Valsalva maneuver at the time of the pelvic examination. Generally, the patient has voided just before the pelvic examination and is asked to cough or perform the Valsalva maneuver to evaluate her pelvic organ support. If the subject demonstrates urine loss under these circumstances, she has a positive supine empty cough stress test. A positive supine empty stress test has correlated strongly with a severe form of stress incontinence referred to as intrinsic sphincter deficiency (47). This entity is further discussed in Chapter 6. These patients generally respond poorly to conservative therapy and often require referral to a specialist for more extensive testing.

The cystometrogram and cough stress test are not essential to the basic evaluation, particularly if one is contemplating conservative nonsurgical therapy. If more invasive therapy is being considered, however, these tests should be performed as indicated.

SUMMARY

The AHCPR, ACOG, and ICI guidelines for evaluation and treatment of urinary incontinence in adults took the initial step in defining those components of a basic evaluation that should be required in the testing of all women with urinary incontinence. For empiric conservative therapy, these guidelines should suffice. However, if more invasive treatment is being considered, a simple cystometrogram and a cough stress test should be included. Finally, Table 5.4 lists several conditions that require special evaluation and should spark concern and referral to a specialist.

REFERENCES

1. Fantl JA, Newman DK, Colling J, et al. *Urinary incontinence in adults: acute and chronic management.* Clinical Practice Guideline, No. 2, 1996 Update. Rockville, MD: U.S. Department of Health and Human Services. Public Health Service, Agency for Health Care Policy and Research. AHCPR Publication No. 96-0682, March 1996.
2. Handa VL, Jensen JK, Ostergard DR. Federal guidelines for the management of urinary incontinence in the United States: which patients should undergo urodynamic testing. *Int Urogynecol J Pelvic Floor Dysfunct* 1995;6:198–203.
3. American College of Obstetricians and Gynecologists, Committee on Quality Assessment, ACOG Criteria Set. *Surgery for genuine stress incontinence due to urethral hypermobility.* No. 4, 1995.
4. Abrams P, Andersson KE, Brubaker L, et al. Recommendations of the International Scientific Committee. In Abrams P, Cardozo L, Khoury S, Wein A, eds. *Incontinence.* Paris: Health Publications Ltd, 2005:1606–1609.
5. Moolgaoker AS, Ardran GM, Smith JC, et al. The diagnosis and management of urinary incontinence in the female. *J Obstet Gynaecol Br Commw* 1972;79:481–497.
6. Harvey MA, Versi E. Predictive value of clinical evaluation of stress urinary incontinence: a summary of the published literature. *Int Urogynecol J Pelvic Floor Dysfunct* 2001;12:31–37.

7. Videla FL, Wall LL. Stress incontinence diagnosed without multichannel urodynamic studies. *Obstet Gynecol* 1998;91:965–968.

8. Diokno AC, Wells TJ, Brink CA. Urinary incontinence in elderly women: urodynamic evaluation. *J Am Geriatr Soc* 1987;35:940–946.

9. Jensen JK, Nielsen FR, Ostergard DR. The role of patient history in the diagnosis of urinary incontinence. *Obstet Gynecol* 1994;83:904–910.

10. Resnick NM, Yalla SV, Laurino E. The pathophysiology of urinary incontinence among institutionalized elderly persons. *N Engl J Med* 1989;320:1–7.

11. Cardozo L, Lose G, McClish D, et al. A systematic review of estrogens for recurrent urinary tract infections: third report of the Hormones and Urogenital Therapy (HUT) Committee. *Int Urogynecol J* 2001;12:15–20.

12. Fantl JA, Cardozo L, McClish DK. Estrogen therapy in the management of urinary incontinence in post menopausal women: a meta-analysis. First report of the Hormones and Urogenital Therapy Committee. *Obstet Gynecol* 1994;83:12–18.

13. Cardozo L, Bachman G, McClish D, et al. Meta-analysis of estrogen therapy in the management of urogenital atrophy in post menopausal women: second report of the Hormones and Urogenital Therapy Committee. *Obstet Gynecol* 1998;92:722–727.

14. Marshall HJ, Beevers DG. Alpha-adrenoceptor blocking drugs and female urinary incontinence: prevalence and reversibility. *Br J Clin Pharmacol* 1996;42:507–509.

15. Fantl JA, Wyman JF, Wilson MS, et al. Diuretics and urinary incontinence in community-dwelling women. *Neurourol Urodyn* 1990;9:25–34.

16. Spence-Jones C, Kamm MA, Henry MM, et al. Bowel dysfunction: a pathogenic factor in uterovaginal prolapse and urinary stress incontinence. *Br J Obstet Gynaecol* 1994;101:147–152.

17. Wyman JF, Choi SC, Harkins SW, et al. The urinary diary in evaluation of incontinent women: a test-retest analysis. *Obstet Gynecol* 1988;71:812–817.

18. Brown JS, McNaughton KS, Wyman JF, et al. Measurement characteristics of a voiding diary for use by men and women with overactive bladder. *Urology* 2003;61:802–809.

19. Wyman JK, Elswick RK, Wilson MS, et al. Relationship of fluid intake to voluntary micturitions and urinary incontinence in women. *Neurourol Urodyn* 1991;10:463–473.

20. Folstein MF, Robins LM, Helzer JE. The Mini Mental State Examination. *Arch Gen Psychiatr* 1983;40:812–816.

21. DeJong RN. *The neurologic examination*. Hagerstown, MD: Harper & Rowe, 1995:439–440.

22. Bump RC, Mattiasson A, Bo K, et al. The standardization of terminology of female pelvic organ prolapse and pelvic floor dysfunction. *Am J Obstet Gynecol* 1996;175:10–17.

23. Swift SE, Herring MD. Comparison of pelvic organ prolapse in the dorsal lithotomy versus the standing position. *Obstet Gynecol* 1998;91:961–964.

24. Brubaker L. *Effects of examination technique modification on pelvic organ prolapse quantification (POP-Q) results*. Abstract presented at the 27th Annual meeting of the International Urogynecological Association. Prague, Czech Republic, August 21–24, 2002.

25. Karram MM, Bhatia NN. The Q-tip test: standardization of the technique and its interpretation in women with urinary incontinence. *Obstet Gynecol* 1988;71:807–811.

26. Walter MD, Shields LE. The diagnostic value of history, physical examination, and the Q-tip cotton swab test in women with urinary incontinence. *Am J Obstet Gynecol* 1988;159:145–149.

27. Fantl JA, Hurt WG, Bump RC. Urethral axis and sphincteric function. *Am J Obstet Gynecol* 1986;155:554–558.

28. Lobel RW, Sand PK, Gore RM. *The cotton swab test in healthy continent women*. Abstract presented at the 22nd Annual International Urogynecologic Association meeting, Amsterdam, The Netherlands, July 30–August 2, 1997.

29. Thorp JM, Jones LH, Wells E, et al. Assessment of pelvic floor function: a series of simple tests in nulliparous women. *Int Urogynecol J Pelvic Floor Dysfunct* 1996;7:94–97.

30. Crystle CD, Charme LS, Copeland WE. Q-tip test in stress urinary incontinence. *Obstet Gynecol* 1971;38:313–315.

31. Montella JM, Ewing S, Cater J. Visual assessment of urethrovesical junction mobility. *Int Urogynecol J Pelvic Floor Dysfunct* 1997;8:13–17.

32. Bent AE, Nahhas DE, McLennan MT. Portable ultrasound determination of urinary residual volume. *Int Urogynecol J* 1997;8:200–202.

33. Stoller ML, Millard RJ. The accuracy of a catheterized residual volume. *J Urol* 1989;141:15–16.

34. Graham CA, Mallett VT, Ransom SB. *Routine urine culture and sensitivity in the evaluation of incontinent women: a utility and cost-effectiveness study*. Abstract presented at the 19th Annual American Urogynecology Society meeting, Washington, DC, November 12–15, 1998.

35. Steele AC, Neff J, Mallipeddi P, et al. *The utility of screening urinalysis in female incontinence and pelvic prolapse*. Abstract presented at 19th Annual American Urogynecology Society meeting, Washington, DC, November 12–15, 1998.

36. van Waalwijk van Doorn ES, Remmers A, Janknegt RA. Extramural ambulatory urodynamic monitoring during natural filling and normal daily activities: evaluation of 100 patients. *J Urol* 1991;146:124–131.

37. Ouslander J, Leach G, Abelson S, et al. Simple versus multichannel cystometry in the evaluation of bladder function in an incontinent geriatric population. *J Urol* 1988;140:1482–1486.

38. Parsons CL. Interstitial cystitis: clinical manifestations and diagnostic criteria in over 200 cases. *Neurourol Urodyn* 1990;9:241–250.

39. Swift SE. The reliability of performing a screening cystometrogram using a fetal monitoring device. *Obstet Gynecol* 1997;89:708–712.

40. Sand PK, Brubaker LT, Novak T. Simple standing incremental cystometry as a screening method for detrusor instability. *Obstet Gynecol* 1991;77:453–457.

41. Kadar N. The value of bladder filling in the clinical detection of urine loss and selection of patients for urodynamic testing. *Br J Obstet Gynaecol* 1988;95:698–704.

42. Swift SE, Ostergard DR. Evaluation of current urodynamic testing methods in the diagnosis of genuine stress incontinence. *Obstet Gynecol* 1995;86:85–91.

33. Scotti RJ, Myers DL. A comparison of the cough stress test and single-channel cystometry with multichannel urodynamic evaluation in genuine stress incontinence. *Obstet Gynecol* 1993;81:430–433.

44. Summitt RL, Stovall TG, Bent AE, et al. Urinary incontinence: correlation of history and brief office evaluation with multichannel urodynamic testing. *Am J Obstet Gynecol* 1992;166:1835–1844.

45. Swift SE, Yoon EA. The test-retest reliability of the cough stress test in women with urinary incontinence. *Obstet Gynecol* 1999;94:99–102.
46. Weidner AC, Myers ER, Visco AG, et al. Which women with stress incontinence require urodynamic evaluation? *Am J Obstet Gynecol* 2001;184:20–27.

47. McClennan MT, Bent AE. Supine empty stress test as a predictor of low Valsalva leak point pressure. *Neurourol Urodyn* 1998;17:121–127.

CHAPTER 6

Urodynamics

Victor W. Nitti and Melissa C. Fischer

INTRODUCTION

The lower urinary tract is responsible for the storage and evacuation of urine. Storage should occur at low pressure in order to ensure continence and protection of the kidneys, and evacuation should be voluntary. However, a variety of problems may arise that interfere with these two basic functions. Urodynamics (UDS) is the dynamic study of the transport, storage, and evacuation of urine by the urinary tract. It is comprised of a number of tests which individually or collectively can be used to gain invaluable information about lower urinary tract function.

The term "urodynamics" was first described by Davis in 1953, but the study of bladder pressure began in earnest in the late 19th century (1,2). Components of UDS include simple, noninvasive tests such as uroflowmetry to more sophisticated, invasive multichannel pressure–flow studies with sphincter electromyography and videofluoroscopy (videourodynamics). The following is a comprehensive review of UDS as it relates to the evaluation of the female patient. Furthermore, an emphasis will be placed on the diagnostic evaluation of urinary incontinence and pelvic floor prolapse. The terminology used conforms to the standards recommended by the International Continence Society (ICS), except where specifically noted (3).

INDICATIONS FOR URODYNAMICS

The initial evaluation of any patient includes a thorough history and physical and formulation of a differential diagnosis. While there have been many technological advances in the field of UDS, clinical expertise in deciding when, why, and how to perform the study is critical to the accurate interpretation and ultimate utility of the test. In general, UDS is indicated when the information and diagnosis provided will guide patient treatment.

Examples of indications are an inconclusive diagnosis after simpler tests, a poor response to empiric therapy, presence of a condition with known deleterious effects (e.g., spinal cord injury or multiple sclerosis), or when a proposed treatment has significant risks. Women who have a combination of stress- and urge-related symptoms, who can poorly characterize their incontinence by history, who have undergone prior surgical procedures, or those in whom neurologic disease is suspected should strongly be considered for UDS prior to intervention. Studies have demonstrated that UDS may also be beneficial in women who report pure stress urinary incontinence prior to surgical intervention, as only 51% had pure urodynamic stress incontinence on urodynamic evaluation (4).

UDS is just one tool that can be used to assist in the diagnosis of genitourinary abnormalities and is best utilized when the clinician has specific questions to be answered. UDS is an interactive test between the clinician and the patient and should attempt to reproduce the patient's symptoms. Often the objective data obtained is influenced by the circumstances and conditions of the test. Therefore, the ultimate interpretation of the data is subjective, requiring experience and an understanding of the patient's history. Three general principles should always be remembered: (a) a study that does not reproduce the patient's symptoms is nondiagnostic; (b) failure to record an abnormality does not rule out its existence; and (c) not all abnormalities are clinically significant (5).

A basic understanding of the physiology of urine storage and voiding and the pathophysiology of voiding dysfunction is required to formulate appropriate questions to be answered by an urodynamic study. However, all too often clinicians become caught up in the intricate neurophysiologic aspects of voiding and storage dysfunction and fail to think in practical terms. One should always focus on the possible urodynamic findings in a given case and how each of the findings may ultimately affect treatment. The functional classification system described by Wein is a useful framework with which to conceptualize voiding dysfunction and characterize it based on urodynamic findings (6). Of equal importance is that treatment options can be guided by this system. The functional classification system is based on the simple concept that the lower urinary tract (comprising the bladder and the bladder outlet) must store and empty urine. For normal storage and emptying to occur, the bladder and bladder outlet must function in a proper and coordinated fashion. Hence, lower urinary tract dysfunction can be classified under the following rubrics: "failure to store," "failure to empty," or a combination of both. Urodynamic abnormalities may result from bladder dysfunction, bladder outlet dysfunction, or a combination of both.

URODYNAMIC TESTING

Uroflowmetry

Uroflowmetry is a noninvasive means of quantifying the general effectiveness of voiding. The information may be used as an initial screening test or for comparison to monitor therapy but is not diagnostic as a single tool. Uroflowmetry is simple, noninvasive, and inexpensive. The test relies on the bladder being filled to normal capacity until the patient is comfortably full and has a normal desire to void. The patient is encouraged to sit and void as usual in a private setting. Prior to interpretation the patient should be asked whether the void was typical for her. We have found uroflowmetry particularly useful in women with significant voiding symptoms (decreased force of stream, hesitancy, straining to void) and incomplete bladder emptying.

The flow rate is directly related to the intravesical volume. The ideal volume for uroflowmetry is dependent upon the individual, but generally the volume should be greater than 150 mL for accurate interpretation (7). While we agree with the statement that a voided volume of 150 mL or more is optimal, we also realize that some patients cannot hold such a volume, and in these cases, the knowledge that the study was "typical" is important. Low-volume voids can be correlated with voiding diaries.

The urinary flow pattern is the result of the expulsion pressure, both detrusor and abdominal, and the outlet resistance. The following parameters can be measured during a noninvasive uroflow:

1. Flow rate: the volume of urine expelled via the urethra per unit time (mL/sec)
2. Voided volume: total volume expelled via the urethra (mL)
3. Maximum flow rate (Q_{max}): the maximum measured flow rate after correction for artifact (mL/sec)
4. Voiding time: the total duration of micturition, including interruptions (sec)
5. Flow time: the time over which measurable flow actually occurs (sec)
6. Average flow rate (Q_{ave}): voided volume divided by flow time (mL/sec)
7. Time to maximum flow: elapsed time from onset of flow to maximum flow (sec)
8. Postvoid residual volume (PVR) may be determined after uroflowmetry to assess how well the patient emptied her bladder. PVR may be measured by a bladder ultrasound or catheterization.

When interpreting an uroflow tracing, it is important to look at not only the objective parameters listed above but also the shape of the flow curve, which can give insight into the way the patient voids. The pattern of flow can be described as continuous or intermittent, smooth or fluctuating (3). A typical flow is a continuous, smooth, bell-shaped curve with high amplitude. A decreased detrusor contraction and/or increased outlet resistance will result in a lower flow rate and a smooth flat curve (8). Characteristic uroflow patterns are shown in Figure 6.1 (9,10).

How can uroflowmetry be applied to clinical practice? If a woman with significant voiding symptoms has a completely normal uroflow (rate and pattern) and a low PVR, then more invasive urodynamic testing may initially be deferred. Conversely, an abnormal uroflow might prompt further testing. An abnormal uroflow indicates that emptying is altered but is not diagnostic of etiology. Emptying abnormalities that affect uroflowmetry include impaired contractility and increased outlet resistance (obstruction) (11). A formal pressure–flow study is necessary to distinguish between the two. Uroflowmetry is particularly useful to evaluate a patient after an intervention that can affect emptying, such as anti-incontinence or prolapse surgery or urethrolysis for obstruction.

Cystometry

A cystometrogram (CMG) is a measure of the bladder's response to being filled. It allows the clinician to determine the pressure–volume relationship within the bladder during bladder filling and

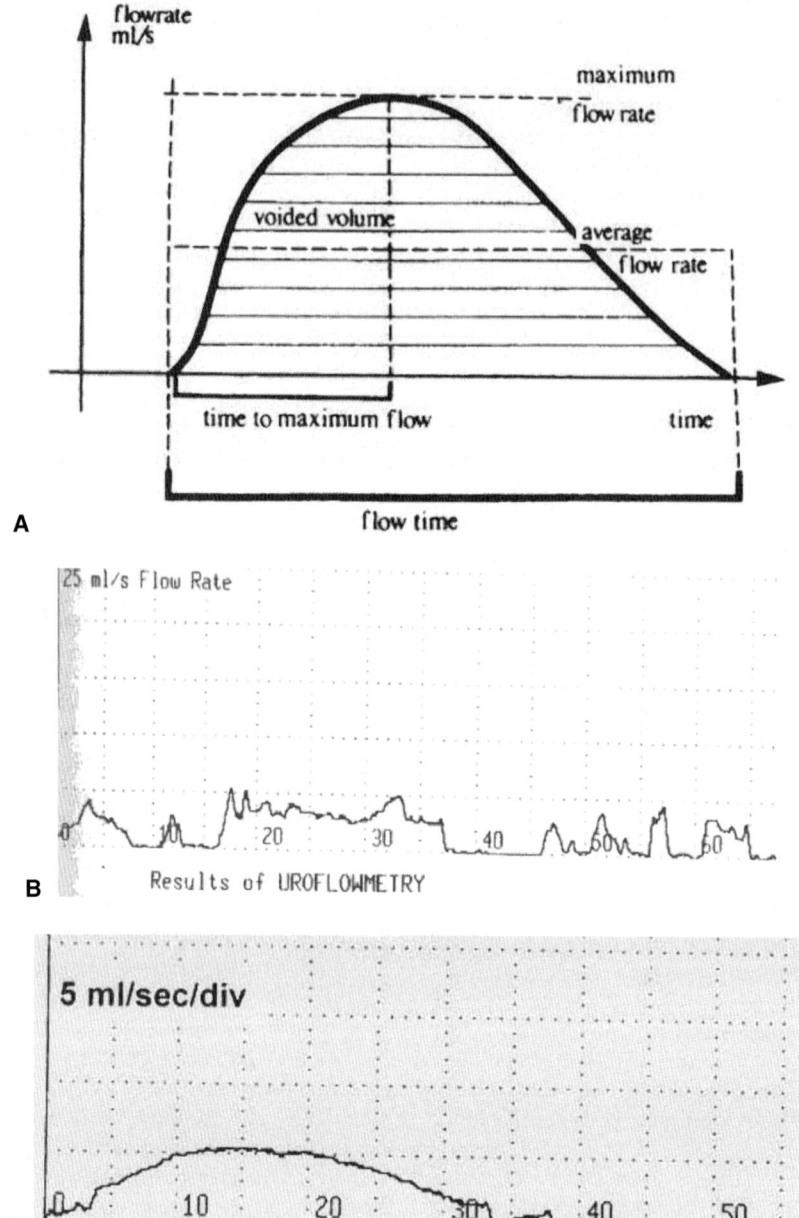

FIGURE 6.1 ● **(A)** Normal flow curve and pattern depicting the terminology of the International Continence Society relating to the urodynamic description of urinary flow. (From Wein AJ, English WS, Whitmore K. Office urodynamics. *Urol Clin North Am* 1988;15:609–623.). **(B)** Interrupted flow curve pattern is consistent with intermittent flow in which downward deflection reaches 2 mL/sec or lower, leading to several separate micturitions separated by 2 to 20 seconds, commonly due to straining in the absence of a detrusor contraction. (From Boone TA, Kim YH. Uroflowmetry. In: Nitti VW, ed. *Practical urodynamics*. Philadelphia: WB Saunders, 1998:28–37.) **(C)** Obstructed flow pattern. Most of the characteristics seen in the flow curve of an obstructed individual can be seen in a person with normal voiding; therefore, flow patterns are not diagnostic of outflow obstruction. However, outflow obstruction is characterized by certain uroflowmetric features, namely prolonged flow time, sustained low flow rate, low Q_{max} and Q_{ave}, and plateau-shaped flow curves. A fixed obstruction like a urethral stricture may give a plateau flow curve with decreased Q_{max} in which the Q_{max} is reached quickly but remains there for most of the micturition. (From Boone TA, Kim YH. Uroflowmetry. In: Nitti VW, ed. *Practical urodynamics*. Philadelphia: WB Saunders, 1998:28–37.)

storage of urine. A function of the bladder is to store increasing volumes of urine at low pressure. In addition, with the cooperation of the patient, it provides a subjective measure of bladder sensation. CMG provides correlation of patient's symptoms with objective measures. Cystometry can be performed as a single-channel study where the bladder pressure (p_{ves}) is measured and recorded during filling and storage or as a multichannel study where abdominal pressure (p_{abd}) is subtracted from p_{ves} to give the detrusor pressure (p_{det}). We believe that cystometry, whether done alone or as part of a pressure–flow study, is ideally done as a multichannel study with subtracted p_{abd} (Fig. 6.2) (12).

It is beyond the scope of this chapter to describe all of the technical nuances of performing proper cystometry and UDS. The reader is referred elsewhere for more detail (13). However, it is important to remember several basic principles. First, the patient should be adequately prepared with an

understanding of what to expect before the study is started. Intravesical catheters (usually 6 to 8 French) should be double- or triple-lumen to allow for both filling and simultaneous pressure measurement (bladder and urethra if desired). Abdominal pressure can be measured by placing a catheter in the rectum, vagina, or an abdominal stoma. Detrusor pressure (p_{det}) cannot be measured directly and therefore is a mathematically generated pressure (p_{ves} minus p_{abd}) calculated automatically by the UDS computer software. The transducers should be at the level of the pubic symphysis, then zeroed to atmospheric pressure. If the transducers are not at the level of the pubic symphysis, then the baseline readings should be adjusted accordingly. At the beginning of the test, the patient is asked to cough to assess accurate transmission of pressure in both p_{abd} and p_{ves}. If there is unequal transmission, then the catheters need to be adjusted or recalibrated prior to initiating the study. Typically medium fill is recom-

Single Channel CMG

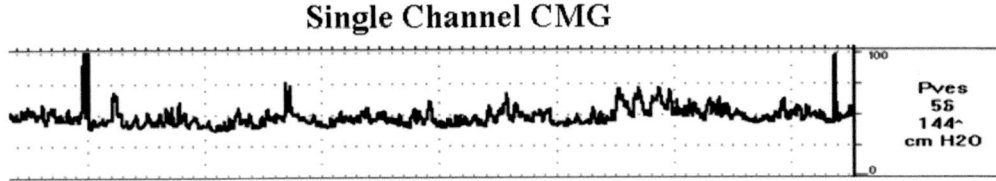

Multichannel Urodynamics

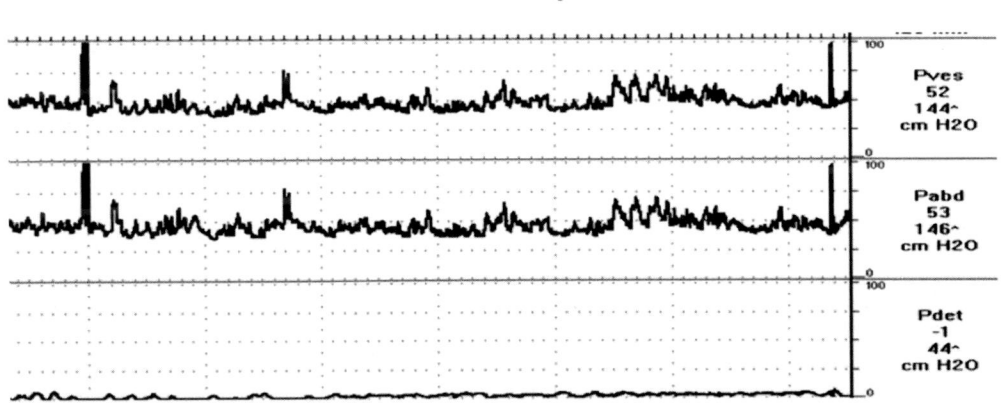

FIGURE 6.2 ● Adding intra-abdominal pressure monitoring gives a better representation of the true detrusor pressure. The top tracing is a single-channel CMG with measurement of only total vesical pressure (p_{ves}). Note the multiple spikes and rises in pressure. Without having simultaneous monitoring of intra-abdominal pressure, it is impossible to determine if these pressure spikes are due to a rise in detrusor or abdominal pressure. The lower tracing depicts the same CMG with intra-abdominal pressure (p_{abd}) monitoring added. The changes in p_{ves} were due to the changes in abdominal pressure. The subtracted detrusor pressure curve (p_{det}) curve is noted to be flat and without any rises in pressure (i.e., a stable and compliant bladder). (From Nitti VW. Cystometry and abdominal pressure monitoring. In: Nitti VW, ed. *Practical urodynamics*. Philadelphia: WB Saunders, 1998:38–51.)

mended (10 to 100 mL/min), and we usually fill between 30 and 50 mL/min with normal saline or radiographic contrast for videourodynamics.

Several parameters may be evaluated during cystometry, including filling pressure, sensation, presence of involuntary or unstable contractions, compliance, capacity, and control over micturition.

Filling Pressure

Normally as the bladder fills it maintains a relatively constant and low pressure. Detrusor pressure usually does not exceed 5 to 10 cmH$_2$O due to the vesicoelastic properties of the bladder; p_{det} remains low until the voluntary voiding phase. Rises in p_{det} may be caused by involuntary detrusor contractions (IDCs) or impaired compliance.

Sensation

Sensation is the part of cystometry that is truly subjective and therefore requires both an alert and attentive patient and clinician. Bladder sensation can be described in many ways. The ICS recommends judging bladder sensation by three defined points: first sensation of bladder filling, first desire to void (the feeling that would lead the patient to pass urine at the next convenient moment, but voiding can be delayed if necessary), and strong desire to void (persistent desire to void without the fear of leakage) (3). Patients can further be described as having normal, increased, reduced, or absent bladder sensation. Also, the ICS has provided terms to describe nonspecific bladder sensations, bladder pain, and urgency (a sudden compelling desire to void). If any of these sensations are experienced, the examiner should ask if they correlate with any of the patient's symptoms.

Capacity

Cystometric capacity is the bladder volume at the end of the filling cystometrogram. The end point should be specified (e.g., the patient had a normal desire to void, a void was precipitated by detrusor overactivity, or the study was terminated for another reason). Maximum cystometric capacity is the volume at which a patient feels she can no longer delay micturition because of a strong desire to void (3). If during the study there is a question as to the bladder volume, the recorded instilled volume can be verified by adding the measured voided volume to the residual, which can be estimated by fluoroscopy or measured with ultrasound or a catheter.

Compliance

Bladder compliance is the change in bladder volume over a change in bladder pressure expressed in mL/cmH$_2$O. Compliance is generally calculated by subtracting the baseline p_{det} from the premicturition pressure (p_{det} just prior to the initial isovolumetric contraction, also termed end-filling pressure) divided by the change in volume. Compliance is a reflection of the viscoelastic properties of the bladder, which normally allow storage of increasing volumes of urine at low pressures (see Fig. 6.2) (12). Abnormal or decreased compliance (increased pressure for a given volume) usually occurs in patients with underlying neurologic conditions, chronic catheterization, or certain inflammatory states. Decreased compliance is generally accepted to be less than 20 mL/cmH$_2$O, which implies a poorly accommodating bladder (14). The absolute value of compliance is probably less important than premicturition pressure. Typically, p_{det} at the end of filling is 6 to 10 cmH$_2$O (15). Clinically, it is most important to decide if the bladder is storing urine at elevated pressures for prolonged periods of time. An example of impaired compliance is shown in Figure 6.3.

Detrusor Contractions

The urodynamic observation of IDCs during the filling or storage phase is termed detrusor overactivity (DO) (Fig. 6.4) (16). DO may be phasic or terminal (occurring at maximum cystometric capacity). DO is usually, but not always, associated with an urge to void and may be associated with urgency or incontinence (DO incontinence). If an IDC is present, then the following should be noted: the volume at which the contraction occurred, the amplitude of the contraction, and if there was an associated leak. Furthermore, DO and DO incontinence are urodynamic observations, and the clinician must interpret the significance of these findings within the clinical context. Unequal transmission of p_{abd} and p_{ves} or rectal contractions may falsely suggest an IDC. Careful attention to the tracings, patient activity, and associated rise in p_{abd} should help delineate the situation.

According to the ICS, DO may also be described according to cause: neurogenic DO, when there is a relevant neurologic condition, and idiopathic DO, when there is no defined cause (3). The term "idiopathic" is a bit of a misnomer in that the cause of DO in a nonneurogenic patient may be readily apparent (e.g., bladder outlet obstruction or inflammatory process) versus truly "unknown." Thus, from a practical standpoint, the terms "neurogenic DO" and "nonneurogenic DO" should be used.

Urodynamic stress incontinence is the involuntary leakage of urine during increased abdominal pressure in the absence of a detrusor contraction

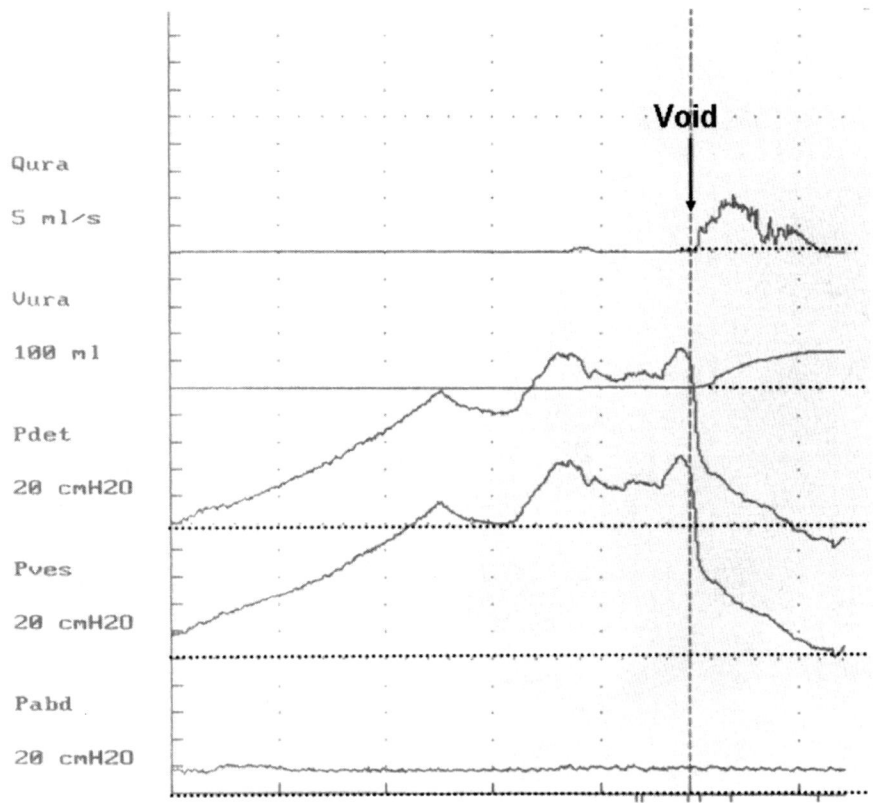

Void

Qura

5 ml/s

Uura

100 ml

Pdet

20 cmH20

Pves

20 cmH20

Pabd

20 cmH20

FIGURE 6.3 ● An example of severely impaired compliance in a woman with incontinence, hydronephrosis, and renal insufficiency after high-dose radiation for a pelvic malignancy. Baseline p_{det} is zero; however, with slow filling there is a steady rise in p_{det} to over 100 cmH$_2$O. When the patient is allowed to void, there is an immediate drop in pressure with the voluntary release of outlet resistance. This represents a dangerous situation, and impaired compliance is responsible for hydronephrosis and renal insufficiency.

(3). There are various urodynamic measurements of sphincteric function (see below), but the diagnosis of urodynamic stress incontinence per se can be made without any such measurements. During cystometry, filling can be stopped and the patient is asked to increase abdominal pressure by progressive Valsalva maneuvers or coughing. The demonstration of leakage with such maneuvers, in the absence of a detrusor contraction, confirms the diagnosis of urodynamic stress incontinence. Typically we start stress testing with cough or Valsalva at 150 mL of bladder volume and progress at 50-mL increments until stress incontinence is demonstrated or capacity is reached. The patient is asked to perform progressively forceful Valsalva maneuvers (Fig 6.5) followed by coughing (or other activity known to produce incontinence in a particular patient). Abdominal pressure at which leakage occurs is the abdominal leak point pressure (ALPP), but measurement of ALPP is not essential to make the diagnosis of urody-

namic stress incontinence. In some cases it may be necessary to remove the urethral catheter in order to demonstrate stress incontinence.

Leak Point Pressures

There are two distinct types of leak point pressures that can be measured in the incontinent patient. The two are independent of each other and represent completely different pathologic conditions. ALPP is a measure of sphincter strength (its ability to resist changes in abdominal pressure) (17). ALPP is defined as the intravesical pressure at which urine leakage occurs due to increased abdominal pressure in the absence of a detrusor contraction (see Fig. 6.5) (3,16). This measure of intrinsic urethral function is applicable to patients with stress incontinence. ALPP cannot be determined if the patient does not demonstrate urodynamic stress incontinence. Conceptually, the lower the ALPP, the weaker the sphincter. There is no normal ALPP, as patients without stress inconti-

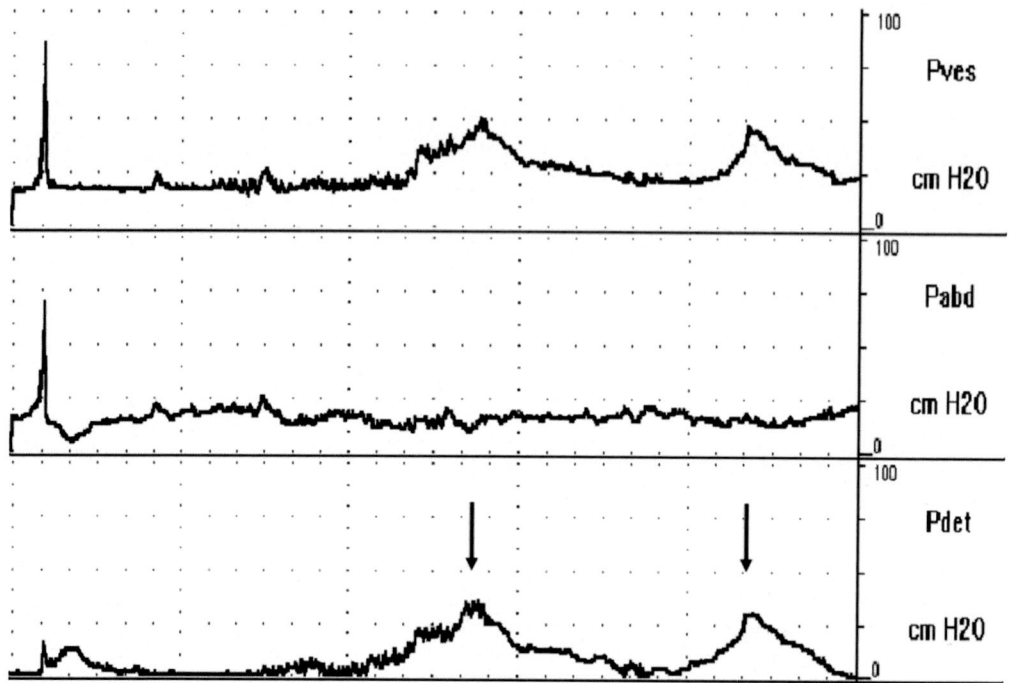

FIGURE 6.4 ● Detrusor overactivity. Note the rises in p_{ves} and p_{det} (*arrows*) with no rise in p_{abd}. (From Kelly CE, Nitti VW. Evaluation of neurogenic bladder dysfunction: basic urodynamics. In: Corcos J, Schick E, eds. *Textbook of the neurogenic bladder*. London: Martin Dunitz, 2004:415–423.)

nence will not leak at any physiologic abdominal pressure.

Attempts have been made to classify stress incontinence and intrinsic sphincter deficiency (ISD) based upon the ALPP. For example, ALPP less than 60 cmH$_2$O is evidence for ISD, ALPP of 60 to 90 cmH$_2$O is equivocal, and greater than 90 cmH$_2$O is suggestive of minimal or no ISD (17). Contemporary theories suggest that all patients with sphincteric incontinence have some degree of ISD, whether it is accompanied by a urethral support defect (urethral hypermobility) or not. The fact that the normal urethra is intended to remain closed no matter what the degree of stress or rotational descent supports this theory. Furthermore, many women with urethral hypermobility remain continent (18). Finally, urethral hypermobility and ISD may and often do coexist in the same patient, and we believe that they do not necessarily define discrete classes of patients (19). Thus, ALPP and urethral hypermobility may be used to characterize incontinence but not necessarily classify patients. Furthermore, there is not an absolute ALPP at which certain treatments fail. Rather than "classifying" stress incontinence as ISD or no ISD, it makes more sense to simply characterize it by two parameters: the degree of urethral mobility (e.g.,

as determined by the Q-tip test) and sphincter strength (e.g., ALPP). In cases of pelvic organ prolapse, ALPP can be measured after reduction of the prolapse to simulate surgical repair.

The second type of leak point pressure is detrusor leak point pressure (DLPP), which is a measure of detrusor pressure in the setting of decreased bladder compliance. It is defined as the lowest detrusor pressure at which urine leakage occurs in the absence of either a detrusor contraction or increased abdominal pressure (Fig. 6.6) (3). The higher the DLPP, the higher the urethral resistance. From a clinical perspective, DLPP is most useful in patients with lower motor neuron disease affecting the bladder (e.g., spina bifida, spinal cord tumors, or after radical pelvic surgery) and in nonneurogenic patients with low bladder compliance (e.g., multiple bladder surgeries, radiation, or tuberculous cystitis). The higher the DLPP, the more likely upper tract damage can occur as intravesical pressure is transmitted to the kidneys (see Fig. 6.3). McGuire documented the deleterious effects that a high leak point pressure has on the upper urinary tracts: leak point pressures greater than 40 cmH$_2$O result in hydronephrosis or vesicoureteral reflux in 85% of myelodysplastic patients (20).

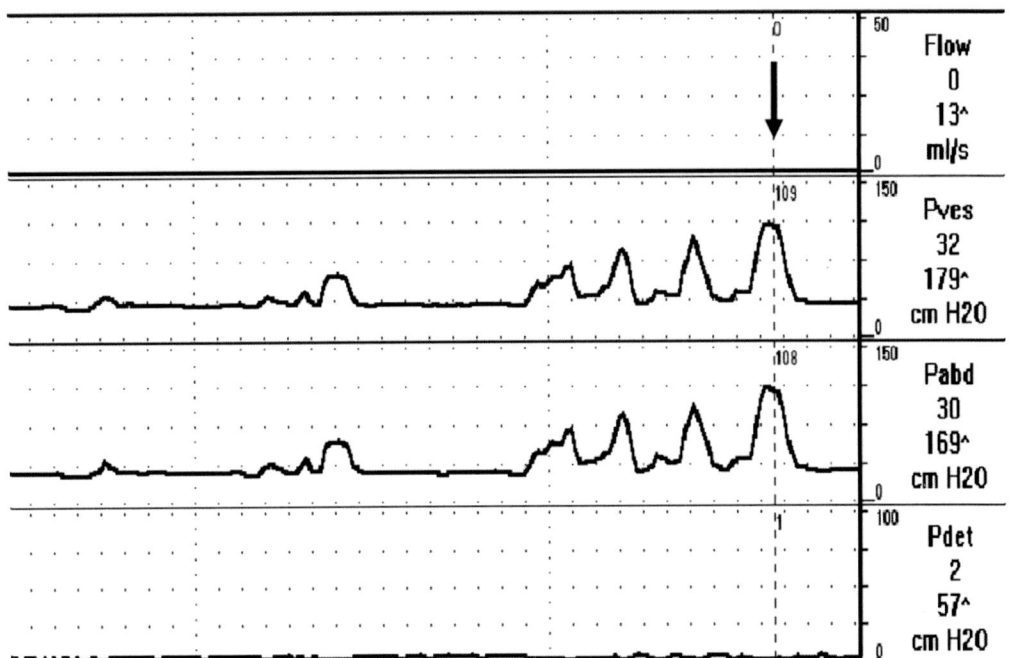

FIGURE 6.5 ● Abdominal leak point pressure (ALPP). At a fixed volume (usually 150 to 200 mL), the patient is asked to perform progressive Valsalva maneuvers until leakage is demonstrated. In this case leakage occurs at the *arrow* and the p_{ves} at that point is 109 cmH$_2$O, which is the ALPP. Note the equal rise in p_{abd} and p_{ves}. If there is no leakage demonstrated at the fixed volume, the patient can be retested at 50-mL increments until leakage is demonstrated. If leakage does not occur with a slow Valsalva, then the patient may be asked to cough. It is often necessary to perform ALPP testing in the standing position. If incontinence is not demonstrated with a urethral catheter in place in patients in whom stress urinary incontinence is suspected, stress maneuvers should be repeated without the catheter in place and the ALPP can be determined from the p_{abd} curve. (From Kelly CE, Nitti VW, Evaluation of neurogenic bladder dysfunction: basic urodynamics. In: Corcos J, Schick E, eds. *Textbook of the neurogenic bladder.* London: Martin Dunitz, 2004:415–423.)

Urethral Pressure Profilometry

Despite an abundant literature on urethral profilometry, its clinical relevance is controversial. The urethral pressure profile (UPP) represents the intraluminal pressure along the length of the urethra in graphic form. Several parameters can be obtained from the UPP. The urethral closure pressure profile is given by the subtraction of intravesical pressure from urethral pressure. The maximum urethral pressure is the highest pressure measured along the UPP, while the maximum urethral closure pressure is the maximum difference between the urethral pressure and the intravesical pressure. Maximum urethral closure pressure (MUCP) is the measure commonly used to evaluate urethral function. Functional profile length is the length of the urethra along which the urethral pressure exceeds intravesical pressure in women. In most continent women, the functional urethral length is approximately 3 cm and the MUCP is 40 to 60, but normal values vary widely from study to study (21).

One caveat of UPP is that it does not diagnose stress incontinence. Many authors have advocated that an MUCP of less than 20 cmH$_2$O correlates with ISD. Unlike ALPP, the demonstration of stress incontinence is not necessary to obtain an MUCP. Several techniques that measure pressure transmission ratios from bladder to urethra during increases in intra-abdominal pressure have been described, but their clinical applicability has yet to be proved (22–25). In 2002, the ICS Standardization Subcommittee concluded that the clinical utility of urethral pressure measurement is unclear (26). Furthermore, there are no urethral pressure measurements that (a) discriminate urethral incompetence from other disorders; (b) provide a measure of the severity of the condition; and (c) provide a reliable indicator to surgical success and return to normal after surgical intervention (26). In our opinion, further investigation is needed to determine the applicability of UPP and MUCP for the diagnosis and treatment of stress incontinence.

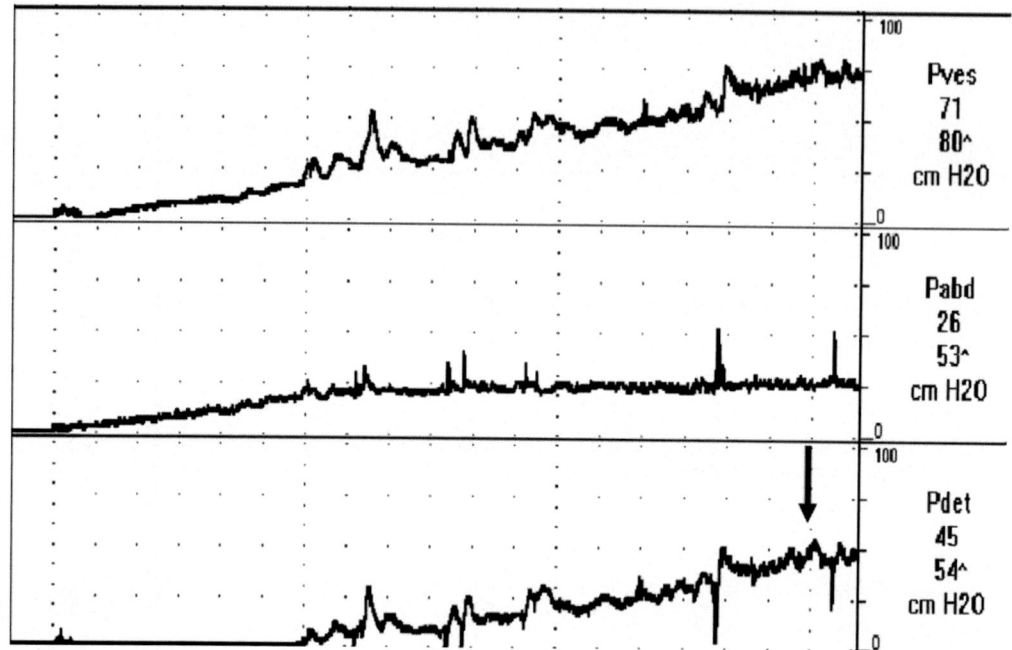

FIGURE 6.6 ● Detrusor leak point pressure (DLPP). Urodynamic tracing of an incontinent patient with neurogenic bladder secondary to myelomeningocele. There is impaired compliance (steady rise in p_{det}) and incontinence is demonstrated at the *arrow*, where p_{det} is 45 cmH$_2$O, which is the DLPP. Note that there is no rise in p_{abd}.

Voiding Pressure–Flow Studies

Multichannel invasive assessment of pressure–flow during the voiding phase of micturition can precisely define voiding dynamics and evaluate for abnormalities in contractility and/or outlet resistance (e.g., obstruction). Normal voiding starts by voluntary relaxation of the striated urethral sphincter, followed by a detrusor contraction, opening of the bladder neck, and initiation of urine flow. UDS allows investigation of each of these phases. During the voiding phase the parameters that were described for uroflowmetry are measured (Q_{max}, Q_{ave}, voided volume, etc.), as well as p_{det} at Q_{max} ($p_{det}Q_{max}$) and maximum detrusor pressure (p_{det}max). Voiding phase abnormalities occur when there are problems with detrusor contractility, increased outlet resistance, or abnormal coordination between the detrusor and sphincters. It is well known that abnormalities of storage are associated with abnormalities of emptying (e.g., association of detrusor overactivity with outlet obstruction or the association of incontinence with incomplete emptying). We believe that routine evaluation of the voiding phase is important for women undergoing UDS. In a study of women presenting with a variety lower urinary tract symptoms, we found that 34% had some abnormality of

the voiding phase (27). Patients should be carefully questioned about voiding symptoms, especially when such symptoms are not the primary presenting symptom.

The ICS defines normal detrusor function as a voluntarily initiated continuous contraction that leads to complete bladder emptying within a normal time span (3). The degree of amplitude and duration of the contraction is dependent upon outlet resistance. The greater the outlet resistance, the greater the detrusor pressure required to empty the bladder. A contraction that is of reduced strength and/or duration is termed "detrusor underactivity." In women it is important to note that in some cases, especially when outlet resistance is low, a low-pressure detrusor contraction can result in normal voiding and emptying and should not be considered a detrusor of reduced strength (Fig. 6.7) (28). An acontractile detrusor is one that does not demonstrate any contractility during UDS. An examiner should be careful not to erroneously diagnose detrusor acontractility. For example, if a patient does not void during the study but does void in daily life, then the diagnosis should not be made because the UDS was not representative of the clinical situation. This often happens when patients are inhibited in the clinical setting and are unable to relax the striated sphincter and initiate

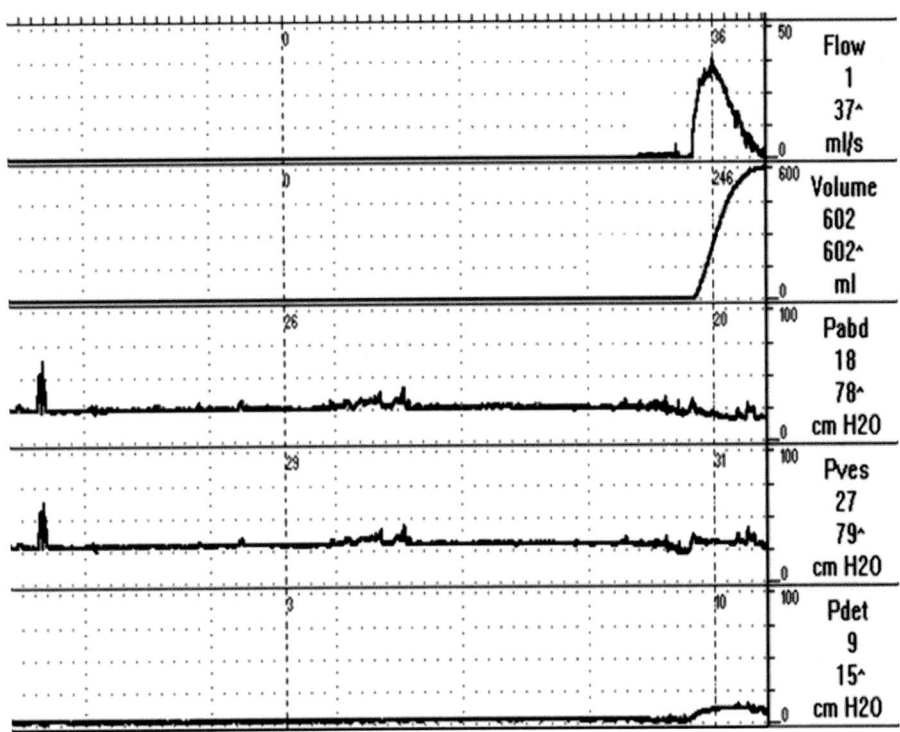

FIGURE 6.7 ● Multichannel UDS tracing of a 72-year-old woman with stress incontinence and low-pressure voiding. Note the minimal rise in p_{det} (most of which is actually a fall in p_{abd} with very little rise, about 2 cmH₂O, in p_{ves}) associated with a "superflow" rate of more than 35 mL/sec and complete bladder emptying. Although this patient voids with a low detrusor pressure, she does not have impaired contractility. (From Nitti VW. Bladder outlet obstruction in women. In: Nitti VW, ed. *Practical urodynamics.* Philadelphia: WB Saunders, 1998:197–210.)

the micturition reflex. In our experience, approximately 24% of women are unable to void characteristically during urodynamic testing (27).

Bladder outlet obstruction (BOO) is a generic term for obstruction during voiding and is classically diagnosed by synchronous comparison of p_{det} and flow rate (3). In men there are a number of nomograms that express the pressure–flow relation and allow for the diagnosis of obstruction and/or impaired contractility (29–31). In men, the model of BOO secondary to benign prostatic enlargement provides a highly prevalent condition with predictable outcomes after treatment. BOO in women is far less common than in men but is probably more prevalent than previously suspected. Furthermore, nomograms derived for men cannot be applied to women, as voiding dynamics differ. In addition, anatomic differences allow many women to empty their bladders by simply relaxing the pelvic floor, and some will augment voiding by abdominal straining. Minor elevations in detrusor pressure or decreases in flow rate, which might be considered insignificant in the male population, might signify obstruction in women. Accordingly,

clinicians must have a high index of suspicion based on lower urinary tract symptoms, incomplete emptying, persistent urinary tract infections, and a history of anti-incontinence surgery, prolapse, or other conditions.

There are a variety of causes of BOO in women, including anatomic and functional etiologies (Table 6.1) (32). Anatomic causes are more obvious than functional causes and are often suspected prior to UDS. Functional causes, conversely, require UDS (and often videourodynamics in women) to make a precise diagnosis. Recent interest in female BOO has resulted in the publication of several unique proposals of diagnostic urodynamic criteria. Chassange et al used the cut-off values for maximum flow rate (Q_{max}) and detrusor pressure at maximum flow rate ($p_{det}Q_{max}$) to define obstruction using a group of clinically obstructed women (post-incontinence surgery, prolapse, and other causes), comparing them to clinically unobstructed women with stress incontinence (33). In 2000, with an expanded database, the authors revised these values and found the best pressure–flow combination to predict obstruction was a Q_{max} of 11 mL/sec and

TABLE 6.1

Anatomic and Functional Causes of Bladder Outlet Obstruction in Women (32)

Anatomic Obstruction	Functional Obstruction
A. Inflammatory processes	A. Detrusor–sphincter dyssynergia
1. Bladder neck fibrosis	
2. Urethral stricture	
3. Meatal stenosis	
4. Urethral caruncle	
5. Skene's gland/cyst abscess	
6. Urethral diverticulum	
B. Pelvic prolapse	B. Dysfunctional voiding
1. Anterior vaginal wall	
2. Posterior vaginal wall	
3. Apical (uterine prolapse/enterocele)	
C. Neoplastic	C. Primary bladder neck obstruction
1. Urethral carcinoma	
2. Bladder carcinoma	
D. Gynecologic (extrinsic compression)	
1. Retroverted uterus	
2. Vaginal carcinoma	
3. Cervical carcinoma	
4. Ovarian mass	
E. Iatrogenic obstruction	
1. Anti-incontinence procedures	
2. Multiple urethral dilatations	
3. Urethral excision/reconstruction	
F. Miscellaneous	
1. Urethral valves	
2. Ectopic ureterocele	
3. Bladder calculi	
4. Atrophic vaginitis/urethritis	

$p_{det}Q_{max}$ of 21 cmH$_2$O (34). In 2004, using asymptomatic controls (instead of women with stress incontinence), they made further revisions to a Q_{max} *of* 12 ml/sec or less and $P_{det}Q_{max}$ of 25 cmH$_2$O or more (35). In 1999, Nitti et al described videourodynamic criteria to diagnose female BOO (36). In this model obstruction is defined as radiographic evidence of an obstruction between the bladder neck and distal urethra in the presence of a sustained detrusor contraction of any magnitude during voiding. Lastly, Blaivas and Groutz designed a nomogram based on the noninvasive Q_{max} and the maximum detrusor pressure during voiding ($p_{det-max}$) (Fig. 6.8) (37).

Each of these proposed criteria has merit and none is perfect in diagnosing obstruction. The videourodynamic criteria and the cut-off values proposed by Chassange et al and Lemack and Zimmern have the highest concordance with a suspicion of clinical obstruction (38). The Blaivas–Groutz nomogram also categorizes degree of obstruction (clinical relevance has not been determined). The nomogram overestimates obstruction compared to other criteria (38). Clearly,

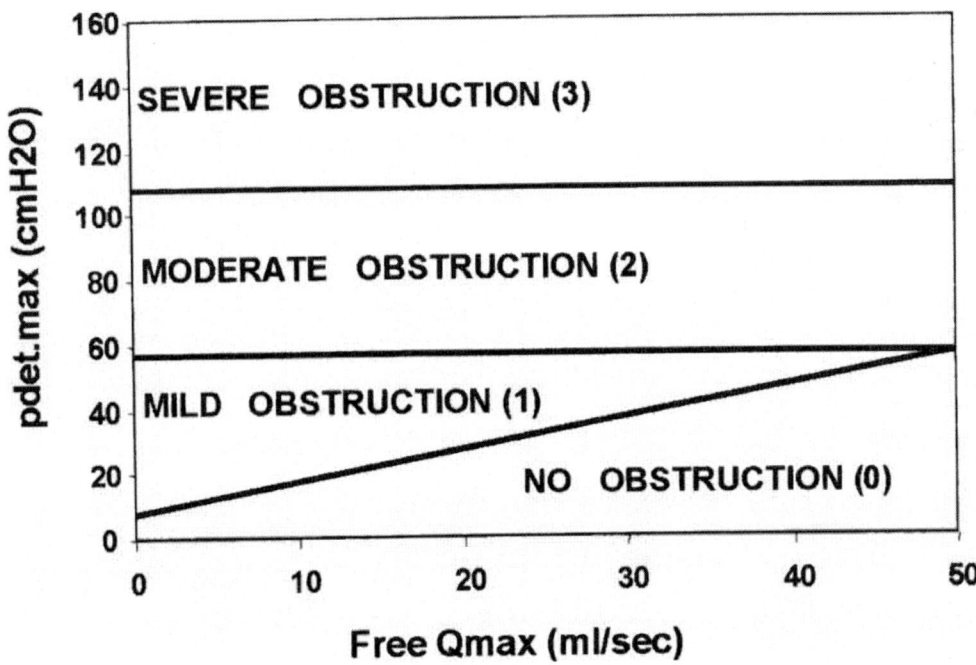

FIGURE 6.8 ● The Blaivas–Groutz nomogram. (From Blaivas JG, Groutz A. Bladder outlet obstruction nomogram for women with lower urinary tract symptomatology. *Neurourol Urodynam* 2000;19:553–564.)

there are cases where obstruction is suspected clinically but is ruled out with UDS, and vice versa. We believe that a combination of clinical parameters and urodynamic findings is currently the best way to diagnose obstruction in women.

Sphincter Coordination and Electromyography

Coordination refers to the bladder–urethral sphincter mechanism relationship during voiding. Normally, during voiding the urethra is open and is continually relaxed to allow for effective emptying. Sphincteric electromyography (EMG) studies the bioelectric potentials of the external urethral sphincter complex. Surface or needle electrodes may be used. Surface electrodes are placed on the skin overlying the muscle of interest and detect potentials for a group of muscles in the area. The electrodes should be placed near the periurethral or perianal area. Needle electrodes are more precise, measuring the potential of one motor unit, but are invasive. Generally, surface electrodes are accurate in providing the necessary information (39). The EMG tracing should be assessed at various points during filling to ensure

proper lead placement and recording prior to the voiding phase. At the beginning of the study, the patient should be asked to contract and relax the sphincter. Also, during the initial cough test and subsequent stress maneuvers there are often increases in the EMG recording. Furthermore, a normal response to bladder filling is a gradual and sustained rise in the EMG potential. During the voiding phase, the first action is relaxation of the external urethral sphincter complex, measured as silence of the EMG (39). The external urethral sphincter complex should remain relaxed until voiding is completed.

EMG is useful in patients with suspected pelvic floor dysfunction or neurogenic voiding dysfunction. The goal of EMG during UDS is to determine whether the external urethral sphincter complex is coordinated or discoordinated with the bladder during voiding (15). If an abnormality is present, the examiner will observe a failure of the sphincter to appropriately relax during voiding. If the patient has a known neurologic condition, the phenomenon is termed detrusor–external sphincter dyssynergia; usually the disease affects the suprasacral spinal cord (Fig. 6.9) (16). If there is no known neurologic abnormality, the discoordi-

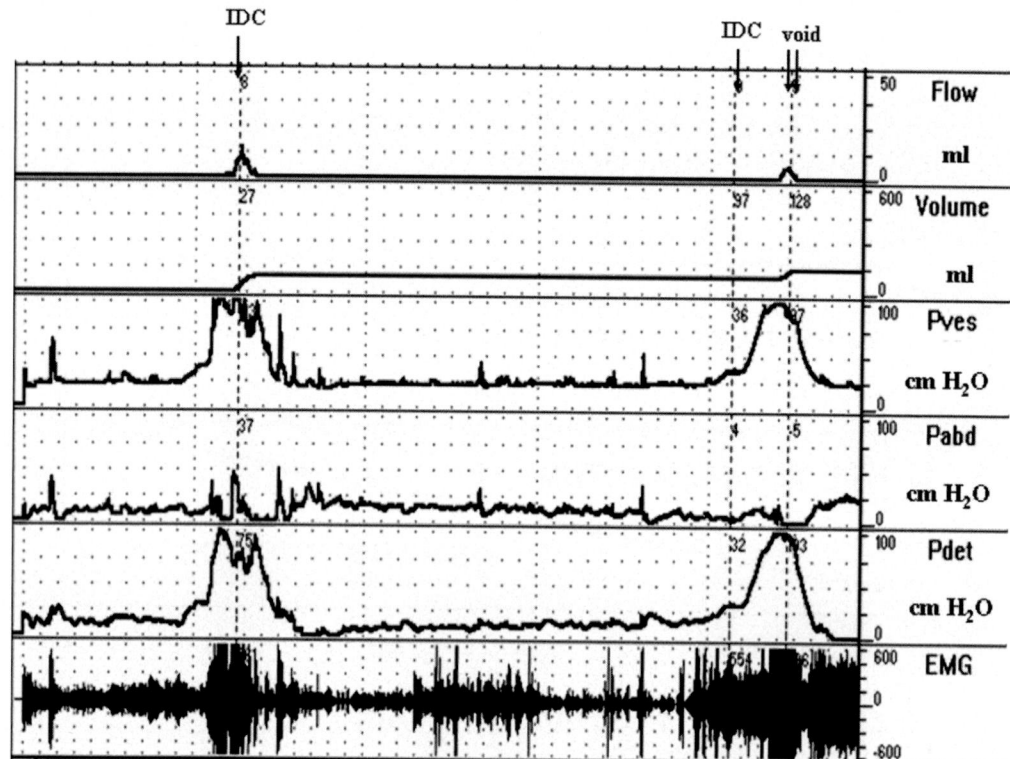

FIGURE 6.9 ● Detrusor overactivity with detrusor–external sphincter dyssynergia. Urodynamic tracing of an 18-year-old woman with frequency, urgency, and urge incontinence who was diagnosed with a tethered cord. Note the IDC (*arrow*) associated with high-volume urine loss as registered in the flowmeter. There is increased sphincter activity, as demonstrated by increased EMG activity consistent with detrusor–external sphincter dyssynergia. On the second fill there is again an IDC, but this time the patient is instructed to void (*double arrow*). Note that there is increased EMG activity throughout the IDC and "voluntary void." Detrusor pressures with IDCs are quite high because of the resistance of the contracting striated sphincter. (From Kelly CE, Nitti VW. Evaluation of neurogenic bladder dysfunction: basic urodynamics. In: Corcos J, Schick E, eds. *Textbook of the neurogenic bladder.* London: Martin Dunitz, 2004:415–423.)

nation is likely a learned behavior and the term "dysfunctional voiding" should be applied (40).

Imaging of the bladder outlet during voiding allows for assessment of the bladder neck–internal sphincter coordination (see below). Failure of the bladder neck to open in the face of a sustained detrusor contraction is abnormal. In cases of neurogenic voiding dysfunction, especially with lesions above the lower thoracic cord, true internal sphincter dyssynergia can occur. Primary bladder neck obstruction has a similar radiographic appearance as internal sphincter dyssynergia and is the diagnosis if there is no known neurologic disease.

Videourodynamics

Videourodynamics involves simultaneous fluoroscopy images of the lower urinary tract and urodynamic studies. The filling solution contains radiographic contrast, which allows for visualization of the lower urinary tract during storage and voiding. Most systems allow for imaging and urodynamic recordings on one monitor, as well as recording of the image with the simultaneous urodynamic tracing. Images may be obtained with the patient supine, seated, or standing. Often in clinical practice, office videourodynamics is not practical and not necessary for an accurate diagnosis in many patients. Furthermore, images of the lower urinary tract may be obtained separate from UDS, but there are several situations in which simultaneous imaging and UDS is crucial. Videourodynamics provides the clinician with the essential ability to correlate anatomy with function at a specific moment in time.

Imaging can assist with the diagnosis of complex incontinence cases by demonstrating involuntary loss of urine with an IDC or with stress maneuvers (39). Fluoroscopy greatly improves the accuracy of determining VLPP, as it is often easier to visualize the flow of contrast on video rather than on examination (15). Video also allows for assessment of urethral hypermobility and degree of cystocele. In women who demonstrate bladder outlet obstruction on pressure–flow studies, imaging allows for determination of the level of obstruction. Videourodynamics is critical to make the diagnosis of bladder neck obstruction versus detrusor internal sphincter dyssynergia and is especially helpful when high-pressure, low-flow voiding is not demonstrated (Fig. 6.10) (36). Cases of complex voiding dysfunction may be less common, but it is precisely those patients in whom videourodynamics is invaluable. Simultaneous fluoroscopy can also identify vesicoureteral reflux, prominent bladder diverticula, or urinary fistulae.

SUMMARY

UDS can be an invaluable part of the diagnosis and management of pelvic floor dysfunction. Prior to the termination of the study, the clinician must assess if all posed questions have been adequately answered (8). If the study is inconclusive with regards to pivotal issues, then every effort should be made to better elucidate the pathology. This may require adjustments, repetition, and creativity. Current technology provides accurate and precise information detailing the storage and emptying dynamics of the lower urinary tract that can be used to guide therapy and properly counsel patients. The relevance of the study is dependent upon appropriate patient selection, proper technique, and experienced interpretation.

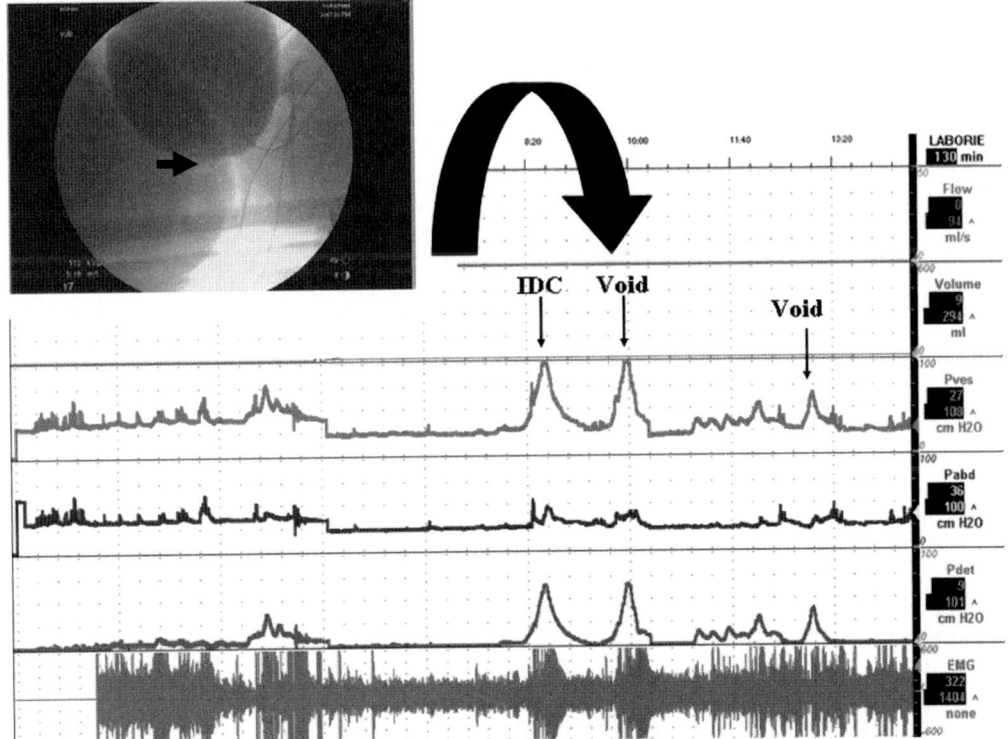

FIGURE 6.10 ● Primary bladder neck obstruction. Videourodynamic tracing of a healthy 37-year-old woman with urinary retention. The filling phase shows detrusor overactivity (IDC), and attempts to void show adequate pressure but no flow. With attempts to void, simultaneous fluoroscopic imaging shows no opening of the bladder neck (*horizontal arrow*). There is some increase in EMG activity, but failure of the bladder neck to open in the face of a sustained detrusor contraction is diagnostic of primary bladder neck obstruction. The patient subsequently underwent a transurethral incision of the bladder neck and now voids and empties normally.

REFERENCES

1. Davis DM. *The mechanism of urology diseases.* Philadelphia: WB Saunders, 1953.
2. Kraklau DM, Bloom DA. The cystometrogram at 70 years. *J Urol* 1998;160:316–319.
3. Abrams P, Cardozo L, Fall M, et al. The standardization of terminology in the lower urinary tract function: report from the standardization subcommittee of the International Continence Society. *Urology* 2003;61:37–49.
4. Weidner AC, Myers ER, Visco AG, et al. Which women with stress incontinence require urodynamic evaluation? *Am J Obstet Gynecol* 2001;184(2):20–27.
5. Nitti VW, Coombs AJ. Urodynamics: when, why, and how. In: Nitti VW, ed. *Practical urodynamics.* Philadelphia: WB Saunders, 1998:15–26.
6. Wein AJ. Classification of neurogenic voiding dysfunction. *J Urol* 1981;125:605–609.
7. Golomb J. Uroflometry. In: Raz S, ed. *Female urology,* 2nd ed. Philadelphia: WB Saunders, 1996:97–105.
8. Schafer W, Abrams P, Liao L, et al. Good urodynamic practices: uroflowmetry, filling cystometry, and pressure–flow studies. *Neurourol Urodyn* 2002;21:261–274.
9. Wein AJ, English WS, Whitmore K. Office urodynamics. *Urol Clin North Am* 1988;15:609–623.
10. Boone TA, Kim YH. Uroflowmetry. In: Nitti VW, ed. *Practical urodynamics.* Philadelphia: WB Saunders, 1998:28–37.
11. Chancellor MB, Blaivas JG, Kaplan SA, et al. Bladder outlet obstruction versus impaired detrusor contractility: the role of outflow. *J Urol* 1991;145:810–812.
12. Nitti VW. Cystometry and abdominal pressure monitoring. In: Nitti VW, ed. *Practical urodynamics.* Philadelphia: WB Saunders, 1998:38–51.
13. Schafer W, Abrams P, Liao L, et al. Good urodynamic practices: uroflowmetry, filling cystometry, and pressure–flow studies. *Neurourol Urodyn* 2002;21:261–274.
14. Stohrer M, Goepel M, Kondo A, et al. The standardization of terminology in neurogenic lower urinary tract dysfunction with suggestions for diagnostic procedures. *Neurourol Urodyn* 1999;18:139–158.
15. Webster GD, Guralnick ML. The neurourologic evaluation. In: Walsh PC, Retik AB, Vaughan ED, et al, eds. *Campbell's urology,* 8th ed. Philadelphia: Saunders, 2002:905–928.
16. Kelly CE, Nitti VW. Evaluation of neurogenic bladder dysfunction: basic urodynamics. In: Corcos J, Schick E, eds. *Textbook of the neurogenic bladder.* London: Martin Dunitz, 2004:415–423.
17. McGuire EJ, Fitzpatrick CC, Wan J, et al. Clinical assessment of urethral sphincter function. *J Urol* 1993;150:1452–1454.
18. Versi E, Cardozo L, Studd JW, et al. Internal urinary sphincter in maintenance of female continence. *Br Med J* 1986;292:166–167.
19. Fleischman N, Flisser AJ, Blaivas JG, et al. Sphincteric urinary incontinence: relationship of vesical leak point pressure, urethral mobility, and severity of incontinence. *J Urol* 2003;169:999–1002.
20. McGuire EJ, Woodside JR, Borden TA, et al. Prognostic value of urodynamic testing in myelodysplastic patients. *J Urol* 1981;126:205–209.
21. Steele GS, Sullivan MP, Yalla SV. Urethral pressure profilometry: vesicourethral pressure measurements under resting and voiding conditions. In: Nitti VW, ed. *Practical urodynamics.* Philadelphia: WB Saunders, 1998:108–130.
22. Versi E. Discriminant analysis of urethral pressure profilometry data for the diagnosis of genuine stress incontinence. *Br J Obstet Gynaecol* 1990;97:251–259.
23. Rosenzweig BA, Bhatia NM, Nelson AL. Dynamic urethral pressure profile transmission ratio: What do the numbers mean? *Obstet Gynecol* 1991;77:586–590.
24. Sorensen S, Waechter PB, Constantinou CE, et al. Urethral pressure and pressure variations in healthy fertile and postmenopausal women with unstable detrusor. *Neurourol Urodyn* 1991;10:483–492.
25. Richardson DA, Ramahi A. Reproducibility of pressure transmission ratios in stress incontinent women. *Neurourol Urodyn* 1993;12:123–130.
26. Lose G, Griffiths D, Hosker G, et al. Standardization of urethral pressure measurement: report from the Standardization Subcommittee of the International Continence Society. *Neurourol Urodynam* 2002;21:258–260.
27. Carlson KV, Fiske J, Nitti VW. Value of routine evaluation of the voiding phase when performing urodynamic testing on women with lower urinary tract symptoms. *J Urol* 2000;164:1614–1617.
28. Nitti VW. Bladder outlet obstruction in women. In: Nitti VW, ed. *Practical urodynamics.* Philadelphia: WB Saunders, 1998:197–210.
29. Griffiths D, Hofner K, van Mastrigt R, et al. Standardization of terminology of lower urinary tract function: pressure–flow studies of voiding, urethral resistance, and urethral obstruction. International Continence Society Subcommittee on standardization of terminology of pressure–flow studies. *Neurourol Urodyn* 1997;16:1–18.
30. Schafer W. Analysis of bladder outlet function with the linearized passive urethral resistance, linPURR, and a disease-specific approach for grading obstruction from complex to simple. *World J Urol* 1995;13:47–58.
31. Abrams P. Bladder outlet obstruction index, bladder contractility index, and bladder voiding efficiency: three simple indices to define bladder voiding function. *BJU Int* 1999;84:14–15.
32. Nitti VW, Raz S. Urinary retention. In: Raz S, ed. *Female urology,* 2nd ed. Philadelphia: WB Saunders, 1996:197–213.
33. Chassange S, Bernier PA, Haab F, et al. Proposed cutoff values to define bladder outlet obstruction in women. *Urology* 1998;51:408–411.
34. Lemack GE, Zimmern PE. Refinement and application of cut-off values for bladder outlet obstruction in women. *J Urol* 2000;163:1823–1828.
35. Defreitas GA, Zimmern PE, Lemack GE, et al. Refining diagnosis of anatomic female bladder outlet obstruction: Comparison of pressure–flow study parameters in clinically obstructed women with those of normal controls. *Urology* 2004;64:675–679.
36. Nitti VW, Tu LM, Gitlin J. Diagnosing bladder outlet obstruction in women. *J Urol* 1999;161:1535–1540.
37. Blaivas JG, Groutz A. Bladder outlet obstruction nomogram for women with lower urinary tract symptomatology. *Neurourol Urodynam* 2000;19:553–564.
38. Akikwala TV, Fleischman N, Nitti VW. Comparison of diagnostic criteria for female bladder outlet obstruction. *J Urol* 2006;176:2093–2097.
39. Rovner ES, Wein AJ. Practical urodynamics. *AUA Update Series,* Lessons 19–20, Vol. XXI, 2002.
40. Carlson KV, Rome S, Nitti VW. Dysfunctional voiding in adult females. *J Urol* 2001;165:143–147.

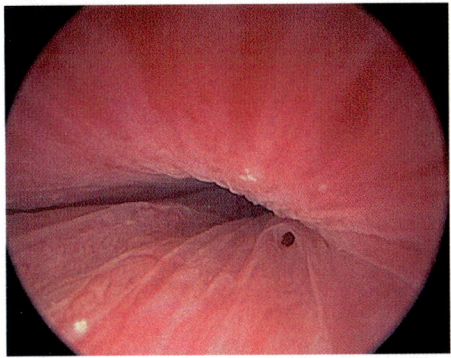

Color Plate 1. Normal urethra. There is pink, lush epithelium in folds. (See Figure 7.5.)

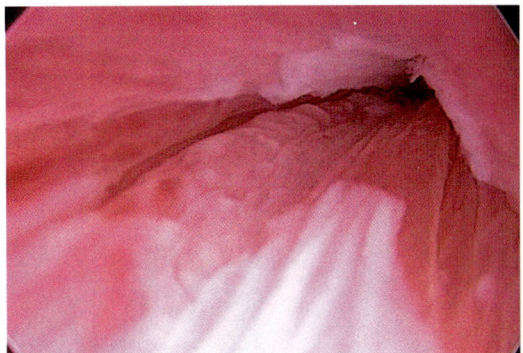

Color Plate 2. Urethral crest and squamous epithelium of normal urethra. The urethral crest runs posteriorly as a longitudinal ridge, and over it is white epithelium. (See Figure 7.6.)

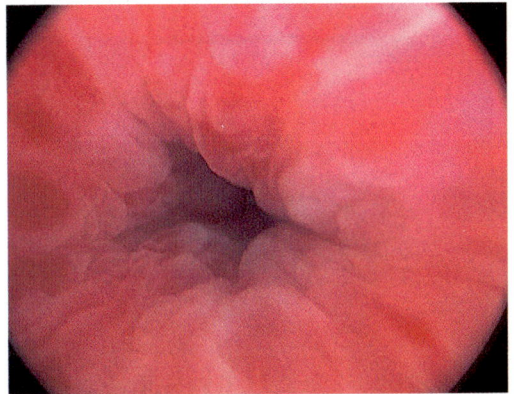

Color Plate 3. Acute urethritis. The urethra is reddened along its length. (See Figure 7.7.)

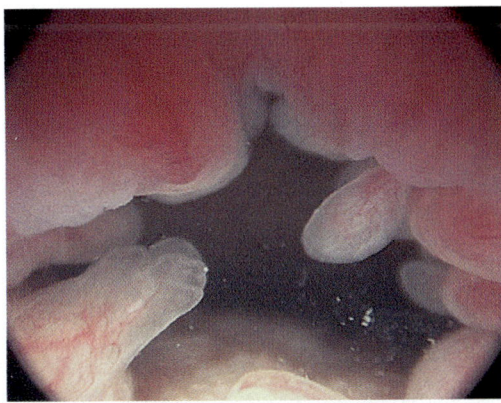

Color Plate 4. Polyps at the urethrovesical junction. (See Figure 7.8.)

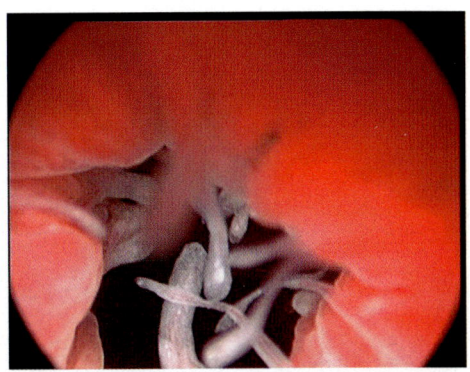

Color Plate 5. Fronds at the urethrovesical junction. (See Figure 7.9.)

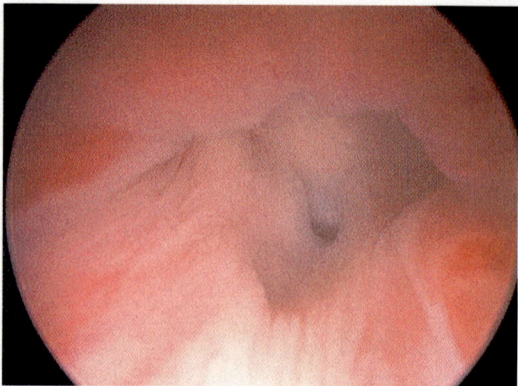

Color Plate 6. Urethrovaginal fistula. The urethral canal is in the upper right of the photograph, and the opening from the urethra to the vagina is clearly seen as a small opening in the center of the picture. (See Figure 7.10.)

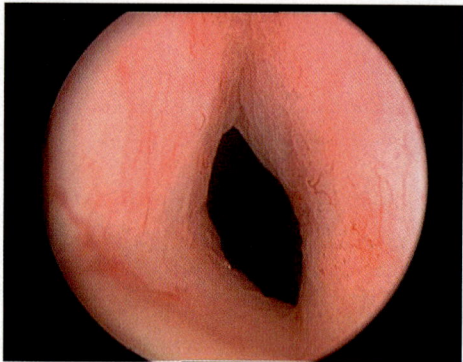

Color Plate 7. Functionless urethra. The urethra is very short and remains passively open, with the urethroscope barely inside the meatus. The epithelium is smooth, and there is no movement with hold or strain maneuvers. (See Figure 7.11.)

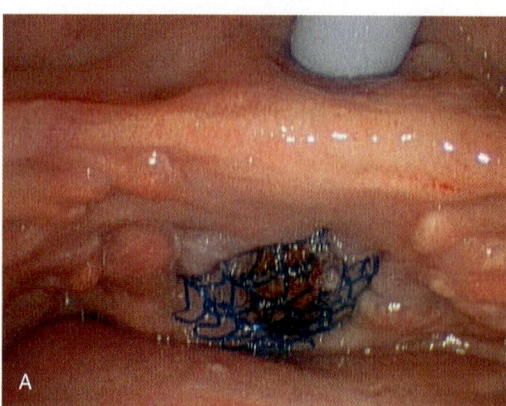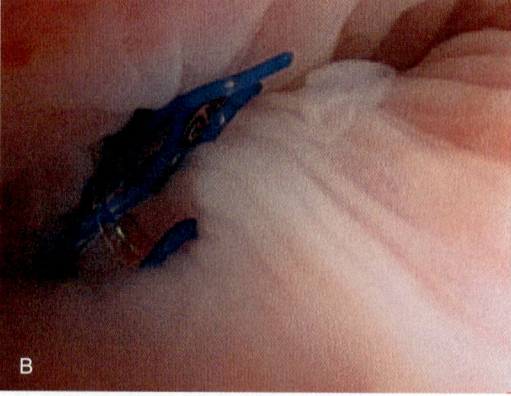

Color Plate 8. Eroded tension-free tape. **(A)** Tape erosion in vagina. **(B)** Tape in urethra. (See Figure 7.12.)

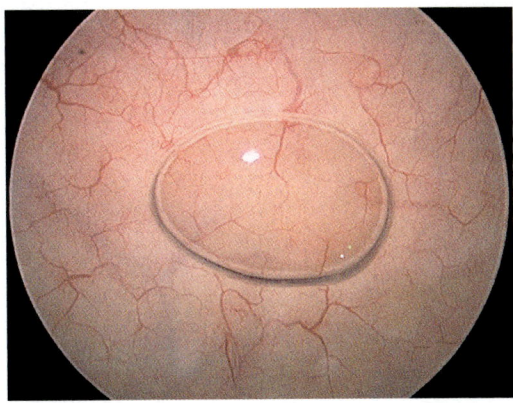

Color Plate 9. Normal bladder. The air bubble at the dome of the bladder serves as a reference marker. The epithelium of the bladder wall is smooth and pale pink and has fine vasculature. (See Figure 7.13.)

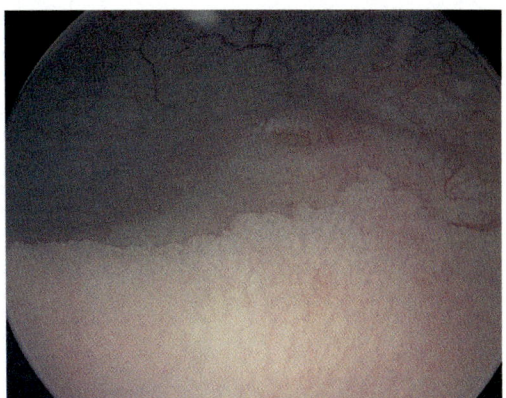

Color Plate 10. Metaplasia of trigone. The white membrane covers much of the trigone leading up to the ureters. Biopsy reveals squamous metaplasia. (See Figure 7.14.)

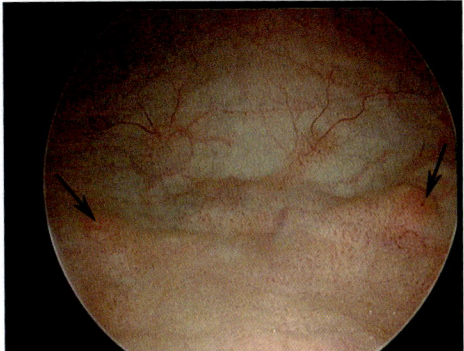

Color Plate 11. Trigone. The trigone is formed by the UVJ inferiorly and the ureteral orifices superiorly. The ureteral openings are marked by *arrows*. The trigone is frequently reddened and granular. (See Figure 7.15.)

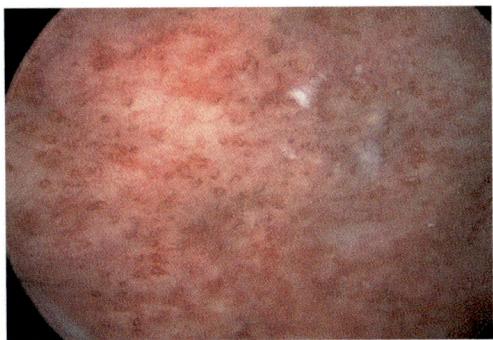

Color Plate 12. Acute cystitis. The bladder mucosa is reddened and edematous, making it difficult to see clearly. There is often active bleeding, further compromising the view. (See Figure 7.16.)

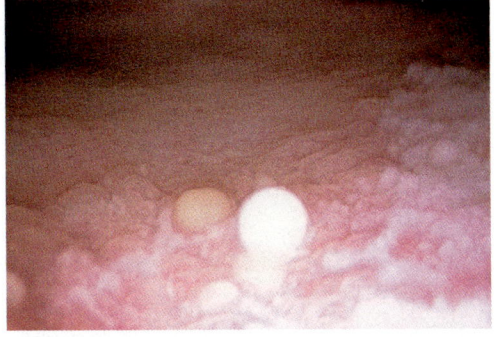

Color Plate 13. Cystitis cystica. The 1- to 2-mm cysts at the bladder base are smooth-walled and are clear or sometimes pigmented. (See Figure 7.17.)

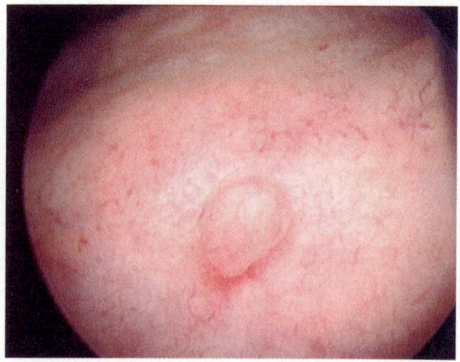

Color Plate 14. Benign bladder polyp. (See Figure 7.18.)

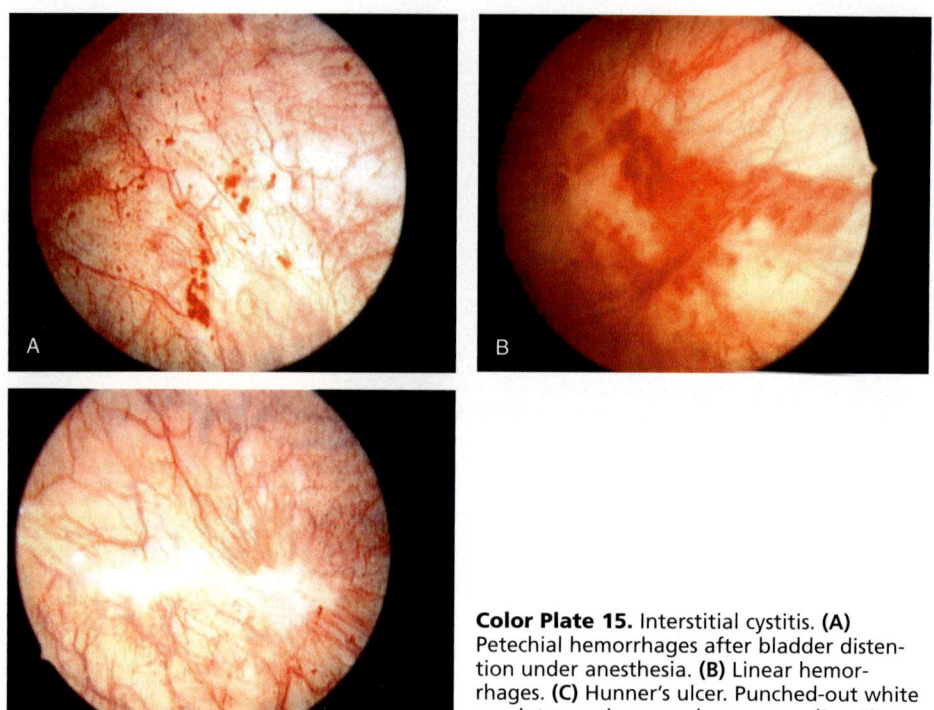

Color Plate 15. Interstitial cystitis. **(A)** Petechial hemorrhages after bladder distention under anesthesia. **(B)** Linear hemorrhages. **(C)** Hunner's ulcer. Punched-out white scar interrupting vascular pattern. (See Figure 7.19.)

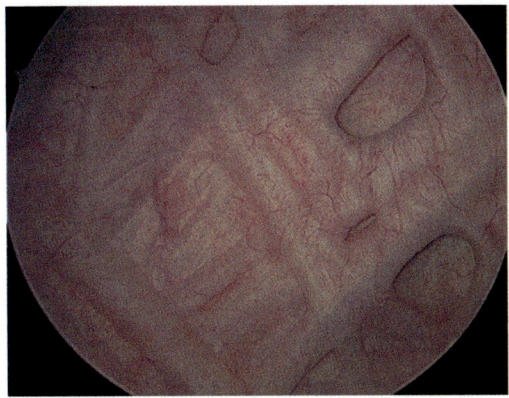

Color Plate 16. Trabeculation. The muscle bundles appear as prominent ridges with intervening pockets or cellules. (See Figure 7.20.)

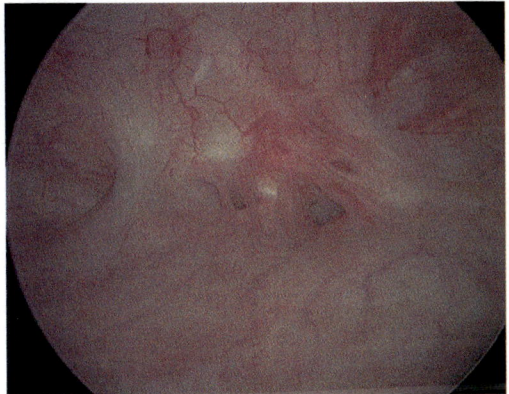

Color Plate 17. Vesicovaginal fistula. The openings in the bladder with a posthysterectomy fistula occur superior to the trigone in the posterior aspect of the bladder, and there are two distinct holes to the vagina in this picture. (See Figure 7.21.)

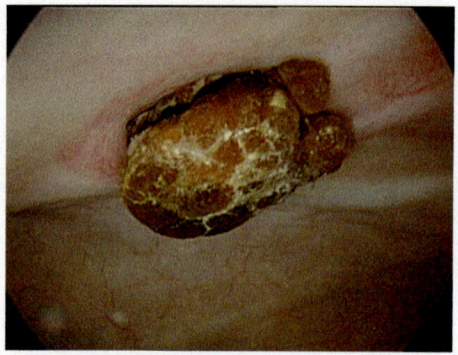

Color Plate 18. Bladder calculus. This usually forms over a suture nidus or some other irritant. (See Figure 7.22.)

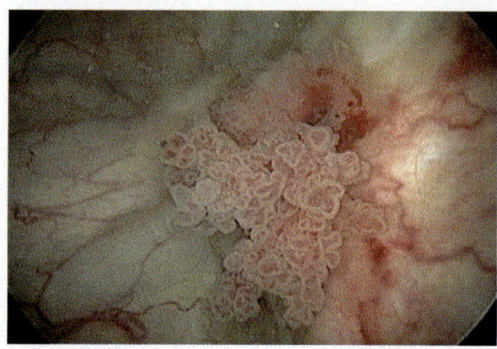

Color Plate 19. Bladder cancer. The pedunculated papillary lesion is a transitional cell carcinoma. (See Figure 7.23.)

CHAPTER 7

Cystourethroscopy

Geoffrey W. Cundiff and Alfred E. Bent

Cystourethroscopy provides a minimally invasive method of visually evaluating the lower urinary tract. It has broad applications in general gynecology and female pelvic surgery (1). The ability to recognize normal and pathologic findings is essential for assessment and surgical correction of female pelvic disorders.

HISTORICAL PERSPECTIVE

Although many credit Kelly with developing the female cystoscope, endoscopy of the female bladder preceded his report by half a century. Bozzini (2) described an endoscopic technique for evaluating the female bladder in the early 19th century. His invention consisted of a stand that supported different-sized hollow funnels, a candle for illumination, and a reflector to direct the light into the funnel when it was placed into the urethra. Desmormeaux (3) introduced a more practical endoscope in 1853 that used different-sized angulated tubes. The tubes increased the surface area of the bladder that could be inspected, and use of an alcohol lamp improved illumination. By 1877, Grünfeld's (4) modification of the endoscope still used a hollow tube but added an obliquely placed glass lens at the vesical end. His endoscope was vastly improved by the adaptation of an electric light source reflected by mirrors. Nitze (5) developed a compound lens system that increased the field of vision and used an incandescent light source to provide illumination.

Kelly's contribution was in overcoming the deficiencies of both Grünfeld's and Nitze's instruments and techniques. The Kelly cystoscope was a hollow tube, without glass, that used an obturator for placement (6). The knee–chest position allowed air to distend the bladder. A head mirror was used to reflect an electric light into the bladder for illumination (Fig. 7.1). The technique was simple yet provided an excellent view.

Modern endoscopy started with the development of the Hopkins fiberoptic telescope in 1954 (7). The use of glass fibers in place of an air chamber dramatically improved light transmission and resolution and also provided a wider viewing angle. The viewing angle could also be changed, which improved the extent of visualization and facilitated more invasive procedures. Later modifications of the Hopkins system incorporated a series of glass rods with optically finished ends separated by intervening spaces.

The improved view of the bladder provided by the Hopkins cystoscope compromised the view of the urethra. An angled telescope is not effective for evaluating the urethral mucosa because most cystoscopic sheaths have a terminal fenestra for use with a catheter deflector mechanism. This design allows the irrigant to escape during its distal location in the urethra. Robertson (8) addressed the compromised view of the urethra by applying fiberoptic technology to a shorter straight-on telescope, later known as the urethroscope.

The most recent development in cystoscopy is the flexible cystoscope. The flexible fiberoptic lens system permits an instrument that bends, thereby increasing the field of view. Comparisons continue regarding resolution and comfort between rigid and flexible instruments (9,10). However, the female urethra is so short that a rigid 17 French sheath with a blunted fenestra can be passed with minimal discomfort, and flexible cystoscopy in the female patient has fewer benefits than in the male patient.

EQUIPMENT

Urethroscopy

The urethroscope is composed of a telescope and sheath. The telescope has a 0-degree (straight-ahead) viewing angle, which provides a circum-

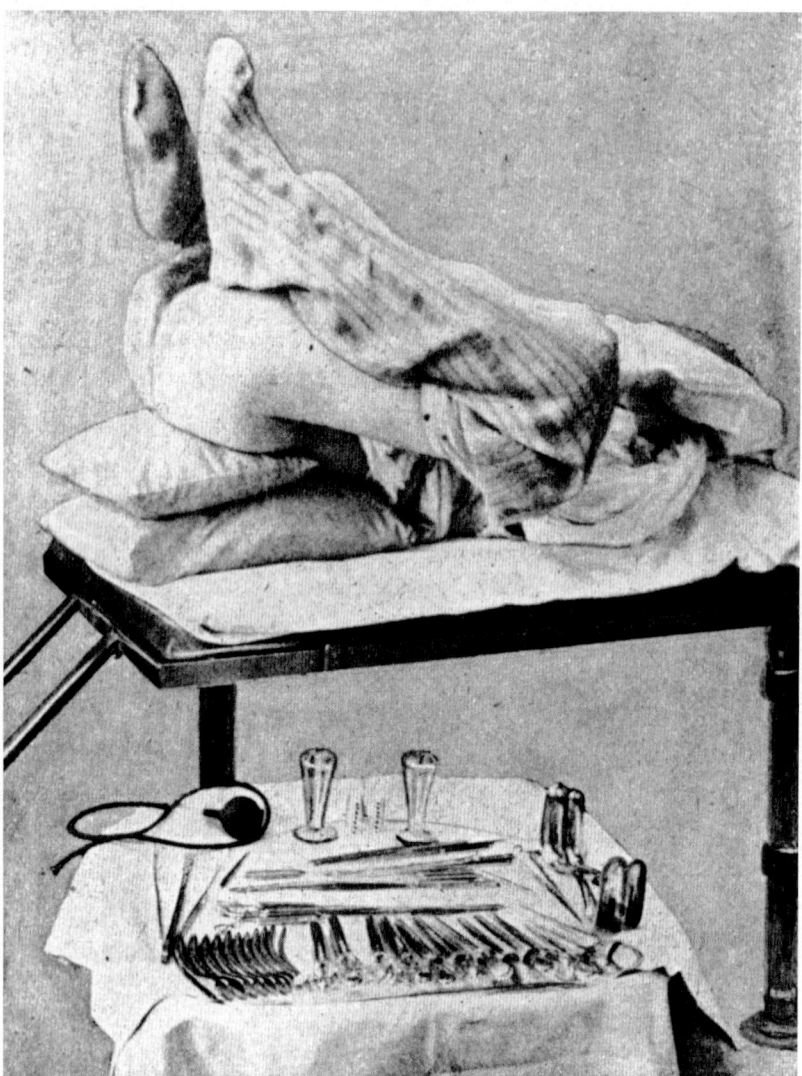

FIGURE 7.1 ● Cystoscopy as described by Kelly used a supine position with the hips elevated. The instruments used by Kelly are arranged in the foreground. (From Kelly HA. The direct examination of the female bladder with elevated pelvis: the catheterization of the ureters under direct inspection, with and without elevation of the pelvis. *Am J Obstet Dis Wom Child* 1894;25:7, with permission.)

ferential view of the urethral lumen as distending medium opens the urethra. The sheath has a port for infusion of medium as well as a valve to initiate flow of medium or allow bladder emptying. Sheath sizes are 15 and 24 French. Fluid flow is minimal with the 15 French sheath, and thus there is minimal urethral distention during its passage. Although the view is minimally compromised using this sheath size, the larger sheath is better for viewing urethral diverticula and fistula. The instrument is also useful for vaginoscopy (Fig. 7.2).

Rigid Cystoscopy

The rigid cystoscope is composed of a telescope, bridge, and sheath (Fig. 7.3). Each component serves a different function and is available with various options to facilitate this role. The telescope transmits light to the bladder cavity and an image to the viewer. Several viewing angles are available, including 0- (straight), 12- (minimal angle for periurethral bulking), 25- or 30- (forward-oblique), 70- (lateral), and 120-degree (retro view) angles. The angled telescopes have a field marker

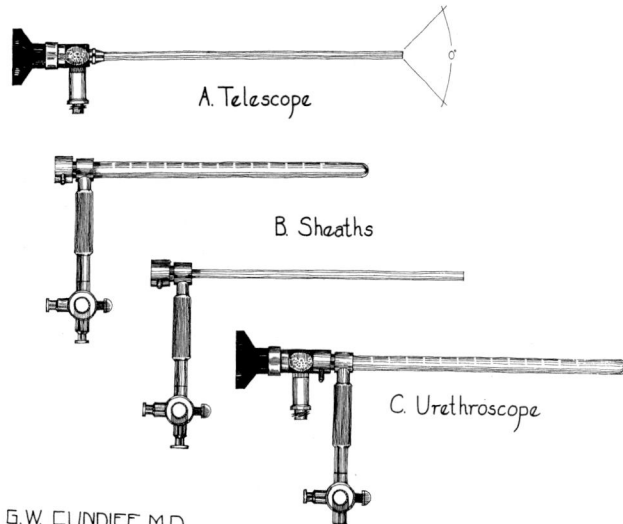

FIGURE 7.2 ● Components of a rigid urethroscope. **(A)** Telescope, 0-degree. **(B)** Sheaths, 15 and 24 French. **(C)** Assembled urethroscope.

that assists the viewer with orientation. It is visible as a blackened notch at the outside of the visual field and opposite the angle of deflection. It points in the same direction as the light post.

The 30-degree lens provides the best view of the bladder base and posterior wall, whereas the 70-degree lens permits inspection of the anterolateral walls. The retro view of the 120-degree lens is not usually necessary for cystoscopy of the female bladder but can be useful for evaluating the urethral opening into the bladder. A 70-degree telescope is perhaps the best general-use cystoscope for viewing the bladder and is essential in the presence of fixation of the bladder neck (urethrovesical junction [UVJ]) and when performing operative cystoscopy at the time of surgery.

The cystoscope sheath provides a vehicle for introducing the telescope and distending medium into the bladder. It is available in various calibers, from 15 to 28 French. The telescope partly fills the lumen of the sheath, leaving room for an irrigation/working channel. The smallest-diameter sheath is useful for diagnostic purposes, whereas larger-caliber sheaths allow instruments to be placed in the working channel. The proximal end of the sheath has two irrigating ports: one for introduction of the distending medium and the other for removal. The distal end of the cystoscope sheath is fenestrated to permit the use of instrumentation in the angled field of view. It is also beveled, opposite the fenestrae, to increase comfort on introduction into the urethra. Larger-diameter sheaths may require an obturator for placement. Most diagnostic work is performed with the 17 French sheath, especially in the awake patient. The sheath size for

operative applications depends on the type of instrumentation.

The bridge serves as the connector between the telescope and sheath and forms a watertight seal with both. It may have one or two ports for introduction of instruments into the working channel. The Albarrán bridge is a variation of the bridge that has a deflector mechanism at the end of an inner sheath (Fig. 7.4). When placed in the cystoscopic sheath, the deflector mechanism is located at the distal end of the inner sheath within the fenestra of the outer sheath. At this location, the elevation of the deflector mechanism assists the manipulation of instruments within the field of view.

Flexible Cystoscopy

The flexible cystoscope combines the optical systems and irrigation/working channel in a single unit. The optical system consists of a single image-bearing fiberoptic bundle and two light-bearing fiberoptic bundles. The fibers of these bundles are coated parallel coherent optical fibers that transmit light even when bent. This permits incorporation of a distal-tip deflecting mechanism that will deflect the tip 290 degrees in a single plane. A lever at the eyepiece controls the deflection. The optical fibers are fitted to a lens system that magnifies and focuses the image. A focusing knob is located just distal to the eyepiece. The irrigation/working port enters the instrument at the eyepiece opposite the deflecting mechanism. The coated tip is 15 to 18 French in diameter and 6 to 7 cm in length, with the working unit constituting half the length. The image may appear somewhat granular, but tech-

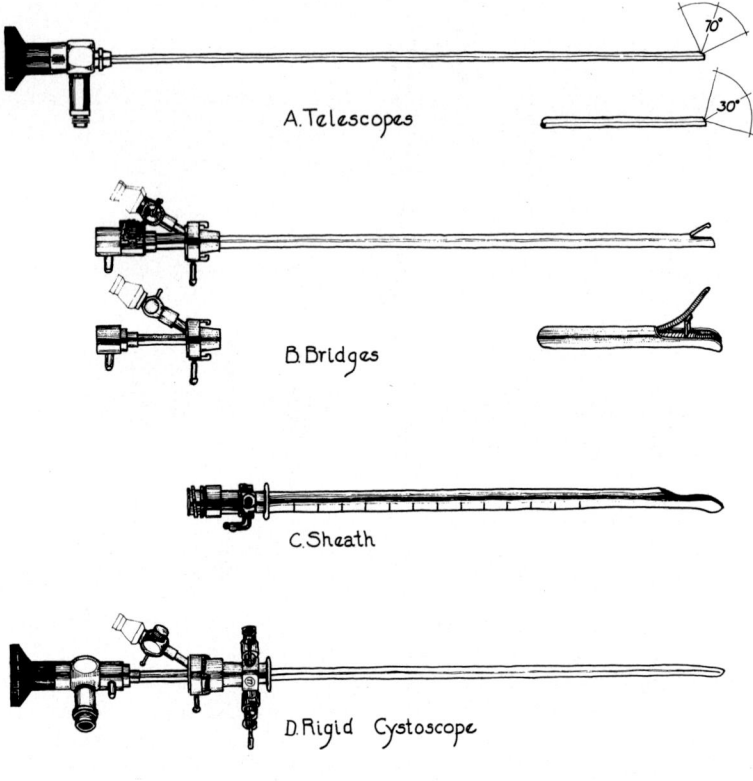

FIGURE 7.3 ● Components of a rigid cystoscope. **(A)** Telescopes. The 70-degree lateral angled-view telescope *(above)* and the 30-degree forward-oblique telescope *(below)*. **(B)** Bridges. Single-port bridge *(below)* and dual-port bridge with an Albarrán deflecting mechanism *(above)*. The position of the deflecting mechanism within the fenestra of the operating sheath is shown. **(C)** Sheath, 22 French operating. **(D)** Assembled cystoscope with a diagnostic 17 French sheath.

nology is rapidly closing the gap with the image produced by rigid instrumentation. The flow rate of the working channel is slower than that of rigid instruments, and this may be further curtailed by passage of instruments down the channel. Use of the instrument channel may also limit some of the movement at the tip of the deflector mechanism. Flexible cystoscopes are more comfortable, especially for male patients. As mentioned previously, the short length of the female urethra and ease of passing the rigid cystoscope may offset perceived advantages of flexible instrumentation in the female patient.

Light Sources and Video Monitors

A high-intensity (xenon) light source is recommended for use in video monitoring and photography. The light cable must be checked periodically for transmission properties. Video monitoring eliminates awkward positioning of the operator and improves teaching abilities. It may also help to distract the patient, while allowing her to see important findings.

Distending Medium

Water or saline is generally used as a distending medium. The fluid is instilled by gravity through a standard intravenous infusion set, with the bag height about 100 cm above the patient's symphysis to provide adequate flow. Pressurized flow is not required.

Instrumentation

A wide range of instrumentation is available for use through the cystoscope sheath. Those most commonly used in female patients are grasping forceps with either rat-tooth or alligator jaws. They are available in flexible or rigid styles and come in varying diameters (1). A monopolar ball

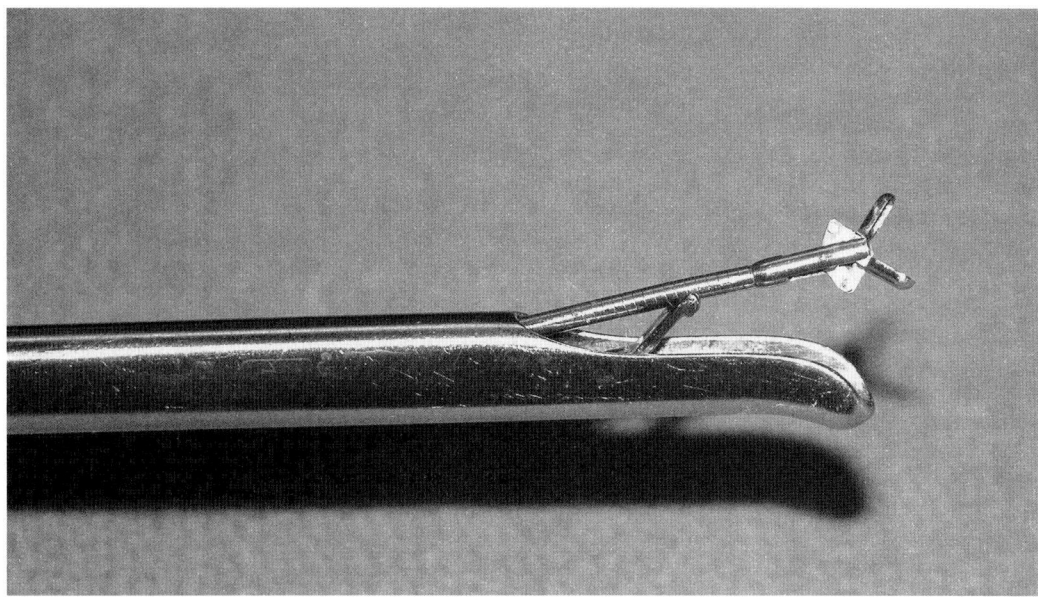

FIGURE 7.4 ● Cystoscope with Alberrán bridge and biopsy forceps in place.

electrode is useful for electrocautery during operative cystoscopy. With the improvement in imaging and photography, biopsy of an obvious tumor may not be necessary, and the picture can be passed along to a consulting urologist for biopsy and transurethral resection of the abnormality.

CYSTOURETHROSCOPY TECHNIQUES: DIAGNOSIS

Diagnostic cystourethroscopy in women is easily performed as an office procedure and is well tolerated without anesthesia in most cases. Lignocaine gel is useful in the female patient who has apprehension regarding pain (11). Most indications for endoscopy warrant evaluation of both the bladder and urethra (Table 12.1).

Urethroscopy

The urethroscope is placed into the urethra with the fluid infusion flowing in order to distend the urethra and facilitate both the view and the passage of the instrument to the bladder. The 24 French sheath allows optimal visualization, although it may be too large in 10% to 20% of patients. Comfort is essential, and the 15 French sheath should be used in these latter patients. The view is not as good with the smaller sheath as with the larger sheath, but it is adequate. The urethra could be dilated to allow passage of the larger sheath,

and in this case topical anesthesia should be used for patient comfort. Topical anesthetic or dilation irritates the urethral mucosa, giving a false impression of inflammation, which should be considered in the final interpretation.

The urethral mucosa is viewed as the instrument is passed slowly to the bladder neck and into the bladder. This causes a small amount of burning-type discomfort. The trigone and ureters may be observed by angling the telescope toward the bladder base and, in some cases, by elevating the trigone with a vaginal finger. The UVJ is observed during the following commands: "hold your urine," "squeeze your rectum," "strain down like having a bowel movement," and "cough." The hold and squeeze commands are performed with the urethroscope withdrawn enough to allow the UVJ to close two thirds of the way. Movement can then be observed as the UVJ closes during the maneuver. The strain and cough commands are performed with the urethroscope withdrawn enough to allow the UVJ to close two thirds of the way. In this manner, opening of the UVJ can be observed. After modest bladder filling, the vaginal finger compresses and massages the urethra over the end of the urethroscope as the instrument is withdrawn. This allows observation for urethral glands, exudate, fistula, and diverticular openings. The patient has somewhat more discomfort during digital compression of the urethra and should be forewarned concerning this 5 to 10 seconds of discomfort.

Cystoscopy

Cystoscopy is generally performed using a 70-degree telescope with 17 French sheath and with some topical anesthetic on the sheath to facilitate movement in and out of the urethra. The cystoscope is placed into the urethral meatus with the bevel directed posteriorly and is advanced directly into the bladder, aiming at the patient's umbilicus. An obturator is not necessary with a small sheath such as 17 French, but the fluid flow during insertion facilitates passage. A volume of 250 mL or greater is desirable for bladder inspection unless the patient has discomfort before this volume, and a slow trickle is maintained if needed for optimum view. The air bubble is identified at the bladder dome, and this serves as a landmark for the rest of the examination. The examination begins at the bladder dome, making full sweeps with the instrument at each hour of an imaginary clock, going from 12 to 4 o'clock, then 11 to 8 o'clock, and then observing the posterior bladder wall between 5 to 7 o'clock. Orientation is maintained by placing the field marker directly opposite the area of the bladder to be inspected. The bladder base may require digital vaginal elevation for complete assessment. The bladder volume can be assessed at the end of the inspection by filling the bladder to patient fullness and then measuring the amount of fluid by emptying the bladder through the sheath, or by measuring the volume voided by the patient after the procedure.

Antimicrobial Prophylaxis

A concern after cystourethroscopy is the prevention of infection, which may occur in up to 5% of cases. A number of these patients may have infection at the time of the examination, even with a recent negative urine culture, but it is best to avoid instrumentation in the presence of a known infection. Prophylaxis is practiced by many, but recent reports cite no difference in infection rates between patients treated with placebo and nitrofurantoin (12,13). If prophylaxis is used, only a 1- or 2-day course is suggested, and a urinary analgesic (e.g., phenazopyridine) may also be administered for one or two doses at 3-hour intervals. Patients may experience dysuria, urgency, frequency, and hematuria for several hours after the examination, but most have minimal postprocedure discomfort.

Operative Cystoscopy

Most minor procedures, such as biopsy of mucosal lesions, removal of small foreign bodies, and cutting and removal of suture material, can be performed in an office setting. These procedures require a larger cystoscope sheath (22 French) and may be associated with discomfort. Lidocaine gel 2% or a mixture of lidocaine 2% and benzocaine 20% may be placed into the urethra for 5 minutes. Bladder anesthesia may be induced by instillation of 50 mL of a 4% lidocaine solution for 5 minutes. A bladder pillar block may augment the anesthesia but is seldom required. It is performed by injecting 5 mL of 1% lidocaine solution at each bladder pillar. After placement of a bivalve speculum, the bladder pillars are located at 2 and 10 o'clock with respect to the cervix. If the uterus is absent, a Sims speculum is used to expose the anterior vaginal wall, and the pillars are just superior and lateral to the UVJ (14).

The best view for operative procedures is immediately in front of the telescope. A 30-degree telescope allows angulation to see the abnormality but also allows visualization of the instrument being used. With the cystoscope in the bladder, the operative instrument is introduced into the operative port and advanced until it is visible just at the end of the cystoscope. Gross movements are made with the cystoscope as the instrument is brought into apposition with the lesion. Minor adjustments are made by moving the instrument within the cystoscope sheath. Bleeding is self-limited in most cases, although a ball electrode can be used if needed.

Intraoperative Cystoscopy

Cystoscopy is an important adjuvant to surgery of the female genitourinary system. It is commonly used to judge coaptation during periurethral collagen injections, to facilitate safe placement of suprapubic catheters, and to evaluate the ureters and bladder mucosa for inadvertent damage. The approach to assessment of the integrity of bladder mucosa after pelvic surgery is similar to the approach described for diagnostic cystoscopy. A thorough survey of the bladder is made, with special attention to the portions of the bladder potentially jeopardized by the specific procedure. Inspection of the anterolateral aspects of the mucosa is important after a bladder suspension procedure, whereas inspection of the trigone is especially important after a difficult vaginal hysterectomy or dissection of an anterior enterocele sac from the bladder. The retropubic passage of a tension-free tape requires confirmation of bladder integrity to be sure the needle insertion devices have not penetrated the plane of the bladder. It is also a good plan to observe the tape indentation on the bladder wall as the insertion needles with attached tape are pulled through the retropubic space to the abdominal incision. The dyed tape shows up against the bladder mucosa as a sling arm has been passed through the bladder. An assessment of ureteral integrity is warranted after every pelvic reconstructive surgery, all bladder suspension procedures, and suspected injury to the bladder or ureter. Visualization of efflux of solution from the ureteral orifice is adequate to demonstrate patency, and this is facilitated by injection of 2.5 to 5 mL of indigo carmine dye intravenously 5 to 10 minutes before cystoscopy. The absence of efflux is an indication for passage of ureteral catheters or other measures to evaluate potential obstruction.

Ureteral Catheterization

Catheterization of the ureteral orifices has been practiced since cystoscopes were first introduced. In gynecology, the primary indications for ureteral catheterization are to evaluate potential ureteral obstruction and to place ureteral markers. Ureteral markers may be useful in radical or extensive pelvic surgery and in cases with abnormal pelvic anatomy. Ureteral catheters are available in various sizes, with a number of specialized tips. Although available from 3 to 12 French, the most useful are 4 to 6 French. The most commonly used catheters are the general-purpose and whistle-tip catheters. Specialized tips include spiral filiform for negotiating strictures and curves and the acorn tip for retrograde studies. Catheters are fabricated from plastic or Dacron and are generally radiopaque. They have graduated centimeter markings for judging depth of insertion.

Once the ureteral orifice is located, the ureteral catheter is advanced into the field of view just outside the fenestrated portion of the cystoscope, with the catheter tip orientated in the axis of the ureteral lumen. The tip is threaded into the first part of the ureteral lumen by advancing the entire cystoscope. Once the tip passes the ureteral orifice, the catheter is gently threaded along the ureter until resistance is met at the renal pelvis, which is about 25 cm. This is done by grasping the catheter manually proximal to its entry point into the operative channel of the sheath or bridge and gently pushing the catheter into the ureter. The deflecting mechanism of the Albarrán bridge may facilitate initial introduction into the ureter. Difficulty in passing the catheter may be due to an anatomic variation such as a stenotic orifice, mucosal fold, or ureteral tortuosity. A stenotic orifice is suspected in the presence of immediate resistance to the catheter tip, and a smaller catheter is selected. A mucosal fold may be managed by repositioning the patient, bladder, or cystoscope. Placing the patient in the Trendelenburg position helps to alter the position of the intramural ureter, as does further filling or emptying of the bladder. A filiform-tip catheter is also valuable for negotiating strictures and tortuosities. If the catheter is to be left in place, it should be secured to a transurethral catheter and connected to a drainage device. Gentle technique is required to prevent hematuria and ureteral spasm.

Suprapubic Teloscopy

Transurethral cystoscopy is applicable during a vaginal surgical approach. Suprapubic teloscopy provides a method to perform cystoscopy from an abdominal approach (15). This may also be accomplished during laparoscopic surgery by passing the telescope through a suprapubic catheter introducer sheath (16). These techniques are seldom used since most patients having reconstructive pelvic surgery are either operated from a vaginal approach or are placed in Allen stirrups, so there is always access to the bladder through the urethra.

CYSTOURETHROSCOPIC FINDINGS

Normal Urethra

The normal urethra has a lush, pink epithelium (Fig. 7.5), and periurethral gland openings may be seen posteriorly along the length of the urethra. There is often a central posterior ridge called the urethral crest, and there may be white epithelium, especially in the posterior wall of the urethra (Fig. 7.6). The UVJ is slightly irregular but rounded in shape. It should normally close with hold maneuvers.

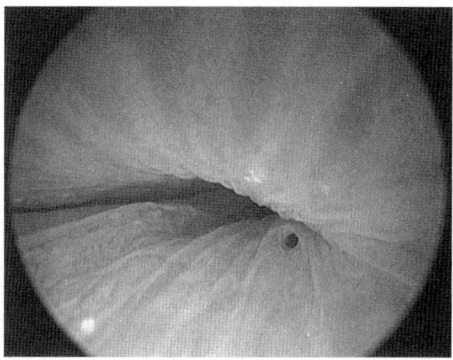

FIGURE 7.5 ● Normal urethra. There is pink, lush epithelium in folds.

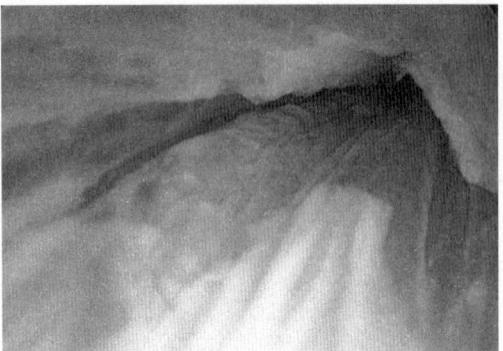

FIGURE 7.6 ● Urethral crest and squamous epithelium of normal urethra. The urethral crest runs posteriorly as a longitudinal ridge, and over it is white epithelium.

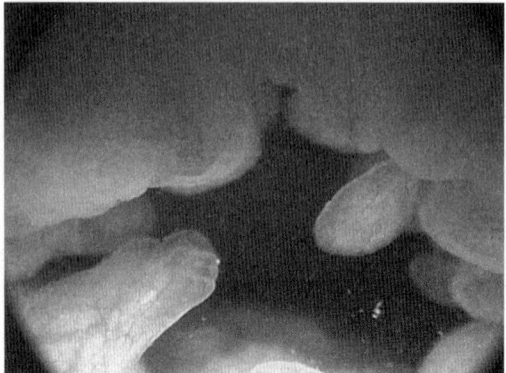

FIGURE 7.8 ● Polyps at the urethrovesical junction.

Abnormal Urethroscopic Findings

Acute urethritis is usually caused by infection, trauma, or irritation (Fig. 7.7). Findings include inflamed, reddened urethral mucosa, bleeding areas, superficial ulceration, and exudate on the mucosal surface. Polyps and fronds may be seen at the UVJ, but their significance is uncertain, and treatment is almost never required (Figs. 7.8 and 7.9). Palpation over the end of the urethroscope may reveal exudate from urethral glands or may facilitate identification of exudate or pus from a urethral diverticulum. A fistula is an opening usually in the posterior aspect of the urethra, and urine or irrigating fluid may be seen escaping into the vagina (Fig. 7.10). A frozen or scarred, functionless urethra may appear pale, may be fixed in an open position, and will have no response to hold or strain maneuvers (Fig. 7.11). With the large number of tension-free tape procedures now performed, there are cases of vaginal erosion at times with urethral penetration of the tape (Fig. 7.12).

Normal Bladder

The bladder has a smooth surface with a pale pink to glistening white hue. The translucent mucosa affords easy visualization of the branched submucosal vasculature. Infusion of fluid is always accompanied by an air bubble, which marks the dome of the bladder (Fig. 7.13). The trigone appears reddened and granular and may have a thickened white membrane with a villous contour (Fig. 7.14). Histologic evaluation of this layer reveals squamous metaplasia, and it is usually referred to simply as metaplasia.

The trigone is triangular, with the inferior apex directed toward the UVJ and the ureteral orifices forming the superior apices (Fig. 7.15). As the cystoscope is advanced past the UVJ, the trigone is apparent at the bottom of the field. The interureteric ridge is a visible elevation that forms

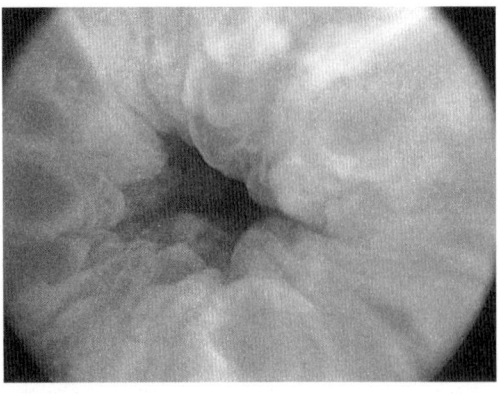

FIGURE 7.7 ● Acute urethritis. The urethra is reddened along its length.

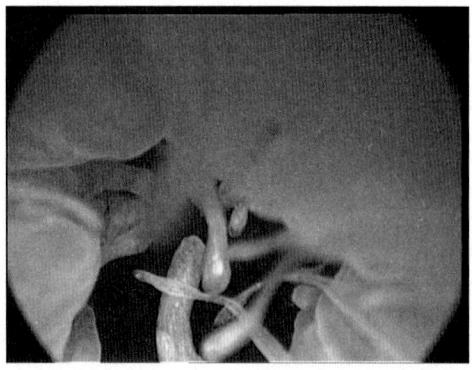

FIGURE 7.9 ● Fronds at the urethrovesical junction.

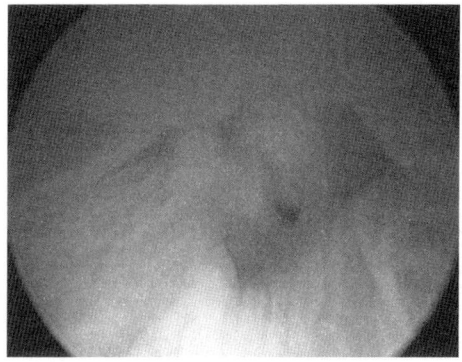

FIGURE 7.10 ● Urethrovaginal fistula. The urethral canal is in the upper right of the photograph, and the opening from the urethra to the vagina is clearly seen as a small opening in the center of the picture.

the superior boundary of the trigone and runs between the ureteral orifices. There is marked variation in the ureteral orifices, but they are usually circular or slitlike and located on the apex of a small mound lateral to the midline of the bladder base. With urine efflux, the ureter opens and the mound retracts in the direction of the intramural ureter. The distended bladder is roughly spherical, but numerous folds of mucosa are evident in the empty or partially filled bladder. The uterus and cervix can be seen indenting the posterior wall of the bladder. Bowel peristalsis may be seen through the bladder wall.

Abnormal Cystoscopic Findings

Bladder pathology either is located in the mucosa or is structural. Mucosal lesions are either inflam-

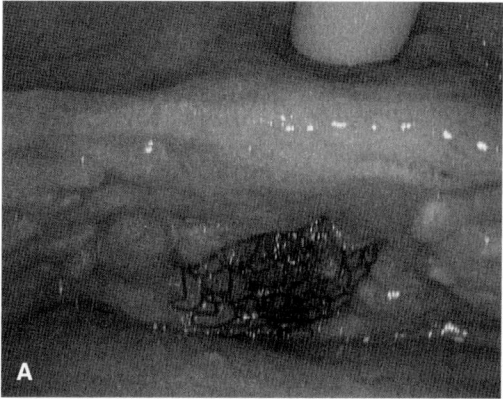

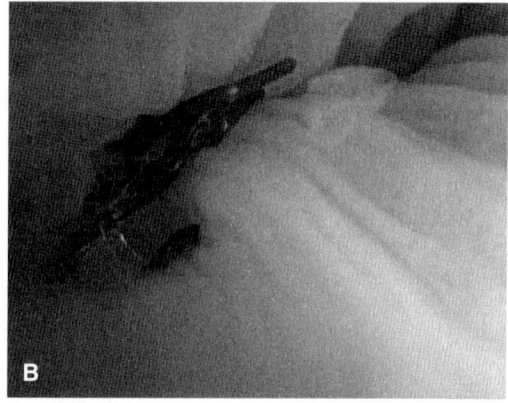

FIGURE 7.12 ● Eroded tension-free tape. **(A)** Tape erosion in vagina. **(B)** Tape in urethra.

matory or neoplastic, although the two may coexist. Cystitis refers to inflammation of the bladder, and generally cystoscopy should be avoided until

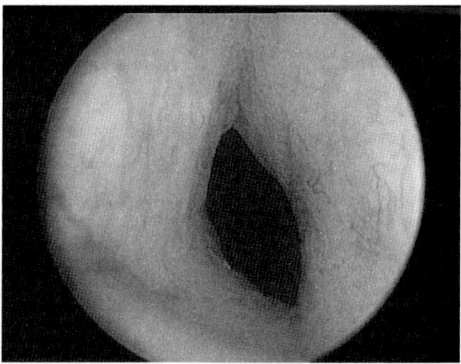

FIGURE 7.11 ● Functionless urethra. The urethra is very short and remains passively open, with the urethroscope barely inside the meatus. The epithelium is smooth, and there is no movement with hold or strain maneuvers.

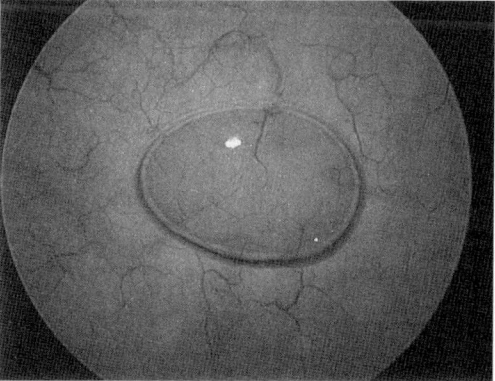

FIGURE 7.13 ● Normal bladder. The air bubble at the dome of the bladder serves as a reference marker. The epithelium of the bladder wall is smooth and pale pink and has fine vasculature.

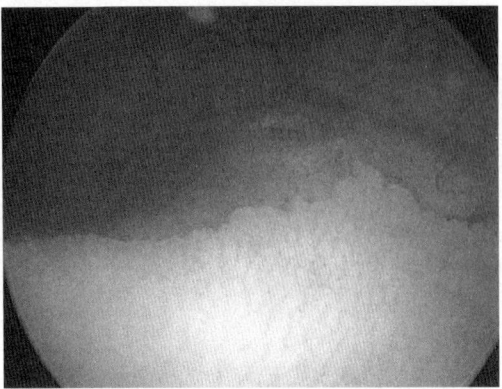

FIGURE 7.14 ● Metaplasia of trigone. The white membrane covers much of the trigone leading up to the ureters. Biopsy reveals squamous metaplasia.

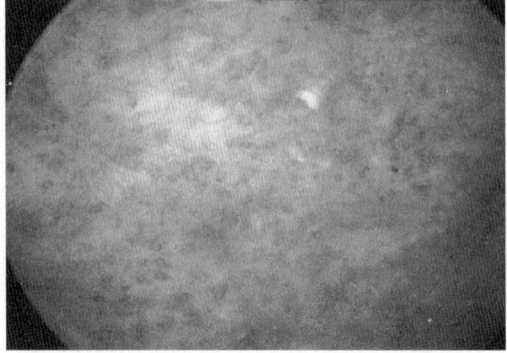

FIGURE 7.16 ● Acute cystitis. The bladder mucosa is reddened and edematous, making it difficult to see clearly. There is often active bleeding, further compromising the view.

the infection is treated. Cystitis may manifest as pink or peach-colored macules or papules. As severity intensifies, the mucosa becomes edematous and hypervascular (Fig. 7.16). In hemorrhagic cystitis, there may be individual or confluent mucosal hemorrhages, and the patient complains of hematuria. The hemorrhagic cystitis that follows bladder infusion with toxins such as cyclophosphamide is characterized by diffuse mucosal hemorrhages. In radiation cystitis, areas of hemorrhage are surrounded by pale mucosa, which may be fibrotic or hypovascular. An indwelling catheter produces an inflammatory reaction of the mucosa in contact with the catheter. There may be associated pseudopapillary edema and submucosal hemorrhages and vesical fibrosis.

Cystitis cystica consists of clear mucosal cysts, which are usually found on the bladder base and are often found in multiples (Fig. 7.17). The cysts are formed by single layers of subepithelial transitional cells, which degenerate with central liquefaction. These are benign findings and do not require investigation. Cystitis glandularis has an appearance similar to cystitis cystica, but the cysts are not clear and have a less uniform contour. There may be associated inflammation. The association of cystitis glandularis with adenovillous carcinoma of the bladder has led to the belief that cystitis glandularis may be a precursor of adenocarcinoma (17). Work-up for this condition is controversial but initial washings and cystoscopy are recommended, with periodic follow-up with one or the other after that. A benign polyp on the bladder wall has a smooth contour and maintains the pink color of the bladder lining (Fig. 7.18).

Interstitial cystitis is suspected in patients with severe frequency, urgency, and suprapubic pain re-

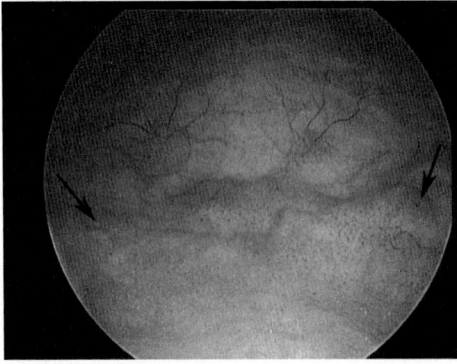

FIGURE 7.15 ● Trigone. The trigone is formed by the UVJ inferiorly and the ureteral orifices superiorly. The ureteral openings are marked by *arrows*. The trigone is frequently reddened and granular.

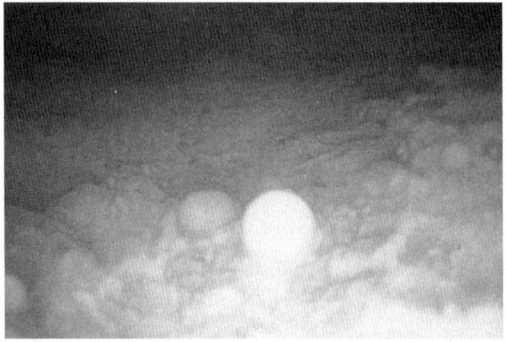

FIGURE 7.17 ● Cystitis cystica. The 1- to 2-mm cysts at the bladder base are smooth-walled and are clear or sometimes pigmented.

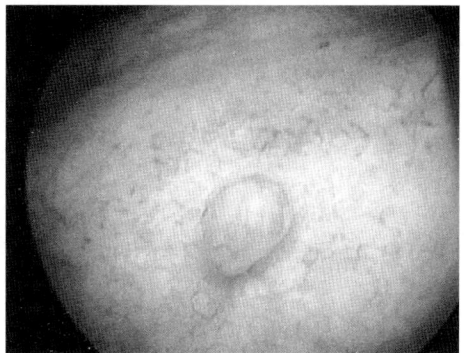

FIGURE 7.18 ● Benign bladder polyp.

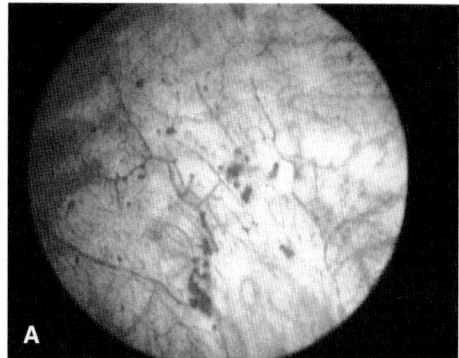

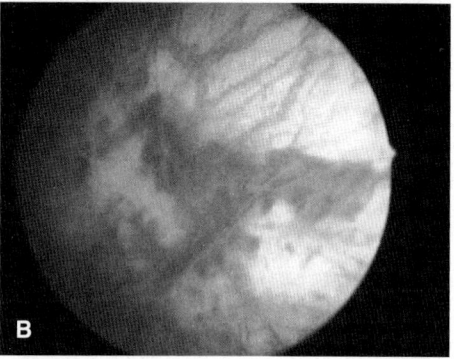

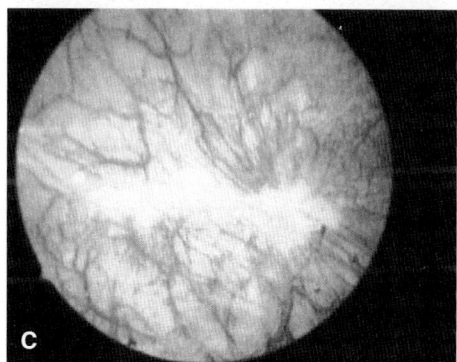

FIGURE 7.19 ● Interstitial cystitis. **(A)** Petechial hemorrhages after bladder distention under anesthesia. **(B)** Linear hemorrhages. **(C)** Hunner's ulcer. Punched-out white scar interrupting vascular pattern.

lieved temporarily by voiding. Cystoscopic examination is usually performed under anesthesia. The pathognomonic lesions appear after filling and then refilling of the bladder to capacity. Glomerulations are petechial hemorrhages or small red dots and are visible in mild cases. Larger hemorrhagic areas may be seen, and severe areas have linear hemorrhages. Petechiae may be seen in normal patients on the posterior bladder wall and trigone. Patients with interstitial cystitis have glomerulations throughout the bladder. Hunner's ulcers are areas of scarring that interrupt the normal vascular pattern of the bladder wall. They occur in fewer than 10% of cases (Fig. 7.19).

Trabeculations are smooth ridges that become evident with distention of the bladder to volumes approaching maximum cystometric capacity. They appear as interlaced cords of different diameters with intervening sacculations (Fig. 7.20). They represent hypertrophied detrusor musculature associated with detrusor instability and functional or anatomic obstruction. A bladder diverticulum can occur when high intravesical pressure produces an enlargement of the intervening sacculations. The thick muscular band that creates the neck varies in diameter and gives way to an outpouching of bladder mucosa. The interior of the diverticulum may harbor a neoplasm and must be examined carefully.

Fistulas may also be encountered at cystoscopy (Fig. 7.21). Posthysterectomy fistulas are usually located in the bladder base superior to the interureteric ridge, corresponding to the level of the vaginal cuff. The fistula openings range in size from small to several centimeters in diameter. In the immediate postoperative state, the surrounding mucosa is edematous and hyperemic, whereas in later stages, the mucosa has a typical smooth appearance. In contrast, vesicoenteric fistulas uniformly have a surrounding inflammatory reaction, often with bullous edema, and the fistula tract is not discernible in two thirds of cases (18).

Bladder calculi may result from urinary stasis or the presence of a foreign body, or an inflammatory exudate may coalesce and serve as a nidus for stone formation. Stones have an extremely variable cystoscopic appearance in terms of color, size, and shape but generally have an irregular surface (19). Foreign bodies and stones are usually accompanied by varying degrees of general or lo-

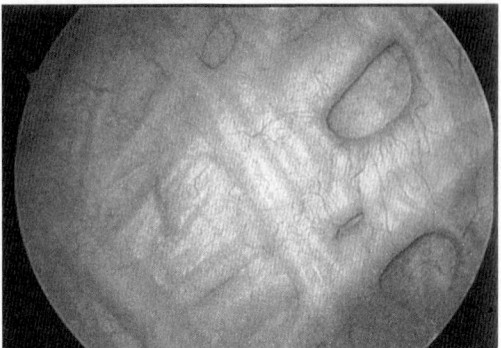

FIGURE 7.20 • Trabeculation. The muscle bundles appear as prominent ridges with intervening pockets or cellules.

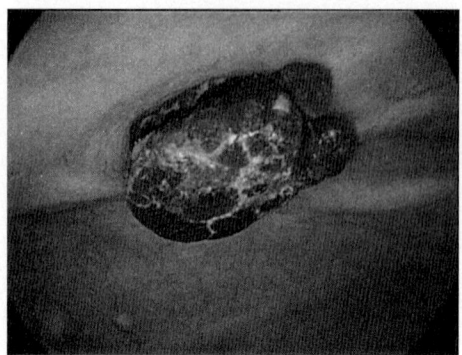

FIGURE 7.22 • Bladder calculus. This usually forms over a suture nidus or some other irritant.

calized inflammatory reaction. A permanent suture may be a nidus for a stone or may remain in its original state (Fig. 7.22).

Bladder cancer is less common in women than in men, but it still may occur, especially after the fifth decade. Transitional cell carcinoma is the most common type, followed by adenocarcinoma and squamous cell carcinoma. Appearance on cystoscopy is variable but usually shows a raised lesion with a villous feathery or papillary appearance (Fig. 7.23). Superficial transitional cell carcinoma may be multicentric or may have associated carcinoma *in situ*. Carcinoma *in situ* may be inconspicuous, mimicking the macules or plaques of cystitis.

Auxiliary ureteral orifices indicate renal collecting abnormalities. When present, they often enter the vesical wall slightly superior to the trigone in proximity to the other ureteral orifice. In a duplicated collecting system, the upper pole kidney drains into the more distal ureteral opening. A ureterocele is caused by laxity of the distal ureteral lumen with herniation into the vesical cavity during efflux.

SUMMARY

Urethrocystoscopy allows visualization of the lower urinary tract. Instrumentation is available with many modifications that increase the applications of the technique. Cystourethroscopy is valuable for diagnosing anatomic lesions of the lower urinary tract that are commonly overlooked by other diagnostic modalities. Cystoscopy is essential to assess ureteral function and vesical integrity during pelvic surgery.

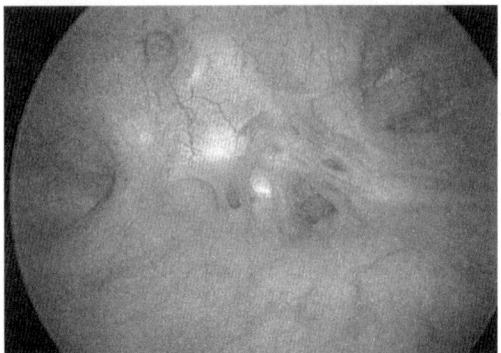

FIGURE 7.21 • Vesicovaginal fistula. The openings in the bladder with a posthysterectomy fistula occur superior to the trigone in the posterior aspect of the bladder, and there are two distinct holes to the vagina in this picture.

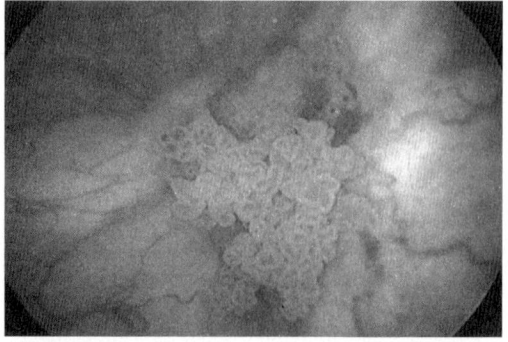

FIGURE 7.23 • Bladder cancer. The pedunculated papillary lesion is a transitional cell carcinoma.

REFERENCES

1. Cundiff GW, Bent AE. *Endoscopic diagnosis of the female urinary tract.* London: WB Saunders, 1999.
2. Bozzini P. Lichteiter, eine erfindung zur anschung innerer theile, und krukheiten nebst abbildung. *J Pract Arzeykunde* 1805;24:107.
3. Desmormeaux AJ. *Transactions of the Societé Chirurgie, Paris.* Gazette des Hop, 1865.
4. Grünfeld I. *Der harnröhrenspiegel (das endoscop), seine diagnostische und therapeutische anwendung.* Vienna: Deutsch Chirugie, 1881.
5. Nitze M. Eine neue balbachtungs-und untersuchunigsmethods fur harnrohre, harnbiase and rectum. *Wien Med Wochenschr* 1879;24:649.
6. Kelly HA. The direct examination of the female bladder with elevated pelvis: the catheterization of the ureters under direct inspection, with and without elevation of the pelvis. *Am J Obstet Dis Wom Child* 1894;25:1–19.
7. Hopkins HH, Kopany NS. A flexible fiberscope, using static scanning. *Nature* 1954;179:39–41.
8. Robertson JR. Air cystoscopy. *Obstet Gynecol* 1968;32: 328–330.
9. Clayman RV, Reddy P, Lange PH. Flexible fiberoptic and rigid-rod lens endoscopy of the lower urinary tract: a prospective controlled comparison. *J Urol* 1984;131: 715–716.
10. Yoshimura R, Wada S, Kishimoto T. Why the flexible cystoscope has not yet been widely introduced? A questionnaire to Japanese urologists. *Int J Urol* 1999;6: 549–559.
11. Choong S, Whitfield HN, Meganathan V, et al. A prospective, randomized, double-blind study comparing lignocaine gel and plain lubricating gel in relieving pain during flexible cystoscopy. *Br J Urol* 1997;80:69–71.
12. Cundiff GW, McLennan MT, Bent AE. Randomized trial of antibiotic prophylaxis for combined urodynamics and cystourethroscopy. *Obstet Gynecol* 1999;93: 749–752.
13. Kraklau DM, Wolf JS Jr. Review of antibiotic prophylaxis recommendations for office-based urologic procedures. *Tech Urol* 1999;5:123–128.
14. Ostergard DR. Bladder pillar block anesthesia for urethral dilatation in women. *Am J Obstet Gynecol* 1980; 136:187–188.
15. Timmons MC, Addison WA. Suprapubic teloscopy: extraperitoneal intraoperative technique to demonstrate ureteral patency. *Obstet Gynecol* 1990;75:137–139.
16. Miklos JR, Kholi N, Sze EH, et al. Percutaneous suprapubic teloscopy: a minimally invasive cystoscopic technique. *Obstet Gynecol* 1997;89:476–478.
17. Edwards PD, Hurm RA, Jaeesehke WH. Conversion of cystitis glandularis to adenocarcinoma. *J Urol* 1972; 108:568–570.
18. Farringer JL, Hrabovsky E, Marsh J, et al. Vesicocolic fistula. *South Med J* 1974;67:1043–1046.
19. Schwartz BF, Stoller ML. The vesical calculus. *Urol Clin North Am* 2000;27:333–346.

CHAPTER 8

Painful Conditions of the Lower Urinary Tract Including Painful Bladder Syndrome

Steven E. Swift, Toby C. Chai, Alfred E. Bent

INTRODUCTION

Chronic pelvic pain is one of the most difficult and frustrating conditions to manage in gynecology. It can result from a multitude of pathologic entities and various pelvic organs can be involved such that there is overlap between pathologic entities and organ systems involved, and the initiating insult is often only distantly related to the patient's current symptom complex. The diagnostic criteria for specific diagnoses are usually vague and response to therapy is disappointing. Painful conditions of the lower urinary tract are no different and make up a subset of these complaints. Similar to their counterparts elsewhere in the pelvis they represent a very difficult and frustrating series of disease entities. Another complicating factor involves the role of external pathology affecting symptoms and function of the lower urinary tract so as to further confuse the clinical picture. Diseases such as endometriosis and pelvic inflammatory disease can present within the context of lower urinary tract symptoms. For clarity this chapter will limit its focus on those pathologic entities that are intrinsic to the bladder and urethra. Chapters 9 and 10 will cover pelvic floor myalgia and urinary tract infections, respectively.

PAINFUL BLADDER SYNDROME/ INTERSTITIAL CYSTITIS

Currently there is a great deal of debate centered around the diagnosis of interstitial cystitis (IC), making it difficult to comment on its definition. The standard definition that has been recommended for years (for research protocols) comes from the National Institute of Diabetes and Digestive and Kidney Diseases (NIDDK) branch of the National Institutes of Health (NIH). This definition involves both bladder pain and evidence of bladder abnormalities (glomerulations or Hunner's ulcers) upon cystoscopic examination (1). The original intent of this criteria list was to ensure maximal objective standardization of patients enrolled into NIH-sponsored IC studies. These criteria were not designed as a diagnostic tool (Table 8.1). Painful bladder syndrome (PBS), on the other hand, was first defined by the International Continence Society (ICS) in 2002 and is defined as the complaint of suprapubic pain related to bladder filling, accompanied by other symptoms such as increased daytime and nighttime frequency, in the absence of proven urinary infection or other obvious pathology (2). The ICS further defined the "symptom" of bladder pain as pain felt suprapubically or retropubically that usually increases with bladder filling, though it may persist after voiding. This is slightly different from the definition of IC as defined by the NIDDK guidelines. The ICS definition defines the location of the pain as suprapubic (and/or retropubic if you use the ICS symptom definition) and also ties in the pain to bladder filling. It specifically does not require evidence of bladder abnormalities (glomerulations) upon cystoscopic examination. The ICS, in their document defining PBS, acknowledged that it would be used as an alternative to IC in a footnote:

> The ICS believes this to be a preferable term to "interstitial cystitis." Interstitial cystitis is a spe-

cific diagnosis and requires confirmation by typical cystoscopic and histological features. In the investigation of bladder pain it may be necessary to exclude conditions such as carcinoma in situ and endometriosis.

So while the two terms PBS and IC may not be identical, readers should recognize that in the literature the two will often be used interchangeably. In a recent study of IC patients, only 105 of 138 of those defined as having IC reported suprapubic

TABLE 8.1

NIDDK Definition of Interstitial Cystitis

Inclusion Criteria

1. Cystoscopy—glomerulations and/or classic Hunner's ulcer
2. Symptoms—bladder pain and/or bladder urgency

Exclusion Criteria

1. Bladder capacity greater than 350 cc on awake cystometry
2. Absence of an intense urge to void with the bladder filled to 100 cc during cystometry using a fill rate of 30 to 100 cc/min
3. Demonstration of phasic involuntary bladder contractions on cystometry using the fill rate described in number 2
4. Duration of symptoms less than 9 months
5. Absence of nocturia
6. Symptoms relieved by antimicrobials, urinary antiseptics, anticholinergics, or antispasmodics
7. Frequency of urination while awake of less than eight times a day
8. Diagnosis of bacterial cystitis or prostatitis within a 3-month period
9. Bladder or ureteral calculi
10. Active genital herpes
11. Uterine, cervical, vaginal, or urethral cancer
12. Urethral diverticulum
13. Cyclophosphamide or any type of chemical cystitis
14. Tuberculous cystitis
15. Radiation cystitis
16. Benign or malignant bladder tumors
17. Vaginitis
18. Age less than 18 years

pain with a relationship to bladder filling status, which led these investigators to question the sensitivity of the ICS definition of PBS in identifying IC patients (3). In order to lessen the confusion for the reader, for the remainder of this chapter we will use the term "interstitial cystitis." This section of the chapter will focus on IC, as this terminology and definition have been in use longer and the literature to date conforms predominantly to this standard.

Epidemiology

IC is best described as a chronic hypersensory bladder condition manifested by urinary frequency, urgency, and bladder pain without an identifiable etiology. This disease mainly afflicts women in their 30s and 40s (4). However, it is being more frequently recognized in males, and the female-to-male ratio is 5:1 (5). This remains a disease more common in females, and because females commonly have acute bacterial cystitis, the diagnosis of IC is often delayed. The primary care physician often treats IC with oral antibiotics because IC symptoms mimic acute bacterial cystitis and urine cultures are not typically sent before treatment of acute bacterial cystitis. The current estimated prevalence of IC in the United States is between 66 and 197 per 100,000 (5,6). The estimation of the number of females afflicted with IC in the United States is between 450,000 and 700,000. Recently, investigators mailed a validated IC symptoms questionnaire (O'Leary-Sant questionnaire; see later section for description) to be completed by 5,000 females in a health maintenance organization (7). This study found that prevalence of IC symptoms is 30- to 50-fold higher in women than the prevalence of a coded physician diagnosis of IC in the same population. The authors concluded that IC may be significantly underdiagnosed.

The etiology of IC remains unclear; however, several causes, such as mast cell activation, neurogenic inflammation, and transitional epithelial dysfunction, have been proposed (8). The most frequently discussed pathologic abnormality used to explain IC is a defect of the transitional epithelium, and specifically the glycosaminoglycan (GAG) layer that separates and protects the transitional epithelium from urine. The rationale that the bladder urothelium is "leaky" in IC patients because of a proposed deficiency in the GAG layer (a proteoglycan or glycoprotein) was derived from several observations. First, in animal models, application of protamine sulfate, which purportedly "strips" the GAG layer, increased bladder permeability in rabbit bladder urothelium (9). Furthermore, the protamine-induced increased permeability was reversed by the addition of sodium pentosan polysulfate, a GAG. Second, protamine placed into normal human volunteers induced pain, urinary frequency, urinary urgency, and increased bladder permeability to urea similar to IC (10). Third was the finding of increased urea uptake by the IC bladders (when exogenous urea was introduced intravesically) compared with control bladders, suggesting increased bladder permeability with IC (11). Finally, there was clinical evidence that sodium pentosan polysulfate (a GAG) alleviates some of the symptoms of IC (12,13). While this theory may explain some cases of IC, the disease is probably multifactorial, which may explain why its etiology remains elusive.

It is also thought that IC may be genetically inherited. This is based on twin studies demonstrating a greater rate of concordance of IC among monozygotic twins than dizygotic twins (14). In addition, there is a 17-fold increase, over the general population, in the incidence of IC in first-degree relatives of patients with IC (15). Future epidemiologic and genetic studies may help pinpoint etiologic mechanisms and also determine the natural history of this puzzling disease.

Clinical Diagnosis

Currently there are no proven etiologies for IC, and defining the disease clinically remains a challenge. The diagnosis is most often made on the grounds of symptoms in the absence of other pathologic entities. There are no classic physical findings, blood tests, histopathology, or radiologic tests for IC. The presentation of symptoms in IC is highly variable, and some have proposed that IC is a complex of diseases with multiple etiologies rather than just a single entity. Because bladder pain is a prominent symptom component of IC, some have included IC in the disease complex of chronic pelvic pain. When IC is better understood from the pathophysiologic standpoint, a more specific terminology may be developed.

Patients who with IC have the prototypical symptom complex of urinary frequency, urinary urgency, and bladder pain without a definable etiology and have had these chronic symptoms for longer than 9 months. The intensity of these symptoms typically waxes and wanes during the course of the disease. Because of the imprecise nature of these symptoms, IC patients are frequently thought to have recurrent urinary tract infection, urethritis, urethrotrigonitis, trigonitis, urethral pain syndrome, urethral stenosis, endometriosis, vulvodynia, vulvar vestibulitis, or pelvic congestion syndrome. A few studies have also found an association between IC, vulvodynia, and chronic pelvic pain, further suggesting that there may be overlap in both symptoms and organs affected (16,17).

Recently, it has been speculated that IC may be a systemic disease because of its association with other conditions, such as irritable bowel disease, allergies, sensitive skin, inflammatory bowel disease, fibromyalgia, chronic fatigue syndrome, and systemic lupus erythematosus (18–21). Whether these associations represent common pathophysiologic mechanisms or spurious associations may relate to the relatively nonspecific diagnostic criteria for all of these conditions and the potential for selection bias of cases and controls in these studies. Recently, a validated questionnaire for non–bladder-related symptoms was given to 35 IC patients and 35 age-matched controls, and it was found that the IC patients did not have more nonbladder symptoms than the controls (22).

Therefore, the diagnosis of IC remains primarily a process of exclusion and clinical suspicion. A list of exclusionary conditions has been set forth by the NIH and the NIDDK (see Table 8.1).

The pain component of IC can be difficult for patients to describe. Because the bladder is autonomically innervated, it is classified as a visceral organ. From a neuroanatomic perspective, this simply means that there is an intervening synapse (ganglia) between the autonomic motor (preganglionic) neuron and the end effector organ (the bladder). However, from a sensory standpoint, patients often have difficulty localizing or describing visceral sensations. The pain may be referred to other areas of the pelvis. Besides the typical pain over the suprapubic (bladder) area, which may be relieved by voiding, IC patients may complain of referred urethra-based pain, such as dysuria, stranguria, or constant burning. They may also complain of low back pain, vulvar pain, rectal pain, and dyspareunia. Quantitation of the severity of pain is quite difficult because of the waxing–waning presentation of symptoms, and there are no formal quantitative objective measures of bladder or pelvic pain.

Urinary urgency is another symptomatic component of IC that can be difficult to separate from pain in some patients. IC patients may describe a constant strong urge to void, despite low bladder volumes, that when severe is described as pain. Urinary frequency is a manifestation of the actual act of voiding, but IC patients have been known not to void because they realize that frequent void- ing does not necessarily lead to relief of pain and urge sensations. From the standpoint of quantifica- tion of IC symptoms, measurement of voiding fre- quency may be the best objective parameter.

In summary, the clinical presentation of IC is characterized by chronic urinary frequency, ur- gency, and pelvic pain in the absence of precise identifiable etiologic features. These symptoms do not necessarily follow a set pattern and may be quite different from one patient to another. IC pa- tients may have one symptomatic component that predominates over the others. Finally, IC symptoms typically wax and wane, which further complicates the evaluation and treatment of this condition. The key is to rule out identifiable and potentially re- versible causes of the bladder symptoms.

Symptom Quantitation

Because IC symptoms are variable, it becomes im- portant to quantitate these symptoms as objec- tively as possible. This is especially important for clinical researchers examining treatment options for IC. Two sets of validated instruments have been described in the literature. One questionnaire instrument was developed by O'Leary et al in 1997 specifically to assess IC patients (23). The questionnaire had two subscales to quantify symp- toms and their impact on quality of life: the Interstitial Cystitis Symptom Index (ICSI) and Interstitial Cystitis Problem Index (ICPI) (Table 8.2). These questionnaires were administered to a group of women with chronic pelvic pain before undergoing laparoscopy and cystoscopy with hy- drodistention to determine whether these instru- ments can detect IC in this patient population. Using positive findings from cystoscopy and hy- drodistention as objective criteria for IC, these in- vestigators determined that the sensitivity, speci- ficity, positive predictive value, and negative predictive value of these indices were 94%, 50%, 53%, and 93%, respectively (24). Furthermore, they found that 38% of these patients with chronic pelvic pain had IC.

A second symptom measurement instrument, the University of Wisconsin IC Scale (UW-ICS), has also been developed and validated (25). The UW-ICS is a 7-point, 0-to-6 rating scale with each item anchored between the extremes of 0 (not at all) and 6 (a lot) (Fig. 8.1). The scale is completed by the patient within the context of reporting the symptoms as, "How much have you experienced the following symptoms today?" Seven items are defined to characterize the IC patient, with a sum-

mary score being the sum of the seven individual items. This summated UW-ICS score will have a value ranging from 0 to 42.

Any of these validated instruments should be administered to the patient with IC to quantitate her symptoms during the course of evaluation and treatment. It is important to use these standardized instruments so that changes in a patient's symp- toms and quality of life can be followed as objec- tively as possible.

Diagnosis
Cystoscopy with Hydrodistention

Cystoscopy with hydrodistention of the bladder under anesthesia is the standard method for the objective diagnosis of IC according to the NIDDK recommendations. The conventional wisdom is that IC bladders have the appearance of glomeru- lations (or petechiae) after bladder hydrodisten- tion (nonulcerative form of IC). However, glomerulations are often not found in subjects with symptomatic IC and are noted in up to 45% of normal subjects without symptoms of IC (26,27). The appearance of classic Hunner's ul- cers is uncommon in IC, although it has been sug- gested that the appearance of Hunner's ulcers is a more specific sign for IC (ulcerative form of IC). Anesthetic bladder capacity of IC patients may also be reduced, although typically IC patients have normal anesthetic capacity. The presumed diagnostic specificity of appearance of postdisten- tion bladder glomerulations or Hunner's ulcers re- sulted in the NIDDK using this as the only objec- tive criterion in classifying a patient as having IC. Although this single criterion is not uniformly ac- cepted by all clinicians, its main purpose is to standardize IC patients enrolled in NIH-sponsored studies.

Description of Hydrodistention

Hydrodistention is performed with the patient under general or regional anesthesia. A full cysto- scopic examination of the bladder is performed first. Patients with IC can have a completely nor- mal-appearing bladder without evidence of uroep- ithelial lesions. Cystoscopic irrigant, water or saline, is then infused at a pressure of 80 to 100 cmH$_2$O into the bladder until filling stops (pres- sure cut-off). The bladder is distended for 2 to 5 minutes before all the irrigant is released from the bladder. Terminal bloody efflux of irrigant sug- gests the diagnosis of IC. The bladder epithelium is re-examined with the cystoscope during repeat filling. Glomerulations (petechiae) or Hunner's

TABLE 8.2

Interstitial Cystitis Symptoms Quantitation

IC Symptom Index (ICSI)	IC Problem Index (ICPI)

1. During the past month, how often have you felt the strong urge to urinate with little or no warning?
0____not at all
1____less than 1 time in 5
2____less than half the time
3____about half the time
4____more than half the time
5____almost always
	During the past month, how much has each of the following been a problem for you?
	1. Frequent urination during the day
	  0____no problem
	  1____very small problem
	  2____small problem
	  3____medium problem
	  4____big problem

2. During the past month, have you had to urinate less than 2 hours after you finished urinating?
0____not at all
1____less than 1 time in 5
2____less than half the time
3____about half the time
4____more than half the time
5____almost always
	2. Getting up at night to urinate
	  0____no problem
	  1____very small problem
	  2____small problem
	  3____medium problem
	  4____big problem

3. During the past month, how often did you most typically get up at night to urinate?
0____not at all
1____less than 1 time in 5
2____less than half the time
3____about half the time
4____more than half the time
5____almost always
	3. Need to urinate with little warning
	  0____no problem
	  1____very small problem
	  2____small problem
	  3____medium problem
	  4____big problem

4. During the past month, have you experienced pain or burning in your bladder?
0____not at all
1____less than 1 time in 5
2____less than half the time
3____about half the time
4____more than half the time
5____almost always
	4. Burning pain, discomfort, or pressure in your bladder
	  0____no problem
	  1____very small problem
	  2____small problem
	  3____medium problem
	  4____big problem

ulcers, appearing as fissures or cracks in the epithelium, are consistent with IC (Fig. 8.2).

Potassium Sensitivity Test

The potassium sensitivity test (PST) was developed as a method to diagnose IC in a relatively noninvasive manner (as compared with cystoscopy and hydrodistention under anesthesia) (28). The rationale for this test is based on the assertion that the bladder urothelium is "leaky" in IC patients because of a proposed deficiency in the GAG layer (a proteoglycan or glycoprotein) on the luminal surface of the bladder uroepithelium. If urothelial leak were the pathophysiologic mechanism in IC, urinary potassium in the urine would cross the leaky IC urothelial barrier to activate (depolarize) the sensory nerve endings in the suburothelium.

How much have you experienced the following symptom today?	0 (not at all)	1	2	3	4	5	6 (a lot)
1. bladder pain							
2. bladder discomfort							
3. getting up at night to go to the bathroom							
4. going to the bathroom frequently in the day							
5. urgency to urinate							
6. difficulty sleeping because of bladder problems							
7. burning sensation in the bladder							

FIGURE 8.1 ● The University of Wisconsin Interstitial Cystitis scale.

The patient is awake and without anesthesia for the PST. The test is performed by infusing 40 mL of solution 1 (sterile water) into the bladder over 2 to 3 minutes. After 5 minutes, the patient rates her pain and urgency using a visual scale from 0 to 5, with 5 being worst. She voids the contents of her bladder. Next, 40 mL of solution 2 (0.4 molar potassium chloride [KCl]) is instilled into the bladder and left for 5 minutes. The patient rates her pain and urgency and voids the solution. A score of at least 2 in either pain or urgency is considered a positive PST, provided the patient does not respond to solution 1. It was shown in this same study that 75% of patients with IC have a positive PST, as compared with 4% of controls. Neither IC nor control subjects had a positive test with 40 mL of water infusion. Parsons observed that there was an 85% positive test when the KCl was administered to gynecologic patients with chronic pelvic pain, leading him to conclude that most gynecologic patients with chronic pelvic pain have IC (29). This is compared with a rate of 38% as determined by cystoscopy and hydrodistention in patients with chronic pelvic pain (9).

However, the ability of the PST to diagnose IC has been questioned. Other investigators have

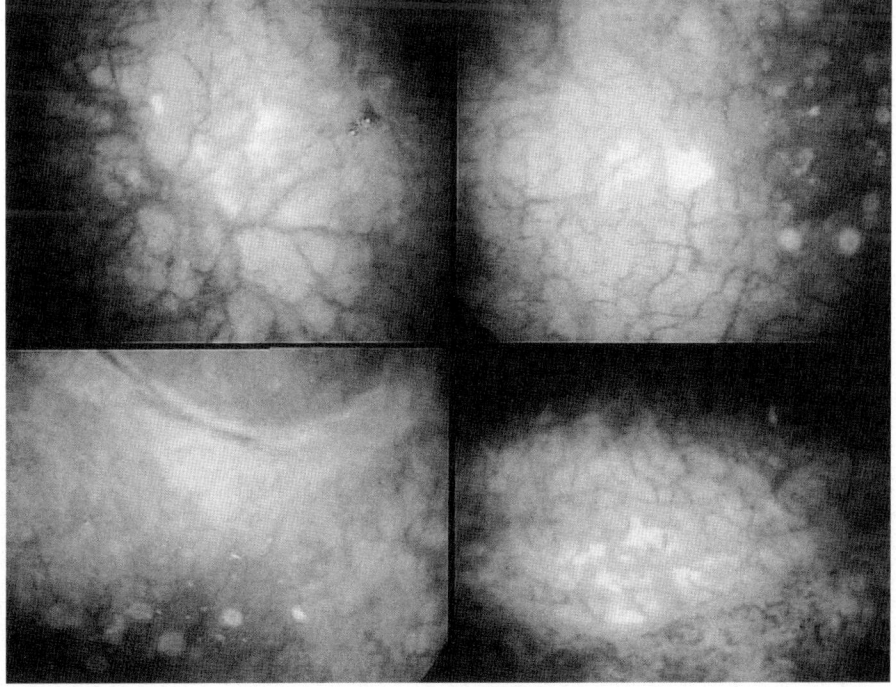

A

FIGURE 8.2 ● **(A)** IC before hydrodistention. The initial filling of the bladder appears normal. *(continued)*

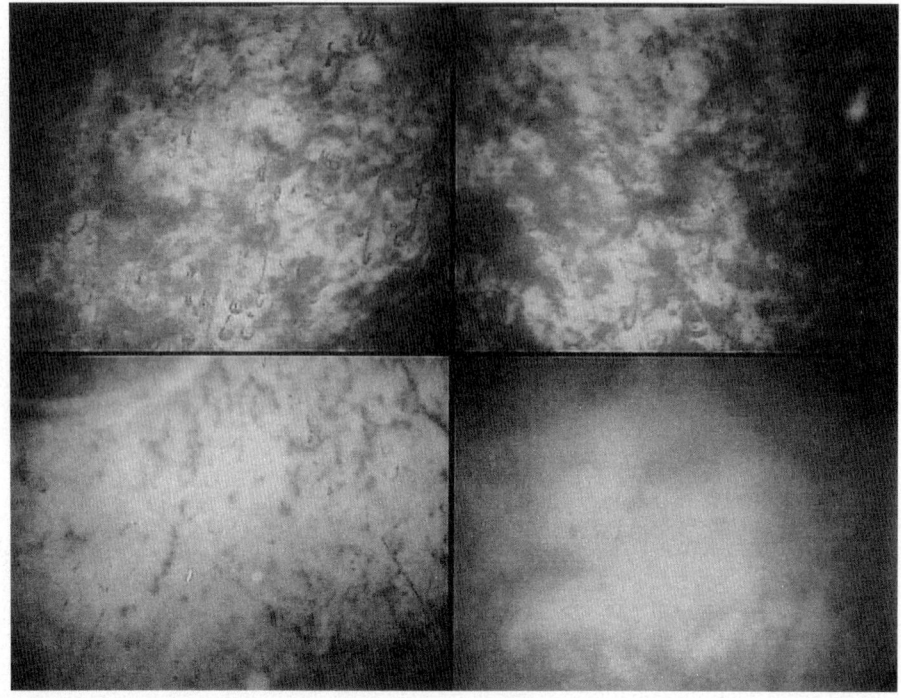

B

FIGURE 8.2 ● *(continued)* **(B)** IC after hydrodistention in same patient. Numerous petechiae and-glomerulations appear after the bladder has been distended and emptied, then refilled, indicating a diagnosis of IC. Eventually, enough blood accumulates to cloud the picture in the bottom right of figure.

noted that up to 25% of women with strict NIDDK criteria–positive IC had a negative PST and 36% of men without symptoms of IC had a positive PST (30,31). Finally, when the PST was compared with cystoscopy and hydrodistention as a diagnostic test, it fared no better in terms of positive predictive value (59% and 66%, respectively) in a population who had symptoms suggestive of IC (32). These investigators concluded that the general use of the PST is not validated and that we must continue to depend on cystoscopy and hydrodistention for the diagnosis of IC.

Finally, the PST does not discriminate between patients with IC and other forms of cystitis (bacterial, radiation, etc.), further limiting its role in diagnosis.

The PST has also been evaluated as a prognostic tool. Teichman found that a positive PST predicted better response to oral sodium pentosan polysulfate than occurs in patients with a negative PST (33). In this study, the complete NIDDK criteria were not used for the diagnosis of IC. Specifically, not all patients received cystoscopy and hydrodistention to look for glomerulations or Hunner's ulcers. Therefore, most patients had an IC diagnosis based solely on symptoms and exclusionary criteria. Interestingly, the IC patient population in this study had a 34% negative PST rate. The investigators gave sodium pentosan polysulfate to all patients regardless of whether their PST was positive or negative. Those who had a positive PST fared better than those who had a negative PST. However, the predictive value of a positive PST was not consistent across all improvement categories (i.e., greater than 25% improvement, greater than 50% improvement).

In conclusion, both "objective" diagnostic tests, hydrodistention under anesthesia and PST, have advantages and disadvantages. Hydrodistention has been traditionally used to categorize patients in NIH-funded studies. The anesthetic capacity of the bladder can be measured, and other potential anatomic abnormalities of the bladder can be cystoscopically assessed. Some patients may symptomatically benefit from hydrodistention, although some also have a temporary worsening of symptoms. PST is a noninvasive test meant to induce temporary pain in IC patients. It might also help to predict those who will respond to sodium pentosan polysulfate.

Taken in whole, the utility of these two tests requires further investigation. It also shows that until the pathophysiology of IC can be proved, a better diagnostic test (such as urine markers, discussed subsequently) awaits.

Role of Urinary Markers

Because of the dilemma that exists in the diagnosis of IC, many investigators have sought urine markers that might serve as noninvasive diagnostic surrogates. Finding a highly sensitive and specific urine marker will also serve to provide insights into the pathophysiologic mechanisms, which may eventually lead to specific targeted treatments. Many urinary substances have been described as increased or decreased in patients with IC compared with controls. These substances, such as histamine, interleukins, GAGs, hyaluronic acid, epithelial growth factors, nerve growth factor, and others, were selected based on theorized etiologies for IC. One of the major problems in using many of these substances as a diagnostic marker is that although the levels may be statistically significantly higher or lower in the IC population when averaged, there is significant overlap of values among control and IC subjects. The reasons for this may be that IC is multifactorial in etiology and that subgroups of IC patients exist depending on the cause. A more extensive review of urine markers has been recently published.

Two markers that have shown particular potential in diagnostic capability are glycoprotein-51 (GP-51) and antiproliferative factor (APF) (34,35). GP-51 levels in urine were examined in controls and those who met NIDDK criteria for IC (36). There was no overlap in urinary GP-51 concentration between those control and IC individuals. APF is a low-molecular-weight protein present in IC urine that is able to inhibit the ability of cultured normal bladder urothelial cells to incorporate ^{3}H-thymidine (37). Recently, both the molecular structure of APF and the receptor for APF have been identified (38,39). Therefore, the development of a clinical diagnostic kit and/or treatment aimed at APF–APF receptor interaction may be possible. The levels of APF activity in patients who meet NIDDK criteria for IC and in control urine specimens do not overlap (40). Both of these markers were based on the gold standard NIDDK objective criteria of presence of glomerulations on cystoscopy or hydrodistention, which may not be a specific finding. It is unknown how these urinary markers are altered in patients with painful bladder symptoms who do not fulfill the NIDDK criteria

for IC. Nevertheless, these two markers provide the foundation for elucidation of the pathophysiologic mechanisms involved in IC and may ultimately serve to be a diagnostic marker for IC.

Urodynamics

The use of urodynamics in the management of IC is also debated. The IC Database Study Group analyzed urodynamic data and compared them to data collected from voiding diaries (41). It was not surprising that urodynamic data closely correlated with the findings of the voiding diaries. Patients with low-volume, high-frequency voiding as recorded in a voiding diary had decreased cystometric capacity and decreased volume of first sensation. Therefore, it has been suggested that urodynamics are unnecessary in the evaluation of IC because the voiding diary, which is noninvasive, would capture the necessary information. However, some believe that urodynamics will allow discrimination between those patients with IC who have bladder symptoms and those with nonbladder symptoms (42). Patients who show motor instability on urodynamics are considered not to have IC and are treated with antimuscarinics.

Summary of Diagnostics

The diagnosis of IC remains a clinical one, and therefore the diagnosis of PBS carries a lot of credibility. The presence of small, frequent, painful voids in the absence of other potential pathologic etiologies is all that is required by most clinicians to render the diagnosis of IC. This criterion can be met employing a voiding diary, urine cultures, and clinical acumen. Cystoscopy, the PST, and urinary markers may eventually find a role in routine clinical practice, but currently they remain research tools for confirming the diagnosis of IC that is clinically suspected.

Treatment of Symptoms

After the diagnosis of IC has been made, a cornucopia of therapies exists. Unfortunately, many of these therapies have not been tested in a rigorous, randomized, blinded fashion using standardized data collection techniques and standardized questionnaire instruments. Part of the difficulty with treatment studies relates to the subjective nature of this condition. Additionally, the typical waxing–waning course of IC makes assessment of treatment modalities more difficult. Finally, because of the lack of understanding of the precise etiology of IC, there does not exist a highly effective treatment, and currently there is no cure for this disease. These reasons make it imperative to assess the outcomes of the available treatments scientifically so that clinicians can counsel patients on the best form of therapy. To date there are only a few prospective randomized clinical trials, with relatively small numbers (Table 8.3).

The NIH, in its commitment to understanding the pathophysiology and treatment of IC, is currently conducting multicenter clinical trials examining outcomes of different IC treatments in a prospective, randomized manner that addresses all these problematic issues. These clinical centers compose the NIH Interstitial Cystitis Clinical Trials Group (ICCTG). The ICCTG recently completed a four-arm blinded, prospective, randomized study comparing sodium pentosan polysulfate plus placebo, hydroxyzine plus placebo, sodium pentosan polysulfate plus hydroxyzine, and placebo plus placebo. Results from this study suggest that there was no benefit of sodium pentosan polysulfate or hydroxyzine over placebo, and therefore a larger trial was abandoned (43). There were many difficulties with this trial, including low patient recruitment, that led to smaller-than-anticipated patient numbers. Nevertheless, the results were not promising. A second clinical trial studying the effectiveness of intravesical bacille Calmette-Guérin (BCG) was recently completed by the same group, with similar findings of no significant efficacy of BCG over placebo (44). Currently, the ICCTG (renamed ICCRN [Interstitial Cystitis Clinical Research Network]) is conducting several other clinical trials in PBS/IC. However, until precise pathophysiologic mechanisms are identified, IC treatments will continue to be empiric (Table 8.4).

Oral-Based Therapies

Oral pharmacologic treatments remain a mainstay of therapy. Each of the following agents has been used with a specific targeted pathway in mind, and most are used in other diagnoses besides IC.

1. Sodium pentosan polysulfate (Elmiron): This medication was developed as a specific treatment for IC based on the theory that IC is due to a leaky urothelium because of the deficiency of the GAG layer in the bladder. Sodium pentosan polysulfate, a weak heparinoid, supposedly replenishes the GAG layer and thus makes the urothelium less leaky. This is the first oral medication for IC that has undergone randomized, placebo-controlled clinical trials (45–48). These studies have shown that sodium pentosan polysulfate can significantly decrease certain IC symptoms. Several caveats should be discussed. First, there seemed to be a period of time (3 to 6 months) before maximal beneficial effect was seen, and this was found in an open-label continuation of the initial clinical trials. Second, differences between control and treated patients in the early trials, although statistically significant, were not dramatically different from a clinical standpoint (28% of sodium pentosan polysulfate treated patients had more than 25% improvement versus 13% of placebo-treated patients). If IC is truly due to only a GAG deficiency that is readily reversible with sodium pentosan polysulfate, a high concentration of sodium pentosan polysulfate introduced intravesically should ameliorate all the symptoms of IC (because only

TABLE 8.3

Randomized Controlled Clinical Trials of IC Therapies

Drug	#RCTs	% improved with drug	% improved with placebo	p value
Amitriptyline (47) (n = 50)	1	63%	4%	<0.001
Pentosanpolysulphate (PPS) (40,42–45) (n = 62–248)	5	~30%	~15%	NS; 0.01
Hydroxyzine (49) (n = 121)	1	31%	20%	NS
Cyclosporine A (49) (n = 64)	1	40%	19% (comparator was PPS)	0.001
Intravesical DMSO (50) (n = 33)	1	40%	18%	Significant
Intravesical BCG (41) (n = 265)	1	21%	12%	0.062

TABLE 8.4

Interstitial Cystitis Therapies

"Standard" oral therapies	"Standard" intravesical therapies
Sodium pentosan polysulfate (Elmiron)	Dimethyl sulfoxide (DMSO)
Amitriptyline (Elavil)	Steroids (methylprednisolone)
Hydroxyzine (Atarax)	Heparin
Gabapentin (Neurontin)	Local anesthetics (Lidocaine, Marcaine)
Antimuscarinics (Detrol, Ditropan)	Sodium pentosan polysulfate (Elmiron)
Alpha-blockers (Hytrin)	Astringents (Chlorpactin, silver nitrate)

3% of the oral dose is excreted into the urinary tract). Empirically, this is not the case. There are some preliminary reports of combining pentosan polysulfate or heparin with lidocaine and sodium bicarbonate and administering it intravesically to provide acute relief (49).

2. Amitriptyline (Elavil): This tricyclic antidepressant has been used to decrease the chronic pain associated with IC. This medication is given once daily at about 6 p.m. and may also have a beneficial effect on sleep disturbances and decrease nocturia. The medication is titrated to effect until the side effects are intolerable (starting at 10 to 25 mg daily). This is one of the few medications studied that appears highly effective at reducing pain scores and alleviating bladder symptoms (50). Other investigators will need to confirm these results. The ICCRN is currently conducting a multi-institutional placebo-controlled randomized trial of amitriptyline for PBS, specifically for patients who have not been treated previously with other oral agents.

3. Hydroxyzine (Atarax): One of the theories for IC involves degranulation of mast cells with release of neuroactive and vasoactive chemicals. To prevent mast cell degranulation, antihistamines such as hydroxyzine have been suggested (51). Hydroxyzine also has a central nervous system effect, giving this medication sedative as well as anxiolytic effects. This medication was dosed at 25 mg given at bedtime and titrated up to 75 mg total (50 mg during the day and 25 mg at bedtime). However, the recent prospective, placebo-controlled randomized study demonstrated no statistically significant benefit over placebo (43). The possible synergy between hydroxyzine

and sodium pentosan polysulfate was also evaluated by this study, and still no effect over placebo was identified.

4. Cyclosporine A: Cyclosporine A is a calcineurin inhibitor that inhibits T-cell activation and stabilizes mast cells. It is a potent inhibitor of the immune system, used frequently to prevent graft rejection, and has been studied in IC patients because of the theory that IC is an autoimmune phenomenon. It has shown promise in one small randomized clinical trial using pentosan polysulfate as a comparator (52). The dose employed was 50 mg bid and had to be cut by 50% in roughly a third of subjects due to side effects.

5. Gabapentin (Neurontin): This is an antiepileptic medication that has gained popularity in the treatment of chronic pain disorders. Gabapentin is a neuronal stabilizer and thus can possibly hyperpolarize those neurons involved in pain transduction and increase sensory thresholds. Because chronic pelvic pain is a major component of IC symptoms, this medication is also being used clinically in IC patients (53). Because IC has a waxing–waning course and there are no objective markers for IC-related pain, studies on the efficacy of gabapentin in IC can prove to be difficult.

6. Antimuscarinics (oxybutynin, tolterodine, solafenacin, darifenacin, trospium): These agents have been developed as the primary agents to treat overactive bladder. Because the symptoms of overactive bladder overlap with IC, the use of these agents in IC is understandable. Antimuscarinics work by blocking the effect of acetylcholine at the neuromuscular junction in the detrusor smooth muscle. The efficacy of these medications is somewhat limited because both IC and overactive bladder are primarily

hypersensory conditions of the bladder. Blocking the motor end of the pathway does not prevent the afferent signal (bladder pain, urinary urgency) from being relayed to the higher neural centers, such as the brain.

Intravesical Therapy

Intravesical therapy allows the introduction of medications directly into the bladder. There are potentially fewer side effects with intravesical administration, primarily because of the lack of systemic absorption if the dwell time of the intravesical agent used is kept short. If the pathophysiology of IC is related directly to urothelial abnormalities, intravesical therapy makes more sense because these agents can directly target the urothelium. Intravesical therapy typically involves the mixture of multiple medications (as a "cocktail"). Again, as for the oral agents, no large prospective, randomized, and blinded trial has been performed for any of these agents, either singly or as a mixture. The following list includes the most commonly used agents.

1. Dimethyl sulfoxide (DMSO): This agent is probably the most used intravesical agent in the treatment of IC. The mechanism of action is thought to be anti-inflammatory. Another described mechanism is depletion of sensory neuropeptides from afferent nerves over a period of time, which leads to a salutary response of decreased pain, voiding frequency, and urgency. The initial release of sensory neuropeptides may help explain the pain that DMSO causes during initial intravesical administration. Another potential mechanism of DMSO is mast cell inhibition. The dose of DMSO used intravesically is 50 mL of a 50% solution. There is one small prospective randomized study to suggest it does have some efficacy (54).

2. Steroids (methylprednisolone): Steroids can also be given intravesically. From 500 mg to 1 g of methylprednisolone can be reconstituted in a small volume (10 to 15 mL) and mixed with DMSO. The rationale for using this agent relates to its anti-inflammatory actions.

3. Heparin: One of the etiologies of IC is theorized to be a decrease in the GAG layer of the uroepithelium. Heparin, which is a GAG derivative, is thought to help replenish this diminished layer. Typically 10,000 to 20,000 U of heparin in 2 to 5 mL of solution is used intravesically.

4. Local anesthetic: Lidocaine (1%) or bupivacaine (Marcaine) (0.5%) may be used. Usually, 20 to 30 mL of local anesthetic is sufficient.

These agents are mixed as a cocktail, infused into the bladder through a urethral catheter, and left to dwell for 30 to 60 minutes (or as long as patients can tolerate). Patients usually undergo one treatment per week for a 6-week period. The selection of this regimen is purely empiric. Some patients have more durable responses when a maintenance schedule of intravesical treatment is given (such as a biweekly or monthly treatment after the initial 6-week treatment).

Other agents that have been used intravesically include silver nitrate and Clorpactin. Both work as bladder astringents. Essentially, these agents coagulate the surface proteins on the urothelium and induce a regenerative reaction of the urothelium. Because of the nature of these agents, they cause pain when infused and thus are typically given under anesthesia in the operating room. These agents have fallen out of favor, not because of clinical data, but because they cause intense pain when infused and require anesthesia to administer.

Other intravesical therapies that are being studied and contemplated include several new agents. One is resiniferatoxin (RTX), a suprapotentanalogue of the hot-pepper derivative capsaicin. RTX works by releasing sensory neuropeptides such as substance P and calcitonin gene-related peptide (CGRP). Over an extended time, RTX should desensitize the sensory nerve of the bladder. An initial study in very few IC patients revealed that RTX was effective (55).

Along these same lines (e.g., modulating the bladder sensory response), some have theorized that the phenotype and function of the sensory nerves can be modulated with gene therapy by introducing a vector through intravesical injection of a herpes simplex type 1 virus. This concept has been proved possible because a gene product (nerve growth factor) has been delivered to and expressed by the dorsal root ganglia neurons (sensory neurons) from intravesical injection of the herpes simplex virus carrying the *NGF* gene (56). Therefore, the theory is that the virus can be engineered to carry a destructive gene that will knock out the sensory function of the dorsal root ganglia neurons and thus render the bladder asensate, and that this could be used to treat a hypersensory disorder such as IC.

A recent study by the ICCTG involved intravesical BCG bacilli. BCG is currently approved by the U.S. Food and Drug Administration (FDA) for treating bladder cancer (carcinoma *in situ*). In a small prospective, randomized, blinded, placebo-controlled trial, intravesical BCG has shown efficacy in reducing IC symptoms; however, these results were not replicable by another group of investigators (57,58). Therefore, the ICCTG replicated these studies using a multi-institutional prospective, randomized, placebo-controlled trial, which did not demonstrate any significant efficacy over placebo (59).

Surgical Therapies to Reduce Symptoms

Major surgical intervention is not the mainstay in treatment of IC symptoms. Nevertheless, cystectomy or bladder augmentation has been described to treat IC (60–62). These aggressive interventions are typically reserved for those patients with a small contracted bladder as measured during cystoscopy and hydrodistention under general anesthesia. One would think that cystectomy with urinary diversion would alleviate these patients' symptoms, but there are anecdotal reports that symptoms persist despite urinary diversion. Although all these studies examining major surgical intervention in IC report excellent outcomes, these studies suffer the same methodologic flaws as all studies on IC—namely, too few patients with no standardized outcome parameters. Clearly, aggressive approaches to treating IC must be applied to carefully selected patients with clearly documented small, contracted bladders during cystoscopy under anesthesia.

Less invasive surgical approaches to treat IC include chronic sacral neuromodulation (InterStim, Medtronic Corporation, Minneapolis, MN). This therapy involves chronic electrical stimulation (by an implanted pulse generator) of the S3 nerve root through an implanted lead placed through the S3 foramen (see Chapter 12 for a full discussion).

The use of the neodymium:YAG laser to fulgurate Hunner's ulcers to alleviate IC symptoms has also been described (63). Twenty-four patients underwent this procedure and had a mean follow-up time of 23 months. There was documented effectiveness in decreasing IC symptoms, but about half of the patients required one to four retreatments with repeat laser fulgurations during the mean 23 months of follow-up. Although this is a relatively noninvasive technique, most IC patients do not have Hunner's ulcers, which makes this therapy not widely applicable. Finally, as in most IC therapies, there has not been a randomized trial comparing outcomes of laser fulguration and cystoscopy alone.

Future Directions

It is obvious that the major goal in IC is to understand the pathophysiology of this disease. Many theories have been proposed, each based on some supporting experimental data. However, a consistent theme is that IC is a result of bladder urothelial abnormalities. Increased permeability of the bladder urothelium due to a deficient GAG layer was one of the early hypotheses that ultimately led to the use of sodium pentosan polysulfate for treatment and to the development of the PST for diagnosis of IC. It is unclear whether this is the ultimate pathway in the development for IC.

Altered peptide growth factor production by the urothelial cells is another pathogenic hypothesis that has received much attention because of the strength of the literature supporting this theory. Studying biochemical alterations in IC urothelial cells will prove to be valuable for understanding the pathophysiology of IC and is hoped to lead to a noninvasive diagnostic test with high sensitivity and specificity. The growth factors that seem the most promising are heparin-binding epidermal growth factor (HB-EGF) and APF (36,64). It has been shown that the IC urothelium produces APF, which inhibits the growth of normal bladder urothelium and thus may inhibit the IC urothelium from regenerating properly, either in the course of normal bladder homeostasis or in response to some insult such as acute bacterial cystitis. APF, furthermore, inhibits the production of other growth factors required for epithelial growth, such as HB-EGF. The abnormalities of these growth factors are providing the basis to develop a urinary test that can be performed in an office setting to diagnose IC. Additionally, another theory is that reversal of these growth factor abnormalities might ameliorate IC symptoms or even cure IC.

Recently, the bladder urothelium has been determined to have a sensory role in bladder function from experimental animal models, which represents a new paradigm for bladder urothelial function (65–67). Traditionally, the urothelium has been thought to serve only a protective function for the bladder, but several intriguing laboratory findings have suggested that the bladder urothelium may be crucial in relaying the sensation of bladder fullness to the brain. When the bladder urothelial cells are stretched during bladder filling, they release adenosine triphosphate, which then acts as a sensory neurotransmitter by binding to sensory nerve terminals located histologically just below the bladder urothelium. It has been shown that this process is augmented in IC, thus possibly explaining the hypersensory defect in IC (68). The vanilloid receptor TRPV1 has been detected in the bladder urothelial cells and, when activated, causes a release of nitric oxide, which can activate suburothelial nerves (69). These data, taken together, strongly suggest that the urothelium may serve as a sensory transducer for the bladder in addition to providing a barrier function. Currently, no medications are available to increase sensory thresholds of the bladder. Development of a bladder-specific analgesic agent could provide an effective treatment for IC.

As discussed previously, the concept of gene therapy using a gene product delivered by a virus introduced into the bladder is also being actively studied (53). The goal of gene therapy would be to deliver a gene to the dorsal root ganglia cells or possibly the bladder uroepithelial cells that would interfere with the sensory function of the bladder or reverse the pathophysiologic defect identified (Table 8.5).

Summary

IC is a disease complex with a core problem that involves the bladder. The epidemiology, genetics, diagnosis, and treatment of IC are still undergoing evolution. The key to IC undoubtedly is determining the etiology. It is probable that ultimately IC is multifactorial and therefore has different etiologies in different patients. However, our current diagnostic abilities cannot separate IC patients into different subcategories, except for perhaps ulcerative (Hunner's ulcer) versus nonulcerative IC. There is no cure for this debilitating problem, and current treatments only alleviate symptoms. To understand this disease will require a new paradigm in which sequential advances that characterize study of other diseases will apply to IC. Advances in IC will occur in parallel in different arenas, including epidemiology, genetics, diagnosis, and treatment, which should all converge on the etiologies of this enigmatic disease.

PAINFUL DISORDERS OF THE URETHRA

Similar to painful conditions of the bladder, painful conditions of the urethra can be difficult to define and manage. These urethral conditions are often mislabeled and treated as a simple lower urinary tract infection that responds poorly to antimicrobial agents and delay diagnosis. As will be noticed, many of the complaints overlap those of PBS or IC, making it difficult to differentiate the two on history. In addition, there are those who ascribe all urethral complaints to PBS or IC. However, there are some findings that distinguish the painful conditions of the urethra from the bladder, and there are many patients who can benefit from reasonable treatment of a variety of urethral conditions. The sections discussed in this chapter include the following:

- Urethral pain syndrome
- Atrophic urethritis
- Acute urethritis
- Meatal abnormalities
- Urethral diverticulum

Urethral Pain Syndrome

Sensory disorders of the urethra are both distressing and disabling conditions. They can be defined as a symptom complex including urinary frequency, urgency, dysuria, suprapubic pain, postvoid fullness, urinary hesitancy, dyspareunia, and urge incontinence, in the absence of significant bacteriuria or structural urinary tract abnormality. Most patients think they have a urinary tract infection, and many have been treated on several occasions for this problem, either without resolution or with rapid recurrence. Often, the patient responds after 1 or 2 days of antibiotic therapy and then relapses very soon after the course is complete. Other patients present with a history of recurrent yeast infections, for which they now self-medicate almost weekly with very poor relief. Many patients have a combination of recurrent antibiotic therapy, followed by a history of recurrent yeast infections. Many physicians still use the term "urethral syndrome," as devised by Gallagher et al, to describe the condition; however, this condition has had many pseudonyms, including nonbacterial urethritis and external urethral sphincter spasticity to name a few (70). The most recent terminology, adopted by the ICS, is "urethral pain syndrome," which is defined as the occurrence of persistent or recurrent episodic urethral pain usually on voiding,

TABLE 8.5

Potential Future Therapies (Symptom Relief or Cure)

Gene therapy delivered intravesically
Sensory modulators (e.g., resiniferatoxin)
Botulinum toxin
Growth factor regulators
Sacral neuromodulation

with daytime frequency and nocturia, in the absence of proven infection or other obvious pathology (2). The diagnosis implies longevity of symptoms, and 6 months is a minimal duration of the problem.

However, despite this new definition of an old problem, there is very little literature on urethral pain syndrome outside of prostatitis. A PubMed search failed to reveal any literature on this condition in women, and the majority of the literature continues to use the term "urethral syndrome."

Incidence

The incidence and prevalence of the condition are not known, but of patients presenting with lower urinary tract symptoms in the absence of infection, 15% to 30% were diagnosed with urethral syndrome (71,72). A more likely number is in the range of less than 5%. In a questionnaire to 792 members of the American Urogynecologic Society, with a 31% response rate, most practitioners saw zero to five patients per month with this condition. The age groups more commonly affected are 20 to 30 years and 50 to 60 years.

Etiology

The etiology has previously been explored, and in the numerous explanations of causality, the pathophysiology has been developed for each proposed cause. The etiology at best is unclear. The more common factors implicated are as follows: (a) infectious—low growth of common organisms often detectable only in the urethra (73); (b) fastidious organisms—*Chlamydia trachomatis, Mycoplasma hominis, Ureaplasma urealyticum* (74,75); (c) early manifestation of IC (76,77); (d) response to stress (78,79); (e) hypersensitivity dysfunction (80,81); and (f) levator myofascial syndrome (82–84). Other causes include allergy, trauma, anatomic features, coexisting medical conditions, urethral instability, external urethral spasm, and urethral obstruction (85–88).

Evaluation

The evaluation requires the basic evaluation for an incontinent patient, which includes history, physical examination, urinalysis and culture, residual urine determination, and 24-hour voiding diary (89). The rest of the workup is a means to exclude other causes of the irritation. The differential diagnosis includes urethral pain syndrome, urinary tract infection, and vaginitis. Other conditions to be ruled out include atrophic urethral changes, acute or subacute urethritis, unstable or overactive bladder, local urethral anatomic pathology, suburethral diverticulum, bladder stone, bladder cancer, and PBS (IC). Additional studies may include wet preparations for vaginal infections, urethral culture, cervical culture for sexually transmitted disease, cystourethroscopy, and cystometrogram.

Treatment

The treatment for urethral pain syndrome is not specific and requires a persistent approach with frequent patient follow-up and reassessment of progress. Most patients are improved over time, with a treatment course lasting up to 2 years for resolution. Much effort is expended in explanation of the condition, its interaction with many body functions, and its gradual road to recovery given the duration of its course to this point. Although many patients have had several years of discomfort before commencing therapy, the treatment course is productive, and there is little connection of this specific focus of urethral pain with the more profound diagnosis of IC.

Because much of this process is trial and error, and there is considerable difference of opinion regarding efficacy, the treatment approaches are described in a logical order in which to proceed in dealing with a refractory patient. Less well-defined modalities are included (Table 8.6).

The first step is to explain that the nerve endings supplying sensation of pain and discomfort to

TABLE 8.6

Treatment of Urethral Pain Syndrome

Extensive explanation of the condition and potential etiology

Dietary changes

Fluid intake

Manage acute or subacute urethral infection

Treat documented urinary tract infection

Prophylaxis against recurrent urinary tract infections

Antispasmodic/analgesic

Anti-inflammatory medication trial

Pain modulation: antidepressant medication

Urethral muscle relaxants

Pelvic floor muscle rehabilitation

Urethral dilation and massage

Steroid periurethral injection

Acupuncture

Overactive bladder medication

Sacral nerve neuromodulation

Urethroplasty

TABLE 8.7

Pharmacologic Management of Urethral Pain Syndrome

Antibiotics
  Subacute
    Azithromycin (Zithromax), 500 mg/d for 6 d
    Doxycycline, 100 bid for 14 d
  Chronic (suppression)
    Nitrofurantoin, 50 mg/d
    Trimethoprim/sulfamethoxazole (TMP/SMZ) (40/200), 1 tablet daily
    Cephalosporin, 250 mg/d
    Norfloxacin (Noroxin), 400 mg/d
Antispasmodic/analgesic
  Pyridium plus 1 tablet tid
  Methenamine hippurate (Urised), 1 or 2 tablets qid
Anti-inflammatory
  Celecoxib (Celebrex), 200 mg bid
  Ibuprofen (Motrin), 800 mg tid
Antidepressants—chronic pain modulators
  Amitriptyline HCl (Elavil), 12.5 to 100 mg/d at 6 p.m.
  Doxepin HCl, 12.5 to 100 mg/d
  Nortriptyline HCl, 12.5 to 100 mg/d
  Selective serotonin reuptake inhibitors (SSRIs), usual antidepressant dose
Urethral smooth muscle relaxants
  Doxazosin mesylate (Cardura), 1 to 8 mg/d
  Prazosin HCl (Minipress), 1 to 2 mg bid
  Terazosin HCl (Hytrin), 1 to 5 mg once daily
  Phenoxybenzamine HCl (Dibenzyline), 10 to 20 mg once or twice daily
Urethral skeletal muscle relaxant
  Diazepam (Valium), 2 to 5 mg tid
Anticonvulsant
  Gabapentin (Neurontin), 300 to 1,200 mg tid
Frequency–urgency symptoms (overactive bladder)
  Oxybutynin chloride (Ditropan XL), 5 to 30 mg/d
  Tolterodine tartrate (Detrol LA), 4 mg/d

the urethra and pelvic area have probably been hypersensitized by some process, and these patients have a low sensation threshold (90). The source of this inciting agent may never be determined, but the important treatment theory is to interrupt the cycle of pain or discomfort and allow the patient to return gradually to normal function. There is no question regarding the validity, severity, and physical nature of the symptoms. The treatment may take as long to reverse the process as the process itself has been present. A lot of effort is expended in how the patient can assist her own recovery by doing certain things, or avoiding certain things, during an exacerbation. The most comprehensive approach is a multidisciplinary one that includes pain medication, local treatment regimens, physical therapy, and psychological support. However, the patient does best in a single-office setting with an understanding therapist (physician) who is able to direct management in all these areas while being the major support figure for the patient.

The importance of diet and fluid intake is difficult to determine, and most of the time this has already been modified by patient experimentation. Generally, caffeine products and alcoholic beverages should be avoided. The effect of high-acid or spicy foods is uncertain. A modest fluid intake is desirable, and water is best because it is devoid of additives.

Many of the inciting factors for initiating the disease process are infection-related, with a subsequent poor resolution of accompanying symptoms. Patients often report quick response with antibiotic therapy the first several times they had what they thought was an infection, but gradually the treatment courses are less effective and the episodes are more frequent. It is still important to be certain that there is no residual acute or subacute infective source, and at least one full course of doxycycline or azithromycin should be considered (Table 8.7). If this has been done previously, there is no need to repeat an adequate course of therapy unless the patient found the previous treatment effective in correcting symptoms for an extended time period.

The next object of therapy is to prevent recurring urinary tract infections, particularly if these have been documented and considered causal in the disease process. If the patient was treated for infections that were not proven by microscopy or culture, the first two episodes should be managed by seeing the patient and obtaining urine for microscopy and culture. Treatment of documented infection with a standard 5-day course of trimethoprim–sulfamethoxazole, nitrofurantoin (Macrobid), or cephalosporin is adequate.

The patient will need something for days when symptoms are increasing in severity with evidence of negative microbiology. The antispasmodic–analgesic preparations may be administered for a 1- to 3-day course to get over this episode and then reserved for future need. Some patients can get through the day with only one dose of the medication, but they require it each day. This is appropriate therapy for a few months while awaiting the impact of other definitive therapy. Concurrently, a course of an anti-inflammatory such as celecoxib (Celebrex) or ibuprofen (Motrin) may be initiated.

The selection of the next agent carries a wide array of opinions. Amitriptyline is a tricyclic antidepressant from a generation ago that has been found to have pain-modulating effects and is extensively used in chronic pain syndromes, IC, and urethral pain syndrome (91). The medication must be given at the time of the evening meal or earlier to avoid the severe drowsiness that ordinarily hits the next morning. It should be commenced in a very low dose of 10 to 12.5 mg and increased in 2- to 6-week intervals to ensure lack of serious side effects. Efficacy cannot usually be determined for at least 6 to 8 weeks. Patients still get dry mouth and may have some alteration or slowing of bowel function. After 3 months of therapy, the side effects become much less pronounced, although a prolonged low-dosage level may be required before increasing the dose to determine efficacy. The course duration is 1 to 3 years. Some patients sensitive to amitriptyline are able to tolerate doxepin, and some therapists prefer the latter agent. The selective serotonin reuptake inhibitors have been suggested and used, but the effect may be more for the antidepressant properties and perhaps even the mood-elevating properties associated with some of these preparations.

The combination of urethral skeletal and smooth muscle relaxants has been used for a long time, and many physicians find this effective as an initial approach (92). The dose of diazepam should be kept low and the course of therapy not prolonged beyond 1 year because of risk for dependency. The choice of smooth muscle relaxant has some options, and although phenoxybenzamine was originally used, the safer products now are doxazosin mesylate (Cardura), prazosin, and terazosin HCl (Hytrin) (93).

As part of a multidisciplinary approach, pelvic floor muscle exercises and bladder-retraining drills with or without biofeedback may provide a form of bladder physiotherapy to which some patients respond. The bladder retraining is especially helpful in patients with urinary frequency. The pelvic floor exercises are useful for coordinating pelvic floor muscles, but the relaxation component of the exercise program may help with relieving overactive pelvic muscles. The extension of this program is in the area of myofascial trigger points, which can be manually released for symptom relief (see Chapter 9).

The use of urethral dilation and massage is an older technique that can provide immediate relief. The once-common initial treatment is still deemed effective by those trained to use it but is falling out of use (94). There are very few studies to suggest it is an effective therapy, but those who perform it claim excellent results. Another procedure performed infrequently is urethroplasty (95). Acupuncture use may be considered before invasive therapy (96).

Sacral neuromodulation in the treatment of overactive bladder symptoms and some pelvic

TABLE 8.8

Vaginal Estrogen Preparations

Estradiol (Estrace), 0.1 mg/g, 42.5-g tube	1 to 2 g one to three times per week
Premarin, 0.625 mg/g, 42-g tube	1 to 2 g one to three times per week
Estropipate (Ogen), 1.5 mg/g, 42-g tube	1 to 2 g one to three times per week
Estradiol vaginal tablets (Vagifem), 25 μg	1 or 2 tablets weekly
Estradiol vaginal ring (Estring), 2 mg	1 ring every 3 months

pain conditions has been established. The frequency–urgency symptoms of IC have also responded to this intervention. It makes sense that the urethral pain syndrome and its myriad of symptoms may also be treated by this modality (see Chapter 12). There is a paucity of information on neuromodulation for urethral pain syndrome, but the expanded use of this modality and its modifications should provide continuing additions to the literature over the next few years.

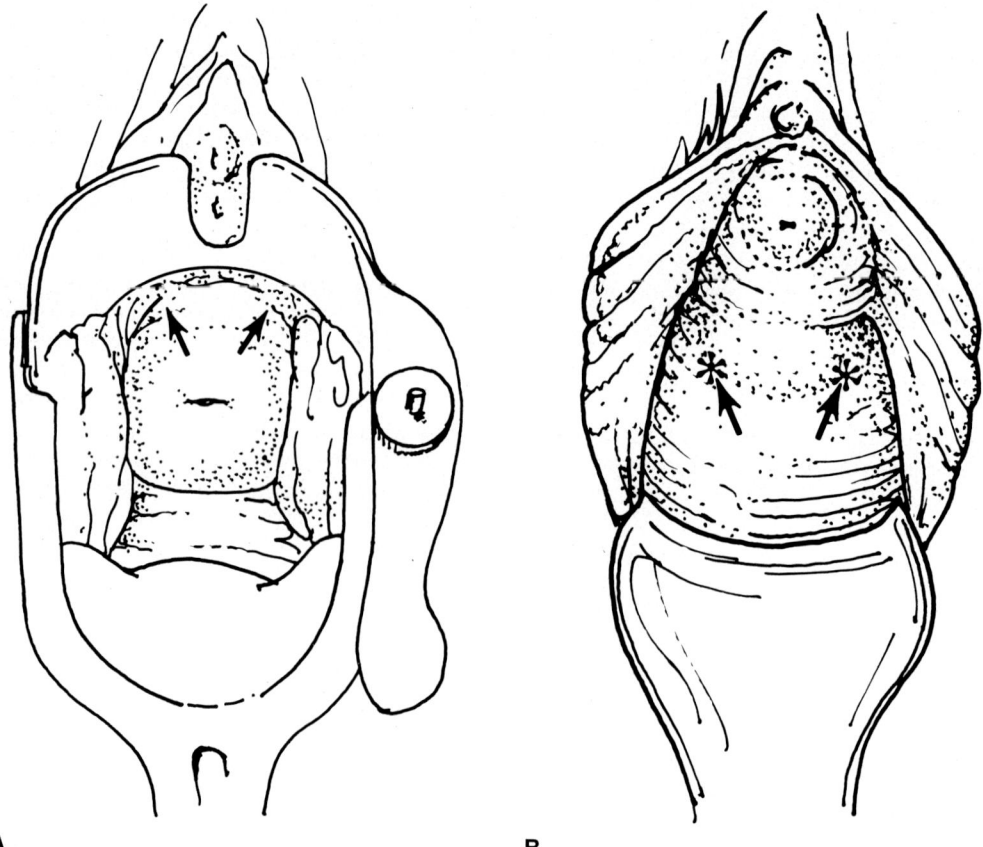

A   **B**

FIGURE 8.3   ●   Bladder pillar block. **(A)** With speculum in place, bladder pillars are at the 2- and 10-o'clock positions (*arrows*), at the attachment to the cervix. **(B)** If there is no cervix, the urethrovesical junction is visualized and the injections are placed at 5 and 7 o'clock (*arrows*). (From Ostergard DR. Bladder pillar block anesthesia for urethral dilatation in women. *Am J Obstet Gynecol* 1980;136:187–188, with permission.)

Atrophic Urethritis

The urethra is an estrogen-sensitive organ (97,98). Atrophic changes result from lack of estrogen, which normally occurs in varying degrees of severity after spontaneous or surgical menopause in the absence of hormone replacement therapy. Sometimes, oral replacement is not sufficient to prevent local vaginal or urethral changes.

Evaluation

Presenting symptoms include dyspareunia, vaginal discharge, urgency, frequency, dysuria, recurrent urinary tract infections, and urinary stress incontinence. Diagnosis is by clinical examination of the vagina and pelvic organs. Saline wet preparations may be prepared from a gentle scrape of the lateral vaginal wall and the slide observed for mature versus immature epithelial cells. Vaginal pH may be increased from a normal of 4 to between 6 and 7. Blood values of follicle-stimulating hormone and estradiol may not reflect local estrogen effects. Urethroscopy may reveal a pale urethra or one that is easily irritated by movement of the scope through it.

Treatment

Urogenital tissues are more sensitive to estrogen than other tissues, and absorption of low-dose topical applications is highest when the vaginal epithelium is atrophic and decreases as the epithelium matures. Oral preparations are used according to appropriate indications and contraindications. Atrophic changes of the bladder and vagina respond to topical therapy, such as one fourth to one third of an applicator of vaginal cream two or three times per week (Table 8.8) (99–101). While there is no data specific to atrophic urethritis, symptoms associated with urogenital atrophy respond to topical estrogen therapy. The medication should be continued indefinitely at a maintenance dose.

Acute Urethritis

This condition is more common in young patients and generally implies one of the sexually transmitted disease entities. The onset of symptoms is recent, and the duration of the problem is generally less than 1 month before consultation. The incubation period for gonorrhea is as short as 1 day and usually within 2 weeks, whereas the incubation period for chlamydia is 1 to 2 weeks and may be up to 5 weeks. Occasionally a low-grade infection may persist, and symptoms may suggest the urethral pain syndrome. The infection may also persist in an asymptomatic state.

Evaluation

Symptoms are usually dysuria, urgency, and frequency. Urethral discharge is uncommon in female patients. The differential diagnosis must include urinary tract infection, vulvovaginal inflammation, primary and recurrent herpes simplex virus inflammation, and local trauma. Vaginal examination is performed. Wet preparations are made for trichomonal infections, yeast, and clue cells. Primary herpetiform lesions are cultured. Specimens are taken for chlamydia and gonorrhea isolation. Urine microscopy or culture is performed to rule out urinary tract infection. Patients diagnosed with a sexually transmitted disease should have serologic testing for syphilis. Cystourethroscopy is indicated for treatment failures and persisting symptoms.

Treatment

Gonorrhea is managed according to Centers for Disease Control and Prevention recommendations, which can be a single dose of cephalosporin or fluoroquinolone followed by 7 days of doxycycline to cover chlamydia, or a single dose of azithromycin, 1 g given orally. The usual recommendation for nongonococcal urethritis is treatment for 7 days with tetracycline, 500 mg given four times a day, or doxycycline, 100 mg twice daily. Alternative therapies include azithromycin, 1 g as a single dose; erythromycin, 500 mg four times daily for 7 days or 250 mg four times daily for 14 days; and ofloxacin, 300 mg twice daily for 7 days. More recent information suggests that a 6-day course of azithromycin, 500 mg once daily, or a 14-day course of doxycycline, 100 mg twice daily, is more effective (102).

Meatal Abnormalities

The urethral lesions that are often disturbing to the patient include caruncle, prolapse, and polyps.

A caruncle is an inflammatory lesion on the posterior aspect of the urethral meatus. It is red and measures 5 to 10 mm in size. Symptoms may not be present or may include pain and bleeding. Treatment includes topical estrogen therapy and occasionally local removal using cryosurgery, laser, or excision. A pillar block is useful analgesia for doing the procedure in the office or clinic setting (Fig. 8.3) (103).

Urethral prolapse is a circumferential red mucosal eversion extending outside the urethral meatus. It is seldom painful but may bleed, especially in children. Treatment is by topical estrogen application for a 2- to 3-month course. It is seldom necessary to perform surgical removal, but the techniques described previously can be used.

Urethral polyps are virtually always benign, but occasionally they protrude from inside the urethra canal and present as a lump or with bleeding. Urethroscopy is used to determine the extent of the abnormality. Treatment is seldom required, but usually an endoscopic maneuver is required to sever the polyp at the base.

Urethral Diverticulum

A diverticulum is a branch or sac pouching out from a hollow organ. An urethral diverticulum is generally located posteriorly anywhere along the urethra, and there may be more than one. The etiology is thought to be obstruction of the duct from a paraurethral gland, although congenital defects have been postulated.

Evaluation

Some diverticula are asymptomatic, but common symptoms include recurrent urinary tract infections, suburethral cyst, painful intercourse, and

TABLE 8.9

Clinical Symptoms of Urethral Diverticula

Asymptomatic recurrent urinary tract infection
Vaginal mass
Dyspareunia
Incontinence
Postmicturition dribbling
Dysuria
Hematuria
Frequency, urgency
Pain
Urinary retention

urinary incontinence (Table 8.9) (104). The size of the diverticular ostia may determine symptoms in that large-necked diverticula are more apt to be as-

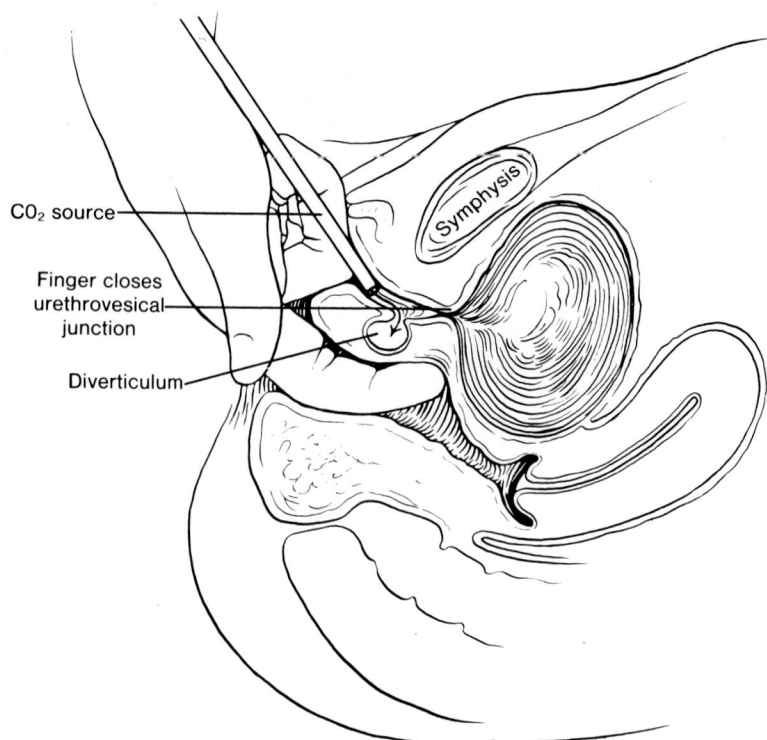

CO$_2$ source

Finger closes urethrovesical junction

Diverticulum

Symphysis

FIGURE 8.4 ● Urethroscopy with occlusion of bladder neck. The bladder is distended with fluid, and the urethrovesical junction is occluded with the examining finger. The fluid is allowed to run briskly, and as the urethroscope is slowly withdrawn, the diverticular opening distends and is visible.

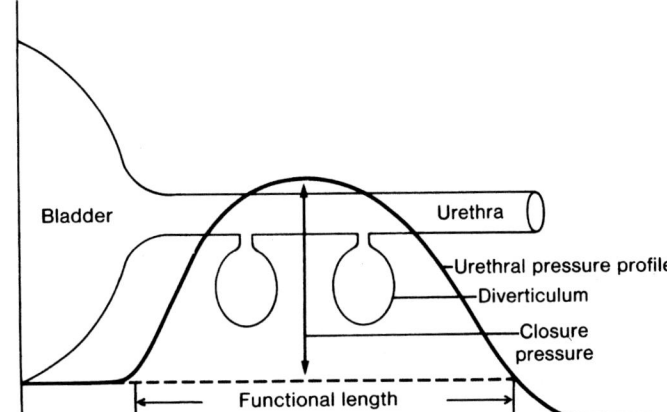

FIGURE 8.5 ● Urethral closure pressure profile with superimposed diverticular orifices proximal and distal to peak urethral closure pressure.

sociated with incontinence, and small-necked diverticula are more frequently associated with pain or recurrent infections. During vaginal examination, a cyst may be seen under the urethra, and pus may be able to be expressed by compression and movement of the examining finger distally along the urethra. A sound or a catheter placed in the urethra may facilitate this examination. Urine is obtained for examination and culture. Frequently, the clinical examination is benign.

Urethroscopy may show one or more posterior openings along the urethra that on compression are associated with extrusion of pus material (Fig. 8.4).

Urodynamics should be performed to determine the concurrent presence of genuine stress incontinence and the quality of the urethral sphinc-ter mechanism. The urethral closure pressure can have a biphasic profile, and the position of the pressure drop reflects the location of the diverticulum related to the high urethral pressure zone (Fig. 8.5). This has been important in determining the type of surgical repair because a distal diverticulum could be treated by a marsupialization procedure; however, the pressure depression in the profile may not accurately indicate the position of the diverticulum opening into the urethra (105).

Transvaginal or endoluminal ultrasonography may accurately predict multiple diverticula (106,107). Positive-pressure urethrography with a Davis or Tratner catheter has been a longstanding technique for identifying urethral diverticula (Figs. 8.6 through 8.8). A voiding cystourethrogram may

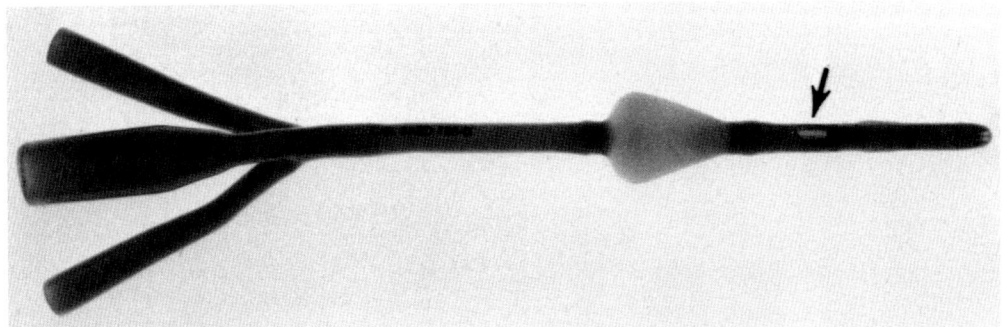

FIGURE 8.6 ● The Tratner catheter. The triple-lumen catheter has a distal balloon that is filled with air to keep it in the bladder by resting against the bladder neck. The proximal balloon is inflated with air and then slides along the catheter to fit snugly against the urethra to prevent escape of dye from the urethral meatus. The third lumen is injected with contrast material, which egresses through an opening between the two air-filled balloons and distends the urethra and urethral diverticulum.

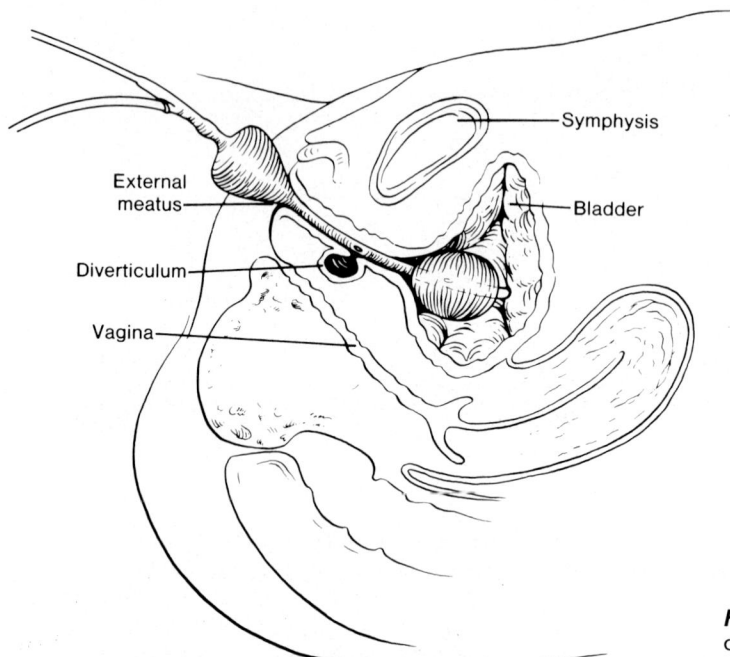

FIGURE 8.7 ● The Tratner catheter in place in the urethra.

also be performed for diagnosis. Recently, magnetic resonance imaging has been used (108). The accuracy of the various methods of diagnosis is summarized in Table 8.10.

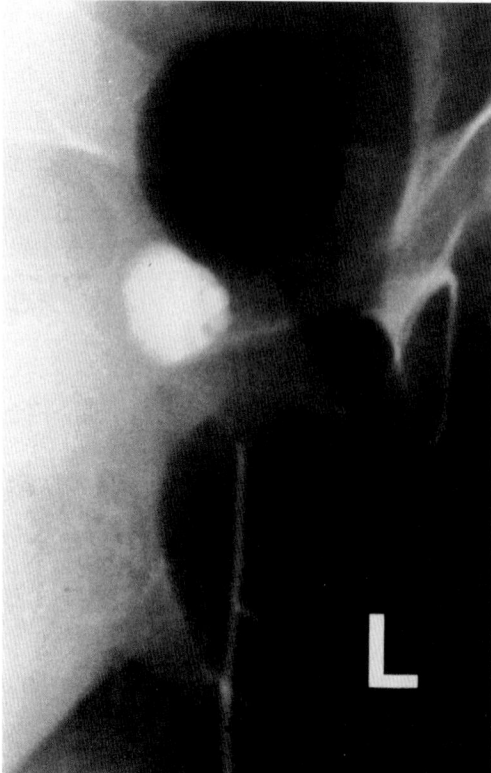

FIGURE 8.8 ● Radiologic view of urethral diverticulum. The diverticulum is filled with contrast material, which shows nicely between the two air-filled balloons.

TABLE 8.10

Efficacy of Diagnostic Modalities in Diagnosing Urethral Diverticula

Technique	Accuracy (%)
Radiologic	
Voiding cystourethrography	65 to 77
Positive-pressure urethrography	90
Ultrasound	
Transvaginal	90
Intraluminal	100
Urodynamics	
Urethral pressure profile	72
Endoscopy	
Urethroscopy	90

From Cundiff DW. Urethral diverticula. In: Cundiff GW, Bent AE, eds. *Endoscopic diagnosis of the female lower urinary tract.* London: WB Saunders, 1999: 43–51, with permission.

Treatment

The Spence procedure is used for diverticula when the sac is located distally below the midurethral pressure peak. The diverticulum is marsupialized and the defect closed with 4-0 polyglycolic acid suture (Fig. 8.9).

A midurethral diverticulum or one located more proximally requires excision (109). The principles are to dissect carefully, creating several layers to be closed later over the repair. A Martius graft may be beneficial to prevent wound breakdown and fistula. Intraoperative urethroscopy is helpful in localizing the diverticulum, and sometimes a Fogarty catheter can be placed transurethrally into

the diverticular opening and inflated, if there is not a palpable cyst structure. An inverted U incision is used over the diverticulum and the vaginal epithelium is reflected inferiorly. A vertical incision is next made in the pubocervical fascia, which is gradually dissected to reveal the cyst. It is often possible to create one vertical and one horizontal tissue planes before entering the cyst structure. The cyst structure is opened and a Foley catheter placed into the bladder to help determine the nature and size of the connection of the diverticulum to the urethra. Sometimes a pediatric Foley catheter can also be placed externally into the diverticular sac to make complete dissection easier. The diverticulum is excised sharply while leaving

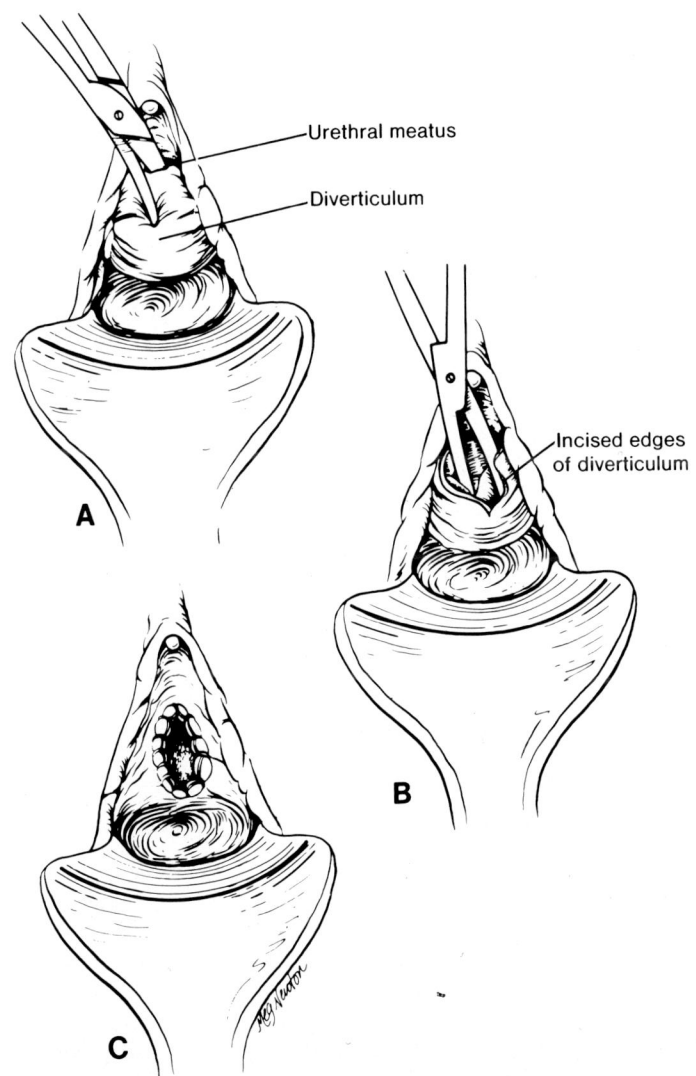

FIGURE 8.9 ● Spence procedure. The scissors are placed into the diverticulum **(A)** and incise full-thickness through to vagina **(B)**. **(C)** A running locked suture secures the edges to prevent bleeding.

the floor of the urethra as undamaged as possible. The urethral defect is closed transversely over the urethral Foley catheter with 4-0 polyglycolic acid suture (Fig. 8.10). The tissue flaps are closed in one or two layers over the repaired defect in the urethra. The vaginal epithelium is then closed. Alternatively, to obtain an extra layer for closure, the excess portion of vaginal epithelium can be used to obtain another tissue layer by stripping off the epithelial covering, either in a transverse or longitudinal incision. If an inverted U incision was made, the fascia can be folded under the remaining epithelium. If a vertical incision was made in the

vaginal epithelium, the tissue layer from one flap can be sutured over the urethra and the full-thickness flap pulled over the top of it (Fig. 8.11). The catheter is left in place for 1 week and removed in an office setting to be sure the patient is able to void.

The partial ablation technique is commenced in similar fashion to the previous description. The diverticular sac is opened longitudinally, and excess sac tissue is excised (110). The sac is then sutured side-to-side to cover the urethral defect using fine suture. A second imbricating layer is placed. The remaining diverticular wall is closed in double-

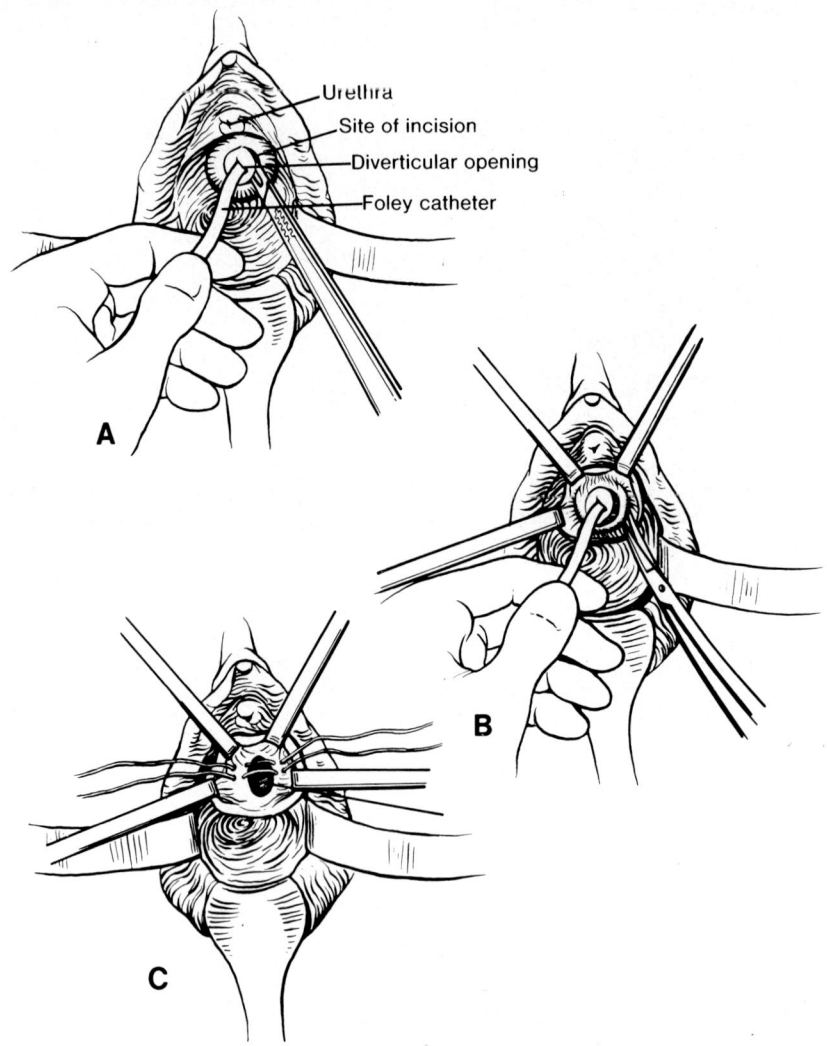

FIGURE 8.10 ● Excision of urethral diverticulum. **(A)** The vaginal incision has been made and dissection of fascia completed to expose the diverticulum sac, which has been opened and a pediatric Foley catheter placed for traction. **(B)** The diverticular sac is sharply dissected free from surrounding attachments and the urethra mucosa. **(C)** Closure of the urethral defect is started, generally a transverse closure, to prevent urethral stricture. (From Glenn JF. *Urologic surgery.* Hagerstown, MD: Harper & Row, 1975, with permission.)

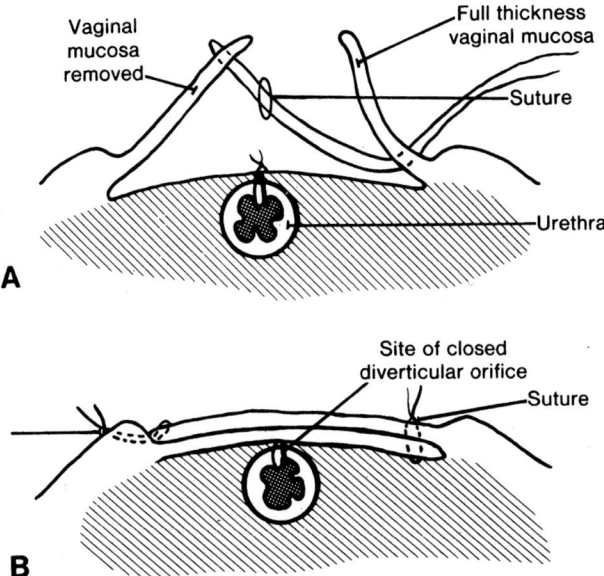

FIGURE 8.11 ● Vaginal flap technique for closure over urethral defect. **(A)** One vaginal flap is denuded of epithelium and sutured underneath the full-thickness flap. **(B)** The full-thickness flap then is sutured over top of the first flap. (From Judd GE, Marshall JR. Repair of urethral diverticulum or vesicovaginal fistula by vaginal flap technique. *Obstet Gynecol* 1976;47:627–629, with permission.)

breasted fashion. The vaginal mucosa is closed, and usually a gentle pack is placed overnight to prevent hematoma under the incisions (Fig. 8.12).

If stress incontinence has been identified preoperatively or if the diverticulum is very large or is located near the bladder neck, a concomitant sub-urethral fascial sling should be performed to prevent stress incontinence (110).

Complications include urethral stricture and urethrovaginal fistula. Antibiotic therapy is recommended intraoperatively and during initial healing while the catheter is in place. Patient stay is gener-

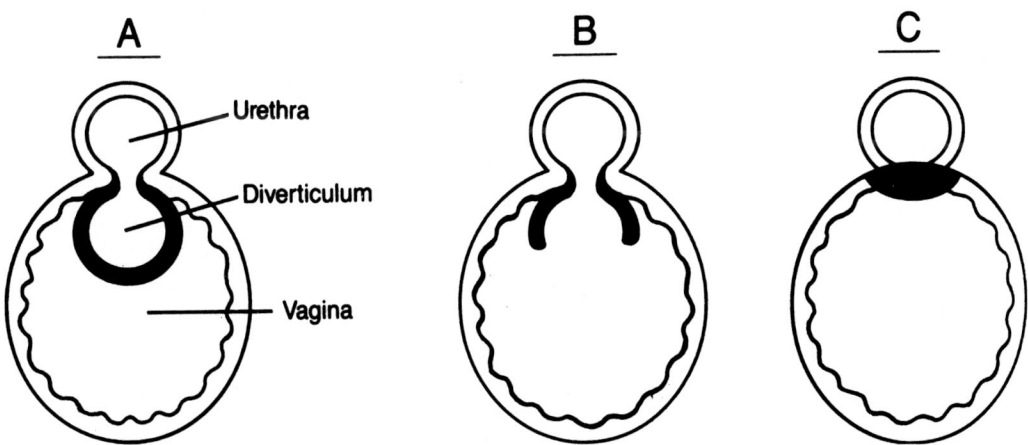

FIGURE 8.12 ● Partial ablation of diverticulum. **(A)** The technique is especially useful when there is considerable inflammation in the tissues. The diverticulum is exposed and isolated from surrounding structures. **(B)** The sac is opened and excess amount of tissue removed. **(C)** The urethral defect is closed by suturing the opening in the sac side to side. The diverticular wall is closed and the vaginal mucosa closed. (From Sanz L. *Gynecologic surgery.* Oradell, NJ: Medical Economics Company, Inc. Copyright 1988. All rights reserved.)

ally limited to 1 day unless sling surgery or other procedures are performed. Catheter drainage is for 1 week. Successful outcome is the rule.

REFERENCES

1. Gillenwater JY, Wein AJ. Summary of the National Institute of Arthritis, Diabetes, Digestive, and Kidney Diseases Workshop on Interstitial Cystitis, National Institutes of Health, Bethesda, Maryland, August 28–29, 1987. *J Urol* 1988;140(1):203–206.
2. Abrams P, Cardozo L, Fall M, et al. The standardization of terminology in lower urinary tract function: report from the Standardization Subcommittee of the International Continence Society. *Neurourol Urodyn* 2002;21:179–183.
3. Warren JA, Meyer WA, Greenberg P, et al. Using the International Continence Society's definition of painful bladder syndrome. *Urology* 2006;67:1138–1143.
4. Simon LJ, Landis JR, Erickson DR, et al. The Interstitial Cystitis Data Base Study: concepts and preliminary baseline descriptive statistics. *Urology* 1997;49[Suppl 5A]:64–75.
5. Clemmons JQ, Meenan RT, Rosetti MCO, et al. Prevalence and incidence of interstitial cystitis in a managed care population. *J Urol* 2005;173:98–102.
6. Curhan GC, Speizer FE, Hunter DJ, et al. Epidemiology of interstitial cystitis: a population-based study. *J Urol* 1999;161(2):549–552.
7. Clemens JQ, Meenan RT, O'Keeffe Rosetti MC, et al. Prevalence of interstitial cystitis symptoms in a managed care population. *J Urol* 2005;174(2):576–580.
8. Lundeberg T, Liedberg H, Nordling L, et al. Interstitial cystitis: correlation with nerve fibres, mast cells, and histamine. *Br J Urol* 1993;71:427–429.
9. Parsons CL, Boychuk D, Jones S, et al. Bladder surface glycosaminoglycans: an epithelial permeability barrier. *J Urol* 1990;143(1):139–142.
10. Lilly JD, Parsons CL. Bladder surface glycosaminoglycans is a human epithelial permeability barrier. *Surg Gynecol Obstet* 1990;171(6):493–496.
11. Parsons CL, Lilly JD, Stein P. Epithelial dysfunction in nonbacterial cystitis (interstitial cystitis). *J Urol* 1991;145(4):732–735.
12. Hanno PM. Analysis of long-term Elmiron therapy for interstitial cystitis. *Urology* 1997;49[Suppl 5A]:93–99.
13. Mulholland SG, Hanno P, Parsons CL, et al. Pentosan polysulfate sodium for therapy of interstitial cystitis: a double-blind placebo-controlled clinical study. *Urology* 1990;35(6):552–558.
14. Warren JW, Keay SK, Meyers D, et al. Concordance of interstitial cystitis in monozygotic and dizygotic twin pairs. *Urology* 2001;57[6 Suppl 1]:22–25.
15. Warren JW, Jackson TL, Langenberg P, et al. Prevalence of interstitial cystitis in first-degree relatives of patients with interstitial cystitis. *Urology* 2004;63:17–21.
16. Gunter J, Clark M, Weigel J. Is there an association between vulvodynia and interstitial cystitis? *Obstet Gynecol* 2000;95[4 Suppl 1]:S4.
17. Clemons J, Arya LA, Myers DL. Diagnosing interstitial cystitis in women with chronic pelvic pain. *Obstet Gynecol* 2001;97(4):S7.
18. Pang X, Boucher W, Triadafilopoulos G, et al. Mast cell and substance P–positive nerve involvement in a patient with both irritable bowel syndrome and interstitial cystitis. *Urology* 1996;47(3):436–438.
19. Alagiri M, Chottiner S, Ratner V, et al. Interstitial cystitis: unexplained associations with other chronic disease and pain syndromes. *Urology* 1997;49[Suppl 5A]:52–57.
20. Clauw DJ. The pathogenesis of chronic pain and fatigue syndromes, with special reference to fibromyalgia. *Med Hypoth* 1995;44(5):369–378.
21. Monga AK, Marrero JM, Stanton SL, et al. Is there an irritable bladder in the irritable bowel syndrome? *Br J Obstet Gynaecol* 1997;104(12):1409–1412.
22. Erickson DR, Morgan KC, Ordille S, et al. Nonbladder related symptoms in patients with interstitial cystitis. *J Urol* 2001;166(2):557–562.
23. O'Leary MP, Sant GR, Fowler FJ Jr, et al. The interstitial cystitis symptom index and problem index. *Urology* 1997;49:58–63.
24. Clemons J, Arya LA, Myers DL. Diagnosing interstitial cystitis in women with chronic pelvic pain. *Obstet Gynecol* 2001;97(4):S7.
25. Goin JE, Olaleye D, Peters KM, et al. Psychometric analysis of the University of Wisconsin Interstitial Cystitis Scale: implications for use in randomized clinical trials. *J Urol* 1998;159(3):1085–1090.
26. Awad SA, MacDiarmid S, Gajewski JB, et al. Idiopathic reduced storage versus interstitial cystitis. *J Urol* 1992;148:1409–1412.
27. Waxman JA, Sulak PJ, Kuehl TJ. Cystoscopic findings consistent with interstitial cystitis in normal women undergoing tubal ligation. *J Urol* 1998;160:1663–1667.
28. Parsons CL, Greenberger M, Gabal L, et al. The role of urinary potassium in the pathogenesis and diagnosis of interstitial cystitis. *J Urol* 1998;159(6):1862–1867.
29. Parsons CL, Bullen M, Kahn BS, et al. Gynecologic presentation of interstitial cystitis as detected by intravesical potassium sensitivity. *Obstet Gynecol* 2001;98(1):127–132.
30. Gregorie M, Liandier F, Naud A, et al. Does the potassium stimulation test predict cystometric, cystoscopic outcomes in interstitial cystitis? *J Urol* 2002;168:556–559.
31. Hanno P, Landis JR, Mathews-Cook Y, et al. The diagnosis of interstitial cystitis revisited: lessons learned from the National Institutes of Health interstitial cystitis database study. *J Urol* 1999;161:553–556.
32. Chambers GK, Fenster HN, Cripps S, et al. An assessment of the use of intravesical potassium in the diagnosis of interstitial cystitis. *J Urol* 1999;162(3 Pt 1):699–701.
33. Teichman JM, Nielsen-Omeis BJ. Potassium leak test predicts outcome in interstitial cystitis. *J Urol* 1999;161(6):1791–1796.
34. Erickson DR, Xie SX, Bhavanandan VP, et al. A comparison of multiple urine markers for interstitial cystitis. *J Urol* 2002;167:2461–2469.
35. Byrne DS, Sedor JF, Estojak J, et al. The urinary glycoprotein GP51 as a clinical marker for interstitial cystitis. *J Urol* 1999;161(6):1786–1790.
36. Byrne DS, Sedor JF, Estojak J, et al. The urinary glycoprotein GP51 as a clinical marker for interstitial cystitis. *J Urol* 1999;161(6):1786–1790.
37. Keay S, Zhang CO, Trifillis AL, et al. Decreased ^{3}H-thymidine incorporation by human bladder epithelial cells following exposure to urine from interstitial cystitis patients. *J Urol* 1996;156(6):2073–2078.
38. Keay SK, Szekely Z, Conrads TP, et al. An antiproliferative factor from interstitial cystitis patients is a frizzled 8 protein–related sialoglycopeptide. *Proc Natl Acad Sci USA* 2004;101(32):11803–11808.

39. Keay SK, Zhang C, Shoenfelt J, et al. Sensitivity and specificity of antiproliferative factor, heparin-binding epidermal growth factor-like growth factor and epidermal growth factor as urine markers for interstitial cystitis. *Urology* 2001;57(6A):9–14.

40. Kirkemo A, Peabody M, Diokno AC, et al. Associations among urodynamic findings and symptoms in women enrolled in the Interstitial Cystitis Data Base (ICDB) Study. *Urology* 1997;49[Suppl 5A]:76–80.

41. Teichman JM, Nielsen-Omeis BJ, McIver BD. Modified urodynamics for interstitial cystitis. *Techniques Urol* 1997;3(2):65–68.

42. Sant GR, Propert KJ, Hanno PM, et al. A pilot clinical trial of oral pentosan polysulfate and oral hydroxxyzine in patients with interstitial cystitis. *J Urol* 2003; 170:810–815.

43. Mayer R, Propert KJ, Peters KM, et al. A randomized controlled trial of intravesical bacillus Calmette-Guérin for treatment refractory interstitial cystitis. *J Urol* 2005; 173:1186–1191.

44. van Ophoven A, Pokupic S, Heinecke A, et al. A prospective, randomized, placebo-controlled, double-blind study of amitriptyline in the treatment of interstitial cystitis. *J Urol* 2004;172:533–536.

45. Parsons CL, Mulholland SG. Successful therapy of interstitial cystitis with pentosanpolysulfate. *J Urol* 1987;138(3):513–516.

46. Mulholland SG, Hanno P, Parsons CL, et al. Pentosan polysulfate sodium for therapy of interstitial cystitis: a double-blind placebo-controlled clinical study. *Urology* 1990;35(6):552–558.

47. Holm-Bentzen M, Jacobsen F, Nerstrom B, et al. A prospective double-blind clinically controlled trial of sodium pentosanpolysulfate in the treatment of interstitial cystitis and related painful bladder disease. *J Urol* 1987;138:503–507.

48. Parsons CL. Current strategies for managing interstitial cystitis. *Expert Opin Pharmacother* 2004;5:287–293.

49. van Ophoven A, Pokupic S, Heinecke A, et al. A prospective, randomized, placebo-controlled, double-blind study of amitriptyline in the treatment of interstitial cystitis. *J Urol* 2004;172:533–536.

50. Theoharides TC. Hydroxyzine for interstitial cystitis. *J Allergy Clin Immunol* 1993;91(2):686–687.

51. Perez-Marrero R, Emerson LE, Feltis JT. A controlled study of dimethyl sulfoxide in interstitial cystitis. *J Urol* 1988;140:36–39.

52. Sasaki K, Smith CP, Chuang YC, et al. Oral gabapentin (Neurontin) treatment of refractory genitourinary tract pain. *Techniques Urol* 2001;7(1):47–49.

53. Sairanen J, Teuvo LJ, Temmela M, et al. Cyclosporine A and pentosan polysulfate sodium for the treatment of interstitial cystitis: a randomized comparative study. *J Urol* 2005;174:2235–2238.

54. Lazzeri M, Beneforti P, Spinelli M, et al. Intravesical resiniferatoxin for the treatment of hypersensitive disorder: a randomized placebo-controlled study. *J Urol* 2000;164(3 Pt 1):676–679.

55. Goins WF, Yoshimura N, Phelan MW, et al. Herpes simplex virus mediated nerve growth factor expression in bladder and afferent neurons: potential treatment for diabetic bladder dysfunction. *J Urol* 2000; 165(5):1748–1754.

56. Peters K, Diokno A, Steinert B, et al. The efficacy of intravesical Tice strain bacillus Calmette-Guérin in the treatment of interstitial cystitis: a double-blind, prospective, placebo-controlled trial. *J Urol* 1997;157(6): 2090–2094.

57. Peeker R, Haghsheno MA, Holmang S, et al. Intravesical bacillus Calmette-Guérin and dimethylsulfoxide for treatment of classic and nonulcer interstitial cystitis: a prospective, randomized double-blind study. *J Urol* 2000;164(6):1912–1915.

58. Keay S, Zhang CO, Trifillis AL, et al. Decreased ^{3}H-thymidine incorporation by human bladder epithelial cells following exposure to urine from interstitial cystitis patients. *J Urol* 1996;156(6):2073–2078.

59. Peeker R, Aldenborg F, Fall M. The treatment of interstitial cystitis with supratrigonal cystectomy and ileocystoplasty: difference in outcome between classic and nonulcer disease. *J Urol* 1998;159(5):1479–1482.

60. Christmas TJ, Holmes SA, Hendry WF. Bladder replacement by ileocystoplasty: the final treatment for interstitial cystitis. *Br J Urol* 1996;78(1):69–73.

61. Linn JF, Hohenfellner M, Roth S, et al. Treatment of interstitial cystitis: comparison of subtrigonal and supratrigonal cystectomy combined with orthotopic bladder substitution. *J Urol* 1998;159(3):774–778.

62. Rofeim O, Hom D, Freid RM, et al. Use of the neodymium:YAG laser for interstitial cystitis. A prospective study. *J Urol* 2001;166(1):134–136.

63. Keay S, Zhang CO, Kagen DI, et al. Concentrations of specific epithelial growth factors in the urine of interstitial cystitis patients and controls. *J Urol* 1997; 158(5):1983–1988.

64. Cook SP, McCleskey EW. ATP, pain, and a full bladder. *Nature* 2000;407(6807):951–952.

65. Cockayne DA, Hamilton SG, Zhu QM, et al. Urinary bladder hyporeflexia and reduced pain-related behavior in P2X3-deficient mice. *Nature* 2000;407(6807): 1011–1015.

66. Vlaskovska M, Kasakov L, Rong W, et al. P2X3 knockout mice reveal a major sensory role for urothelially released ATP. *J Neurosci* 2001;21(15):5670–5677.

67. Sun Y, Keay S, De Deyne PG, et al. Augmented stretch activated adenosine triphosphate release from bladder uroepithelial cells in patients with interstitial cystitis. *J Urol* 2001;166:1951–1956.

68. Birder LA, Apodaca G, De Groat WC, et al. Adrenergic- and capsaicin-evoked nitric oxide release from urothelium and afferent nerves in urinary bladder. *Am J Physiol* 1998;275(2 Pt 2):F226–229.

69. Gallagher DJ, Montgomery JZ, North JD. Acute infections of the urinary tract and the urethral syndrome in general practice. *Br Med J* 1965;543:622–626.

70. Tait J, Peddie BA, Bailey RR, et al. Urethral syndrome (abacterial cystitis): search for a pathogen. *Br J Urol* 1985;57:522–526.

71. Gurel H, Gurel SA, Atilla MK. Urethral syndrome and associated risk factors related to obstetrics and gynecology. *Eur J Obstet Gynecol Reprod Biol* 1999;83: 5–7.

72. Cox CE. The urethra and its relationship to urinary tract infection: the flora of the normal female urethra. *South Med J* 1966;59:621–626.

73. Mutlu B, Mutlu N, Yucesoy G. The incidence of *Chlamydia trachomatis* in women with urethral syndrome. *Int J Clin Pract* 2001;55:525–526.

74. Vitoratos N, Gregoriou O, Papadias C, et al. Sexually transmitted diseases in women with urethral syndrome. *Int J Gynaecol Obstet* 1988;27:177–180.

75. Parsons CL, Zupkas P, Parsons JK. Intravesical potassium sensitivity in patients with interstitial cystitis and urethral syndrome. *Urology* 2001;57:432–433.

76. Bologna RA, Tu LM, Whitmore KE. Hypersensitivity disorders of the lower urinary tract. In: Walters MD,

Karram MM, eds. *Urogynecology and reconstructive surgery.* St. Louis: Mosby, 1999:320–321.

77. Baldoni F, Ercolani M, Baldaro B, et al. Stressful events and psychological symptoms in patients with functional urinary disorders. *Percept Mot Skills* 1995; 80:605–606.

78. McCauley AJ, Stern RS, Nomes DM, et al. Micturition and the mind: psychological factors in the etiology and treatment of urinary symptoms in women. *Br Med J* 1987;294:540–543.

79. Wesselmann U, Burnett A, Heinberg LJ. The urogenital and rectal pain syndromes. *Pain* 1997;73:269–294.

80. Price WE. The urethral syndrome: myth or reality? A commentary. *Minn Med* 1990;73:33–34.

81. Summit RL. Urogynecologic causes of chronic pelvic pain. *Obstet Gynecol Clin North Am* 1993;20:685–698.

82. Weiss JM. Pelvic floor myofascial trigger points: manual therapy for interstitial cystitis and the frequency–urgency syndrome. *J Urol* 2001;166:2226–2231.

83. Bernstein AM, Phillips HC, Linden W, et al. A psychophysiological evaluation of female urethral syndrome: evidence for a muscular abnormality. *J Behav Med* 1992;15:299–312.

84. Hamilton-Miller JM. The urethral syndrome and its management. *J Antimicrob Chemother* 1994;33[Suppl A]:63–73.

85. Paira SO. Fibromyalgia associated with female urethral syndrome. *Clin Rheumatol* 1994;13:88–89.

86. Barbalia G, Meares E. Female urethral syndrome: clinical and urodynamic perspectives. *Urology* 1984; 23:208–212.

87. Lyon RT, Smith DR. Distal urethral stenosis. *J Urol* 1963;8:414–421.

88. Urinary Incontinence Guideline Panel. *Urinary incontinence in adults: clinical practice guideline update.* AHCPR Pub. No. 96-0686. Rockville, MD. Agency for Health Care Policy and Research, Public Health Service, U.S. Department of Health and Human Services, March 1996.

89. Kellner R. Psychosomatic syndromes, somatization, and somatoform disorders. *Psychother Psychosom* 1994;61:4–24.

90. Pranikoff K, Constantino G. The use of amitriptyline in patients with urinary frequency and pain. *Urology* 1998;51[Suppl 5A]:179–181.

91. Raz S, Smith RB. External sphincter spasticity syndrome in female patients. *J Urol* 1976;115:443–446.

92. Serels S, Stein M. Prospective study comparing hyoscyamine, doxazosin, and combination therapy for the treatment of urgency and frequency in women. *Neurourol Urodyn* 1998;17:31–36.

93. Lemack GE, Foster B, Zimmern PE. Urethral dilation in women: a questionnaire-based analysis of practice patterns. *Urology* 1999;54:37–43.

94. Richardson FH. External urethroplasty in women: technique and clinical evaluation. *J Urol* 1969;101: 719–721.

95. Zheng H, Wang S, Shang J, et al. Study on acupuncture and moxibustion therapy for female urethral syndrome. *J Tradit Chin Med* 1998;18:122–127.

96. Youngblood VH, Tomlin EM, Williams JO, et al. Exfoliative cytology of the senile female urethra. *J Urol* 1958;79:110–113.

97. Ingleman-Sundberg A, Rosen J, Gustafsson SA, et al. Cytosol estrogen receptors in the urogenital tissues in stress-incontinent women. *Acta Obstet Gynaecol Scand* 1981;60:585–586.

98. Manonai J, Theppisai U, Suthutvoravut S, et al. The effect of estradiol vaginal tablet and conjugated estrogen cream on urogenital symptoms in postmenopausal women: a comparative study. *J Obstet Gynaecol Res* 2001;27:255–260.

99. Bernier F, Jenkins P. The role of vaginal estrogen in the treatment of urogenital dysfunction in postmenopausal women. *Urol Nurs* 1997;17:92–95.

100. Stenberg A, Heimer G, Ulmsten U. The prevalence of urogenital symptoms in postmenopausal women. *Maturitas* 1995,22[Suppl]:S17–S20.

101. Skerk V, Schonwald S, Strapac Z, et al. Duration of clinical symptoms in female patients with acute urethral syndrome caused by *Chlamydia trachomatis* treated with azithromycin or doxycycline. *Chemotherapy* 2001;13:176–181.

102. Ostergard DR. Bladder pillar block anesthesia for urethral dilatation in women. *Am J Obstet Gynecol* 1980; 136:187–188.

103. Cundiff GW. Urethral diverticula. In: Cundiff GW, Bent AE, eds. *Endoscopic diagnosis of the female lower urinary tract.* London: WB Saunders, 1999:43–51.

104. Summitt RL, Stovall TG. Urethral diverticula: evaluation by urethral pressure profilometry, cystourethroscopy, and voiding cystourethrogram. *Obstet Gynecol* 1992;80:695–699.

105. Lee TG, Keller FS. Urethral diverticulum: diagnosis by ultrasound. *AJR Am J Roentgenol* 1977;128: 690–694.

106. Chancellor MB, Liu JB, Rivas DA, et al. Intraoperative endoluminal ultrasound evaluation of urethral diverticula. *J Urol* 1995;153:72–75.

107. Nezu FM, Vasavada SP. Evaluation and management of female urethral diverticulum. *Tech Urol* 2001;7: 169–175.

108. Fortunato P, Schettini M, Gallucci M. Diagnosis and therapy of the female urethral diverticula. *Int Urogynecol J Pelvic Floor Dysfunct* 2001;12:51–57.

109. Tancer ML, Mooppan MM, Pierre-Louis C, et al. Suburethral diverticulum: treatment by partial ablation. *Obstet Gynecol* 1983;62:511–513.

110. Faerber G. Urethral diverticulectomy and pubovaginal sling for simultaneous treatment of urethral diverticulum and intrinsic sphincter deficiency. *Tech Urol* 1998; 4:192–197.

CHAPTER 9

Pelvic Floor Tension Myalgia

Richard P. Marvel

INTRODUCTION

Pain has been defined by the International Association for the Study of Pain as "an unpleasant sensory and emotional experience associated with the actual or potential tissue damage, or described in terms of such damage" (1). It is always subjective, unpleasant, and an emotional experience. It cannot be confirmed or refuted by a physical test. Patients must be taken at their word that they are in pain.

Pelvic floor myalgia literally means muscular pain emanating from the muscles of the pelvic floor or in their attachments to the sacrum, coccyx, ischial tuberosity, and pubic rami. Pelvic floor tension myalgia is a chronic pain condition related to chronically increased tone and tenderness of one or several of the muscles that compose the pelvic floor. It is a poorly recognized, underdiagnosed, but common problem existing as a component of chronic pelvic pain. It has been recognized as a cause of pelvic pain in women for over a century (2), but only more recently in men (3).

Myofascial pain of the muscles of the pelvic floor has been referred to by several other names, including coccydynia, levator ani syndrome, and proctalgia fugax. Each of the terms have a unique definition appearing in the literature (Table 9.1). The most widely used terms related to pelvic floor dysfunction and pain come form the Rome diagnostic criteria for the functional bowel disorders. These criteria were developed by the Committee on Functional Bowel Disorders, Multinational Working Teams to Develop Diagnostic Criteria for Functional Gastrointestinal Disorders (4). The functional bowel disorders require that organic causes of the pain be ruled out and are based solely on the history of symptoms.

One of the cornerstones in the evaluation of women with chronic pelvic pain is the ability to recreate the pain on physical examination. This makes the functional gastrointestinal disorders less useful in evaluating women with chronic pelvic pain.

HISTORY

One of the first reports in the medical literature of pain involving the pelvic floor was by Sir J. Y. Simpson in 1859, when he described a case of a woman with unrelenting chronic pain after she was thrown from her horse. After recovering from her injuries, she developed severe pain with sitting. She continued with pain for 2 years and had a "miserable and wretched existence." In 1855, after conservative treatments failed to bring relief, Simpson performed the first reported coccygectomy, which led to complete resolution of her pain. Simpson coined the term "coccygodynia" after the leading symptom of pain in the region of the coccyx, acknowledging that the pain was emanating from the pelvic floor muscles and their attachments. He noted that injuries such as a hard fall backwards or sitting down forcibly on a chair or angled body could bring about the painful syndrome. Patients suffering from coccygodynia were noted to have pain with sitting, reclining, and rising from the sitting position. He believed that the pain occurred from the action of the muscles causing motion of the coccyx, with possible inflammation (2).

The first concise description of the syndrome, including the muscular origin of the pain, is credited to Dr. George Thiele in 1936 (5). He described 38 cases with confirmed presence of tonic spasm of the levator ani and coccygeus muscles by his own examination. After pooling patients from

TABLE 9.1

Definitions of Pelvic Floor Pain Disorders

Diagnostic Term	Definition
Pelvic floor dyssynergia (previously "anismus")	Paradoxical contraction of the pelvic floor with defecation (39)
Levator ani syndrome	Chronic anal pain lasting more than 20 minutes in absence of organic disease (39)
Proctalgia fugax	Fleeting severe rectal pain lasting several seconds to minutes, especially at night (39)
Pelvic floor tension myalgia	Pain due to tension of the pelvic floor musculature with pain in the muscles themselves or emanating from the areas of attachment such as the sacrum, coccyx, ischial tuberosity, and pubic rami (24)
Dyspareunia	Recurrent or persistent genital pain associated with sexual intercourse, divided into entry and deep components (40)
Vaginismus	Recurrent or persistent involuntary spasm of the outer third of the vagina interfering with vaginal penetration and causing personal distress (40)
Levator syndrome	Symptom complex of pain, pressure, or discomfort in the region of the rectum, sacrum, and coccyx, with tenderness and spasm of the levator muscles (41)
Coccydynia	A symptom of pain in or around the coccyx, usually reproduced with palpation or movement of the coccyx (2,25)

other colorectal surgeons, he reviewed 87 patients from nine practices. None had a history of recent injury of the coccyx or fracture. The duration of symptoms ranged from 3 days to 32 years, with an average of 2 years. Of these patients, 19 of 87 (21.8%) had a history of trauma, including "falls, parturition, and long automobile rides." Tonic spasm was reported in 64 of 69 cases. He also described a group of 33 patients with piriformis spasm and tenderness and noted a consistent history of supragluteal pain and pain radiating down the posterior thigh(s). He developed the first recognized treatment, still known as Thiele's massage (described later in this chapter).

CHRONIC PELVIC PAIN

Chronic pelvic pain is a common clinical condition encountered by gynecologists, urogynecologists, and primary care physicians. It was most recently defined as noncyclic pain of 6 or more months' duration that localizes to the anatomic pelvis, anterior or abdominal wall at or below the umbilicus, the lumbosacral back, or the buttocks and is of sufficient severity to cause functional disability or

lead to medical care (6). It is a common problem, especially among women in the reproductive years. In Great Britain, chronic pelvic pain was found to have a community-based prevalence of 3.8% in women aged 15 to 73 , higher than migraine headache (2.1%) and asthma (3.7%) (7). In a U.S. phone survey, a prevalence of 14.7% was reported over a 3-month time period (8). It accounts for 10% of referrals to gynecologists, 40% of gynecologic diagnostic laparoscopies, and 12% of all hysterectomies (9). Chronic pelvic pain has a significantly negative impact on quality-of-life factors, with 26% of women reporting being bedridden due to pain within a 2-week period of time (8).

The evaluation of chronic pain of any location is complex. In the acute pain model, the pain is usually due to an isolated factor that can be diagnosed and managed, leading to alleviation of the pain, such as in acute appendicitis. Chronic pain is very different. In chronic pelvic pain, the pain is usually due to a combination of painful stimuli that as a whole compose their pain syndrome. An exhaustive search for "the" cause of the pain is generally fruitless and frustrating for patient and physician alike. A completely different approach is necessary using a rehabilitation model, improving each component of the pain over time to achieve the goal of improved function.

Pain is a very individual experience and is based on a multitude of factors, including past experiences, culture, genetics, injury, trauma, abuse, personality, and support systems. The vast majority of women have multiple components related to the etiology of their pain involving many aspects of the human mind and body. It is not uncommon for women with chronic pelvic pain to have endometriosis, interstitial cystitis, myofascial pain, peripheral neuropathy, depression, anxiety, a history of abuse (physical, emotional, or sexual), and poor coping skills. All of these and many undetermined factors play a part in their overall pain and illness. Diagnosing and treating one component (e.g., endometriosis) will many times be unsuccessful in alleviating the pain and suffering of this population of women. It is within this concept of the genesis of chronic pelvic pain that evaluation and management of all components, among them pelvic floor myalgia, is the cornerstone in helping women with chronic pelvic pain.

ANATOMY

The pelvic floor is made up of a system of muscles and fascial attachments in the shape of a bowel inside the true pelvis (Fig. 9.1). The muscles of the pelvic floor include the levator ani, comprised of the puborectalis, iliococcygeus, pubococcygeus, and coccygeus. Some authors also include the muscles of the urogenital triangle, including the is-chiocavernosus, bulbospongiosus, and superficial transverse perinei muscles, which lie inferior to the true pelvic floor (Fig. 9.2). It is important to realize that within this group of muscles, the boundaries of individual muscles are difficult to distinguish. Although a common cause of deep pelvic pain, the piriformis muscle is actually part of the posterior wall of the pelvis. The piriformis muscle originates from the anterior and lateral surfaces of the sacrum, portions of the ilium, and sacroiliac joint capsule. It forms the posterolateral border of the pelvis. It traverses the greater sciatic foramen, the main space-filling muscle, inserting into the medial side of the upper border of the greater trochanter of the femur. It is innervated from branches from the L5, S1, and S2 nerve roots. Its action is to laterally rotate the extended thigh and abduct the flexed thigh and is thus an external rotator of the thigh.

The coccygeus, sometimes referred to as the ischiococcygeus, attaches to the lateral border of the coccyx and lower sacrum, with the apex of this triangular muscle attached to the ischial spine. It may be mostly tendinous and fused with portions of the sacrospinous ligament, which it covers. Its function may have been related to movement of the residual tail of other species. It is innervated by branches from the S2, S3, and S4 nerve roots. The iliococcygeus is more inferior and medial to the ischiococcygeus. It originates from the white line (arcus tendineus fascia pelvis) of the pelvic sidewall and fascia of the obturator internus muscle. Most of the fibers attach in the midline to the anococcygeal ligament or raphe, thus fusing with muscles fibers from the contralateral side. The

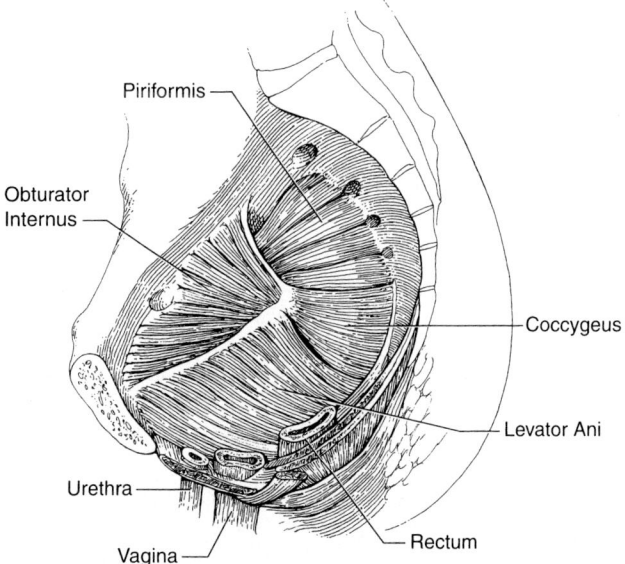

FIGURE 9.1 ● Muscles of the pelvic floor and sidewall, demonstrating the proximity to the vagina and rectum and slinglike support of the pelvic organs. (From Howard FM. *Pelvic pain: Diagnosis and management.* Philadelphia: Lippincott Williams & Wilkins, 2000:36.)

Piriformis

Obturator Internus

Coccygeus

Levator Ani

Urethra

Rectum

Vagina

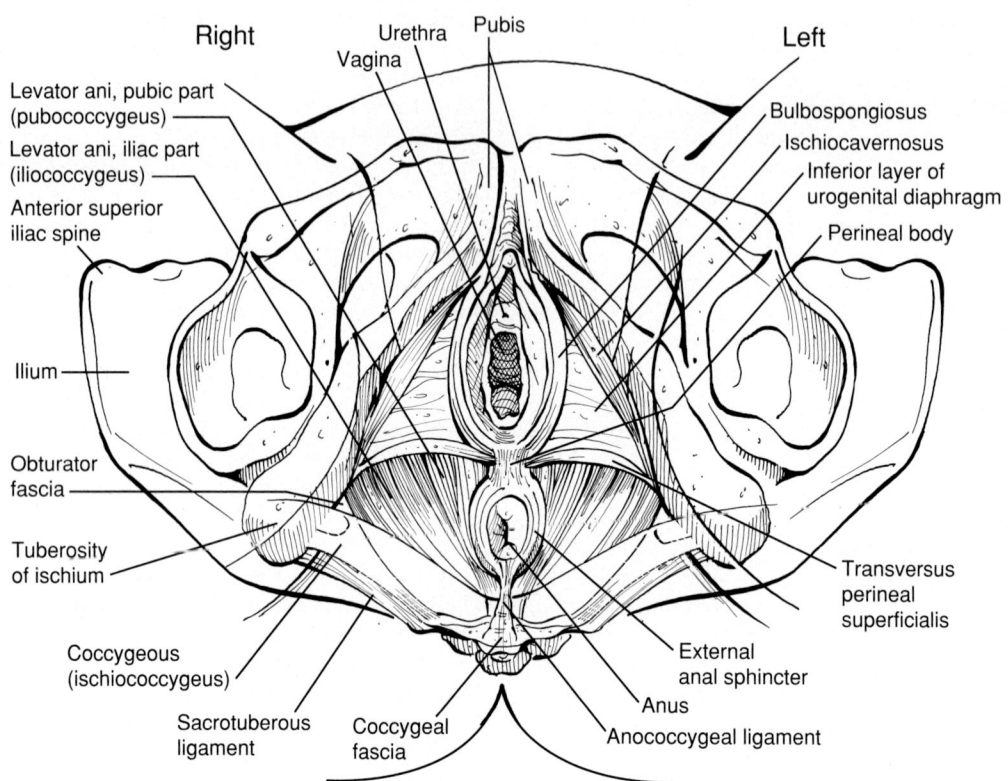

Right — Urethra, Pubis — *Left*
Vagina

Levator ani, pubic part
(pubococcygeus)
Levator ani, iliac part
(iliococcygeus)
Anterior superior
iliac spine

Ilium

Obturator
fascia

Tuberosity
of ischium

Coccygeous
(ischiococcygeus)

Sacrotuberous
ligament

Coccygeal
fascia

Bulbospongiosus
Ischiocavernosus
Inferior layer of
urogenital diaphragm
Perineal body

Transversus
perineal
superficialis

External
anal sphincter
Anus
Anococcygeal ligament

FIGURE 9.2 ● Pelvic floor muscles as seen from below in the supine female subject. (Illustration by Barbara D. Cummings. From Travell JG, Simons DG. Myofascial pain and dysfunction. *The trigger point manual, volume 2: The lower extremities.* Baltimore: Williams & Wilkins, 1983:113.)

pubococcygeus muscle originates from the posterior pubic ramus. Some fibers branch off from the main body of the muscles to encircle the urethra and vagina. These portions are sometimes referred to as the pubourethralis and pubovaginalis muscles. The main body of the muscle then passes posteriorly around the rectum, joining with fibers from the contralateral side. This forms a sling of muscle that maintains the rectoanal angle. This portion of the muscle pulls the rectum anteriorly towards the pubic symphysis and is important in maintaining the anorectal angle and fecal continence (10).

The innervation of the pelvic floor has been debated. It is well accepted that branches of the pudendal nerve innervate the external anal sphincter, ischiocavernosus, bulbocavernosus, and external urethral sphincter. Some authorities believe that the puborectalis also has some innervation from the pudendal nerve (11). In a cadaveric study with histologic confirmation, Barber et al found no branches of the pudendal nerve leading to the puborectalis muscle. In fact, they found a separate nerve from either the S3 and S4 or the S4 and S5

nerve roots (not all three), which they named the levator ani nerve (12). The muscles of the urogenital diaphragm, superficial and deep perinei, bulbospongiosus, and ischiocavernosus, are innervated by branches of the pudendal nerve. The internal anal sphincter is innervated by the autonomic nervous system via the inferior hypogastric plexus, which occupies the 2 and 10 o'clock positions along the rectum and extends onto the lateral walls of the proximal and midvagina. The proximal urethral sphincter component is also innervated from this plexus, while the external urethral sphincter is innervated by a branch of the pudendal nerve (13).

PELVIC FLOOR FUNCTION

The pelvic floor serves a variety of functions. It is part of the support system for the pelvic organs, including the rectum, cervix, vagina, and bladder, helping to maintain normal anatomic relationships and actively participating in the storage function of these organs. The maintenance of some tone in the puborectalis is part of the anal continence mechanism, specifically for solid stool. The puborectalis and external anal sphincter maintain a constant tone and relax at the time of defecation. The resting tone pulls the anorectal junction anteriorly to create a 90-degree angle between the rectal and anal canals. The musculature has a normal baseline tone eloquently described by Simmons (14).

> Muscle tension depends on the viscoelastic properties of the tissues in the muscle as well as the degree of activation of the contractile apparatus of the muscle. Muscle stiffness, meaning the resistance to movement with palpation, is a combination of these two properties. A variety of factors, such as radiation, can alter the elasticity of the tissues, leading to increased stiffness, absent of significant increases in contractility of the muscle fibers themselves. Electromyographic recording identifies only the electrogenic contraction of the muscle (i.e., the contraction elicited by electrical activity of the motor nerve and muscle cell). Pelvic floor musculature has a baseline resting tone defined as the viscoelastic stiffness in the absence of contractile activity (motor unit activity and/or contracture).

Defecation is initiated by voluntary relaxation of the puborectalis. The puborectalis also functions in the prevention of incontinence. With an effort to prevent involuntary loss of stool or gas, the anal canal constricts concentrically and pulls in, the latter a function of the puborectalis. A reflexive contraction of the pelvic floor during Valsalva helps to maintain the bladder neck in an intra-abdominal position, helping to maintain urinary continence.

The pelvic floor also has a role in sexual function. Contraction of the pelvic floor plays an important role in the sensation of the female orgasmic response.

Emotional Control of Pelvic Floor Function

One of the more fascinating aspects of pelvic floor function is the emotional motor control via the limbic system. The emotional motor system consists of a medial and a lateral component. The lateral component of the emotional motor system consists of a set of cell groups in the fore and midbrain, involved in a number of specific motor activities generally related to survival mechanisms, including defensive postures, vocalization, mating, and continence (15). Holstege has demonstrated an output system in the feline in which the nucleus retroambiguus (NRA) projects to a distinct set of motoneuronal cell groups in the lumbosacral cord (15). These cell groups are thought to participate in the posturing necessary for mating. In females, the strength of this NRA motoneuronal projection pattern appeared to depend strongly on the estrous cycles and was almost nine times as strong in the estrous as in the nonestrous females.

A common, well-known example of an emotional motor component is seen in the canine. Tail wagging and other tail movements have a strong emotional basis. With happiness or elation, the tail wags back and forth, a maneuver of the sacrococcygeus ventralis muscle. When threatened, the tail is brought between the legs, protecting the genitals, a function of the coccygeus muscles, much more developed in canine species. These are emotionally driven conditioned motor responses well documented in animal species.

As some of the more important functions of the pelvic floor involve continence of urine and stool, it is logical that some control of the pelvic floor should be activated in the fight-or-flight response (i.e., when threatened). This aspect of pelvic floor function was investigated in studies of vaginismus. Vaginismus is an involuntary contraction of the muscles of the urogenital diaphragm and perhaps the puborectalis muscle in response to attempted penetration. Van der Velde et al investigated pelvic floor muscular activity in women who were exposed to several different film segments, namely threatening, erotic, neutral, or sexually threatening (16). They measured surface electromyographic activity during a baseline period of rest and during the film segments. Pelvic floor muscle activity was correlated with the threatening aspect of the film segments rather than the sexual content. In fact, the sexually threatening segment led to less pelvic floor activity than the threatening segment. They concluded that the increase in pelvic floor muscle activity was related to a generalized defense mechanism to a threatening situation rather to a sexually threatening situation. In addition, there was no difference between the vaginismistic subjects and the control subjects in response to the films, both groups tightening their pelvic floors similarly.

They subsequently repeated the study while measuring emotional responses to the film segments measured on a 7-point Likert scale, including enjoyment, fright, sexual arousal, disgust, relaxation, threat, and powerlessness. They concluded that the involuntary muscle contractions of vaginismus occur as an automatic defensive reaction in situations where conditioning of an emotion–symptom relationship had been established. Of the vaginismistic women, seven had a history of negative sexual experiences. This subgroup of women showed more muscle activity during the erotic segment. They concluded that in these women the vaginismistic reactions may be explained by the fact that based on earlier experiences, erotic situations always have a threatening component (17). This evidence gives an anatomic and functional basis to an emotional component of pelvic floor dysfunction and myalgia. With a history of exposure to a consistently threatening environment, pelvic floor dysfunction, tension, and myalgia can develop due to a prolonged sustained guarding posture. Over time, this leads to continued shortening of the muscles, overload, hypoxia, muscle dysfunction, and pain. This necessitates psychotherapy as a component of therapy to alleviate the threat, break the guarding posture, and enable the pelvic floor to exist in a more relaxed state. This again substantiates the notion of an interdisciplinary approach to chronic pain syndromes including physical therapy, psychotherapy, medical and possibly surgical interventions.

PATHOGENESIS

Our current understanding of myofascial pain is largely based upon the work of Travell and Simmons (18). Spasticity is associated with hyperactive stretch reflexes and tendon jerks and is related to a loss of supraspinal inhibition. Muscle spasm is an involuntary muscle contraction caused by contractile activity and documented by electromyographic findings. Pain is due to muscle ischemia and the releasing of pain-producing substances due to the ischemia. If the muscle contracts at or above 30% of maximal contraction, compression of intramuscular blood vessels leads to further ischemia. In addition, the entire muscle need not be in spasm to cause pain: pain can emanate from only a segment of the muscle that is overloaded. This type of spasm is likely to occur when the muscle has remained for some time in the shortened position. It can be induced by voluntarily contracting the muscle when in the shortened position (14).

Myofascial trigger points are self-sustaining, hyperirritable foci located in skeletal muscle or its associated fascia. These trigger points are initiated and maintained by different factors. Trigger points can exist in both active and latent states. Characteristics of an active trigger point are listed in Table 9.2. A latent trigger point is a focus of hyperirritability in muscle or its fascia that is clinically quiescent with respect to spontaneous pain; it is painful only when palpated (18). Normal muscles do not exhibit these phenomena. These taut bands can entrap or irritate a peripheral nerve in or near the muscle, further complicating the pattern of pain. Acute strain due to sudden muscle overload or overstretching activates a trigger point, which has the ability to heal in several days. In the presence of perpetuating factors, however, the activated trigger point becomes a self-sustaining focus of neuromuscular hyperirritability and a continuing source of referred pain. Chronic strain can both activate and perpetuate trigger points.

With activation of a trigger point, pain is referred in an identifiable fashion not associated with dermatomes or peripheral nerve distributions. Trigger points in the anal sphincter, levator ani muscles, and coccygeus do not have as well-documented referral patterns as other trigger points; however, they can be a cause of groin pain and pain that radiates across the lower abdomen and the low back in a bandlike distribution. They classically refer pain to the sacral area (see Fig. 9.2). In the presence of sufficiently severe perpetuating factors, the active trigger points persist and may propagate as secondary and satellite trigger points, leading to a progressively severe and widespread chronic myofascial pain syndrome (18).

The onset of pelvic floor tension myalgia is generally multifactorial and related to multiple pain components that coexist together. The initiat-

TABLE 9.2

Characteristics of an Active Myofascial Trigger Point

1. Referred pain (usually the chief complaint)
2. Decreased range of motion
3. Shortened firm bands of fibers within muscle containing spots of deep tenderness capable of producing referred pain
4. Local twitch response: brief contraction within the band in response to sudden change in pressure with snapping or pressure
5. Pressure on the active trigger point evokes the referred pain in the typical pattern.

ing event can be related to an inflammatory process, such as an abscess, fistula, severe vaginitis, acute cystitis, or anal fissure. Trauma related to a direct fall or childbirth can precipitate the condition. Many patients readily recall an injury to the coccyx when questioned. The classic type of injury is a fall onto the coccyx on a hard surface when one's feet slip out from under one, such as stepping onto an icy surface or falling off the edge of a chair. Such a traumatic injury to the coccyx can lead to fracture or sprain; however, this is unusual. The resultant inflammatory reaction can lead to reflex tension of the pelvic floor, which can then continue long after healing of the initial coccygeal injury. Trauma can also occur at the time of vaginal delivery with cephalopelvic disproportion or abnormal presentations. Prolonged pushing on a hard surface limits the extension of the coccyx, preventing an increase in the AP diameter of the pelvic outlet. This can lead to trauma to the coccyx itself or the sacrococcygeal ligament. Sustained hypertonus of the pelvic floor can then lead to trigger points in the muscle. The focal localized spasm of the muscle in the trigger point leads to focal hypoxia and the release of algesic substances, activating nociceptors and maintaining pain.

A cascading effect then takes place with the onset of other painful conditions, each related to the other and each contributing further pain and dysfunction to the overall syndrome. Pelvic floor pain can lead to painful defecation. Fear of pain with defecation has a further impact on muscle dysfunction, leading to increased tension and worsening constipation. Hard stools can then lead to anal fissures and chronic anal pain. Worsening anxiety and depression can occur, further decreasing descending inhibitory effect on dorsal horn neurons and increasing pain from all sources. Increased muscle tone and hypoxia leads to altered vascular function, increased blood flow, and symptoms of pelvic congestion. Dyspareunia develops, leading to personal and marital distress. Splinting of tender muscles to avoid pain leads to worsening sitting and standing posture, furthering musculoskeletal dysfunction, trigger points, and pain. It is easy to see that regardless of the entry point, a vicious cycle ensues leading to a multitude of symptoms, crossing specialty boundaries, that are nonresponsive to the usual interventions and are frustrating to patient and clinician alike.

RISK FACTORS

A variety of factors can lead to the development of pelvic floor tension myalgia. One of the best ex-

amples of chronic pelvic pain due primarily to pelvic floor myofascial pain occurs in adolescents or young adults with a leg-length discrepancy. An anatomic leg-length discrepancy leads to a lateral pelvic tilt, hip height discrepancy, functional scoliosis, and pelvic floor tension myalgia. They classically present with incapacitating chronic pelvic pain and a completely normal standard workup. These women have generally had an extensive evaluation with laboratory studies, pelvic ultrasound, computed tomography scans, and generally a negative laparoscopy. Careful physical examination reveals a leg-length discrepancy associated with a pelvic floor that is contracted and tender upon palpation, which reproduces their pain. An anatomic or functional leg-length discrepancy leads to a pelvic tilt and functional scoliosis, changing the normal anatomic relationships of many axial and pelvic muscles. This leads to ongoing muscle tension, shortening, trigger points, dysfunction, and pelvic pain. Physical therapy, orthotics, and changes in posture and positioning can lead to alleviation of the pain (19).

Several other postural abnormalities can also be both an initiating and perpetuating factors leading to chronic overload and shortening of the pelvic floor musculature. One such posture is the typical pelvic pain posture described by King et al (20). In their study of 132 patients with chronic pelvic pain, 75% were found to have an exaggerated lordotic posture of the lumbar spine, anterior tilt of the pelvis, and kyphosis of the thoracic spine. This leads to weakening and stretching of the abdominal wall muscles and shortening of the iliopsoas and piriformis muscles. Poor posture or sitting habits can also be a factor. Thiele in 1963 identified a slouched sitting posture as "the most important traumatic factor in coccydynia" and referred to it as "television disease." He noted the severity of pain is in direct proportion to the amount of time sitting. In his review of 324 patients, etiologies were felt to be anorectal inflammation in 43%, poor sitting posture in 32%, acute trauma in 20%, and parturition in 4.4% (5). Poor sitting posture with less weight supported on the ischial tuberosities and more pressure on the sacrum leads to shortening of the levator ani musculature. Prolonged sitting in this position can then lead to adaptive changes in the pelvic floor muscles and lead to the typical pelvic pain posture described by Baker (21).

Chronic constipation is another condition that puts extra stress on the pelvic floor. Significant straining can be required to pass hard stools. This leads to a combination of strain on the muscle, muscle pain, muscle trigger points, and increasing tone of the muscle. With increased tone, the defecatory angle is increased and the normal rectoanal reflex relaxation of the puborectalis muscle is lessened, worsening constipation. Prolonged straining and difficulty passing stools then can lead to traumatic injury to the pudendal nerve and pudendal neuralgia. This also can then lead to increasing dysfunction and pain of the pelvic floor.

Birth trauma can also be a factor predisposing women to pelvic floor tension myalgia. In a comprehensive review of pelvic floor morbidity related to deliveries, Liebling found that in labors with a prolonged second stage, instrumented delivery was associated with an increase in pain significant enough to lead to interruption of intercourse. When cesarean section after an attempted instrumented delivery was compared to immediate cesarean without attempted operative vaginal delivery, the rate of pain leading to the discontinuation of intercourse was significantly higher: 18% versus 9% ($p = 0.01$) (22). In the study of coccydynia by Wray, 30 of 120 patients (25%) had a history of a fall, 14/120 cases started after childbirth, 15/120 patients reported repetitive trauma such as cycling or rowing, and 6/120 cases occurred following a surgical procedure.

Some systemic factors, including enzyme dysfunctions, nutritional dysfunctions, and metabolic and endocrine dysfunctions, can be related to perpetuation of active trigger points. Some recommended laboratory studies to investigate these causes are thyroid function tests, ionized calcium, B-complex vitamins, particularly B_1, B_6, B_{12}, folic acid, zinc, copper, iron, electrolytes, and antithyroid antibodies (23).

CLINICAL PRESENTATION

Increased tension of the pelvic floor can exist in women who are completely asymptomatic. In fact, it is likely that increased tone exists for quite some time prior to the onset of symptoms and pain. When patients do become symptomatic they generally complain of a dull, aching, heavy type of discomfort. It can be unilateral or bilateral, diffuse or localized, or alternating from side to side. Sometimes it is described as a sensation of something "falling out." In a review by Sinaki (24), common symptoms included low back pain, leg pain, dyschezia, constipation, and dyspareunia (Table 9.3). It is generally worsened with activity, prolonged standing, sitting for more than 30 minutes, and stress. It is improved by heat, a hot bath and relaxation, sedatives, and muscle relaxants (Table 9.4). Pain commonly can radiate into the sacral area, hip, and thigh. It can vary with time of day, being absent or less significant in the morning and worse in the afternoon and at the end of the day. It can last for days or, in the most severe state, be an ongoing severe unrelenting pain.

Most women do not complain of pain with intercourse, but postcoital aching is a common symptom. Similarly, defecation and orgasm can lead to a flare of symptoms. Pain associated with or after orgasm is common. In some cases this pain can be quite severe. With severe pelvic floor tension myalgia, intercourse is precluded due to a constant spasm and tenderness of the pelvic floor muscles.

While pelvic floor tension myalgia is clinically distinct from the functional bowel disorders, there

TABLE 9.3

Most Common Symptoms in 94 Patients with Pelvic Floor Tension Myalgia

Symptoms	Patients	
	No.	%
Low back pain	77	82
"Heavy feeling in the pelvis"	60	64
Leg pain (unilateral or bilateral)	45	48
Pain with defecation	31	33
Constipation	24	26
Coccyx pain	18	19
Dyspareunia	10	13*

*Out of 78 women

TABLE 9.4

Factors Affecting Symptoms

Factors	Patients	
	No.	%
Alleviating Factors		
Medications (analgesics, muscle relaxants, sedatives)	57	61
Lying position	30	32
Relaxation	21	22
Hot tub bath	21	22
Exacerbating Factors		
Sitting for a long time (more than 30 minutes)	83	88
Tension	46	49
Physical activity	28	30
Prolonged standing	15	16
Sexual intercourse	14	15

is likely considerable overlap. The functional bowel disorders are a subgroup of functional gastrointestinal disorders as defined by the Rome diagnostic criteria. This group of conditions, with symptoms attributable to the mid or lower gastrointestinal tract, include diagnoses such as irritable bowel syndrome, levator ani syndrome, pelvic floor dyssynergia, and proctalgia fugax (4). These disorders are diagnosed solely on the basis of symptoms, with the assumption that an organic cause for the pain has been excluded. The criteria for the diagnosis of some of the relevant functional bowel disorders are contained in Table 9.5.

EVALUATION

Evaluation of the pelvic floor is a difficult task. In order to become proficient, one must carefully evaluate the state of the pelvic floor in normal women who are asymptomatic. Nulliparous women presenting for contraception are an ideal population in whom the clinician can become accustomed to the normal examination. On initial observation in the lithotomy position, some of the distal vaginal mucosa is visible. In the normal state, the pelvic floor musculature is nontender, soft, without taut bands, and in a relaxed state.

Patients have the ability to contract and relax the pelvic floor on digital examination.

DIAGNOSIS

Diagnosis is made based on history and physical examination. A careful musculoskeletal examination is the most enlightening. The examination generally starts with evaluation of sitting and standing posture. The classic typical pelvic pain posture with kyphosis/lordosis is common. A leg-length discrepancy can be screened for by having the patient standing in front of and facing away from the examiner. The examiner places the hands on the iliac crests with thumbs medially and palms down. A hip-height difference of 1 cm is considered significant.

During the pelvic examination, the first clue to the diagnosis is narrowing of the introitus. The hymeneal ring appears to be pulled into the vaginal canal and the vaginal canal is hidden. When asked to contract, there is minimal if any elevation of the anus or perineal body. A careful single-digital examination is then confirmatory. The examiner's finger is carefully inserted into the vaginal canal. First, posterior pressure on the rectum can palpate the portion of the puborectalis that encircles the

TABLE 9.5

Diagnostic Criteria Based on the Rome II Criteria of Functional Bowel Disorders

Functional Abdominal Pain Syndrome (4)

At least 6 months of:

1. Continuous or nearly continuous abdominal pain; and
2. No or only occasional relation of pain with physiological events (e.g., eating, defecation, or menses); and
3. Some loss of daily functioning; and
4. The pain is not feigned (e.g., malingering); and
5. Insufficient criteria for other functional gastrointestinal disorders that would explain the abdominal pain.

Irritable Bowel Syndrome (4)

At least 12 weeks, which need to be consecutive, in the preceding 12 months of abdominal discomfort or pain that has two of three features:

1. Relieved with defecation; and/or
2. Onset associated with a change in frequency of stool; and/or
3. Onset associated with a change in form (appearance) of stool.

Levator Ani Syndrome (39)

At least 12 weeks, which need not be consecutive, in the preceding 12 months of:

1. Chronic or recurrent rectal pain or aching; and
2. Episodes last 20 minutes or longer; and
3. Other causes of rectal pain such as ischemia, inflammatory bowel disease, cryptitis, intramuscular abscess, fissure, hemorrhoids, prostatitis, and solitary rectal ulcer have been excluded.

Proctalgia Fugax (39)

1. Recurrent episodes of pain localized to the anus or lower rectum; and
2. Episodes last from seconds to minutes; and
3. There is no anorectal pain between episodes.

Pelvic Floor Dyssynergia (39)

1. The patient must satisfy diagnostic criteria for functional constipation.
2. There must be manometric, EMG, or radiologic evidence for inappropriate contraction or failure to relax the pelvic floor muscles during repeated attempts to defecate;
3. There must be evidence of adequate propulsive forces during attempts to defecate; and
4. There must be evidence of incomplete evacuation.

lower rectum. The finger is then swept along the puborectalis and iliococcygeus muscle. The levator ani can be palpated without conscious contraction of the pelvic floor. In more severe states, taut bands of muscle or areas of nodularity can be palpated. Palpation of the muscle reproduces a significant component of the patient's pain. In some cases, palpation of trigger points can lead to pain in the classic referral zones noted by Travell (Fig. 9.3).

In a prospective study by Wray, 50 consecutive patients referred for coccydynia, defined as pain in and around the coccyx, were extensively investigated, including full clinical examination; plain radiographs of the lumbosacral spine, pelvis, and coccyx; computed tomography scans of the lumbosacral spine; isotope bone scans of the sacrococcygeal area; and a comprehensive personality/behavioral assessment. They found that plain radiographs, isotope bone scans, and computed tomography scans were of no benefit in the evaluation. Only 3/50 patients had an abnormal finding on personality/behavioral assessment, which did not correlate with success or failure of any treatment (25). In men with chronic pelvic pain syndrome, Hetrick evaluated patients and controls and found that pelvic floor hypertonicity and instability, measured as a coefficient of variance of the surface electromyographic signal, reliably differentiated men in the study and control groups (26). Many women however, can have similar findings on electromyography but experience pain. It remains a clinical diagnosis.

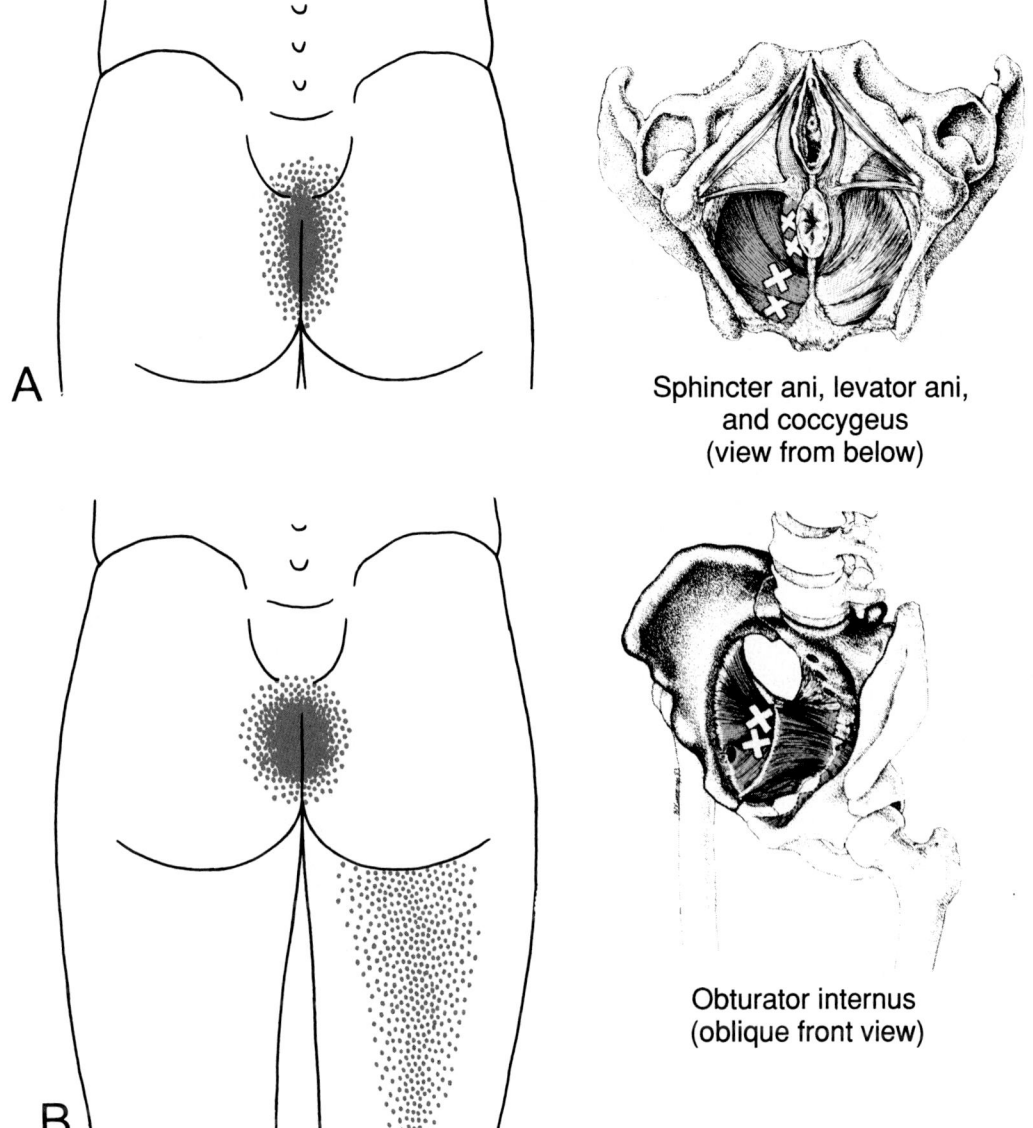

FIGURE 9.3 ● Referred pain patterns generated by trigger points (X) in the right sphincter ani, levator ani, and coccygeus muscles. (Illustration by Barbara D. Cummings. From Travell JG, Simons DG. Myofascial pain and dysfunction. *The trigger point manual, volume 2: The lower extremities.* Baltimore: Williams & Wilkins, 1983:112.)

TREATMENT

In approaching the treatment of women with pelvic floor tension myalgia, it is essential to consider the multifactorial nature of chronic pain. Initially, medical and physical therapies are instituted to alleviate the spasm and discomfort. This is, however, only the initial phase. In order to maintain the improvement, perpetuating factors need to be altered to give long-term relief.

Ongoing physical therapy to optimize posture, gait, sitting, and other habits altering myofascial function is essential. An evaluation of the workspace to optimize chair height, monitor positioning, and other factors in the work environment can be extremely helpful. Psychotherapy to alleviate depression and anxiety and improve coping skills is important to minimize these perpetuating factors. Evaluation of other pain-generating pelvic disorders should be investigated and all factors optimally managed. An evaluation for the presence of endometriosis, interstitial cystitis, and neuropathy is necessary. All pain components should be managed concurrently over time to lead to progressive improvement in the clinical situation.

Pelvic Floor Massage

The first treatment approach utilized specifically for pelvic floor tension myalgia was reported by Thiele and consisted of levator ani muscle massage, commonly referred to as Thiele's massage (5). His treatment consisted of lateroposterior pressure across the levator ani and coccygeus muscles at almost right angles to the fibers. He used lateral motion with strokes along the fibers in the same way as "a strop is stroked by a razor." Massage was done lightly at first, with increasing pressure with consecutive visits. The massage lasted 1 to 2 minutes and patients got an average of 11 treatments over 11 weeks. He reported a cure rate of 61.3% (19/31), with 35.5% (11/31) being improved and 3.2% (1/31) unimproved. Time of follow-up was not reported. In a subsequent follow-up report in 1963, Thiele reported on 224 patients. Of this cohort, 142 (63.7%) were cured and 60 (27%) were significantly improved. In this report "cured" was defined as "completely and permanently relieved of pain" with 10-year follow-up, while "significant relief" was defined as completely comfortable under all ordinary circumstances. He also believed strongly that improved sitting posture and eliminating slouching was a critical part of the therapy.

McGiveny treated a cohort of 64 patients, 48 women and 16 men, with a combination of physical therapy and diazepam. Treatments lasted from 3 weeks to 6 months. In this study, 51/64 (79%) had complete or marked resolution of symptoms, while 13/64 (21%) had minimal or no relief (27).

Pelvic Floor Stimulation

Electrogalvanic stimulation of the pelvic floor has been studied by multiple investigators. The mechanism of action is believed to be due to sustained contraction of the muscles leading to muscle fatigue and release of spasm. In a study by Fitzwater (28), 34 of 66 (52%) patients had an indication of improvement with therapy. Survival analysis revealed that in 51% of these patients the benefit was maintained for at least 30 weeks following therapy. In a series by Billingham, 40% rated the outcome excellent or good, while 60% rated it fair or poor (29). Morris reported a 75% response rate after four to eight 1-hour treatments (30). Neither

of these studies reported long-term follow-up. This was subsequently investigated by Hull, who found that with an average follow-up of 28 months involving 52 patients with levator ani syndrome, the cure rate was only 19%, with 57% of patients reporting no relief at all (31). This approach has been largely abandoned.

Biofeedback

Biofeedback in patients with levator ani syndrome was studied by Heah in a group of 16 patients with no evidence of organic disease on anoscopy, colonoscopy, or computed tomography scan. Biofeedback was performed for four 1-hour sessions over a 4-week period using a manometric biofeedback apparatus. The study group improved from a median pain score of 8/10 prior to biofeedback to a post-treatment median of 2/10. There was also a significant decrease in nonsteroidal anti-inflammatory analgesic requirements from all 16 patients to only 2. There were no recurrences in 12 months of follow-up (32,33).

In a prospective controlled study in patients with chronic idiopathic anal pain, Grimaud evaluated 12 patients with colonoscopy and gynecologic and proctologic investigations that found no organic cause for the pain. They then underwent defecography and anal manometry. A control group of 12 healthy pain-free volunteers were then studied with anal manometry. They found that the study group had a significantly higher resting anal pressure: $67 +/- 4.4$ mmHg (50 to 90) versus $44 +/- 3$ mmHg (30 to 70); $p <0.01$. Also, 42% of the study group had an abnormal anal inhibitory rectoanal reflex. Patients were then treated with anal manometry-based biofeedback. All patients had alleviation of their pain with an average of eight biofeedback sessions. Following treatment all patients had a significant reduction in anal resting pressure, with a mean of $42.5 +/- 2.4$ mmHg ($p <0.01$). One relapse was observed 2 months after cessation of therapy. Patients were followed from 10 to 24 months (34).

Trigger Point Injections

Pelvic floor trigger point injections can be helpful when physical therapy alone fails. The classic therapy with trigger point injections involves dry needling of the trigger point or injection with local anesthetic followed by stretching of the muscle. With many muscles, this can be accomplished by external movements and stretching. With the pelvic floor, however, stretching must be accomplished with direct pelvic floor massage.

A randomized, nonblinded study by Park compared electrogalvanic stimulation and pelvic floor injections in patients with levator ani syndrome according to the Rome II criteria (35). They enrolled 53 patients after eliminating organic conditions such as ischemia, inflammatory bowel disease, abscess, fissure, and rectal ulceration. Patients were randomized to local injection with injection of 40 mg of Kenalog in 1 cc of lidocaine into the maximally tender point on examination biweekly until the patient had no pain for 2 weeks. In this group 2 patients received one injection, 26 patients had two injections, and 3 patients had three injections. The second group of 22 patients received electrogalvanic stimulation for 15 to 30 minutes one or two times a week for six or more times. Both groups continued medical therapy, sitz baths, and digital massage. Patients were followed up 1 week after the last treatment, then at 1, 3, 6, and 12 months after therapy. At 12 months levator injections were more successful in maintaining relief, with complete relief in 8 (25.8%) versus 2 (9.1%), partial relief in 16 (51.8%) versus 8 (36.4%), and little or no relief in 7 (22.6%) versus 12 (54.5%), which was statistically significant ($p = 0.04$). Of interest, when comparing a visual analog scale score for pain, there was no significant difference between the groups.

One of the more recent treatments for pelvic floor tension myalgia is the injection of botulinum toxin type A into the muscles of the pelvic floor. The first report for its use in chronic pelvic pain due to pelvic floor myalgia was by Thomson. A patient developing severe pain after a complicated termination of pregnancy requiring hysterectomy was found to have increased perineometry readings and failed multiple treatments, including multiple medical therapies, relaxation techniques, laparoscopy, pelvic floor trigger point injections, physical therapy, and psychotherapy. After 9 years of symptoms she received pelvic floor injections of botulinum type A, with a total dose of 80 units in divided doses to the levator ani. Postinjection improvements were seen in pain, urinary symptoms, quality of life, and sexual function questionnaires. The benefit peaked at 8 weeks, with gradual return of symptoms to pretreatment levels.

In patients with anismus, inappropriate contraction of the pelvic floor during attempts at defecation, Botox injected into the puborectalis achieved relaxation and short-term improvement in 75%; however, after 6 months of follow-up, there was no improvement in pain scores (36). To achieve long-term results, Botox needs to be injected every 3 months or improved muscle function needs to maintained with comprehensive physical therapy and postural education (12,37).

Neuromodulation

Sacral neuromodulation has also been found to be beneficial for women with pelvic floor myalgia. In a study of 64 patients (54 women), Aboseif found that 80% of patients had a greater than 50% improvement in symptoms with a fall in the visual analog scale score for average pain from 5.8/10 to 3.7/10 ($p < 0.05$) (38). He found that severe spasticity and hyperactivity were associated with urinary retention and hesitancy. After treatment with sacral nerve stimulation, the voided volume increased from 1.5 to 6.6 oz ($p < 0.05$) and the postvoid residual volume declined from 11 to 2.0 oz ($p < 0.05$). Out of 20 patients who required intermittent self-catheterization prior to therapy, 18/20 (90%) could void spontaneously during therapy. He concluded that idiopathic urinary retention with obstruction was due to overactivity of the guarding reflexes, leading to detrusor sphincter dyssynergia (38).

Multidisciplinary management was investigated by Wray et al and published in 1991 (25). They prospectively followed a cohort of 50 patients with a four-step sequential therapeutic program. The patients progressed to the next step because of failure of the prior treatment in alleviating their symptoms. Patients initially underwent physiotherapy with 2 weeks of daily pelvic floor ultrasound followed by 2 weeks of short-wave diathermy. If not improved, they received injection therapy with bupivacaine and Depo-Medrone into the soft tissues around the sides and tip of the coccyx, without injection into the sacrococcygeal joint. Injection was repeated after 1 month if necessary. The next step was manipulation of the coccyx under general anesthesia with repetitive flexion and extension over a minute with repeat injection. If after 6 weeks the patient was still in significant pain, coccygectomy was performed. All patients were followed for 1 year. They found that only 16% of patients were cured by physiotherapy. (It is important to realize that the physiotherapy included ultrasound and diathermy but not manual pelvic floor therapy or postural education, as is currently recommended.) Local injection alone led to a cure rate of 38% at 1 year of follow-up, and 71% for those who went on to manipulation of the coccyx under general anesthesia with injection.

Subsequently, 70 patients were randomized to local injection versus manipulation and local injection. In this part of the study, injection had a 60% success rate, while injection and manipulation led to relief in 85% of subjects. Recurrences occurred in 21% of the injection group and 28% of the manipulation group over the course of several years, most in the first year after treatment. Twenty-three patients went on to coccygectomy, of whom 21/23 had complete and sustained relief of pain (25).

All of these studies suggest that different physical or medical interventions can lead to temporary relief of symptoms, but improvement is generally not maintained over time. Success of therapy depends on the chronicity of the problem and the associated perpetuating factors, without correction of which relief will be temporary at best. With resolution of the perpetuating factors, however, the involved muscles become increasingly responsive to appropriate therapy (18). Consistent pelvic floor physical therapy, preferably with internal manual myofascial release, over a period of time has the best chance of alleviating the pain. This may need to be repeated, depending on patient compliance with posttreatment recommendations. As chronic pelvic pain is generally a combination of pain components, ongoing evaluation and therapy of all associated pain factors is required for the individual to reach therapeutic potential, whatever that may be for each individual. Postural training with the elimination of poor sitting and standing posture, while commonly overlooked, is of great importance. A comprehensive approach to managing the entire patient with sleep restoration, cognitive-behavioral therapy, treatment of anxiety disorders and nutritional deficiencies, and starting a therapeutic exercise program can lead to ongoing improvement and rehabilitation over time.

SUMMARY

Chronic pelvic pain is a common and serious clinical condition in women with a significant negative effect on quality of life and a high cost to society. The primary goal of the clinician involved in the management of these women is the alleviation of suffering. It is generally associated with a combination of components that can be diagnosed and managed over time to allow the woman to live a normal life. Pelvic floor tension myalgia is a common component of chronic pelvic pain, although the prevalence in unknown. Development of pelvic floor tension myalgia occurs over time due to a combination of initiating and perpetuating factors. Poor posture, both sitting and standing, and injury to the coccyx or pelvic floor are significant contributors to the initiation of the dysfunction. The diagnosis is made with a careful history and physical examination. The emotional motor system exerts some control over pelvic floor muscle function and dysfunction, necessitating a psycho-

logical evaluation. An interdisciplinary approach involving not only physical therapists but also gynecologists, psychologists, primary care clinicians, gastroenterologists, as well as other clinicians is necessary for optimal outcomes. This is a true clinical disorder that needs to be brought into the mainstream of understanding in the clinical care of the women we treat.

REFERENCES

1. Lindblom U, Merskey H, Mumford J. Pain terms: a current list with definitions and notes on usage. *Pain* 1986; S215–S221.
2. Simpson JY. Coccygodynia, and the diseases and deformities of the coccyx. *Medical Times and Gazette* 1859; 40:1031.
3. *Bottlenose dolphins of Galveston Bay: at the top of the bay's food web.* Galveston Bay Foundation, U.S. Fish and Wildlife Service, 1996, 1997.
4. Thompson WG, Longstreth GF, Drossman DA, et al. Functional bowel disorders and functional abdominal pain. *Gut* 1999;45(Suppl 2):II43–II47.
5. Thiele GH. Coccygodynia and pain in the superior gluteal region and down the back of the thigh: Causation by tonic spasm of the levator ani, coccygeus, and piriformis muscles and relief by massage of these muscles. *JAMA* 1937;109:1271–1275.
6. ACOG Practice Bulletin No. 51. Chronic pelvic pain. *Obstet Gynecol* 2004;103(3):589–605.
7. Zondervan KT, Yudkin PL, Vessey MP, et al. Prevalence and incidence of chronic pelvic pain in primary care: evidence from a national general practice database. *Br J Obstet Gynaecol* 1999;106(11):1149–1155.
8. Mathias SD, Kuppermann M, Liberman RF, et al. Chronic pelvic pain: prevalence, health-related quality of life, and economic correlates. *Obstet Gynecol* 1996; 87(3):321–327.
9. Howard FM. The role of laparoscopy in chronic pelvic pain: promise and pitfalls. *Obstet Gynecol Surv* 1993; 48(6):357–387.
10. True pelvis, pelvic floor, and perineum. In: Standing S, ed. *Gray's anatomy,* 39th ed. Elsevier, 2005:1357–1371.
11. Guaderrama NM, Liu J, Nager CW, et al. Evidence for the innervation of pelvic floor muscles by the pudendal nerve. *Obstet Gynecol* 2005;106(4):774–781.
12. Barber MD, Bremer RE, Thor KB, et al. Innervation of the female levator ani muscles. *Am J Obstet Gynecol* 2002;187(1):64–71.
13. Yucel S, De SA Jr, Baskin LS. Neuroanatomy of the human female lower urogenital tract. *J Urol* 2004;172(1): 191–195.
14. Simons DG, Mense S. Understanding and measurement of muscle tone as related to clinical muscle pain. *Pain* 1998;75(1):1–17.
15. Holstege G. The emotional motor system in relation to the supraspinal control of micturition and mating behavior. *Behav Brain Res* 1998;92(2):103–109.
16. van der Velde J, Laan E, Everaerd W. Vaginismus, a component of a general defensive reaction. An investigation of pelvic floor muscle activity during exposure to emotion-inducing film excerpts in women with and without vaginismus. *Int Urogynecol J Pelvic Floor Dysfunct* 2001;12(5):328–331.
17. van der Velde J, Everaerd W. The relationship between involuntary pelvic floor muscle activity, muscle aware-

ness and experienced threat in women with and without vaginismus. *Behav Res Ther* 2001;39(4):395–408.

18. Travell JG, Simons DG. Myofascial pain and dysfunction. *The trigger point manual, vol. 2, the lower extremities.* Baltimore: Williams & Wilkins, 1983.

19. Defrin R, Ben BS, Aldubi RD, et al. Conservative correction of leg-length discrepancies of 10mm or less for the relief of chronic low back pain. *Arch Phys Med Rehabil* 2005;86(11):2075–2080.

20. King PM, Myers CA, Ling FW, et al. Musculoskeletal factors in chronic pelvic pain. *J Psychosom Obstet Gynecol* 1991;12:87–98.

21. Baker PK. Musculoskeletal origins of chronic pelvic pain: diagnosis and treatment. *Obstet Gynecol Clin North Am* 1993;20(4):719–742.

22. Liebling RE, Swingler R, Patel RR, et al. Pelvic floor morbidity up to one year after difficult instrumental delivery and cesarean section in the second stage of labor: a cohort study. *Am J Obstet Gynecol* 2004;191(1):4–10.

23. Carter J. Abdominal wall and pelvic myofascial trigger points. In: Howard F, Perry C, Carter JE, et al, eds. *Pelvic pain, diagnosis, and management.* Philadelphia: Lippincott Williams & Wilkins, 2000:314–357.

24. Sinaki M, Merritt JL, Stillwell GK. Tension myalgia of pelvic floor. *Arch Phys Med Rehab* 1977;58(11):543.

25. Wray CC, Easom S, Hoskinson J. Coccydynia. Aetiology and treatment. *J Bone Joint Surg [Br]* 1991;73(2):335–338.

26. Hetrick DC, Glazer H, Liu YW, et al. Pelvic floor electromyography in men with chronic pelvic pain syndrome: a case-control study. *Neurourol Urodyn* 2006;25(1):46–49.

27. McGivney JQ, Cleveland BR. The levator syndrome and its treatment. *South Med J* 1965;58:505–510.

28. Fitzwater JB, Kuehl TJ, Schrier JJ. Electrical stimulation in the treatment of pelvic pain due to levator ani spasm. *J Reprod Med* 2003;48(8):573–577.

29. Billingham RP, Isler JT, Friend WG, et al. Treatment of levator syndrome using high-voltage electrogalvanic stimulation. *Dis Colon Rectum* 1987;30(8):584–587.

30. Morris L, Newton RA. Use of high-voltage pulsed galvanic stimulation for patients with levator ani syndrome. *Phys Ther* 1987;67(10):1522–1525.

31. Hull TL, Milsom JW, Church J, et al. Electrogalvanic stimulation for levator syndrome: how effective is it in the long-term? *Dis Colon Rectum* 1993;36(8):731–733.

32. Heah SM, Ho YH, Tan M, et al. Biofeedback is effective treatment for levator ani syndrome. *Dis Colon Rectum* 1997;40(2):187–189.

33. Sinaki M, Merritt JL, Scott SG. Pelvic floor myalgia: outcome of treatment in traumatic and nontraumatic patients. *Arch Phys Med Rehab* 1980;61(10):491.

34. Grimaud JC, Bouvier M, Naudy B, et al. Manometric and radiologic investigations and biofeedback treatment of chronic idiopathic anal pain. *Dis Colon Rectum* 1991; 34(8):690–695.

35. Park DH, Yoon SG, Kim KU, et al. Comparison study between electrogalvanic stimulation and local injection therapy in levator ani syndrome. *Int J Colorectal Dis* 2005;20(3):272–276.

36. Ron Y, Avni Y, Lukovetski A, et al. Botulinum toxin type-A in therapy of patients with anismus. *Dis Colon Rectum* 2001;44(12):1821–1826.

37. Thomson AJ, Jarvis SK, Lenart M,et al. The use of botulinum toxin type A (Botox) as treatment for intractable chronic pelvic pain associated with spasm of the levator ani muscles. *Br J Obstet Gynaecol* 2005;112(2):247–249.

38. Aboseif S, Tamaddon K, Chalfin S, et al. Sacral neuromodulation as an effective treatment for refractory pelvic floor dysfunction. *Urology* 2002;60(1):52–56.

39. Whitehead WE, Wald A, Diamant NE, et al. Functional disorders of the anus and rectum. *Gut* 1999;45(Suppl 2):II55–II59.

40. Weijmar SW, Basson R, Binik Y, et al. Women's sexual pain and its management. *J Sex Med* 2005;2(3):301–316.

41. Grant SR, Salvati EP, Rubin RJ. Levator syndrome: an analysis of 316 cases. *Dis Colon Rectum* 1975;18(2):161–163.

CHAPTER 10

Lower Urinary Tract Infection

Mickey M. Karram and Sam Siddighi

Urinary tract infections (UTIs) in women produce significant health problems. They are among the most common infections dealt with by primary care physicians. Although rarely followed by severe sequelae, sometimes they lead to acute pyelonephritis and bacteremia and become a major cause of morbidity and time lost from work.

The proper management of these patients, although often simple, has recently been challenged by several occurrences: (a) the introduction of new antimicrobial agents, (b) the advent of single-dose therapy, (c) the recognition of additional lower urinary tract pathogens such as *Staphylococcus saprophyticus* and *Chlamydia trachomatis*, (d) the realization that many women with symptomatic cystitis may have less than 10^5 organisms/mL in urine cultures; and (e) the understanding that certain patients with infection-like symptoms will be considered to have urethral syndrome, painful bladder, or even interstitial cystitis because they have no apparent cause for their symptoms.

PREVALENCE

About 5 million cases of acute cystitis occur annually in the United States, resulting in an estimated 6 million office visits (1). The overall expenditure for the treatment of UTIs in women in the United States, excluding outpatient medication prescriptions, was approximately $2.47 billion in the year 2000 (2).

UTIs are much more prevalent among women than men (ratio of 8:1). This is probably secondary to an anatomically short urethra in proximity to a large bacterial reservoir within the introital tract and along the vaginal vestibule (3). The incidence of UTIs rises with age. At 1 year of age, there is an approximately 1% to 2% incidence of bacteriuria

in females; pathology directly correlates with these infections. As many as 50% of patients show abnormalities on intravenous pyelogram (IVP) that is scarring and either ipsilateral reflux or some obstructive disease (4,5). After 1 year of age, the infection rate decreases to about 1% and continues to decrease until puberty. The incidence of urologic pathology associated with these infections also continues to decrease progressively. With the introduction of sexual activity and pregnancy, the incidence starts to rise and continues to increase progressively with age. Between the ages of 15 and 24 years, the prevalence of bacteriuria is about 2% to 3% and increases to about 10% at the age of 60 years, 20% after the age of 65 years, and 25% to 50% after the age of 80 years (6) (Fig. 10.1). Additionally, more than 50% of menopausal women will experience some symptoms of urogenital atrophy and UTI (7).

About 2% of all patients admitted to a hospital acquire a UTI during their stay, which accounts for 500,000 hospital-acquired UTIs per year. One percent (5,000) of these infections become life-threatening. Instrumentation or catheterization of the urinary tract is a precipitating factor in at least 80% of these nosocomial infections (8,9).

DEFINITIONS

Before discussing UTI, an understanding of generally accepted definitions is essential because the commonly used terminology can, at times, be confusing.

Cystitis indicates inflammation of the bladder, whether used as a histologic, bacteriologic, cystoscopic, or clinical description. Most commonly, it produces symptoms of urinary frequency and dysuria. Bacterial cystitis needs to be differentiated from nonbacterial cystitis (e.g., radiation, interstitial).

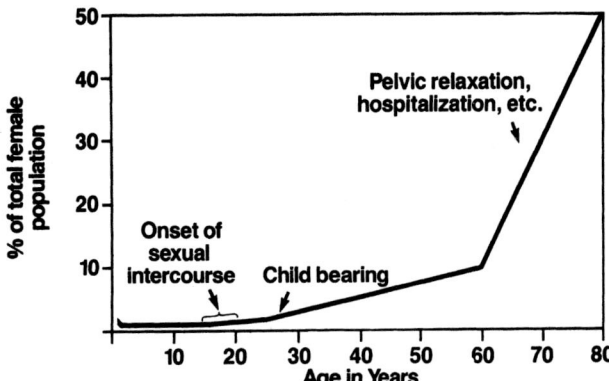

FIGURE 10.1 ● Prevalence of bacteriuria in females as a function of age.

Urethritis refers to inflammation of the urethra and usually requires an adjective for modification (e.g., chlamydial, nonspecific). In female patients, symptoms of urethritis are impossible to distinguish from those of cystitis.

Trigonitis is inflammation or localized hyperemia of the trigone. This term is commonly used to describe the normal cobblestone or granular appearance of the trigone and floor of the vesical neck. The failure to recognize that this epithelium is part of the normal embryologic development and the lack of experience in cystoscopic examinations of normal women without bladder symptoms are probably responsible for the terms "trigonitis" and "granular urethral trigonitis."

Bacteriuria implies the presence of bacteria in the bladder urine and not contaminants that have been added to sterile bladder urine. The term includes both renal and bladder bacteria. Lower UTI can be defined as bacteriuria of greater than 10^2 colony-forming units per milliliter (cfu/mL) in the presence of symptoms, or asymptomatic bacteriuria with the growth of 10^5 cfu/mL or more.

Urethral syndrome is a poorly defined syndrome of frequency, urgency, dysuria, suprapubic discomfort, and voiding difficulties in the absence of any organic pathology. This term needs clarification, and it should not be used to describe urine with bacterial counts of less than 10^5 organisms/mL, chlamydial infection of the urethra, or a hypoestrogenic urethra. When we use the term "urethral syndrome," we have ruled out detrusor and urethral dysfunction as well as any lower UTI. Thus, it is basically a "wastebasket" diagnosis of lower urinary tract symptoms without any discernible pathology (10,11).

PATHOGENESIS

The pathogenesis of UTI in female patients has been postulated to involve three primary mechanisms: hematogenous, lymphatic spread, or ascending extension of organisms directly from the rectum (Fig. 10.2). Retrograde (ascending) infection is the most widely accepted mechanism and appears to be important in the management of infections. Hematogenous dissemination is the principal route by which staphylococcal organisms seed the kidney. This leads to pyelonephritis and may be an important route for patients who do not have vesicoureteral reflux.

The normal female urinary tract is remarkably resistant to infection. Although certain risk factors for developing UTIs have been identified (Table 10.1), it remains unclear why certain women are more prone to infection. Individual differences at the molecular level (i.e., genetic differences and production of inhibitory substances) may account

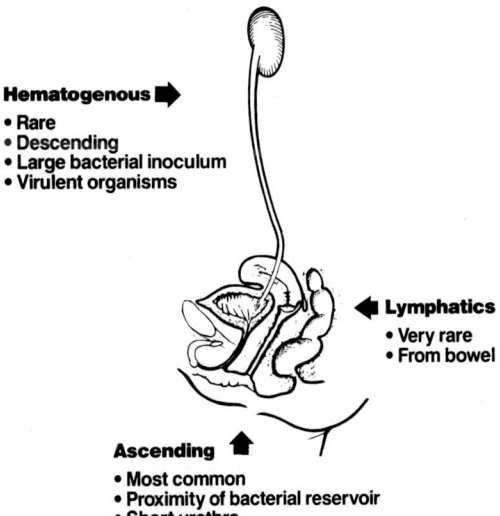

FIGURE 10.2 ● Pathways of bacterial entry into the urinary tract.

TABLE 10.1

Known Risk Factors for UTI

Advanced age
Inefficient bladder emptying
Pelvic relaxation
Large cystocele with high residuals
Uterovaginal prolapse resulting in obstructive voiding
Neurogenic bladder (e.g., diabetes, multiple sclerosis, spinal cord injury)
Drugs with anticholinergic effects
Decreased functional ability
Dementia
Cardiovascular accidents
Fecal incontinence
Neurologic deficits
Nosocomical infections
Indwelling catheters
Hospitalized patients
Physiologic changes
Decreased vaginal glycogen and increased vaginal pH in women

---

for the aforementioned (12). Susceptibility probably also depends on the inoculum size, the virulence properties of the invading microorganism, and, most importantly, the status of the defense mechanisms of the host. These host mechanisms are found in the urine, the vagina, and throughout the female urinary tract.

The Enterobacteriaceae are responsible for about 80% of bacteriuria in UTIs. *Escherichia coli* accounts for the majority of the community-acquired infections; other organisms are responsible for a disproportionate number of infections, considering their frequency in stool flora. *Klebsiella* species cause about 12% of infections, whereas *Enterobacter* and *Proteus* species together account for another 12% of infections outside the hospital. *Serratia marcescens* and *Pseudomonas aeruginosa* are almost always hospital-acquired and are due to omission of infection control practices, usually after urethral catheterization or manipulation. Although anaerobes are present in abundance in the feces of normal individuals, they are rarely the cause of UTI. The oxygen tension in the urine probably prevents their growth and persistence within the urinary tract. *Staphylococcus epidermidis* is also a cause of nosocomial UTI in catheterized patients and is frequently resistant to antibacterial agents (13–18). Other gram-positive organisms, including the group B (*Staphylococcus*

agalactiae) and group D streptococci (*Enterococcus*), cause 1% to 2% of UTIs.

In summary, based on the most recent North American Urinary Tract Infection Collaborative Alliance (NAUTICA) study results, prevalence rates based on outpatient urinary isolates from 41 medical centers are as follows: *E. coli* (57.5%), *Klebsiella pneumoniae* (12.4%), *Enterococcus* spp. (6.6%), *Proteus mirabilis* (5.4%), *P. aeruginosa* (2.9%), *Citrobacter* spp. (2.7%), *Staphylococcus aureus* (2.2%), *Enterobacter cloacae* (1.9%), coagulase-negative staphylococci (1.3%), *S. saprophyticus* (1.2%), other *Klebsiella* spp. (1.2%), *Enterobacter aerogenes* (1.1%), and *Streptococcus agalactiae* (1.0%) (19).

Bacteria are not the only organisms that can infect the lower urinary tract. Yeast can be identified in the urine culture of some hospitalized patients at a concentration of above 10^3 yeast colonies/mL. The most common predisposing factors are antibiotic therapy and an indwelling catheter, but diabetes mellitus and immunocompromised conditions are also strong risk factors. *Candida albicans* is the predominant organism responsible for candiduria in susceptible patients. Other *Candida* spp. as well as *Torulopsis glabrata* may lead to UTI. Rarely, trematodes such as *Schistosoma haematobium* and tapeworms such as *Echinococcus granulosus* (hydatid cysts) may also infect the lower urinary tract, especially the bladder (20).

HOST DEFENSE MECHANISMS

Urine

Urine has certain defense mechanisms against infection. The most important inhibitory factors include a very high osmolality (i.e., high urea concentration) and a high organic acid concentration (i.e., low pH). Both of these reduce bacterial growth by inhibiting phagocytosis and decreasing the reactivity of complement. In general, anaerobic bacteria and other fastidious organisms that make up most of the urethral flora do not multiply in urine. However, urine usually supports growth of nonfastidious bacteria (21,22).

Vaginal, Periurethral, and Perineal Colonization

There is accumulating evidence that the antibacterial defense mechanisms of the vaginal walls and periurethral area are important in preventing the progression of microorganisms from the rectum to the bladder. Normally, this area is colonized by gram-positive bacteria, lactobacillus, and diphtheroids (organisms that grow very poorly in urine and do not cause UTIs). A number of studies have shown that females with recurrent cystitis first colonize their vaginal introitus and periurethral area with enterobacteria before the onset of the symptoms of cystitis and then are at risk for infection until this colonization reverses to a normal situation (4,21,23). Acidity of vaginal secretions may contribute to vaginal resistance to coliform bacteria. In premenopausal females, the vaginal pH is usually near 4.0. This low acidic pH prohibits the growth of organisms such as *E. coli* but promotes the growth of the normally present organisms (e.g., lactobacillus) that will interfere with the growth of uropathogens (24,25). High vaginal pH appears to be associated with the growth of enterobacteria (26). Treatment of menopausal patients with intravaginal estrogen leads to reappearance of lactobacilli, decline in vaginal pH, decrease in growth of uropathogens, and reduction in the incidence of UTI (27,28).

Normal Periodic Voiding

Periodic voiding is one of the most important known bladder defense mechanisms. One study noted the introduction of 10 million bacteria into normal male bladders failed to establish infection because the organisms were rapidly cleared by voiding, diluting with fresh urine, and voiding again (29). Voiding displaces infected urine with sterile urine and flushes out bacteria attached to desquamated uroepithelial cells. In addition, a thin film of urine remains in the bladder after emptying and any bacteria present are removed by the mucosal cell production of organic acids.

Unfortunately, episodic voiding is not enough to prevent infection after sexual intercourse. In case-controlled studies, voiding patterns before and after sexual activity were not associated with recurrent UTIs (30).

Prevention of Bacterial Adherence

The ability of an organism to bind to the epithelial cell has been shown to correlate with its ability to infect the urinary tract. The ascending loop of Henle secretes Tamm-Horsfall protein, which is a uromucoid, rich in mannose. This protein may inhibit bacterial adherence and trap bacteria in the urine, allowing them to be flushed from the urinary tract (31). Also, the presence of urinary immunoglobulin and the lining of the bladder with a glycosaminoglycan may be important factors in the blocking of bacterial adherence. The reduction

of glycosaminoglycan probably plays a role in recurrent cystitis (32,33).

HOST SUSCEPTIBILITY FACTORS

Bacterial Adherence

Adherence of microorganisms to mucosal cells is considered to be a prerequisite for colonization and infection (34). As previously mentioned, when these organisms enter the urethra and bladder in most women, they do not adhere and are easily washed away. In patients who are susceptible to UTIs, the organisms will quickly lock into the defective epithelial cells. The fecal flora is almost invariably the source of the infecting organisms. *E. coli* is the major pathogen, although *S. epidermidis* and *Enterococcus, Klebsiella,* and *Proteus* species can sometimes be identified (Fig. 10.3). The interaction of the mucosal and bacterial cells is probably dependent on both receptors on the mucosa and some type of attachment mechanism used by the bacteria. *E. coli* has been shown to possess surface organelles that mediate attachment to specific host receptors. These structures are called pili and can be present in large numbers on the microbial cell. Two types that appear to be important in urinary infections have been identified. Type I pili seek mannose as a receptor and are isolated from individuals with cystitis. They tend to bind with a low affinity, and their presence is not correlated highly with pathogenicity. Type II pili are mannose-negative or "p pili" and adhere to the P blood group antigens. *E. coli* strains possessing p fimbriae are more virulent and more likely to cause pyelonephritis than strains without them (35–37).

Schaeffer et al (38) studied the adherence of *E. coli* to vaginal epithelial cells in control subjects and in women who had experienced at least three UTIs in the past year. They found adherence to be

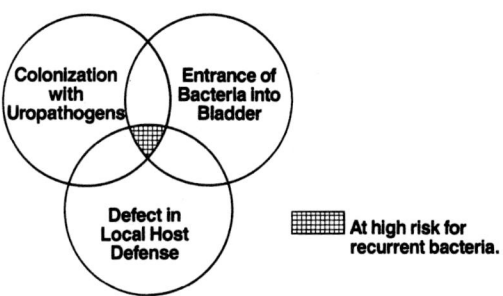

FIGURE 10.3 ● Factors determining host risk and susceptibility to bacterial cystitis in normal females with anatomically normal urinary tracts.

greater in the study patients than in the controls. The vaginal cells of those receiving a sustained course of antimicrobial showed less adherence than the vaginal cells of patients who were not taking antibiotics. If the antibiotics were discontinued, adherence returned, and reinfection usually occurred (39). In another study, Schaeffer et al (40) noted that adherence tended to be higher during the early estrogen-dependent phase of the menstrual cycle.

Furthermore, women at high risk for recurrent UTIs may be more genetically prone to recurrent infection. Although the mechanism is not understood, women who bear human leukocyte antigen A3 subtype (HLA-A3) are more likely to have had recurrent UTIs than those who lack this antigen (41). Other work also suggests that women of blood group B or AB who are nonsecretors of blood group substances are at significantly higher risk for developing infections than are women of other blood groups (42). In addition, patients with Lewis blood group types who are considered secretors have a lower incidence of UTIs. The Lewis blood groups exists at two genetic loci: Le_a and Le_b. Secretors possess the Lewis "b" genetic locus (i.e., $Le_{(a+,b+)}$ and $Le_{(\bar{a},b+)}$, whereas nonsecretors are $Le_{(\bar{a},\bar{b})}$). Evidence suggests that bacteria are unable to adhere to the urothelial cell because of alterations to the uromucoid, which inhibits binding (42–46).

Thus, these genetic differences at the cellular level appear to influence bacterial adherence and make certain women more prone to UTIs.

Sexual Intercourse

In women, sexual intercourse appears to be a major determinant for bacterial entry into the bladder. Prospective studies have shown that many UTIs develop the day after sexual intercourse (47). Both the frequency and recency of sexual intercourse increase the risk for UTI. It has been shown that women who have engaged in sexual intercourse within the prior 48 hours have a risk for infection 60 times greater than women who have not (47). Sexual intercourse with a new partner within the past year is also another independent risk factor.

Infection appears to occur through inoculation of periurethral bacteria into the bladder during active intercourse. Women who have not colonized their vaginal and periurethral areas with coliform bacteria will have introduction of normal vaginal flora (e.g., lactobacillus, diphtheroid, or *S. epidermidis*), which will not produce infection and are rapidly cleared with voiding. However, in the colonized women, the pathogenic organisms, such as

E. coli, will infect the bladder. There is evidence that women who have recurrent UTI have shorter distances from the urethral meatus and posterior fourchette to the anus (48). Another commonly overlooked factor is the use of diaphragms. A number of studies have confirmed that diaphragm users are at increased risk for UTI even after statistically controlling for sexual activity and history of previous UTI (49,50). The mechanism is unknown; it is believed that it may be related to urethral obstruction caused by the diaphragm (51,52). Also, diaphragm users have reduced vaginal colonization with lactobacillus, but coliforms are isolated three times more often than in women using other contraceptive methods (50). Additionally, the spermicidal agent nonoxynol-9 is an independent risk factor for UTIs. Spermicides reduce vaginal lactobacilli, allowing growth of uropathogens.

Systemic Factors

Diabetic patients are prone to develop neurogenic bladder dysfunction and severe vascular disease, both of which can predispose to UTIs. Other genetic problems that are commonly associated with UTIs are gouty nephropathy, sickle cell trait, and cystic renal disease.

It must be understood that the explanations mentioned for the pathogenesis of UTIs apply only to those females who have normal urinary tracts. Bacteria in the presence of obstructions, stones, or a neurogenic bladder do not need to have special invasive properties other than the ability to grow in urine.

CLINICAL PRESENTATION

The signs and symptoms of UTI in females can be diverse. It is helpful to distinguish lower UTI (cystitis) from upper tract infection (pyelonephritis) to aid in the selection of proper antimicrobial therapy and to plan appropriate follow-up.

The most common symptom of uncomplicated UTI is frequency of urination, present in 94% of patients (53). Cystitis is also manifested by lower urinary tract irritative symptoms such as dysuria, urgency, nocturia, suprapubic discomfort, low backache, and even flank pain. Urinary incontinence occasionally may be a symptom of UTI. This may be due to the urethral sphincter relaxation mediated by *E. coli* endotoxin (54). Uncommonly, one can have gross hematuria. Systemic symptoms such as fever and chills are usually absent in lower UTIs. One should be aware that the elderly may have more subtle symptoms such as malaise, mild abdominal pain, nocturia, and urinary incontinence instead of the classic symptoms discussed above.

Upper tract infections involving the renal pelvis, calyces, and parenchyma commonly present with fever, chills, malaise, and occasionally (especially in elderly patients) nausea and vomiting. Costovertebral angle tenderness and flank pain are usually present. However, it should be noted that because of referred pain pathways, lower UTIs may also be accompanied by flank pain and costovertebral angle tenderness. There is colicky pain if acute pyelonephritis is complicated by either a renal calculus or a sloughed renal papilla secondary to diabetic or analgesic nephropathy. More detailed discussion of upper UTI is beyond the scope of this chapter.

DIAGNOSIS OF BACTERIURIA

Before performing tests to document the presence or absence of pathogenic bacteria in the urine, the method of urinary collection must be considered. Considerable care must be taken in the collection of urine from ambulatory females. Kass (55,56) published results demonstrating that one whole voided urine specimen with a colony count of greater than 10^5 cfu/mL has only an 80% chance of representing true infection. Three specimens increased the odds to 95% (55,56). Even when intelligent, educated patients are given clear, detailed instructions for collection of urine, errors can occur. Certain patients, because of physical disability or obesity, are simply unable to obtain a clean voided specimen without assistance. When necessary to avoid these limitations, specimens can be obtained by urethral catheterization. Additionally, the patient can lie in the lithotomy position on an examining table and void after the perineum is cleaned with soap and water while the nurse collects a midstream specimen. Sometimes, bladder urine may need to be aspirated suprapubically (57). Although urethral catheterization is the most time-honored method, it should be kept in mind that catheterization is not without risks. Reports have noted that catheter-induced infection rates range from 1% in young, healthy females to as high as 20% in hospitalized females (58,59).

Urine Microscopy

Microscopic analysis of urine is an easy and valuable method of evaluating women with symptoms of UTI. A thorough microscopic examination of an uncentrifuged sample of urine showing minimal epithelial cells (thus not contaminated), bacteria

moving in the field, and 2 to 6 leukocytes per high-power field correlates with above 10^6 cfu/mL on culture. If infection with greater than 10^4 cfu/mL is present, the finding of one or more bacteria on a Gram-stained specimen of urine correlates highly with the presence of UTI, having a sensitivity of 80% and a specificity of 90% with a positive predictive value of about 85% (60). Gram stain of the urine is useful in detecting abundant bacteriuria but is of little help in infection with colony counts of less than 10^4 cfu/mL.

Fresh, unspun urine should also be quantitatively assessed with a hemocytometer for the number of white blood cells. The hemocytometer is positioned on the microscope stage. The number of leukocytes is counted in each of nine large squares, divided by 9 and multiplied by 10 to yield the number of white blood cells per milliliter. Pyuria is defined as greater than 10 leukocytes/mL. Pyuria is present in nearly all women with acute UTI. Studies note the presence of pyuria to be 80% to 95% sensitive (even when bacteria counts are less than 10^4) and 50% to 75% specific for the presence of UTI. However, a study of pregnant patients presenting acutely to a labor ward showed that only 17% of patients with significant pyuria had a significant urine culture (61). It is also of value to ascertain whether red blood cells are present or to perform a urine dipstick for blood. Microscopic hematuria can be found in about 50% of women with acute UTI and is rarely present in patients who have dysuria from other causes (62,63).

Office Urine Kits

If expertise for office microscopy is not available or feasible, it is reasonable to substitute a rapid diagnostic test for bacteriuria, pyuria, and hematuria, although in general these lead to less accurate results than microscopy.

The most common rapid detection test is the nitrite test. Certain bacteria such as *Proteus* species and occasionally *E. coli* have the enzyme nitrate reductase, which converts dietary nitrates into nitrite; this, in turn, causes the amine-impregnated dipstick to turn pink within 60 seconds of reaction. Numerous commercial urine dip tests are available, and one should check the sensitivity and specificity of the particular test kit used. Generally, a positive nitrite test is highly specific (92% to 100%) for UTI and deserves treatment. However, the test is not sensitive and is not a good screening tool (i.e., only 25% of patients with UTI test positive for nitrites). Lack of dietary nitrate, organisms that lack nitrate reductase, and diuretics can lead to false-negative results.

The nitrite test is often integrated with a test for leukocyte esterase (LE), which is an enzyme found in primary neutrophil granules. When LE reacts with reagents impregnated in the dipstick, a blue color is produced within 1 to 2 minutes, indicating a positive test. The LE test has a specificity of 94% to 98% (64). However, the sensitivity of the LE test is directly related to the bacterial load. Wu et al (65) showed a sensitivity of only 22% in infections with 10^4 to 10^5 cfu/mL versus 60% for those with greater than 10^5 cfu/mL. In other words, low-level pyuria (5 to 20 white blood cells per high-power field microscopy) may be associated with a false-negative LE test. These tests are also best performed on concentrated first-morning voided specimens. It has been suggested that false-negative results are more likely if the test is used as a sampling technique at other times during the day (66). Furthermore, certain dyes such as bilirubin, methylene blue, or phenazopyridine may interfere with interpretation of the test.

Other rapid detection tests, such as filter methods (e.g., Back-T-Screen, Marion Laboratories, Inc., Kansas City, MO), concentrate a specific quantity of urinary sediment on a filter of controlled pore size. One milliliter of urine is mixed with 3 mL of a diluent containing glacial acetic acid and other ingredients that dissolve crystals and increase adherence of bacteria and leukocytes. The diluted mixture is then passed through the filter and rinsed with a diluent. A safranin dye is then used to stain the bacteria and leukocytes, and a decolorizer is added to remove excess dye. Resulting colors are compared with a reference to quantitate the presence of bacteria and leukocytes. The sensitivity of these tests for urine infected with 10^4 to 10^5 cfu/mL is 34% to 65%. As the number of organisms increases to greater than 10^5, the sensitivity also increases to 79% to 85%. The specificity of this test at lower bacterial counts is about 75% (65,67). The main advantage of these tests is a more reliable detection of smaller numbers of bacteria at the expense of lower specificity (68). The test is believed by some to be a good screening method because it detects both bacteria and pyuria.

A symptomatic patient should be treated with antibiotics even if an office urinary kit is negative for both nitrites and leukocytes. Empiric antibiotic use is guided by symptoms because treatment leads to faster resolution of lower urinary tract symptoms and will reduce the median duration of constitutional symptoms (fever and shivers) by 4 days (69). Additionally, treatment can reduce time of restricted activity and leave from work.

Urine Culture

In the patient who has clinical signs of acute lower UTI and is noted to have pyuria, bacteriuria, or hematuria on one of the previously mentioned office tests, it is reasonable to initiate antibiotic therapy without obtaining a urine culture. However, if one of the screening techniques is deemed inappropriate or inconclusive, if the patient has recurrent infection that has not been subjectively relieved with previous antibiotics, or if signs and symptoms are consistent with upper UTI, a bacterial culture and sensitivity should be performed.

The traditional approach to the interpretation of a urinary culture has been that there must be growth of at least 10^5 cfu/mL to consider it positive. This criterion is based on studies demonstrating that the finding of at least 10^5 cfu/mL on two consecutive urine cultures distinguishes women with asymptomatic bacteriuria or pyelonephritis from those with contaminated specimens (55,56,60).

The use of this cutoff, however, has two limitations for the clinician who treats these patients. First, 20% to 24% of women with symptomatic urinary infections present with less than 10^5 bacteria/mL of urine (57,70–72). This is probably secondary to a slow doubling time of bacteria in urine combined with frequent bladder emptying from persistent irritation. Stamm et al (73) proposed that the best diagnostic criterion for culture detection in young symptomatic women is 10^2 cfu/mL, not 10^5 cfu/mL.

The second limitation of the 10^5 cutoff is one of overdiagnosis. In the original studies by Kass (55,56,74), a single culture of at least 10^5 cfu/mL had a 20% chance of representing contamination. Because patients who are susceptible to infection often carry large numbers of pathogenic bacteria on the perineum, contamination of an otherwise sterile urine can occur. For this reason, care in the collection of the urine specimen must again be emphasized. Most health care workers do not spend much time and effort to explain adequately how a patient should collect a midstream urine clean-catch specimen. However, one study showed contamination rates to be similar among patients whose urine samples were collected with traditional instructions (midstream urine sample, perineal cleansing, and spreading of the labia) compared with urine samples of patients told to urinate into a clean container without cleansing (75).

Although methods of obtaining cultures in the office are available, most clinicians use commercial laboratories. One should be familiar with the individual laboratory policy of reporting culture results. Some laboratories report any culture of less than 10^5 cfu/mL as negative and often report only the predominant organism in mixed cultures.

Sensitivity testing is also usually obtained using a commercial laboratory, even though office tests have been described. The disadvantages of sensitivity testing include the time involved, which is typically 24 to 48 hours; the absence of control of processing by the referring physician; and the relatively high cost.

Cystoscopy

Cystitis may appear as diffuse inflammation (non-raised, red areas distributed throughout) on cystoscopy. Occasionally, one may note one or multiple small clear cysts throughout the bladder from a resolved UTI. This is termed "cystitis cystica."

Cystoscopy is not routinely indicated for the evaluation of lower UTI, and routine endoscopic evaluation in females with UTI is a controversial issue. Fowler and Pulaski (76) reported on 74 cystoscopies performed in women with two or more previous infections and noted the only abnormality that altered treatment was the presence of a urethral diverticulum in three cases. Engel et al (77) reviewed 153 women who had undergone cystoscopy for UTI. Although abnormalities were noted in 62% of the cases, 84% of these abnormalities were inflammatory in nature and presumably secondary to prior infection. Only one abnormality, a colovesical fistula, had an effect on treatment (77).

Cystoscopy under local anesthesia has basically no risk and occasionally reveals findings useful in subsequent patient management. Therefore, it should be considered in patients with recurrent or persistent UTI or asymptomatic hematuria.

Radiologic Studies

Although it has long been believed that UTI constitutes one of the important indications for urography, the use of routine IVPs in women with otherwise uncomplicated infection has been challenged. The minimal (1% to 2%) yield of the IVP makes it an inefficient and expensive method of identifying underlying disease (76–81). The cost of detecting a single significant and treatable urologic disorder has been estimated at $9,000 (81). However, the IVP is a valuable diagnostic test when properly indicated. The indications for obtaining an IVP for UTI are (a) a history of previ-

ous upper UTI; (b) a history of childhood UTIs; (c) a history of recurrent infections caused by the same organism, particularly if the organism is urea-splitting, such as *Proteus mirabilis*, because this is frequently associated with infected stones (Fig. 10.4); (d) all cases of infection associated with painless hematuria; (e) women with a history of stones or obstruction; and (f) patients with bacterial evidence of rapid recurrence, suggesting bacterial persistence or the presence of an enterovesical fistula.

A dynamic computed tomography scan (helical CT scan) with thin slices can provide similar or better information than an IVP without the need for dye. Consequently, CT scans also provide information about other structures in the abdomen.

A voiding cystourethrogram, double-balloon catheter study, or magnetic resonance imaging (MRI) study should be performed if a urethral diverticulum is thought to be contributing to recurrent infections. Signs and symptoms of urethral diverticulum include leakage of urine and the finding of pus or pain on palpation and massage of the urethra.

Urodynamic Studies

Urodynamic studies involving a range of procedures from a simple cystometrogram and flow studies to complicated videourodynamic studies are sometimes useful to demonstrate abnormal contraction and emptying of the bladder. A vicious cycle of repeated lower UTIs can lead to an obstructed voiding pattern, with high residuals resulting from spasm of the external striated urethral sphincter secondary to infection or to the pain of the acute cystitis (82). These tests can prove helpful in patients with recurrent UTI who have neurologic disease or a history of pelvic or spinal surgery.

DIFFERENTIAL DIAGNOSIS

In women whose history or laboratory findings are not consistent with UTI, other causes of their lower urinary tract symptoms must be considered.

Vaginitis is a major cause of lower urinary tract symptoms, with *Trichomonas* and *Candida* species being the most commonly implicated organisms. "Nonspecific urethritis" is a term that has been used by some to describe patients with dysuria secondary to what is believed to be an inflamed urethra. Several organisms have been proposed as potential pathogens in such cases. These have included *C. trachomatis*, lactobacilli, *S. sapro-*

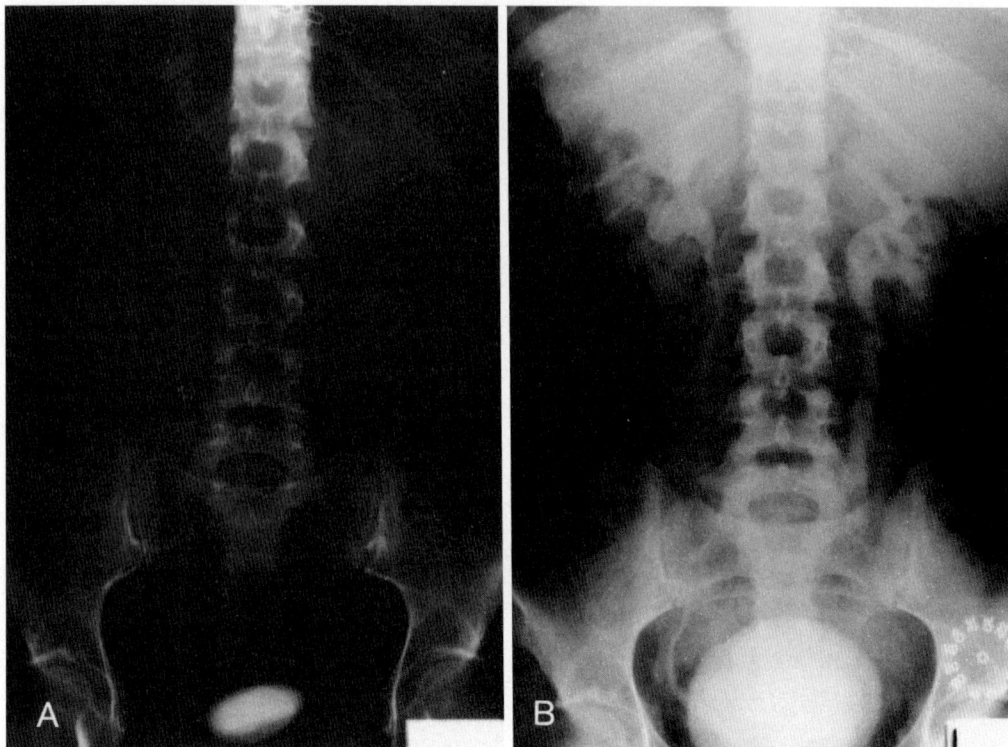

FIGURE 10.4 ● Flat plate and intravenous pyelogram of a young female who presented with persistent UTI secondary to *Klebsiella pneumoniae.* **(A)** Large intravesical bladder calculi. **(B)** Bilateral hydronephrosis and hydroureter.

phyticus, and corynebacteria as well as other fastidious organisms, such as *Ureaplasma urealyticum,* and *Mycoplasma hominis.* However, data to substantiate correlation between clinical symptoms and the presence of these organisms are lacking (83,84). Trauma related to intercourse or other activities may also produce symptoms of UTI. Unfortunately, many of these patients are unnecessarily treated with repetitive courses of antibiotics. Dysuria is also a common presenting symptom in sexually transmitted diseases, particularly *C. trachomatis* and, less commonly, herpes simplex virus or *Neisseria gonorrhoeae.*

Some patients can distinguish internal from external dysuria. Discomfort that is centered inside the body is more commonly associated with UTI or urethritis due to *C. trachomatis;* pain that starts when the urine flows across the perineum is more commonly associated with vaginitis or herpetic infection. Frequency, urgency, and voiding small amounts of urine are common in UTI and in sexually transmitted diseases and rare in vaginitis. Virtually all women with acute symptomatic UTI have pyuria, and about half have microscopic hematuria. Pyuria can also exist in patients with

urethritis secondary to sexually transmitted diseases. It is not present in vaginitis. Hematuria is not a feature of either sexually transmitted diseases or vaginitis; therefore, its presence is a strong clue toward the diagnosis of cystitis. Postmenopausal women may have dysuria secondary to desiccation of the urethra and the vaginal mucosa caused by estrogen deficiency (85).

A group of women exists who are not estrogen-deficient and who complain of persistent lower urinary tract symptoms despite negative urine, vaginal, and urethral cultures. The term "urethral syndrome" (83–86) has been introduced to describe these patients, and a full discussion of this condition is presented elsewhere.

A suggested approach to the evaluation and management of women with dysuria is shown in Figure 10.5.

MANAGEMENT OF LOWER URINARY TRACT INFECTION

General measures, such as rest and hydration, should always be emphasized in women with UTI. Hydration dilutes bacterial counts and may destroy

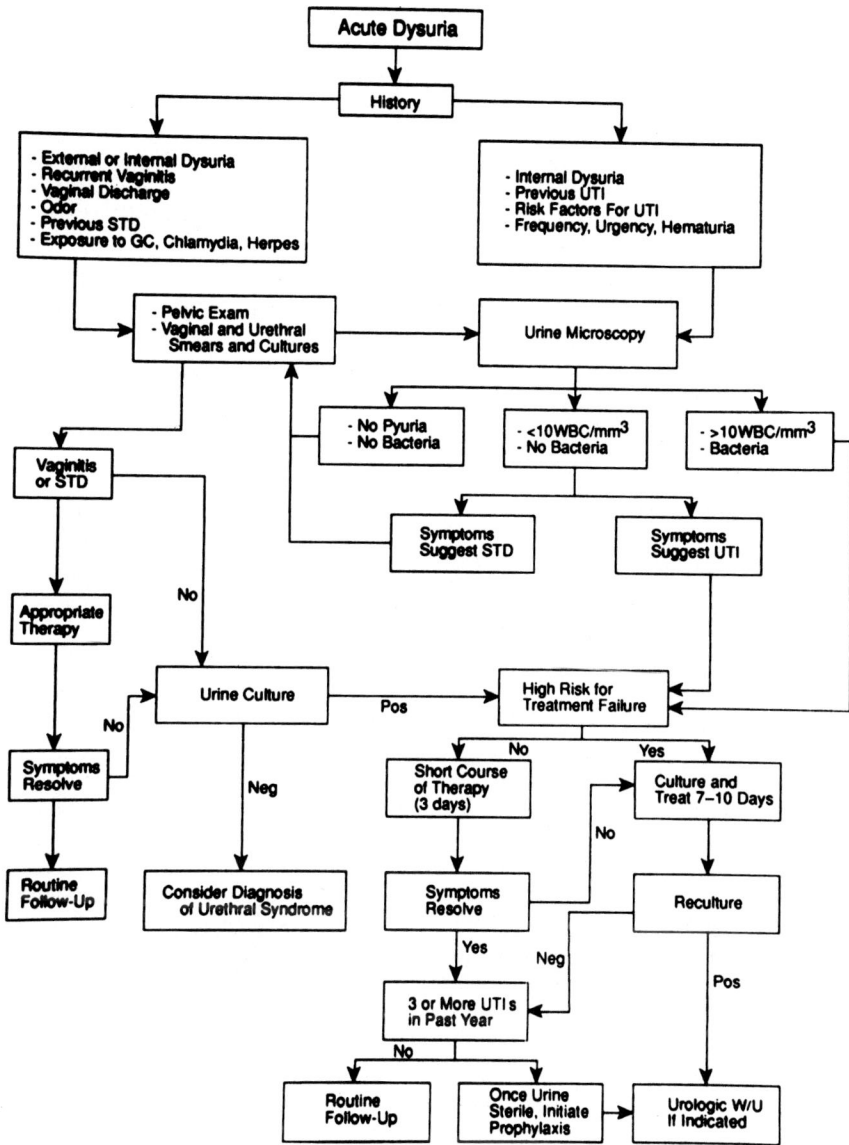

FIGURE 10.5 ● Algorithm for diagnosis and management of females presenting with acute dysuria.

cell wall–deficient bacterial strains. Acidification of the urine is helpful only in recurrent infections and in patients taking methenamine compounds, which demonstrate maximal antibacterial activity at a pH of 5.5 or less. It has also been noted that the ingestion of undiluted cranberry juice or extract may be protective against the development of cystitis by inhibiting bacterial adherence (87).

Typically, a patient waits almost 5 days before seeking medical attention for uncomplicated UTI (88). After taking an oral antibiotic, the vast majority of patients get relief from their symptoms within 24 hours (89). Nevertheless, urinary anal-

gesic agents such as phenazopyridine hydrochloride (Pyridium) can help relieve symptoms sooner. If prescribed, they should be used for a short period of time along with a specific antibacterial agent. Daily, long-term use of Pyridium may lead to lemon-yellow nails, icterus, unconjugated bilirubinemia, methemoglobinemia, and renal failure. Also, one should avoid use of Pyridium if a patient has sulfa allergy (90). Other urinary tract analgesic agents are also available; Urised (a.k.a. Urisept) is a cocktail containing phenyl salicylate, sodium phosphate, hyoscyamine, methenamine, and methylene blue. This agent may turn urine and contact lenses blue and should be avoided with sulfa-containing medications.

With regard to the therapeutic management of this condition, certain factors should be kept in mind. The ideal antibiotic should have a higher concentration in the bladder in comparison to other tissues in the body, such as the bowel and vagina. A drug can alter bacteria in the bowel either directly by passing through the gastrointestinal tract without being absorbed or by having a high serum level. It is also important that a drug maintain a low serum level to avoid disrupting the flora in the vagina. If an antibiotic appropriately matched to bacterial sensitivity causes a yeast vaginitis, the subsequent therapy for the vaginitis will increase patient morbidity and raise the cost of therapy. In addition, the vaginitis created by the antibiotic could lead to a vaginitis–cystitis cycle that may be difficult to treat.

These therapeutic goals should be kept in mind when treating these infections because there are many misconceptions about commonly prescribed antibiotics. For example, ampicillin and tetracycline are both frequently prescribed for simple cystitis, despite the fact that they have an incidence of yeast vaginitis that may approach 25% and 80%, respectively, because both drugs are excreted in the fecal stream unchanged and have a stool concentration three times the urine concentration (91–94). Nitrofurantoin, on the other hand, has excellent activity against *E. coli* and has no significant serum level. It has a 19-minute serum half-life and is metabolized in every tissue in the body, resulting in no significant changes in fecal or vaginal flora, which is why no increase in bacterial resistance to nitrofurantoin is seen after 30 years of use in the United States (94–99).

The most common sulfonamide preparation used in the management of UTI is the combination of trimethoprim and sulfamethoxazole (TMP-SMX, Bactrim, Septra). These agents have been shown to have a moderate effect on bowel and vaginal wall flora (100,101). Furthermore, TMP-SMX has become very popular in the management of UTIs because of its broad range of activity against uropathogens, low incidence of adverse effects, and twice-daily dosage. It should be noted that in a recent study, up to 39% of *E. coli* were resistant to TMP-SMX in a cohort of women with community-acquired UTI in states such as Michigan and California (102).

A group of synthetic quinoline derivatives, which are related chemically to nalidixic acid, has recently been introduced as antibacterial agents for UTI. Derivatives include norfloxacin, ciprofloxacin, lomefloxacin, amifloxacin, fleroxacin, enoxacin, ofloxacin, levofloxacin, and prulifloxacin (103). These agents are more active than nalidixic acid against gram-negative urinary tract pathogens (e.g., *E. coli*). In addition, they have an expanded antibacterial spectrum that includes *P. aeruginosa* and gram-positive bacteria (e.g., staphylococci, enterococci). All of these agents are administered orally, and parenteral formulations are available for some (e.g., ciprofloxacin and levofloxacin). An extended-release formulation of ciprofloxacin is available and is better tolerated than the immediate-release version (104). The cost of fluoroquinolones limits their routine use. These agents are also not appropriate for pregnant women, nursing mothers, and adolescents under the age of 18 as they interfere with bone and cartilage development and may impair growth (105).

Because they have no advantage over more standard agents (e.g., nitrofurantoin, TMP-SMX) for uncomplicated infections, newer-generation quinolones should be reserved for use in patients with resistant infections or as an alternative to parenteral antibiotics in certain complicated infections and cases of pyelonephritis (106–112). Unfortunately, their attractiveness has lead to widespread use, making ciprofloxacin the fourth most commonly prescribed antibiotic in the United States. This overuse has been accompanied by an increase in bacterial resistance; already, strains of *E. coli* are resistant to ciprofloxacin (113).

Based on the most recent NAUTICA study results, resistance rates of outpatient urinary isolates to commonly utilized antibiotics are as follows: ampicillin (45.9%), TMP-SMX (20.4%), nitrofurantoin (14.3%), ciprofloxacin (9.7%), and levofloxacin (8.1%) (19). One should appreciate the fact that antibiotic resistance patterns differ not only between countries, but also between different regions of a country and different hospitals within the same city (114,115).

Listed in Tables 10.2 and 10.3 are the dosage, toxicity, and spectrum of antimicrobial activity of some of the commonly prescribed oral antibiotics.

Asymptomatic Bacteriuria (in Patients Without Catheters)

By definition, asymptomatic bacteriuria is the recovery of at least 10^5 cfu/mL of a single bacterial species in at least two consecutive clean-voided urine specimens in the absence of clinical symptoms (55). Little is known about the natural history of untreated bacteriuria in women because most are treated once the diagnosis is made. Two studies have, however, compared antibiotic treatment with placebo in women with asymptomatic bacteriuria.

TABLE 10.2

Dosage and Toxicity of Antibiotics Commonly Used in the Treatment of UTIs

Drug and Frequency	Minor Toxicity	Major Toxicity
TMP-SMX 1 tablet bid.	Allergic	Serious skin reactions, blood dyscrasia
Nitrofurantoin 50 to 100 mg q6–8h	GI upset	Peripheral neuropathy, pneumonitis
Ampicillin 250 to 500 mg q6h	Allergic candidal overgrowth	Allergic reactions, pseudomembranous colitis
Tetracycline 250 to 500 mg 6qh	GI upset, skin rash, allergic candidal growth	Hepatic dysfunction, nephrotoxicity
Cephalexin 250 to 500 mg q6h	Allergic	Hepatic dysfunction
Norfloxacin 400 mg q12h	Nausea, vomiting, diarrhea, abdominal pain, skin rash	Convulsions, phychoses, joint damage
Levofloxacin 250 to 500 mg q24h	Disturbance of blood glucose, allergic, nausea, headache	Allergic reactions, tendon rupture, photosensitivity, pseudomembranous colitis
Ciprofloxacin 100 to 500 mg q12h	Anosmia, taste loss, myalgia, anaphylactic reaction	Theophylline interactions, dyspepsia, central nervous system effects, pseudomembranous colitis

TABLE 10.3

Spectrum of Antimicrobial Activity Against Common Lower Urinary Tract Pathogens

Organism	TMP-SMX	Nitrofur-antoin	Ampi-cillin	Tetra-cycline	Cepha-lexin	Carbeni-cillin	Genta-micin	Nor-floxacin	Levo-floxacin	Cipro-floxacin
Escherichia coli	++	++	++	±	++	++	++	++	++	++
Pseudomonas sp.	--	--	--	--	--	++	++	++	++	++
Klebsiella sp.	++	±	--	±	++	--	++	++	++	++
Proteus sp.	++	--	++	--	++	++	++	++	++	++
Enterobacter sp.	++	--	--	--	--	++	++	++	++	++
Enterococcus sp.	--	±	++	++	±	--	--	++	±	±
Staphylococcus sp.	--	±	++	+	++	++	+	++	++	++
Serratia marcescens	+	--	--	--	--	--	++	++	++	++

++, excellent; +,good; ±, occasionally effective; --, resistant.

They noted that 60% to 80% of these patients spontaneously clear their infection whether they are treated or receive placebo (116,117). Although the long-term effects of asymptomatic bacteriuria are not completely known, there appears to be no association with renal scarring, hypertension, or progressive renal azotemia.

Screening for asymptomatic bacteriuria has little apparent value in adults, with two exceptions: before urologic surgery and during pregnancy. Postoperative complications, including bacteremia, are reduced by recognizing and treating asymptomatic bacteriuria before urologic surgery (118). All pregnant women should be screened for bacteriuria in the first trimester and should be treated if bacteriuria is present to reduce their markedly increased risk for acute pyelonephritis and the accompanying risks for prematurity and low birthweight in their infants (119,120).

To date, there is no definite advantage to treating asymptomatic bacteriuria in nonpregnant female patients. There are, however, recent studies that have shown a significant association between asymptomatic UTI and overall mortality (121,122). Whether this mortality is a false-positive result or whether the bacteriuria is serving as a marker for a chronic disease that was the actual cause of death needs to be confirmed by further studies.

First Infections or Infrequent Reinfections

Many treatment regimens have been reported for initial therapy of simple cystitis, ranging from one dose to 2 or more weeks of medication. The longer treatment regimens were instituted in an attempt to prevent relapse, which occurs in about 20% of patients treated for cystitis. Almost all of these relapses are attributable to the colonization of the vaginal walls and urethra with gram-negative bacteria that have continued to grow on the perineum or reappeared when the drug was stopped. It does not indicate that the prescribed drug has failed to eradicate the bacteriuria.

There are numerous studies in the literature evaluating single-dose therapy in the management of acute uncomplicated cystitis (123–132). When single-dose therapy was compared with 10 days of TMP-SMX, there was a significantly higher treatment failure rate with single-dose therapy (132). Further concern has been raised that single-dose regimens are less likely to be effective in treatment of infections when an unrecognized complicating factor is present, such as pregnancy, diabetes, or an anatomic or functional abnormality of the urinary tract. Single-dose therapy has also been noted to be suboptimal in the treatment of occult upper UTI (133).

A plethora of studies has been conducted in recent years to define the optimal antimicrobial agent and length of treatment for uncomplicated cystitis in women. With most antimicrobial agents, 3-day regimens appear optimal, with efficacy comparable with 7-day regimens but with fewer side effects and lower cost. Nitrofurantoin, cefadroxil, amoxicillin, and TMP-SMX have been shown to be effective in 3-day regimens, either in open trials or in comparative trials with longer regimens. A recent prospective randomized trial compared these four antimicrobial agents in a 3-day regimen in young women with acute cystitis (134). The findings demonstrated that a 3-day regimen of twice-daily TMP-SMX was more effective than 3 days of nitrofurantoin, cefadroxil, or amoxicillin. Moreover, TMP-SMX was the least expensive of the four regimens, mainly because, compared with the other regimens, patients were less likely to have to return for evaluation of persistent or recurrent UTI or for yeast vaginitis (134). We, therefore, favor the use of TMP-SMX as our first-line agent for empiric treatment of acute uncomplicated cystitis in women.

Alternate regimens that can be used in women who have a history of intolerance to TMP-SMX are nitrofurantoin, 100 mg four times daily, or TMP, 100 mg twice daily. We try to avoid the use of amoxicillin or first-generation cephalosporins because we have experienced a relatively high failure rate with these agents in our clinic. Single-dose therapy or a short course of therapy should be considered only in patients who are at very low risk for treatment failures. Thus, patients who have (a) systemic diseases, such as diabetes mellitus; (b) a history of acute pyelonephritis; (c) a history of a treatment failure in the past 6 months; (d) a history of childhood UTIs; or (e) known structural abnormalities of the urinary tract should be given a longer 7- to 10-day course of therapy.

For patients with acute simple cystitis who have complete resolution of their symptoms, it is not necessary to perform any routine posttreatment urinary assessment. However, in those patients whose urinary symptoms persist beyond the 3 days of therapy, a urine culture and sensitivity should be obtained. Persistence of symptoms should suggest the possibility that either the initial diagnosis of UTI was in error or that the patient's infection is secondary to a resistant organism that was present from the onset of therapy or has developed during initial therapy. In cases of resistance, a 7- to 10-day course of a sensitive antibiotic should then be prescribed.

A recent study evaluated the use of phone triage of patients with symptoms of acute uncomplicated UTI. Eligible patients were offered antibiotics without an office visit, urinalysis, or urine culture. There were no significant increases in potential adverse outcomes, namely subsequent visits for cystitis, sexually transmitted diseases, or pyelonephritis, during the 60 days after diagnosis (135).

Recurrent Infections

About 75% of all women who experience a UTI subsequently experience less than one infection per year (136). However, the other 25% of women develop reinfections at a rate of almost three infections per year. These women compose 50% of all women presenting with acute UTIs (136–139).

Once the urine has been sterilized by appropriate antimicrobial therapy, the pattern of culture-documented reinfection or recurrence is very helpful in the subsequent management of these patients (Fig. 10.6). It can also be used to classify patients with different infectious etiologies to identify those who may be at increased risk or require further urologic evaluation. The most common type of recurrence is reinfection by bacteria different from the initially infecting strain. Even though the infections may be caused by the same species (e.g., *E. coli*), the organisms can usually be differentiated on the basis of colonial morphology and antimicrobial sensitivities. These infections are almost invariably due to a recurrent ascending infection from the vaginal introital area. It has been shown that the same strain can exist in the introital area for many months and cause multiple reinfections. Sexual intercourse and occult urinary tract abnormalities may also facilitate reinfection and must always be considered in these patients.

Relapsing infection from an upper urinary tract source of an infected stone should be suspected if the same organism is repeatedly isolated 7 to 10 days after treatment with an antimicrobial agent to which the organism is sensitive. In many of these patients, one cannot obtain sterile urine, and thus these cases are termed bacterial persistence (causes

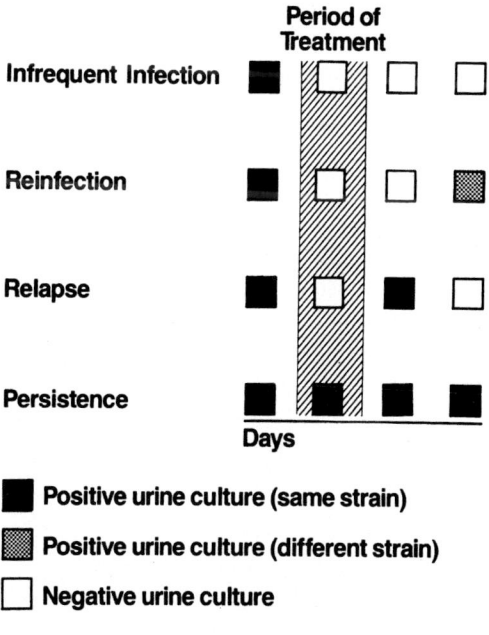

FIGURE 10.6 • Natural history of UTI.

are listed in Table 10.4). Endoscopic and radiographic evaluations must be selectively performed in cases of relapse or persistence of infection.

The goal of the management of reinfected urine is to achieve sterile urine; this is the basis for subsequent successful use of antimicrobial agents. To eradicate UTIs successfully, antimicrobial agents should be administered in sufficient doses to exceed, by a wide margin, the minimal concentration required to inhibit growth. Lower dosages lead to the selection of resistant organisms from the original population in about 10% of the cases, complicating the treatment of these already difficult patients.

Recurrent cystitis should be documented by culture at least once and then managed by one of three strategies: continuous prophylaxis, postcoital prophylaxis, or therapy initiated by the patient (self-start therapy). Continuous prophylaxis has been shown to be highly cost-effective and is recommended as the initial form of therapy in women who have frequent reinfections (140,141). Its success depends on using the minimal dosage of an antimicrobial agent that has minimal or no adverse effect on the fecal flora. Once the urine has been completely sterilized by a full-dose course of therapy, nightly therapy is begun with one of many different drugs (Table 10.5). Nitrofurantoin (140), 100 mg, or cephalexin (141), 250 mg, is effective therapy. These drugs do not cause resistance in the fecal flora; however, vaginal colonization with sensitive bacteria does continue. Their efficacy depends on nightly bactericidal activity in the bladder urine against sensitive reinfecting organisms. The efficacy of cephalexin is dependent on use of a minimal dosage. If it is given four times a day in

TABLE 10.5

Oral Antimicrobial Agents Useful for Prophylactic Prevention of Recurrent UTIs

Nitrofurantatoin 100 mg
Cephalexin 250 mg
TMP-SMX 1 tablet (each regular tablet contains 80 mg trimethoprim and 400 mg sulfamethoxazole)
Cinoxacin 250 to 500 mg

full dosages, it gives rise to resistant strains. When it is given in a dose of 250 mg nightly, it does not. TMP-SMX (142) is active not only because of bactericidal activity against urinary bacteria but also because TMP diffuses into the vaginal fluid at a concentration bactericidal to most urinary pathogens in the vagina (143). Low-dose TMP-SMX or TMP alone causes resistance in about 10% of rectal cultures (142). Most of these patients continue to maintain sterile urine while receiving prophylactic therapy, although breakthrough infections may infrequently occur and should be treated with full-dose sensitive antimicrobial therapy. We empirically continue the prophylactic therapy for about 6 months and, at that time, follow the patient off therapy with frequent cultures. About 30% of women have a spontaneous remission for at least the following 6 months (139). Unfortunately, a remission does not necessarily reflect a complete cure. If reinfection occurs, it must be managed by reinstitution of low-dose nightly prophylaxis.

Self-start intermittent therapy can be an alternative to continuous prophylactic therapy in patients with recurrent UTIs. When this regimen is used, the patient is given a dip-slide device and instructed to perform a urine culture when she has symptoms consistent with a recurrent UTI. She then empirically starts a 3-day course of full-dose antimicrobial therapy, usually with one of the previously mentioned antibiotics. Full-dose nitrofurantoin, cinoxacin, or norfloxacin is usually successful. Norfloxacin appears to be an ideal drug for self-start therapy. It has a broader spectrum of activity than any other oral agent and is comparable with or better than most available parenteral antimicrobial agents. In addition, it has activity against multiple-resistance bacteria, and bacteria

TABLE 10.4

Correctable Urinary Tract Abnormalities Causing Persistent Bacteriuria

Urethral diverticulum
Infected stone
Significant anterior vaginal wall relaxation
Papillary necrosis
Foreign body
Duplicated or ectopic ureter
Atrophic pyelonephritis (unilateral)
Medullary sponge kidney

exposed to this agent have a low rate of spontaneous mutation to resistant organisms. In a multicenter comparative study of more than 350 patients with UTI, the percentage of strains susceptible to norfloxacin was 99%. This was significantly greater than the percentage of strains susceptible to TMP-SMX, which was about 90%. Also, the percentage of bacteriologic cures was significantly higher with the norfloxacin (than TMP-SMX), and side effects were minimal (144). Self-start therapy has proved to be safe, effective, reliable, and economical in women with recurrent UTIs (145,146).

If a patient's history suggests that reinfections are preceded by intercourse, she may take a single antimicrobial tablet before or after intercourse (147). Vosti (148) first demonstrated that nitrofurantoin given after coitus prevented recurrent UTI. More recently, Pfau et al (149) showed that TMP-SMX, nalidixic acid, nitrofurantoin, and sulfonamide were all effective in preventing recurrent UTIs when given to young sexually active women whose infections occurred postcoitally. In a recent study, 135 sexually active premenopausal women with recurrent UTIs were randomly assigned to receive daily prophylaxis of ciprofloxacin, 125 mg, or a single dose of 125 mg after intercourse. Results for the two groups were similar, with the postintercourse group consuming only one-third the amount of drug (150). If feasible, a woman who has recurrent UTIs and uses a diaphragm as her mode of contraception should consider another method. If she is unable or unwilling to change to another method, she should be closely questioned about symptoms of urinary obstruction occurring with the diaphragm in place. If such symptoms occur, it should be ascertained if the fit of the diaphragm is too large. Women in this category of intercourse-related infection should also be advised to void as promptly as possible after intercourse.

Postmenopausal women may also have frequent reinfections. These infections are sometimes attributable to residual urine after voiding, which is often associated with pelvic organ prolapse. In addition, the lack of estrogen causes marked changes in the vaginal microflora, including loss of bacilli and increased colonization by E. coli (151). Antimicrobial prophylaxis or topically applied estrogen cream can be used as an alternative preventive measure in such women. It has been shown that in addition to antibiotic prophylaxis, postmenopausal women with recurrent UTIs using an estradiol-releasing silicone vaginal ring had significantly fewer recurrent UTIs than women

without estrogen treatment (152). Local estrogen therapy leads to increased bladder perfusion; this may be the mechanism behind its protective effect (153).

Complicated Infections

Complicated UTIs occur in patients with a functionally, metabolically, or anatomically abnormal urinary tract or are caused by pathogens that are resistant to antibiotics. It is only safe to assume that a premenopausal, sexually active, nonpregnant woman, with recent onset of symptoms, who was not recently subjected to instrumentation, has an uncomplicated UTI. Complicated infections can range from mild cystitis to life-threatening urosepsis. In addition, there may be long periods of asymptomatic bacteriuria. Urine cultures, therefore, must be obtained in patients suspected of having complicated infection to identify the infecting pathogen and perform susceptibility testing.

The wide variety of underlying conditions and diverse spectrum of possible etiologic agents make generalizing about antimicrobial therapy difficult. For empiric therapy in patients with mild-to-moderate illness who can be treated as outpatients, the fluoroquinolones provide a broad spectrum of antimicrobial activity covering most expected pathogens and achieve high levels in the urine. At least 10 to 14 days of therapy is usually necessary. Pseudomonas and enterococcal infections are especially difficult to treat and may warrant more prolonged therapy. Without correction of the underlying anatomic, functional, or metabolic defect, infection often recurs. For this reason, a urine culture should be repeated 1 to 2 weeks after the completion of therapy.

Catheter-Associated Infection

Catheter-associated UTI is the most common hospital-associated infection and is the most frequent source of bacteremia in hospitalized patients (154). One study showed a threefold increase in mortality in these patients (155). In another study of 1,497 newly catheterized patients at a university hospital, 235 new cases of catheter-associated UTI were discovered. However, greater than 90% of the infected patients were symptom-free, and only one patient developed a secondary bloodstream infection (156). The mechanism through which bacteriuria is related to mortality is uncertain. Risk factors for catheter-associated infection are advanced age, female sex, and an increasing degree of underlying illness (157). The pathogenesis of catheter-associated urinary infection has not been studied as well as UTI of noncatheterized patients. Points of bacterial entry, however, have been well defined and include introduction of bacteria residing in the urethra into the bladder at the time of catheterization, subsequent entry of bacteria colonizing the urethra meatus along the mucus sheath external to the catheter, and ascent of bacteria within the catheter lumen itself. The relative proportions of infections occurring through these different routes of entry have not been clearly defined. Prospective studies demonstrated that organisms causing infection in catheterized patients can be identified in the urethral or rectal flora 2 to 4 days before the onset of bacteriuria in 70% of women (158). Another prospective study of 1,497 newly catheterized patients found 235 new urinary tract infections and determined that 66% were extraluminal and 34% were derived from intraluminal contaminants (159).

Until more is known about the pathogenesis of nosocomial bacteriuria, the bulk of preventive efforts should continue to focus on aseptic care of the urinary catheter (160) (Table 10.6). There has been no demonstrable efficacy of local antimicrobial ointments applied to the meatal junction despite the apparent association of meatal colonization with subsequent infection (161,162). The use of antimicrobial irrigants has also been ineffective in reducing the prevalence of bacteriuria (163). Although systemic antimicrobial agents reduce the occurrence of bacteriuria for the first few days of catheterization, their use cannot be widely recommended at this time because the benefit accrued (that is, reduction of asymptomatic bacteriuria) may not be worth the cost and attendant risk for development of resistant microorganisms (164).

The diagnosis and management of these UTIs in elderly nursing home patients with long-term catheterization (greater than 3 months) can present

TABLE 10.6

Prevention of Bladder Infection in Elderly Long-Term Catheterized Patients

Monitor urine level in bag q4h; exchange catheter if cessation of flow for 4h.
Fluid intake of 1.5L/d
Avoid catheter manipulations.
Exchange catheter if infection is suspected.
Exchange catheter every 8 to 12 weeks.

a challenge. All patients with indwelling catheters for any length of time will develop bacteria in their urine (Fig. 10.7). However, as long as the catheter system is a closed functioning system and the patient has no local or systemic symptoms or signs, there is no advantage to empiric systemic antibiotics. On the other hand, 10% of elderly patients with indwelling catheters develop bacteremia and gram-negative septicemia, a serious disease with a 20% to 50% mortality rate. These patients must be promptly identified because they require hospitalization and vigorous systemic antibiotic therapy. A traumatic event consisting of obstruction, manipulation, or removal of an inflated indwelling bladder catheter often precedes the onset of urosepsis. In addition to antibiotic therapy, it is essential to establish free flow of urine for the catheterized patient with acute urosepsis.

The complications of concomitant bacteremia (shock, adult respiratory distress syndrome, disseminated intravascular coagulation, and gastric hemorrhage) must be readily recognized and managed appropriately. Certain measures can be taken to prevent these life-threatening complications in patients with chronic indwelling catheters (see Table 10.6). Catheters should be checked every 4 hours by experienced personnel to ensure proper drainage and to prevent formation of any encrustation within the tubing of the catheter; indwelling catheters should be changed every 8 to 12 weeks, depending on whether they are silicon- or Teflon-coated catheters.

Lower Urinary Tract Instrumentation

Whether patients undergoing lower urinary tract instrumentation for diagnostic or therapeutic purposes need prophylactic antibiotics is, currently, an unresolved issue. A recent prospective double-blind placebo-controlled study by Cundiff et al (165) compared nitrofurantoin with placebo in patients undergoing urodynamics and cysto-urethroscopy. Although the power of the study was limited, they found no significant difference in bacteriuria between the two groups. Also, the prevalence of significant bacteriuria before instrumentation was low at 5%, and the overall incidence of significant bacteriuria after instrumentation was 6% for both groups (165). For this reason, we do not routinely give antibiotics to low-risk patients after lower urinary tract instrumentation. In patients undergoing intermittent catheterization, bacteriuria may be reduced by bladder irrigation with a solution of neomycin or polymyxin or by oral methenamine, nitrofurantoin, or TMP-SMX prophylaxis (166).

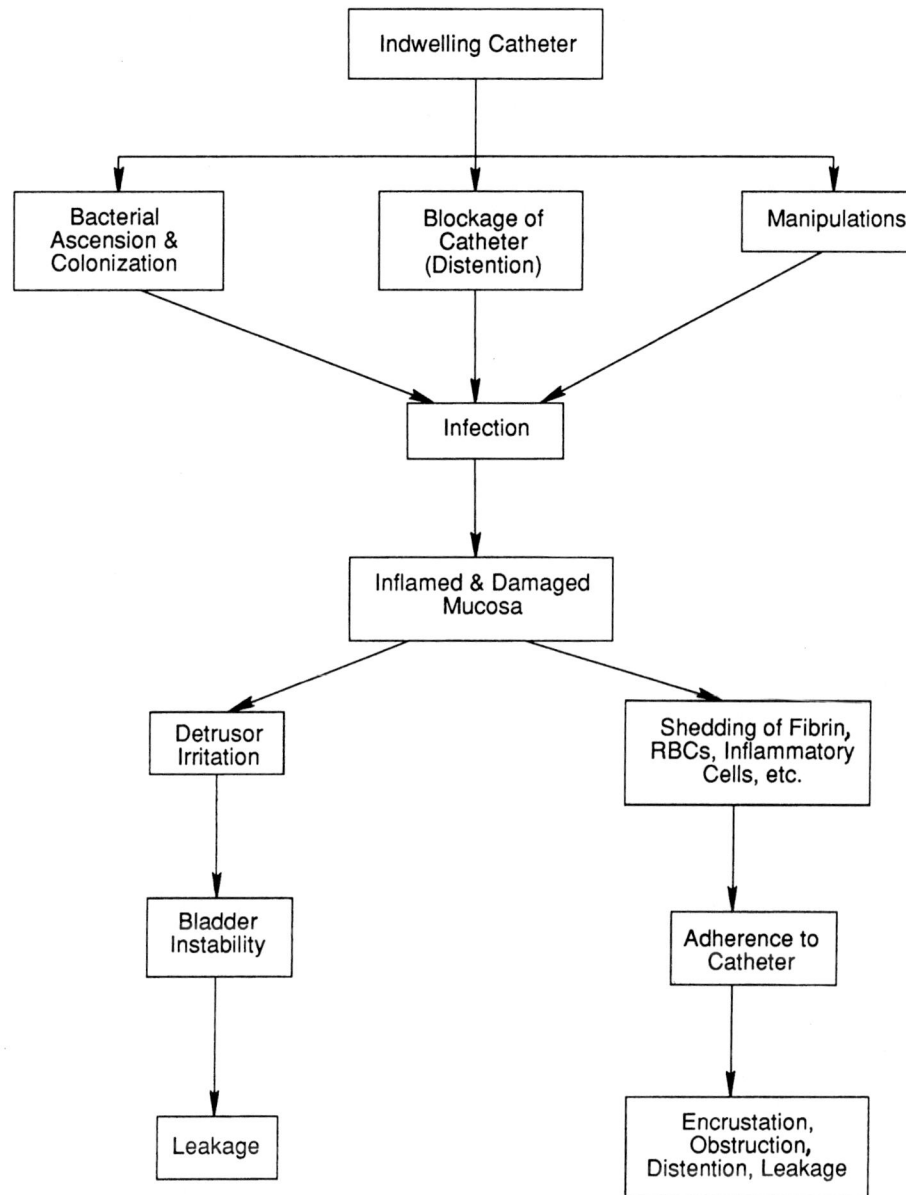

FIGURE 10.7 ● Pathogenesis of infection and clinical picture of females with long-term indwelling catheters. RBC, red blood cell.

REFERENCES

1. National Center for Health Statistics. Ambulatory medical care rendered in physicians offices. United States 1975. *Adv Data* 1977;12:1–8.
2. Gribling TL. Urologic diseases in America project: trends in resource use for urinary tract infections in women. *J Urol* 2005;173:1281–1287.
3. Cox LE, Lacy SS, Hinman F. The urethra and its relationship to urinary tract infection. II. The urethral flora of the female with recurrent urinary tract infection. *J Urol* 1968;99:632–638.
4. Winberg J, Anderson HJ, Bergstrom T, et al. Epidemiology of symptomatic urinary tract infection in childhood. *Acta Paediatr Scand* 1974;252[Suppl]:3–21.
5. Rolleston GL, Shannon FT, Utley WLF. Relationship of infantile vesico-ureteric reflux to renal damage. *Br Med J* 1970;1:460–464.
6. Mulholland SG. Controversies in management of urinary tract infection. *Urology* 1986;27[Suppl]:3–8.
7. Bachmann G. Urogenital ageing: an old problem newly recognized. *Maturitas* 1995;22[Suppl]:1–5.
8. Mayer TR. UTI in the elderly: how to select treatment. *Geriatrics* 1980;35:67–73.

9. Turck M, Stamm W. Nosocomial infection of the urinary tract. _Am J Med_ 1981;70:651–659.

10. Maskell R. Importance of coagulase-negative Staphylococci as pathogens in the urinary tract. _Lancet_ 1974; 1:1155–1159.

11. Sellin M, Cooke DI, Gillespie WA, et al. Micrococcal urinary tract infections in young women. _Lancet_ 1975; 2:570–572.

12. Smyth M, Moore JE, McClurg RB, et al. Quantitative calorimetric measurement of residual antimicrobials in the urine of patients with suspected urinary tract infection. _Br J Biomed Sci_ 2005;62(3):114–119.

13. Hovelius B. Urinary tract infections caused by _Staphylococcus saprophyticus_ recurrences and complications. _J Urol_ 1979;122:645–650.

14. Marrie T, Kwan C, Noble M, et al. _Staphylococcus saprophyticus_ as a cause of urinary tract infections. _J Clin Microbiol_ 1982;6:427–432.

15. Bailey RR. Significance of coagulase-negative Staphylococcus in urine. _J Infect Dis_ 1973;127:179–183.

16. Wallmark G, Arremark I, Telander B. _Staphylococcus saprophyticus_: a frequent cause of acute urinary tract infection among female outpatients. _J Infect Dis_ 1978; 138:791–794.

17. Lewis JF, Brake SR, Anderson DJ, et al. Urinary tract infection due to coagulase-negative Staphylococcus. _Am J Clin Pathol_ 1982;77:736–742.

18. Nicolle LE, Hoban SA, Harding GKM. Characterization of coagulase-negative Staphylococci from urinary isolates. _J Clin Microbiol_ 1983;17:267–271.

19. Zhanel GG, Hisanaga TL, Laing NM, et al. Antibiotic resistance in outpatient urinary isolates: final results from North American Urinary Tract Infection Collaborative Alliance (NAUTICA). _Int J Antimicrob Agent_ 2005;26(5):380–388.

20. Nash TE, Cheever AW, Ottesen EA, et al. Schistosome infections in humans: perspectives and recent findings. NIH conference. _Ann Intern Med_ 1982;97(5):7 40–754.

21. Bryant RE, Sutcliffe MC, McGee FE. Human polymorphonuclear leukocyte function in urine. _Yale J Biol Med_ 1973;46:113.

22. Kaye D. Antibacterial activity of human urine. _J Clin Invest_ 1968;47:2374–2390.

23. Stamey TA. Urinary tract infections in women. In: Stamey TA, ed. _Pathogenesis and treatment of urinary tract infections._ Baltimore: Williams & Wilkins, 1980: 122–209.

24. Eden CS, Eriksson B, Hanson LA. Adhesion of _Escherichia coli_ to human uroepithelial cells in vitro. _Infect Immunol_ 1977;18:767–773.

25. Stamey TA, Timothy MM. Studies of introital colonizations in women with recurrent urinary infections. I. The role of vaginal pH. _J Urol_ 1975;114:261–265.

26. Parsons DL, Schmidt JD. Control of recurrent lower urinary tract infections in the postmenopausal women. _J Urol_ 1982;128:1224.

27. Cardozo L, Lose G, McClish D, et al. A systematic review of estrogens for recurrent urinary tract infections: a report of the Hormones and Urogenital Therapy (HUT) committee. _Int Urogyn J_ 2001;12(1):15–20.

28. Cardozo L, Benness C, Abbott D. Low-dose oestrogen prophylaxis for recurrent urinary tract infections in elderly women. _Br J Obstet Gynaecol_ 1998;105:403–407.

29. Cox CE, Hinman F. Experiments with induced bacteriuria, vesical emptying, and bacterial growth on the mechanism of bladder defense to infection. _J Urol_ 1961;86:739.

30. Foxman B, Somsel P, Tallma P, et al. Urinary tract infection among women aged 40 to 65: behavioral and sexual risk factors. _J Clin Epidemiol_ 2001;54: 710–718.

31. Orskov I, Ferencz A, Orskov F. Tamm-Horsfall protein or uromucoid is the normal urinary slime that traps type I fimbriated _Escherichia coli._ Lancet 1980;1:887–893.

32. Parsons CL. Prevention of urinary tract infection by the exogenous glycosaminoglycan sodium pentosanpolysulfate. _J Urol_ 1982;127:167–169.

33. Parsons CL, Greenspan C, Moore SW, et al. Role of surface mucin in primary antibacterial defense of bladder. _Urology_ 1977;9:48–52.

34. Reid G, Sobol JD. Bacterial adherence in the pathogenesis of urinary tract infection: a review. _Rev Infect Dis_ 1987;9:470–487.

35. Kallonius G, Mollby R, Svenson SB, et al. The P^k antigen as receptor for the haemagglutinin of pyelonephritic _Escherichia coli._ _FEMS Microbiol Lett_ 1980; 7:297.

36. Vaisanen V, Elo J, Tallgreen LG, et al. Mannose-resistant haemagglutination and P antigen recognition are characteristic of _Escherichia coli_ causing primary pyelonephritis. _Lancet_ 1981;2:1366–1371.

37. Iwahi T, Abe Y, Nakao M, et al. Role of type I fimbriae in the pathogenesis of ascending urinary tract infection induced by _Escherichia coli_ in mice. _Infect Immunol_ 1983;39:1307–1315.

38. Schaeffer AJ, Jones JM, Dunn JK. Association of in vitro _Escherichia coli_ adherence to vaginal and buccal epithelial cells with susceptibility of women to recurrent urinary tract infections. _N Engl J Med_ 1981;304: 1062–1066.

39. Schaeffer AJ, Amundsen SK, Schmidt LN. Adherence of _Escherichia coli_ to human urinary tract epithelial cells. _Infect Immunol_ 1979;24:753–757.

40. Schaeffer AJ, Radvany RM, Chmiel JS. Human leukocyte antigens in women with recurrent urinary tract infections. _J Infect Dis_ 1983;148:604–610.

41. Kinane DF, Blackwell CC, Brettle RP, et al. ABO blood group, secretor state, and susceptibility to recurrent urinary tract infection in women. _Br Med J_ 1982; 285:7–11.

42. Gaffney RA, Schaeffer AJ, Anderson BE, et al. Effect of Lewis blood group antigen on antigen expression on bacterial adherence to COS-1 cells. _Infect Immunol_ 1994;62:3022–3026.

43. Hopkins WJ, Heisey DM, Lorentzen DF, et al. A comparative study of major histocompatibility complex and red blood cell antigens phenotypes as risk factors for recurrent urinary tract infections in women. _J Infect Dis_ 1998;177:1296–1301.

44. Jantausch BA, Criss VR, O'Donnell R, et al. Association of Lewis blood groups phenotypes with urinary tract infection in children. _J Pediatr_ 1994;124: 863–868.

45. May SJ, Blackwell CC, Brettle RP, et al. Non-secretion of ABO blood group antigens: a host factor predisposing to recurrent urinary tract infections and renal scarring. _FEMS Microbiol Immunol_ 1989; 1(6–7):383–387.

46. Sheinfeld J, Schaeffer AJ, Cordon-Cardo C, et al. Association of the Lewis blood group phenotype with recurrent urinary tract infections in women. _N Engl J Med_ 1989;320:773–777.

47. Nicolle LE, Harding GKM, Preiksaitis J, et al. The association of urinary tract infection with sexual intercourse. _J Infect Dis_ 1982;146:579–584.

48. Hooton TM, Stapleton E, Roberts PL, et al. Perineal anatomy and urine-voiding characteristics of young women with and without recurrent urinary tract infections. *Clin Infect Dis* 1999;29:1600–1601.

49. Strom BL, Collins M, West SL, et al. Sexual activity, contraceptive use, and other risk factors for symptomatic and asymptomatic bacteriuria. *Ann Intern Med* 1987;107:816–823.

50. Fihn SD, Latham RH, Roberts P, et al. Association between diaphragm use and urinary tract infection. *JAMA* 1985;253:240–244.

51. Foxman B, Frerichs RR. Epidemiology of urinary tract infection. I. Diaphragm use and sexual intercourse. *Am J Public Health* 1985;75:1308–1315.

52. Fihn SD, Johnson L, Pinkstaff C, et al. Diaphragm use and urinary tract infection: analysis of urodynamic and microbiologic factors. *J Urol* 1986;136:853–856.

53. Nickel JC, Lee JC, Grantmyre JE, et al. Natural history of urinary tract infection in a primary care environment in Canada. *Can J Urol* 2005;12(4):2728–2737.

54. Nergardh A, Boreus LO, Holme T. The inhibitory effect of coli endotoxin on alpha-adrenergic receptor functions in the lower urinary tract. An in vitro study in cats. *Scand J Urol Nephrol* 1977;11:219–228.

55. Kass EH. Asymptomatic infections of the urinary tract. *Trans Assoc Am Physicians* 1956;69:56.

56. Kass EH. Bacteriuria and diagnosis of infections of the urinary tract. *Arch Intern Med* 1967;100:709–714.

57. Stamey TA, Govan DE, Palmer JM. The localization and treatment of urinary tract infections: the role of bactericidal urine levels as opposed to serum levels. *Medicine* 1965;44:1–8.

58. Turck M, Goffe B, Petersdorf RG. The urethral catheter and urinary tract infection. *J Urol* 1962;88:834–837.

59. Thiel G, Spuhler O. Urinary tract infection by catheter and the so-called infectious (episomal) resistance. *Schweiz Med Wochenschr* 1965;95:1155.

60. Fihn SD, Stamm WE. Management of women with acute dysuria. In: Rund D, Wolcott BW, eds. *Emergency medicine annual.* Norwalk, CT: Appleton-Century-Crofts, 1983;2:225.

61. MacDermott RJ. The interpretation of midstream urine microscopy and culture results in women who present acutely to the labor ward. *Br J Obstet Gynecol* 1994; 101:712–713.

62. Stamm WE. Measurement of pyuria and its relation to bacteriuria. *Am J Med* 1983;75:53.

63. Johnson JR, Stamm WE. Diagnosis and treatment of acute urinary tract infection. *Infect Dis Clin North Am* 1987;1:773–779.

64. Pappas PG. Laboratory in the diagnosis and management of urinary tract infections. *Med Clin North Am* 1991;75:313–325.

65. Wu TC, Williams EC, Koo SY, et al. Evaluation of three bacteriuria screening methods in a clinical research hospital. *J Clin Microbiol* 1985;21:796–814.

66. Kunin CM. *Detection, prevention, and management of urinary tract infection*, 4th ed. Philadelphia: Lea & Febiger, 1987:195–234.

67. Bixler-Forell E, Bertram MA, Bruckner DA. Clinical evaluation of three rapid methods for the detection of significant bacteriuria. *J Clin Microbiol* 1985;22:62–68.

68. Needham CA. Rapid detection methods in microbiology: are they right for your office? *Med Clin North Am* 1987;71:591–605.

69. Richards D, Toop L, Chamvers S, et al. Response to antibiotics of women with symptoms of urinary tract infection but negative dipstick urine test results: double-blind randomised controlled trial. *Br Med J* 2005; 331(7509):143.

70. Kraft JK, Stamey TA. The natural history of symptomatic recurrent bacteriuria in women. *Medicine* 1977;56:55–61.

71. Mabeck CE. Studies in urinary tract infections. I. The diagnosis of bacteriuria in women. *Acta Med Scand* 1969;186:35–41.

72. Kunz HH, Sieberth HG, Freiberg J, et al. Zur Bedeutung der Blasenpunktion fur den sicheren Nachweis einer Bacteriurie. *Dtsch Med Wochenschr* 1975;100:2252.

73. Stamm WE, Counts GW, Running KR, et al. Diagnosis of coliform infection in acutely dysuric women. *N Engl J Med* 1982;307:463–467.

74. Kass EH. The role of asymptomatic bacteriuria in the pathogenesis of pyelonephritis. In: Quinn EL, Kass EH, eds. *Biology of pyelonephritis.* Boston: Little, Brown, 1960:399.

75. Lifshitz E, Kramer L. Outpatient urine culture: does collection technique matter? *Arch Intern Med* 2000; 160:2537–2540.

76. Fowler JE Jr, Pulaski T. Excretory urography, cystography, and cystoscopy in the evaluation of women with urinary tract infection. *N Engl J Med* 1981;304: 462–468.

77. Engel G, Schaeffer AJ, Grayhack JT, et al. The role of excretory urography and cystoscopy in the evaluation and management of women with recurrent urinary tract infection. *J Urol* 1980;123:190–198.

78. DeLange HE, Jones B. Unnecessary intravenous urography in young women with recurrent urinary tract infections. *Clin Radiol* 1983;34:551–556.

79. Fair WR, McClennan BL, Jost RG. Are excretory urograms necessary in evaluating women with urinary tract infections? *J Urol* 1979;121:313.

80. Mogensen P, Hansen LK. Do intravenous urography and cystoscopy provide important information in otherwise healthy women with recurrent urinary tract infection? *Br J Urol* 1983;55:261.

81. Newhouse JH, Rhea JT, Murphy RX, et al. Yield of screening urography in young women with urinary tract infection. *Urol Radiol* 1982;4:187.

82. Tanagho EA, Miller ER, Lyon HP, et al. Spastic striated external sphincter and urinary tract infection in girls. *Br J Urol* 1971;43:69.

83. Gallagher DJ, Montgomerie JZ, North JD. Acute infections of the urinary tract and the urethral syndrome in general practice. *Br Med J* 1965;1:622.

84. Gillespie WA, Henderson EP, Linton KB, et al. Microbiology of the urethral (frequency and dysuria) syndrome: a controlled study with 5-year review. *Br J Urol* 1989;64:270–274.

85. Bergman A, Karram MM, Bhatia NN. Urethral syndrome: a comparison of different treatment modalities. *J Reprod Med* 1989;34:157–160.

86. Stamm WE, Running K, McKevitt M, et al. Treatment of acute urethral syndrome. *N Engl J Med* 1981;304: 956–960.

87. Kontiokari T, Sundquist K, Nuutenen M, et al. Randomised trial of cranberry-lingoberry juice and Lactobcillus GG drink for the prevention of urinary tract infections in women. *Br Med J* 2001;322:1571–1575.

88. Nickel JC, Lee JC, Grantmyre JE, et al. Natural history of urinary tract infection in a primary care environment in Canada. *Can J Urol* 2005;12(4):2728–2737.

89. Klimberg I, Shockey G, Ellison H, et al. Time to symptom relief for uncomplicated urinary tract infection treated with extended-release ciprofloxacin: a prospective, open-label, uncontrolled primary care study. *Curr Med Res Opin* 2005;21(8):1241–1250.

90. Amit G, Halkin A. Lemon-yellow nails and long-term phenazopyridine use. *Ann Intern Med* 1997;127(12): 1137.

91. Sobota AE. Inhibition of bacterial adherence by cranberry juice: potential use for the treatment of urinary tract infections. *J Urol* 1984;131:1013–1017.

92. Kunin CM, Finland M. Clinical pharmacology of the tetracycline antibiotics. *Clin Pharmacol Ther* 1961;2: 51.

93. Francke EL, Neu HC. Chloramphenicol and tetracyclines. *Med Clin North Am* 1987;71:1155–1168.

94. Parsons CL. Urinary tract infections in the female patient. *Urol Clin North Am* 1985;12:355–361.

95. Reed MD, Blumer JL. Urologic pharmacology in the office setting. *Urol Clin North Am* 1988;15:737–751.

96. Conklin JD. The pharmacokinetics of nitrofurantoin and its related bioavailability. *Antimicrob Agents Chemother* 1978;25:233–237.

97. Mayrer AR, Andriole VT. Urinary tract antiseptics. *Med Clin North Am* 1982;66:199–216.

98. Hoener B, Patterson SE. Nitrofurantoin disposition. *Clin Pharmacol Ther* 1981;29:808–815.

99. Kalowski S, Rudford N, Kincaid-Smith P. Crystalline and macrocrystalline nitrofurantoin in the treatment of urinary tract infection. *N Engl J Med* 1974;290:385–389.

100. Reed MD, Besunder JB, Blumer JL. Sulfonamides. In: Koren G, Prober CG, Gold R, eds. *Antimicrobial therapy in infants and children.* New York: Marcel Dekker, 1988:153–172.

101. Weinstein L, Madoff MA, Samet CM. The sulfonamides. *N Engl J Med* 1960;263:793–801.

102. Manges AR, Johnson JR, Foxman B, et al. Widespread distribution of urinary tract infections caused by multidrug-resistant *Escherichia coli* clonal group. *N Engl J Med* 2001;345:1007–1013.

103. Carmignani G, De Rose AF, Olivieri L, et al. Prulifloxacin versus ciprofloxacin in the treatment of adults with complicated urinary tract infections. *Urol Int* 2005;74(4):326–331.

104. Fourcroy JL, Berner B, Chiang YK, et al. Efficacy and safety of a novel once-daily extended-release ciprofloxacin tablet formulation for treatment of uncomplicated urinary tract infection in women. *Antimicrob Agent Chemother* 2005;49(10):4137–4143.

105. Stahlmann R. Children as a special population at risk: quinolones as an example for xenobiotics exhibiting skeletal toxicity. *Arch Toxicol* 2003;77(1):7–11.

106. Hooper DC, Wolfson JS. The fluoroquinolones: pharmacology, clinical uses, and toxicities in humans. *Antimicrob Agents Chemother* 1985;28:716–722.

107. Neu HC. Quinolones: a new class of antimicrobial agents with wide potential uses. *Med Clin North Am* 1988;72:623–636.

108. Wise R, Griggs D, Andrews JM. Pharmokinetics of the quinolones in volunteers: a proposed dosing schedule. *Rev Infect Dis* 1988;10[Suppl 1]:S83–S89.

109. Wolfson JS, Hooper DC. The fluoroquinolones: structures, mechanisms of action and resistance, and spectra of activity in vitro. *Antimicrob Agents Chemother* 1985;28:581–590.

110. Childs SJ, Goldstein EJ. Ciprofloxacin as treatment for genitourinary tract infection. *J Urol* 1989;141:1–5.

111. Goldstein EJ, Alpert ML, Najem A. Norfloxacin in the treatment of complicated and uncomplicated urinary tract infections: a comparative multicenter trial. *Am J Med* 1987;82:65–69.

112. Lee C, Ronald AN. Norfloxacin: its potential in clinical practice. *Am J Med* 1987;82:27–34.

113. Arslan H, Azap OK, Egonul O, et al. Risk factors for ciprofloxacin resistance among *Escherichia coli* strains isolated from community-acquired urinary tract infections in Turkey. *J Antimicrob Chemother* 2005; 56(5):914–918.

114. Alos K, Serrano MG, Gomez-Garces JL, et al. Antibiotic resistance of *Escherichia coli* from community-acquired urinary tract infections in relation to demographic and clinical data. *Clin Micro Infect* 2005; 11(3):199–203.

115. Astal ZE. Increasing ciprofloxacin resistance among prevalent urinary tract bacterial isolates in the Gaza Strip. *Singapore Med J* 2005;46(9):457–460.

116. Guttmann D. Follow-up of urinary tract infection in domiciliary patients. In: Brumfitt W, Asscher AW, eds. *Urinary tract infection.* London: Oxford University Press, 1973:62.

117. Mabeck CE. Treatment of uncomplicated urinary tract infection in nonpregnant women. *Postgrad Med* 1972;48:69–81.

118. Zhanel GG, Handing GRM, Guay DRP. Asymptomatic bacteriuria: which patients should be treated? *Arch Intern Med* 1990;150:1389–1396.

119. Andreole VT, Patterson TF. Epidemiology, natural history, and management of urinary tract infections in pregnancy. *Med Clin North Am* 1991;75:359–373.

120. Kass EH, Platt R. Urinary tract and genital mycoplasmal infection. In: Wald NJ, ed. *Antenatal and neonatal screening,* 1st ed. New York: Oxford University Press, 1984:345–357.

121. Platt R. Adverse consequences of acute urinary tract infections in adults. *Am J Med* 1987;82[Suppl 6B]:47–52.

122. Evans DA, Kass EH, Hennekens CH, et al. Bacteriuria and subsequent mortality in women. *Lancet* 1982;1: 156–161.

123. Fihn SD. Single-dose antimicrobial therapy for urinary tract infections: "less is more?" or "reductio ad absurdum?" *J Gen Intern Med* 1986;1:62–65.

124. Brumfitt W, Faiers MC, Franklin IN. The treatment of urinary infection by means of a single dose of cephaloxidine. *Postgrad Med* 1970;46:65–72.

125. Buckwold FJ, Ludwid P, Godfrey KM, et al. Therapy for acute cystitis in adult women: randomized comparison of single-dose sulfasoxazole vs trimethoprim-sulfamethoxazole. *JAMA* 1982;247:1839–1843.

126. Rubin RH, Fang LST, Jones SR, et al. Single-dose amoxicillin therapy for urinary tract infection. *JAMA* 1980;244:561–564.

127. Greenberg RN, Sanders CV, Lewis AC, et al. Single-dose cefaclor therapy of urinary tract infection: evaluation of antibody-coated bacteria test and C-reactive protein assay as predictors of cure. *Am J Med* 1981;71: 841–847.

128. Bailey RR, Abbott GD. Treatment of urinary tract infection with a single dose of amoxicillin. *Nephron* 1977;18:316–321.

129. Ireland D, Tacchi D, Bint AJ. Effect of single-dose prophylactic cotrimoxazole on the incidence of gynecological postoperative urinary tract infection. *Br J Obstet Gynaecol* 1982;89:578–585.

130. Tolkoff-Rubin NE, Weber D, Fang LST, et al. Single dose therapy with trimethoprim-sulfamethoxazole for

urinary tract infection in women. *Rev Infect Dis* 1982; 4:443–447.

131. Fang LST, Tolkoff-Rubin NE, Rubin RH. Efficacy of single-dose and conventional amoxicillin therapy in urinary tract infection localized by the antibody-coated bacteria technic. *N Engl J Med* 1978;298: 413–418.

132. Fihn SD, Johnson C, Roberts PL, et al. Trimethoprim-sulfamethoxazole for acute dysuria in women: a double-blind, randomized trial of single-dose versus 10-day treatment. *Ann Intern Med* 1988;108:350–357.

133. Ronald AR, Boutros P, Mourtada H. Bacteriuria localization and response to single-dose therapy in women. *JAMA* 1976;235:1854–1858.

134. Hooten TM, Winter C, Tiu F, et al. Randomized comparative trial and cost analysis of 3-day antimicrobial regiments for treatment of acute cystitis in women. *JAMA* 1995;273:41–45.

135. Saint S, Scholes D, Fihn SD, et al. The effectiveness of a clinical practice guideline for the management of presumed uncomplicated urinary tract infection in women. *Am J Med* 1999;106:636–641.

136. Wathne B, Hovelius B, Mardh PA. Causes of frequency and dysuria in women. *Scand J Infect Dis* 1987;19:223.

137. Kraft JK, Stamey TA. The natural history of symptomatic recurrent bacteriuria in women. *Medicine* 1977; 56:55–64.

138. Stamm WE, McKevitt M, Counts GW, et al. Is antimicrobial prophylaxis of urinary tract infections cost effective? *Ann Intern Med* 1981;94:251–256.

139. Nicolle LE, Ronald AR. Recurrent urinary tract infections in adult women. *Infect Dis Clin North Am* 1987; 1:793–814.

140. Stamey TA, Condy M, Mihara G. Prophylactic efficacy of nitrofurantoin macrocrystals and trimethoprim-sulfamethoxazole in urinary infections: biologic effects on the vaginal and rectal flora. *N Engl J Med* 1977;296:780–788.

141. Martinez FC, Kindrachuk RW, Thomas E, et al. Effect of prophylactic low dose cephalexin on fecal and vaginal bacteria. *J Urol* 1985;133:994–998.

142. Stamm WE, Counts GW, McKevitt M, et al. Urinary prophylaxis with trimethoprim and trimethoprim-sulfamethoxazole: efficacy, influence on the natural history of recurrent bacteriuria, and cost control. *Rev Infect Dis* 1982;4:450–461.

143. Stamey TA, Condy M. The diffusion and concentration of trimethoprim in human vaginal fluid. *J Infect Dis* 1975;131:261–268.

144. Sabbaj J, Hoagland VL, Shih WJ. Multiclinic comparative study of norfloxacin and trimethoprim-sulfamethoxazole for treatment of urinary tract infections. *Antimicrob Agents Chemother* 1985;27:297–302.

145. Schaeffer AJ, Stuppy BA. Efficacy and safety of self-start therapy in women with recurrent urinary tract infections. *J Urol* 1999;161:207–211.

146. Gupta K, Hooton TM, Roberts PL, et al. Patient-initiated treatment of uncomplicated recurrent urinary tract infections in young women. *Ann Intern Med* 2001;135:9–16.

147. Wong ES, McKevitt M, Running K, et al. Management of recurrent urinary tract infections with patient-administered single-dose therapy. *Ann Intern Med* 1985;102:302–309.

148. Vosti KL. Recurrent urinary tract infections: prevention by prophylactic antibiotics after sexual intercourse. *JAMA* 1975;231:934–938.

149. Pfau A, Sacks T, Englestein D. Recurrent urinary tract infections in premenopausal women: prophylaxis based on an understanding of the pathogenesis. *J Urol* 1983;129:1152–1160.

150. Melekos MD, Asbach HW, Gerharz E, et al. Post-intercourse versus daily ciprofloxacin prophylaxis for recurrent urinary tract infections in premenopausal women. *J Urol* 1997;157:935–939.

151. Raz R, Stamm WE. A controlled trial of intravaginal estriol in postmenopausal women with recurrent urinary tract infections. *N Engl J Med* 1993;320:753–756.

152. Eriksen BC. A randomized, open, parallel-group study on the preventive effect of an estradiol-releasing vaginal ring (Estring) on recurrent urinary tract infections in postmenopausal women. *Am J Obstet Gynecol* 1999;180:1072–107.

153. Pinggera GM, Feuchtner G, Frauscher F, et al. Effects of local estrogen therapy on recurrent urinary tract infections in young females under oral contraceptives. *Eur Urol* 2005;47(2):243–249.

154. Kreger DE, Creven DE, Carling PC, et al. Gram-negative bacteremia. III. Reassessment of etiology, epidemiology, and ecology in 612 patients. *Am J Med* 1980;68:332–338.

155. Platt R, Polk BF, Murdock B, et al. Mortality associated with nosocomial urinary tract infection. *N Engl J Med* 1982;307:736–745.

156. Tambyah PA, Maki DG. A prospective study of 1497 catheterized patients. *Arch Intern Med* 2000;160: 678–682.

157. Garibaldi RA, Burke JP, Dickman ML, et al. Factors predisposing to bacteriuria during indwelling urethral catheterization. *N Engl J Med* 1974;291:215–221.

158. Garibaldi RA, Burke JP, Britt MR, et al. Meatal colonization and catheter-associated bacteriuria. *N Engl J Med* 1980;303:316–321.

159. Tambyah PA, Halvorson KT, Maki DG. A prospective study of pathogenesis of catheter-associated urinary tract infections. *Mayo Clin Proc* 1999;74:131–136.

160. Wong ES, Hooton TM. Guidelines to prevention of catheter-associated urinary tract infection. *Infect Control* 1980;2:125–136.

161. Burke JP, Jacobson JA, Garibaldi RA, et al. Evaluation of daily meatal care with polyantibiotic ointment in prevention of urinary catheter-associated bacteriuria. *J Urol* 1983;129:331–334.

162. Burke JP, Garibaldi RA, Britt MR, et al. Prevention of catheter-associated urinary tract infections. *Am J Med* 1981;70:655–661.

163. Warren JW, Platt R, Thomas RJ, et al. Antibiotic irrigation and catheter-associated urinary tract infections. *N Engl J Med* 1978;299:570–576.

164. Britt MR, Garibaldi RA, Miller WA, et al. Antimicrobial prophylaxis for catheter-associated bacteriuria. *Antimicrob Agent Chemother* 1977;11:240–246.

165. Cundiff GW, McLennan MT, Bent AE. Randomized trial of antibiotic prophylaxis for combined urodynamics and cystourethroscopy. *Obstet Gynecol* 1999;93: 749–752.

166. Kuhlemeier K, Stover SL, Lloyd LK. Prophylactic antibacterial therapy for preventing urinary tract infections in spinal cord injury patients. *J Urol* 1985;134: 514–518.

CHAPTER 11

Management of Overactive Bladder

Joseph M. Montella

DEFINITION

As defined by the International Continence Society, overactive bladder (OAB) is the condition in which a patient has symptoms of urgency with or without urge incontinence, usually with frequency and nocturia, in the absence of infection, metabolic disturbance, or other pathologic factors that would account for these symptoms. It is a symptomatic diagnosis and therefore does not require the performance of urodynamic testing or cystometry for confirmation. Urgency is defined as the feeling that the patient must void immediately for fear of losing urine, and frequency is defined as greater than 10 micturitions in a 24-hour period. Urge incontinence describes involuntary loss of urine associated with an urgent, strong desire to void.

The term "detrusor overactivity" (unstable bladder) is more restrictive and describes an OAB caused by detrusor contractions documented by cystometrogram. Detrusor overactivity occurs when the bladder contracts spontaneously, or on provocation, during bladder filling while the patient is attempting to inhibit micturition. Detrusor overactivity is diagnosed during provocative cystometry when one of the following conditions occurs: a true detrusor pressure rise of 15 cmH_2O (motor urge incontinence) or a true detrusor pressure rise of less than 15 cmH_2O in the presence of urgency or urge incontinence (sensory urge incontinence) (1). Subthreshold detrusor contractions of less than 15 cm H_2O may have clinical significance and have been shown to cause urinary incontinence in 10% and urgency in 85% of patients (2).

Additionally, a urodynamic diagnosis associated with the symptom of urge incontinence in a frail elderly patient is detrusor hyperactivity with impaired contractility (DHIC). These patients have involuntary detrusor contractions causing incontinence but are unable to empty their bladders completely, leaving a large postvoid residual (3). A pressure rise during filling may represent decreased bladder compliance or insufficient time to accommodate the increase in volume because cystometry is time dependent (4), and this would not be considered as detrusor overactivity in this context.

Detrusor hyperreflexia is detrusor overactivity secondary to a known neurologic abnormality (1). The term "neurogenic bladder" is reserved for spinal cord injuries and other similar defects and their impact on bladder function.

Incorrect synonyms that have been applied to OAB include bladder dyssynergia and vesical instability. These terms should no longer be used.

PREVALENCE AND IMPACT ON QUALITY OF LIFE

The National Overactive Bladder Evaluation (NOBLE) program estimated the overall prevalence of OAB as 16.9% of women and 16.0% of men, a rate that corresponds to 33.3 million adult Americans, with an impact on quality of life equal to that of urinary incontinence (5,6). The occurrence of involuntary detrusor contractions in infancy is a normal state for bladder emptying and is later controlled by the development of cortical inhibition of reflex bladder activity. Farrar et al (7) described the prevalence of OAB as 8% to 50%, depending on age distribution. In more than 2,000 women studied by Abrams (8), OAB occurred in 38% of those 65 years of age or older and in 27% of those younger than 65 years of age. In institutionalized women, the incidence of urinary incontinence secondary to OAB is greater than 80% (9). Thus, the prevalence of OAB is greatest at the extremes of life; OAB has a 5% to 10% occurrence in premenopausal patients, increasing to as much as 38% in elderly patients and perhaps to more than 80% in institutionalized incontinent elderly patients.

Although the severity of OAB has been measured by outcome variables such as micturition frequency or quantity of urine lost, the impact on quality of life must also be measured in terms of physical and psychological functioning. Psychosocial complications included disturbed sleep, impaired mobility and work productivity, isolation and depression, impaired domestic and sexual functioning, and diminished quality of life (10).

CLINICAL PRESENTATION

The symptoms of OAB include urgency, frequency (greater than 10 micturitions in a 24-hour period), urge incontinence, and nocturia (two times or more). There can also be a history of childhood nocturnal enuresis in some patients (11). OAB may coexist with genuine stress incontinence, and stressful activity may trigger a detrusor contraction causing urge incontinence. In 100 women with the urodynamic diagnosis of detrusor overactivity, Wiskind et al (12) reported that although 86% of patients had symptoms of urge incontinence, 76% also complained of stress incontinence. Sand et al (13) reported on 188 incontinent women, and of those reporting only stress incontinence, 34.9% had detrusor overactivity. Only 32.6% of patients reporting both urge and stress incontinence had detrusor overactivity.

DIFFERENTIAL DIAGNOSIS

Because the symptoms of OAB overlap with those of other lower urinary tract conditions, a number of other diagnoses must be entertained. Table 11.1 lists the differential diagnosis for these symptoms. A special word must be written about urethral instability, which tends to be rather poorly defined. Wise et al (14) investigated the prevalence and significance of urethral instability in a group of women with OAB. This occurred in 42% of patients with OAB and was strongly associated with the sequence of relaxation of the urethra before unprovoked detrusor contraction. Women with OAB and a stable urethra exhibited primary contraction of the detrusor, whereas the symptom of stress incontinence was more common in women with urethral instability. The investigators postulated that women with OAB should be divided into two groups: those with and those without urethral instability, the latter group possibly benefiting from α-agonist therapy. In addition, Petros and Ulmsten (15) found that provocative urethrocystometry re-

TABLE 11.1

Differential Diagnosis of OAB

Severe genuine stress incontinence
Uninhibited urethral relaxation
Urethral diverticulum
Urinary tract fistula
Cystitis
Bladder foreign body (stone, suture, etc.)
Bladder tumor
Urethritis

vealed a rise in detrusor pressure followed by a fall in urethral pressure, both preceded by urge symptoms. They concluded that urethral instability, OAB, and urge incontinence were different manifestations of a prematurely activated micturition reflex. Urethral instability may not be a separate entity but a part of urine loss associated with urge.

PATHOPHYSIOLOGY

Table 11.2 lists the etiologies of OAB. Neurologic diseases (multiple sclerosis, cerebrovascular disease, parkinsonism, Alzheimer's disease), local bladder and urethral irritants (cystitis, foreign bodies, tumors), outflow obstruction (severe cystocele or vaginal vault prolapse), and medications (parasympathomimetics) must be considered as etiologies. Most cases, however, apart from those in very young or elderly patients, are idiopathic in nature. Del Carro et al (16) compared women with idiopathic OAB with age-matched controls using subtracted cystometry and anal sphincter electromyography sacral reflex analysis along with other neurologic tests using evoked potentials. All patients had normal neurophysiologic tests, and there was no significant difference between patients and controls. Because women with OAB do not appear to have either clinical or subclinical damage of central sensory or motor pathways, other investigators have put forth their theories regarding intrinsic bladder abnormalities. The pathophysiology of OAB may be principally neurogenic, myogenic, obstructive, or idiopathic.

Neurogenic

The bladder is never really in a complete resting state. Rather, *in vitro* and *in vivo* studies show that

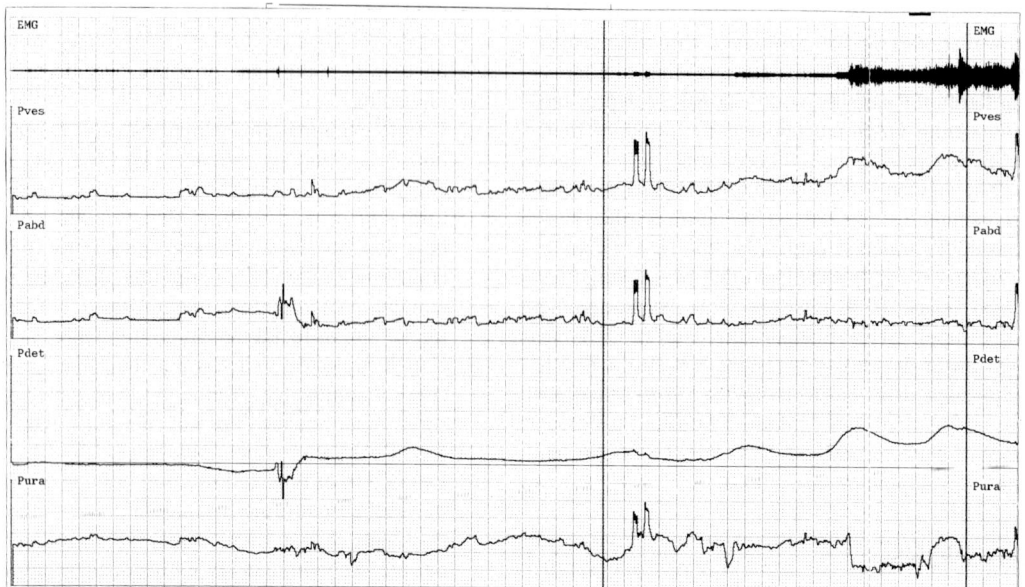

FIGURE 11.1 ● Multichannel cystometrogram illustrating detrusor instability. The patient had a detrusor contraction after she washed her hands. Before provocation, she had no contraction.

In cases in which traditional cystometry fails to produce a diagnosis, alternative methods may be used. One such method is extramural ambulatory urodynamic monitoring. McInerney et al (31) and Webb et al (32), in two separate studies, pronounced ambulatory monitoring as more sensitive in the diagnosis of detrusor overactivity than conventional cystometry. Porru and Usai (33) used this technique in 46 patients with urinary incontinence, 16 of whom had urge incontinence symptoms. Conventional cystometry identified detrusor contractions in only 50% of these patients, whereas ambulatory monitoring identified detrusor contractions in 93%.

Another technique involves diuresis cystometry, in which a patient is given a diuretic to fill the bladder to approximate more closely the anterograde filling phase. Van Venrooij and Boon (34) evaluated women with frequency and urge incontinence with a negative retrograde cystometrogram using diuresis cystometry and noted an increase in the detection of detrusor overactivity.

Finally, although multichannel standing cystometry is considered the gold standard for diagnosis, it may not always be possible to perform this test in patients with poor mobility or in those who are unable to maintain a standing position. Simple cystometry at the bedside was found to have a specificity of 75% and a sensitivity of 88% compared with multichannel testing in the diagnosis of detrusor overactivity (35). This may be an excellent method of diagnosing detrusor overactivity in frail elderly patients using a Toohey syringe attached to a Foley catheter (Fig. 11.2). The bladder is filled in incremental fashion, and a rise in the meniscus represents a detrusor contraction.

MANAGEMENT

Because OAB is a diagnosis based on symptoms, therapy may be instituted without performing any complex testing.

There are several methods of managing OAB, as listed in Table 11.3. Depending on the severity of the problem and its impact on the patient's quality of life and lifestyle, these treatments may be used separately or in tandem.

Bladder Training (Timed Voiding)

There are three main components to bladder training: education, scheduled voiding with systematic delay of voiding, and positive reinforcement. The education portion combines written, visual, and verbal instruction that serves to familiarize patients with the anatomy and physiology of the lower urinary tract. Patients are then asked to resist or inhibit the sensation of urgency, to postpone voiding, and to urinate according to a timetable rather than according to the urge to void (36). Adjustment in fluid loads and delaying voiding to increase bladder volume may be used to augment

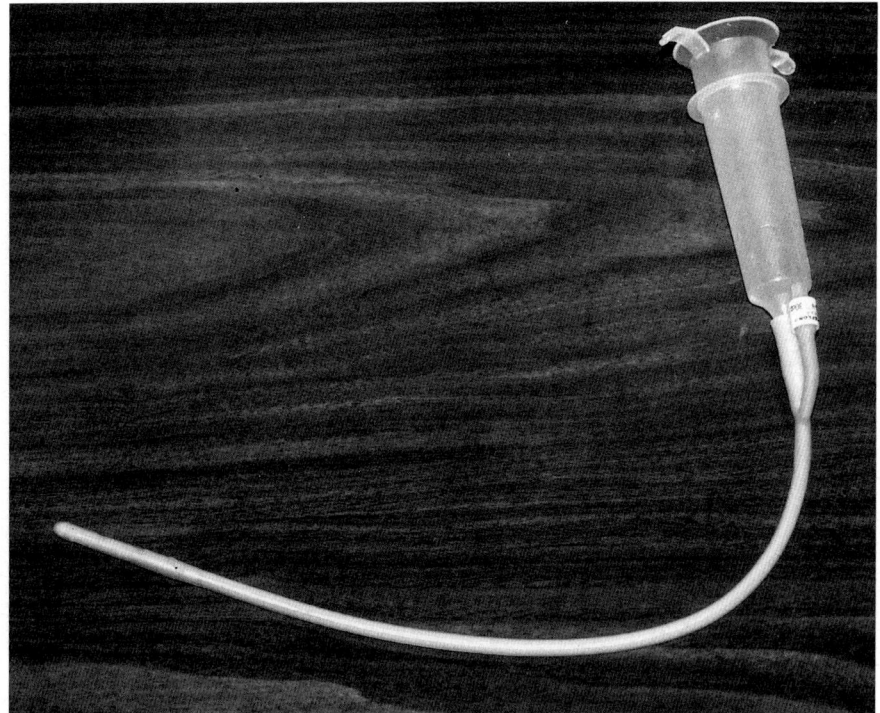

FIGURE 11.2 ● Toohey syringe attached to catheter for bedside cystometrogram.

this therapy (37). The patient is also asked to complete a daily diary, as illustrated in Figure 11.3.

Fantl et al (38) conducted a controlled randomized study of 123 women with unstable detrusor function and sphincteric incompetence who received treatment in the form of behavioral strategies to decrease urge, patient education, and a schedule of voiding. Twelve percent became dry, and 75% had at least a 50% reduction in the number of incontinence episodes, with a greater effect in women with detrusor instability. Although primarily used for treatment of stress incontinence, pelvic floor muscle exercises may augment bladder training (39).

Behavioral Modification Protocol

An effective bladder training program that has produced good results consists of a 6-week outpatient voiding protocol (40). It is presented to the patient as a means of regaining cortical control over the detrusor and is offered as primary management for patients with OAB. Patients are assigned a voiding schedule based on their daily voiding interval; they are usually told to start by voiding every hour while awake for the first 2 weeks. Instructions to the patients include the following:

1. Empty your bladder at the scheduled time whether or not you feel the urge to void.
2. The important aspect is the voluntary initiation of voiding, not the amount voided.
3. Avoid going to the bathroom between scheduled times, and suppress the urge at other times.
4. Do not feel embarrassed if you leak.

The protocol requires follow-up every 2 weeks until the desired effect is obtained. Because this is

TABLE 11.3

Management of OAB

Behavioral (timed voiding)
Electrical stimulation
Medical
   Anticholinergics
   Tricyclic antidepressants
Surgical
   Sacral neuromodulation
   Augmentation cystoplasty
   Bladder denervation

NAME _____   DATE _____

TIME	VOID	TIME	VOID	TIME	VOID
6 AM		2 PM		10 PM	
7 AM		3 PM		11 PM	
8 AM		4 PM		Midnight	
9 AM		5 PM		1 AM	
10 AM		6 PM		2 AM	
11 AM		7 PM		3 AM	
Noon		8 PM		4 AM	
1 PM		9 PM		5 AM	

Please place a check mark next to the time that you void.

FIGURE 11.3 ● Timed voiding record.

a form of behavioral therapy, positive reinforcement is used. The voiding interval is increased by 15 to 30 minutes, depending on how well the patient did in the first 2 weeks. Combining this therapy with Kegel's exercises can increase the patient's ability to be continent because the increase in pelvic floor muscle tone will increase the patient's ability to hold urine. The treatment is considered successful if the patient achieves a voiding interval of 2.5 to 3 hours and is free of OAB symptoms.

Behavioral Modification in Elderly Patients

The overall incidence of OAB increases with age, and in older patients, OAB, cognitive deficits, and decreased mobility are more common causes of urinary incontinence. Hadley (41) described four scheduling regimens (Table 11.4) specifically tailored to the capabilities of the patient. They ranged from behavioral modification, used in cognitively intact ambulatory patients, to prompted voiding, used in patients with severe cognitive and mobility impairments. Hu et al (42) used a randomized prospective protocol to study the efficacy of a prompted voiding regimen in 133 institutionalized women. Using nurses' aides to prompt and assist patients to void every hour for 14 hours of the day, they were able to reduce wet episodes by 0.6 per

day, a reduction of 26% over baseline episodes. Ouslander et al (43) designed a prospective study to look at the combined effects of a timed voiding schedule and oxybutynin chloride in 15 institutionalized patients with detrusor instability. In a longitudinal study design, timed voiding was implemented for the first 2 weeks alone. Oxybutynin was then added to the timed voiding regimen. Timed voiding significantly reduced the episodes of incontinence, and the addition of oxybutynin chloride did not confer any additional benefit. Fantl et al (38) studied 123 community-dwelling women aged 50 years using a standard bladder training protocol. In this group of women they were able to reduce incontinence episodes by 57% and quantity of fluid loss by 54%.

Medication

Table 11.5 lists medications used to treat OAB.

Anticholinergics

Anticholinergic agents are recommended as first-line medical therapy for OAB by working at the ganglionic receptor to block detrusor contractions in both the normal bladder and the OAB. These medications are contraindicated in patients with gastric retention, urinary retention, hypersensitivity to the particular medication, and uncontrolled

TABLE 11.4

Scheduling Regimens for OAB

Regimen	Indication	Principle
Bladder training	Ambulatory, cognitively intact patient	Re-establishment of cortical inhibition of sacral reflexes
Habit training	Ambulatory, cognitively intact patient	Toileting schedule fitted to individual's voiding pattern
Timed voiding	Neurogenic bladder, minor cognitive impairment	Fixed voiding schedule to regularly empty bladder
Prompted voiding	Severe cognitive and mobility deficits	Attention focusing on need to void with assistance to void

narrow-angle glaucoma; however, few patients in the 21st century have this last condition because they have been treated with laser surgery or with medications. If the physician is concerned about prescribing this class of medications in patients with narrow-angle glaucoma, consultation with the patient's ophthalmologist is recommended. The low dosage range is always initially used in elderly patients and titrated according to its effectiveness and side effects. Side effects of this class of medication involve atropine-like side effects, such as dry mouth and dry eyes, the severity of which are dose-dependent; gastroparesis; constipation; gastroesophageal reflux; and somnolence. Less common side effects are headache, dizziness, and peripheral edema.

Based on the strength of scientific evidence through placebo-controlled, double-blinded studies, there are two anticholinergic agents that are recommended as the starting point of medical therapy. In 1997, tolterodine tartrate was introduced to treat OAB. This is available in two forms: an immediate-release preparation and a timed-release preparation. Several placebo-controlled studies have documented the effectiveness of both forms of therapy in terms of significant reduction in urgency, frequency, and number of incontinence episodes (44,45). This medication is metabolized by the CYP2D6 isoform of the cytochrome P-450 system and must be used with caution in patients who are on any medications that competitively inhibit this enzyme, such as oral antifungals and macrolide antibiotics. The recommended dosage is 2 mg twice a day for the immediate-release preparation and 4 mg once a day for the timed-release preparation.

Another anticholinergic agent that has been considered highly effective in the treatment of OAB is oxybutynin chloride. This agent has both anticholinergic and smooth muscle relaxant properties. In five placebo-controlled studies in middle-aged outpatients, oxybutynin reduced incontinence frequency by 19% to 58% over placebo (46–50). Side effects were noted in all studies and included dry skin, blurred vision, nausea, constipation, and marked xerostomia. The severity of side effects increased with increasing dosages, with severe xerostomia occurring in 84% of patients receiving oxybutynin in a dose of 5 mg four times a day. The recommended dosage is 2.5 to 5 mg taken orally three or four times a day (44). Oxybutynin is also available in a timed-release formulation taken once a day in doses of 5, 10, or 15 mg. The side effects with the long-acting medication have been considerably reduced. Oxybutynin is also available in a transdermal form that delivers a dose of 3.9 mg oxybutynin daily over a 3- to 4-day period, bypassing first-pass metabolism. The patch cannot be cut to decrease the dose, and more than one patch cannot be used at a time. Local skin reactions are the most common side effect. Its efficacy is close to that of oxybutynin, although no head-to-head trials have been conducted (51).

Trospium chloride is a quaternary amine compound that acts as a muscarinic receptor antagonist that is hydrophilic and theoretically might not cross the blood–brain barrier and cause central nervous system effects. Only about 10% of the dose is absorbed after oral administration, and absorption is decreased by 70% to 80% if the drug is taken with food. Serum concentrations peak in 3.5 to 6 hours. Clinical studies show that there was a decrease in urinary frequency compared to placebo, with dry mouth being the most common adverse event (20% of patients) (52). It appears to offer no advantage over long-acting anticholiner-

TABLE 11.5

Medications for OAB

Drug	Dosage Forms	Dosage[a]
Tolterodine tartrate	Tablets: 1, 2 mg	1 to 2 mg bid
(Detrol, Detrol LA)	Timecaps: 2, 4 mg	2 to 4 mg qd
Oxybutynin chloride	Tablets: 5, 10 mg	2.5 to 10 mg
(Ditropan, Ditropan XL)	Syrup: 5 mg/5 mL	2.5 to 10 mg
	Timecaps: 5, 10, 15 mg	5 to 15 mg qd
Transdermal oxybutinin (Oxytrol)	39-cm^2 patch	2x/week (3.9 mg qd)
Trospium chloride (Sanctura)	Tablets: 20 mg	20 mg qd to bid
Solifenacin succinate (Vesicare)	Tablets: 5, 10 mg	5 to 10 mg qd
Darifenacin hydrobromide (Enablex)	Tablets: 7.5, 15 mg	7.5 to 15 mg qd
Dicyclomine (Bentyl)	Tablets: 10, 20 mg	20 mg
	Syrup: 10 mg/5 mL	
Hyoscyamine (Levsin)	Tablets: 0.125 mg	0.125 to 0.25 mg
	Timecaps: 0.375 mg	0.375 mg bid
Propantheline (Pro-Banthine)	Tablets: 7.5, 15 mg	7.5 to 15 mg + 30 mg qhs
Flavoxate (Urispas)	Tablets: 100 mg	100 to 200 mg
Imipramine (Tofranil)	Tablets: 10, 25, 50 mg	25 mg

[a]Dosages are three or four times daily, unless otherwise noted.

gics due to its short half-life and poor absorption from the gastrointestinal tract.

Solifenacin succinate and darifenacin hydrobromide are selective M3 muscarinic antagonists with tissue selectivity for the bladder over the salivary glands. The potential selectivity of these agents for muscarinic receptors in the urinary bladder could reduce adverse effects and thus improve compliance; persistent and severe dry mouth and constipation are the principal reasons for noncompliance during therapy with any anticholinergic. Ninety percent of solifenacin is available after oral administration, with a half-life of approximately 50 hours. It is metabolized in the liver by the CYP-450 isoenzyme 3A4 and should be used with caution in the presence of potent CYP-450 inhibitors or in patients with severe hepatic impairment. In one trial, oral solifenacin 5 to 20 mg once daily resulted in a significant decrease in the number of urinary voids per 24 hours, a significant increase in mean volume voided, and a decrease in symptoms of urgency and incontinence. Most of the therapeutic effects were evident at 2 weeks. Solifenacin appears to be as least as effective as, and better tolerated than, tolterodine (53,54). It also has a long half-life, permitting once-daily dosing. However, cost may limit its place in therapy, and additional comparative trials are needed. The metabolism of darifenacin is also through CYP2D6 and CYP2A4, so it should also be used with caution in the presence of potent CYP-450 inhibitors. It has a half-life of 13 to 19 hours. A study by Haab showed darifenacin to be superior to placebo in reducing micturition episodes, with mild-to-moderate dry mouth in 20% of patients (55).

Propantheline is the prototype of anticholinergic agents used for urologic conditions because it best approximates atropine's effect on the bladder *in vitro,* although its central nervous system side effects are less marked. This is recommended as a second-line anticholinergic agent in doses of 7.5 to 30 mg three to five times per day and may need to be given in higher doses of 15 to 60 mg four times daily. Side effects include blurry vision, xerostomia (most common), nausea, constipation, tachycardia, drowsiness, and confusion. Two studies evaluated propantheline use in nursing home patients and found a 13% to 17% reduction of incontinence over placebo, which was statistically significant (56,57).

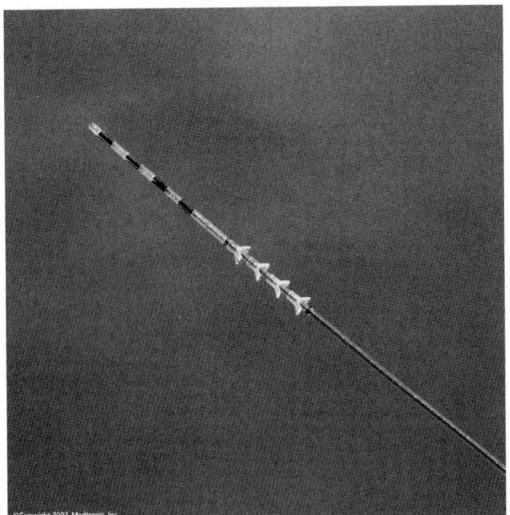

FIGURE 12.4 ● Tined lead.

Attachment to the test stimulator confirms placement, as evidenced by contraction of the anal sphincter with elevation of the pelvis with or without plantar flexion of the great toe. If there is any doubt as to whether it is an S3 response, needles can be placed above or below the initial foramina to determine an S2 response. Fluoroscopy is often useful at this time, especially the lateral view to determine how far up on the sacrum the spinal needles are located.

After confirmation of an S3 response, a wire is then placed down the spinal needle into the foramina. A small incision is placed from the spinal needle down 0.5 cm to allow for easier placement of the plastic introducer. The rest of the placement is very similar to placing a central line (i.e., the use of the Saldinger technique). Once the wire is through the foramina, the spinal needle is removed. A wider introducer with a plastic covering is then inserted over the wire and through the foramina. There is a distinctive "pop" or give as this goes through the foramina. Fluoroscopy confirms that the plastic sheath is deep enough in the foramina. There is a small radiopaque ring at the tip of the sheath, and this should be just beyond the bony plate.

With a twist of the needle, the inside metal introducer is removed, leaving the plastic sheath in place. Through this plastic sheath, a tined lead is passed (Fig. 12.5). The lead has four electrodes similar to the previous one, with the exception that electrode 1 is now wider to compensate for small degrees of lead movement that may occur postoperatively. The lead is passed down through the plastic sheath to the level of the first mark on the lead. This ensures that the electrodes are beyond the end of the plastic sheath but that the barbs of the tined lead are still within the plastic sleeve and not activated.

Progressive stimulation of the four individual electrodes is then performed to determine the optimal position of the lead. The lead can be adjusted deeper or more superficially by gently moving the plastic outer sheath and lead together. It is very important not to move the lead itself; otherwise, the tines may be activated prematurely and the lead cannot be readjusted after that. Ideally, at least two electrodes should give an EMG response. It is preferable to obtain a good motor response from electrode 1, as this is the widest electrode. If anything, the leads tend to be pulled back, so it is preferable to obtain a response from the more superficial leads 3, 2, and 1 as opposed to 0 and 1. This means that in the event that the lead is pulled back slightly, response may be lost in electrodes 2 or 3 but allows for 1 and 0 to pick up.

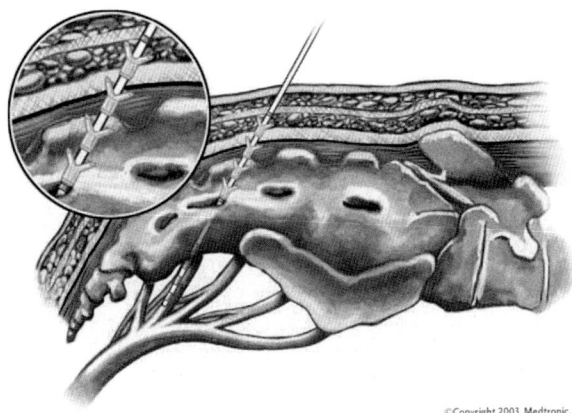

FIGURE 12.5 ● The lead (*left*) is now placed though the introducer (*right*).

When ideal placement is confirmed, a lateral film is taken. This film is then left on the one side of the fluoroscopy viewer and under live view; an attempt is made to remove the outer plastic sheath while leaving the electrode configuration in the same position as the initial film. The lead is then tunneled to the buttock on the side selected for the programmer (IPG). A small pocket is fashioned to accommodate the interconnection piece. A special tunneling device is provided with the kit that enables smooth passage. A boot is placed over this wire, the interconnection lead attached to the electrode, and the boot secured in place with suture to minimize the risk of any fluid leaking into the connection area. The tunneling device is used again to tunnel from the buttock incision to the opposite side where the temporary lead exits. It is important to place the exit site as far away as possible from the future site of the IPG and the lead to minimize the risk of infection.

The operative sites are irrigated with sterile water. The incisions are closed. The buttock incision is typically closed in two layers to minimize the risk of seroma or hematoma, which increases the risk of infection. Sterile dressings are then applied and a large bio-occlusive dressing is placed over the whole area. Patients are typically covered with a broad spectrum of antibiotic for several days to a week after the procedure. The exteriorized wire is then connected to the patient programmer. The handheld temporary programmer is then set to the electrode configuration that was felt to be the optimal response in the operating room. The patient is then allowed to adjust the intensity of stimulation. The temporary programmer does allow for reprogramming between the different electrodes should an optimal response not be obtained initially. Success rates for this test stimulation have typically been higher than for the original PNE (see Table 12.1) (23,24).

Permanent Implantation

Stage 2: Implantation of the IPG

Assuming there is greater than a 50% reduction of symptoms, the patient is eligible for the second stage, which is the much shorter of the two procedures. This can be done with the patient in the prone position but is also easily achieved with the patient in the lateral position. This latter position is quicker, as one can avoid the padding required for the prone position. The site where the buttock incision was made for the first stage is placed uppermost. This incision is then opened, the connection piece disconnected, the bulkier end of the wire cut, and the exteriorized portion of the wire pulled out

through the skin. It is important not to drag the exterior wire back through the pocket. The pocket is then enlarged to accommodate the IPG. Once hemostasis is achieved, the wire is attached to the IPG, which is then placed in the pocket. Impedance values are then obtained to ensure all the connections are appropriate, and the device can then be programmed to the electrode combination that was determined to be the best during the first stage. Ideally, the impedance should be less than 2,000 Ω. The pocket is then closed with a subcutaneous suture and then either subcuticular or interrupted skin sutures (Fig. 12.6).

Postoperative Care

Some physicians will place the patient on broad-spectrum antibiotics for several days up to a week. The patient may adjust the intensity of the stimulation with the telemetry unit (Fig. 12.7). Patients need to be informed that the stimulation may need to be increased or decreased over the next several weeks depending on the amount of edema and trauma to the area. They should avoid twisting or bending and lifting for 4 to 6 weeks to minimize the risk of lead movement.

Predictors for Successful Implantation

Patient selection for permanent implantation is based largely on the successful test stimulation (i.e., successful stage 1 implantation). Several authors have sought to determine if any clinical characteristics are predictive of a successful trial stimulation. Scheepens et al noted that patients who were older, had longer duration of complaints, and a neurogenic bladder were more likely to have an unsuccessful test (25). In addition, patients with urinary retention were less likely to have successful stimulation compared to patients with urge incontinence. The history of disc surgery increased the likelihood of a positive test. The authors, however, concluded by saying that a test stimulation phase is still necessary to determine objectively whether the patient can be successfully implanted.

In a recent study assessing the role of patient age, Amundsen et al noted that cure rates, defined as no daily incontinent episodes, were significantly greater in patients under the age of 55 (65% vs. 37%) (26). Though there was no difference in comorbidities between the two age groups, they noted that individuals with three or more chronic conditions had a lower chance of cure. Both groups, however, had a statistically significant improvement in the number of incontinent episodes, quality of life, pad usage, and voiding frequency. Of note, the two groups may have not been comparable, as detrusor contractions on formal urody-

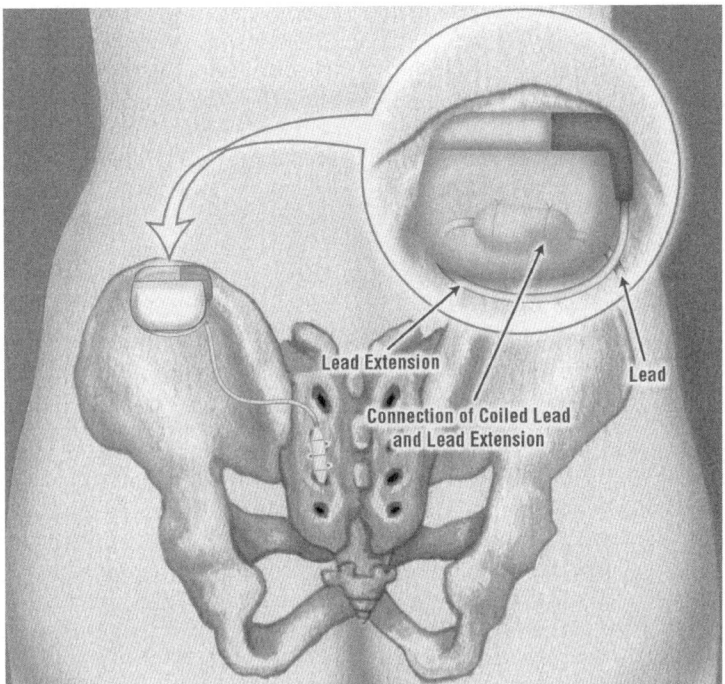

FIGURE 12.6 ● Implantable pulse generator and lead in place.

namic testing were noted in 80% of the younger patients as opposed to 60% in the older patients. These results were reported for the older technique of outpatient test stimulation (PNE) followed by surgical placement of the leads. In their initial study of these older patients, the same group noted a 48% response rate to the test stimulation, which is lower than most reported rates of successful test stimulation (27). It would be interesting to reassess those patients who failed the initial test stimulation with the now two-staged procedure. It is possible that these older patients had more orthopaedic ab-

normalities, which made spinal needle placement more difficult, and fluoroscopy may have been useful. Certainly in other groups, it has been shown that the two-staged approach does result in a greater percentage of successful test stimulations.

Results

Frequency, Urgency, and/or Urge Incontinence

A recent Medline search to 2005 reveals that there continues to be only three randomized control trials evaluating Interstim in patients with frequency, urgency, and/or incontinence (overactive bladder). There have been no additional ones since 2000. Schmidt et al randomized 34 patients with urge incontinence to immediate implantation and 42 patients to delayed implantation (28). At 6 months, 47% of the implanted group were dry and 29% had a greater than 50% improvement. There was a significant reduction in leaks per day and pad usage. Once stimulation was deactivated, the number of incontinent episodes increased back to baseline. Hassouna et al randomized 51 patients with frequency/urgency: 25 to immediate implantation and 26 to delayed implantation (3). At 6 months

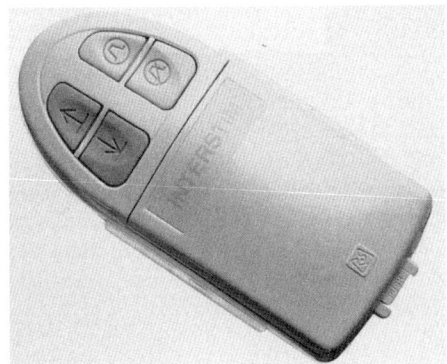

FIGURE 12.7 ● Patient telemetry unit.

there was a statistically significant reduction in number of voids per day (16.9 +/- 9.7 to 9.3 +/- 5.1), volume per void (118 mL +/- 74 to 226 mL +/- 124), and degree of urgency (rank 2.2 +/- 0.6 to 1.6 +/- 0.9). Efficacy was sustained at 12 and 24 months. Weil et al randomized 21 patients to immediate implantation and 23 to continuation of conservative therapy (20). At 6 months the control group was eligible to cross over. Fifty-six percent were dry and 75% had greater than a 90% improvement. Implanted patients exhibited improved quality-of-life measures (physical function and emotional role) compared with controls.

These studies suffer from a number of epidemiological problems, most notably patient dropout. Schmidt initially implanted 86 patients, but 6-month data was reported on only 58 patients (58/86 = 67%) (28). Similarly, Weil et al randomized 21 patients to immediate implantation, but only 16 patients were evaluable at 6 months (20). Long term, the dropout numbers are even greater, with 36% of the original patients evaluable at 18 months (28). This raises the concern about the potential of significant bias, since it is possible that those lost patients represented a disproportionate number of treatment failures.

Observational trials have produced similar results. Cure rates range from 26% to 68%, with greater than 50% improvement in 4% to 85% (Table 12.2) (1,3,13,15,16,19,28–44). Long-term results have typically shown lower success rates, with a certain percentage noting failure with time. At a mean follow-up of 30.8 months, Janknegt et al noted more than 50% improvement in 30% of the 96 patients (37); Siegel 59% at 3 years (41); Elhilali 45% at a mean of 6.45 years (39); and Aboseif 77% at 24 months (42).

With increasing time, it has become obvious that surgical revision rates are higher than initially reported (Table 12.3). Explantation rates range from 1.4% to 22% and replacement/relocation rates range from 1.4% to 54%. Dasgupta noted a 54% revision rate in 26 retention patients, with the most common reasons being loss of efficacy, discomfort, and leg pain (45). The total number of operations often exceeds the numbers of patients in the particular study; for example, Weil reported a total of 57 reoperations in 36 patients (16). Recently Elhilali reported on 41 of 52 patients available for long-term follow-up (39). Of the 22 patients with urgency and frequency, at a mean of 6.45 years, 2/22 (9.1%) had the device removed and 3/22 (13.6%) stopped using it. Of the six urge incontinent patients, 2/6 were explanted and 1/6 stopped using it. Additionally, 1/9 retention patients stopped using the device. Thus, the overall

removal rate was 5/41 (22%), with an additional 22% stopping using the device. This is an important consideration in view of the expense of the device. Therefore, it is important to choose patients well and to stress to them that this is not a "one-shot deal" but a life-long commitment during which time they may require multiple operations and that efficacy may change with time.

In addition, use in the older patient must be approached with caution. The small amount of data available suggests that the success may be lower in older patients and those with multiple comorbidities (25–27).

Retention

Most studies reporting on success with urinary retention have small numbers of patients. This is not surprising, as this condition is typically less common than overactive bladder. In the only randomized control trial, Jonas et al enrolled 177 patients with urinary retention refractory to standard therapy (46). Sixty-eight patients had successful peripheral nerve evaluations; 37 of these patients were randomly assigned to immediate implantation and 31 patients to delayed implantation. Results were reported on 29 of the implanted patients and 22 controls. Of the remaining 17 patients, 6 had not yet been enrolled, 3 were lost to follow-up, and 8 did not complete the voiding diary. At 6 months, 69% of those treated were voiding normally without catheterization and 14% had greater than a 50% reduction in postvoid residual. Results were sustained at 18 months. Observational data has consistently shown higher cure rates for this condition compared to overactive bladder, with cure rates of 65% to 97%. An additional 11% to 33% of patients required minimal catheterization (once per day). The effect appears to be well sustained long term, especially when compared to the long-term results for overactive bladder patients (Table 12.4) (23,30,31,34, 41,42,45–47).

Interstitial Cystitis

Interstitial cystitis is still not an approved indication for implantation. These patients are typically implanted because of their complaints of frequency and urgency. Several small series have been published detailing the success in patients with refractory or end-stage disease. Unlike studies of frequency and urgency, these studies typically report quality-of-life measures, and most use a pain scale assessment (47–52).

The largest study to date, by Whitmore et al, found significant improvement in frequency, pain, and quality-of-life measures (48). More than 76%

TABLE 12.2

Success Rate for Treatment of Urge Incontinence (UI), Frequency, Urgency

Author	Study	Diagnosis	n	Voids/Day	Leaks/Day (pre-/post-surgery)
Elabbady (30)	Observational	Frequency, urge, pain	9	Improved by 37%	Improved by >50%
Schmidt (28)	Randomized	UI	34 Immediate Rx		9.7/2.6
			42 Delayed Rx		9.3/11.3
Bosch (15)	Observational	UI	18		
Thon (29)	Observational	UI	20		
Shaker (31)	Observational	UI	18		6.49/1.98
Weil (16)	Observational	UI	24	13.7/8.7	4.9/1.1
Dijkema (13)	Observational	UI, frequency, urge, pain	23		7.4/1.5
Edlund (18)	Observational	UI	9		5.9/2.8
Weil (20)	Randomized	UI	44		
Bosch (17)	Observational	UI	30	14.1/10.3	7.8/3.3
Tanagho (1)	Observational	UI	97		
Hassouna (3)	Randomized	Urgency, frequency	25 Immediate Rx	16.9/9.3	
			26 Delayed	15.2/15.7	
Bosch (19)	Observational	UI	45		7.1/1.3
Spinelli (34)	Observational	UI	86		5.4/1.1
Chartier-Kastler (33)	Observational	UI	9	16.1/8.2	
Everaert (32)	Observational	UI, retention, pain	53		
Cappellano (35)	Observational	UI	47		5.8/0.9
Heesakkers (36)	Observational	UI	105		10.9/4.3
Janknegt (37)	Observational	UI	96	13.2/9.2	10.9/4.2
Spinelli (38)	Observational	UI	20	10/7.3	4.9/2.5
Elhilali (39)	Observational	Frequency, urgency	22 frequency, urge; 6 UI		
Ruiz-Cerda (40)	Observational	UI	25		4.5/0.8
Siegel (41)	Observational	UI, frequency, urgency	41		
Aboseif (42)	Observational	Frequency, urgency	43	17.9/8.6	6.4/2

Author	Pads	Urgency	>90% Improvement	>50% Improvement	Cure	Criteria	Follow-up
Elabbady (30)	Improved by >50%			9		Diary	3–52 m
Schmidt (28)	6.2/1.1 5.0/6.3			29%	47%	Diary	6 m
Bosch (15)			61%	83%	50%	Diary	29 m

(continued)

TABLE 12.2 *(Continued)*

Success Rate for Treatment of Urge Incontinence (UI), Frequency, Urgency

Author	Pads	Urgency	>90% Improvement	>50% Improvement	Cure	Criteria	Follow-up
Thon (29)				85%		Not stated	Min. 12 m
Shaker (31)				4	44%	Diary/UDS	3–83 m
Weil (16)	6.6/2.3		66%	12%		Diary/UDS	6 m
Dijkema (13)	4.5/1.8		60%	83%		Diary	12 m
Edlund (18)	3/1.9					Diary	8–39 m
Weil (20)			75%	33%	56%	Diary/UDS	6 m
Bosch (17)	6.6/2.4					Diary/UDS	6–68 m
Tanagho (1)					68%	Not stated	Not stated
Hassouna (3)		2.2/1.6				Diary	24 m
Bosch (19)	5.4/1.2		40%	20%		Diary/UDS	
Spinelli (34)					57%	Diary	3 m
					65%	Diary	6 m
					55%	Diary	9 m
					59%	Diary	12 m
					43%	Diary	18 m
Chartier-Kastler (33)			100%	56%	Diary/UDS		7–72 m
Everaert (32)				28%	57%	Diary	13–39 m
Cappellano (35)						Diary	12 m
Heesakkers (36)	6.5/2.4						45 m*
Janknegt (37)	6.6/2.7			30%	26%	Diary	30.8 m*
Spinelli (38)	3.7/2.25					Diary	6 m
Elhilali (39)				45%		Diary	1.3–13.33 y
				17%			6.45 y*
Ruiz-Cerda (40)				66%	55%	Diary	6.8 m
Siegel (41)				59%	40%	Diary	3 y
				56%			2 y
Aboseif (42)	3/1.5			77%		Diary	24 m*

*= mean
UDS, urodynamic study.

of the 33 patients reported more than 50% improvement. Smaller studies have reported similar findings, with all showing a significant decrease in pain and improved quality of life. Improvement rates from 76% to 96% were reported (Table 12.5). Peters at al noted that in 21 narcotic-dependent end-stage patients, 4/18 stopped all narcotics, and the mean decrease in morphine equivalents was from 81.6 to 52.0 mg/day (30%) (52).

Urodynamic Changes

There appears to be a general consensus in the literature that there is an increase in first sensation to void and maximum cystometric capacity for those with frequency, urgency, and urge incontinence. Unfortunately most studies published do not state whether this was a statistically significant change (Table 12.6) (13,15,17,20,30,31,53–55). Of the

TABLE 12.3

Surgical Revision Rates (Long Term)

Author	Explant	Replaced/Relocated	No. of Reoperations
Heesakers (36)	14/105 (13%)		
Ruffion (43)	4/33 (12%)		
Weil (16)	12/36 (33%)		57
Ruiz-Cerda (40)	1/69 (1.4%)	1/69 (1.4%)	5
Spinelli (23)	1/22 (4.5%)		5
Aboseif (42)	1/64 (1.6%)		5
Scheepens (25)	2/15 (13%)	1/15 (6.5%)	5
Bosch (19)		7/45 (15.5%)	25
Koldewijn (44)	6/40 (15%)	9/40 (22%)	26
Shaker (31)	1/18 (5.5%)	2/18 (11%)	7
Dasgupta (45)		14/26 (54%)	21
Janknegt (37)	11/96 (11%)		
Elhilali (39)	5/41 (12%)		
Hijaz (24)	16/130 (12.3%)	26/130 (20%)	

TABLE 12.4

Success with Urinary Retention

Author	Study	n	Self-Cath (Preop/Postop)	Cure	>50% Reduction in PVR	Follow-up
Elabbady (30)	Observational	8	4.2/1.3			3–52 m
Shaker (31)	Observational	20			Decreased from 78.3 to 5.5 mL	1–18 m
Chai (47)	Observational	7		71%		2–48 m
Jonas (46)	Randomized	37 Rx 31 Control		69%	14%	18 m
Spinelli (34)	Observational	45		67%	13% cath 1x/day	6 m
				50%	33% cath 1x/day	12 m
Spinelli (23)	Observational	21	3.96/1.19			6 m
Dasgupta (45)	Observational	26		65%	11% cath 1x/day	2–73 m
Elhilali (39)	Observational	9		78%		1.3–13.3 y
Siegel (41)	Observational	42			70%	1.5 y
Aboseif (42)	Observational	20		90%	>90% improvement in quality of life	6–36 m

PVR, postvoid residual.

TABLE 12.5

Results in Patients with Interstitial Cystitis

Author	Study	n	Frequency	Pain	Improvement	Quality of Life	Follow-up (mean)
Whitmore (48)	Observational—end stage	33	Significant decrease	2.2/1.6 (0–3 scale)	76% >50% improvement	ICSI 16.4/8.6 ICPI 13.8/8.6	During stim 7–14 days
Maher (49)	Observational—end stage	15	47% >50% reduction	8.9/2.4	87% >50% decrease in pain 73% elected for permanent	SUDI 40.7/19.5	After stim 7 days
Comiter (50)	Observational—refractory	17*	24/16.9 day 4.5/1.7 night	5.8/1.6	>94% improved in all areas		14 m
Peters (51)	Observational	26*	24/12 day 5.7/2.3	71% moderate/ marked improvement	96% undergo again	76% improvement	5.6 m

*Permanent implantation
ICPI, interstitial cystitis problem index; ICSI, interstitial cystitis symptom index; SUDI, short urogenital distress inventory.

TABLE 12.6

Urodynamic Changes with Interstim

Author	Indication	n	First Sensation (Pre/Post [mL])	Maximum Capacity (Pre/Post [mL])	Volume at First Contraction (Pre/Post [mL])	Peak Flow Rate (Pre/Post [mL/sec])
Dijkema (13)	Retention, frequency, pain	23		135/227[c]	80/167[c]	
Elabbady (30)	Retention, frequency, pain	17		465/595		7.8/18
Bosch (15)	Urge incontinence	18	204/318[a]	318/402	206/258[b]	
Shaker (31)	Urge incontinence	18	133/203[c]	291/336[c]	80/124[c]	
Bosch (17)	Urge incontinence	24/30	213/291[a]	306/380		
Shaker (53)	Retention	20	204/167	384/381		0/14[a]
Weil (20)	Urge incontinence	21	93/167	266/370[a]	115/370[a]	
Groen (54)	Urge incontinence	26		285/313		
Walsh (55)	Urge incontinence	74	109/167[a]	345/404[a]		

[a]Significant at p <0.05
[b]8/10 patients had no contractions after stimulation.
[c]Significance not reported

two urodynamic reports on retention, there appears to be an increase in peak flow rate after implantation. Shaker's group (53) showed statistical significance but Elabbady et al (30) did not. This may be due to the fact that in the former group no patients voided preoperatively versus the latter, where incomplete voiders were included.

The bottom line is that if a symptom diary shows significant reduction in frequency, urgency, and incontinence and improved voiding in the case of retention, the patient is eligible for implantation irrespective of urodynamic changes.

COMPLICATIONS

Tables 12.7 and 12.8 summarize the adverse events with test stimulation and permanent implantation, respectively (3,6,13,20,24,28,32,34). Revision rates range from 10% to 33%. Common complications are pain at the implant site (4% to 34%) followed by lead migration (4% to 17%). The high prevalence of pain is partially accounted for by the fact that the initial implantation devices (IPG) were placed in the lower abdomen. It is currently standard practice to place these over the buttock; however, Everaert reported pain equally at all sites (32). Patients need to be informed of the relatively high rate of reoperation as discussed above. Explantation rates range from 1.4% to 22% and replacement/relocation rates from 1.4% to 54%. Infection or skin breakdown invariably results in removal. Several authors have noted that no matter how quickly or often you attempt to move the device or reclose the skin, once the skin is breached, removal is inevitable (see Table 12.3) (24).

Recently there have been reports of decreased efficacy or cessation of response with time. Weil et al noted over a 6- to 36-month follow-up, 8/34 (24%) had deterioration in primary outcome measures (20). On logistic regression analysis, they noted no predictors for these treatment failures. Everaert et al reported 6/53 (11%) late device failures. Reoperation resulted in no improvement in 4 and a temporary response in 1, but the ultimate result was failure (32). The authors concluded that revision for late failures in patients with a good S3 response is not successful. This has also been the author's own personal experience.

TABLE 12.7

Complications with Permanent Implantation

Author	Weil (20)	Schmidt (28)	Hassouna (3)	Spinelli (34)	Everaert (32)	Swinn (6)
Number of patients	21	34	219	103	53	38
Complication (%)						
Pain at IPG	29	19.1	15.3	3.9	34	
Lead migration	17	7	8.4		4	8
Lead pain			5.4			
Operative revision		32.5	33.3	9.7		24
Leg pain	17					8
New pain			9		17	
Leg stimulation	5				8	
Change in bowel function	5	2.9			6	
Urinary retention	2					
Vaginal cramps	2					
Anal pain	2					
Skin irritation	2	5.7				
Infection			6.1		2	
Wound problem				1.9		

IPG, initial implantation device.

TABLE 12.8

Complications with PNE

Complication	Multicenter Pooled Data	Dijkema (13)	Schmidt (28)	Hijaz (24)
Lead migration	9.90%	8.60%		
Lead/test stimulator disconnection	2.60%			
Stimulator defect		4.30%		
Temporary pain	2.60%	21.70%	2.9%	
Change in bowel habit	0.60%			
Infection or skin irritation	0.60%		5.70%	4%

PNE, peripheral nerve evaluation.

The use of neurophysiological testing can help to identify true device failures versus those who may benefit from reprogramming or revision. With the stimulator on, those who have a detectable EMG response at the anal sphincter are not reoperation candidates. No EMG response in the setting of normal impedance indicates electrode movement, and reoperation may be successful. It is the only objective means of determining the correct function and position of the lead (56).

Bilateral Chronic Sacral Neuromodulation

As we can see from the results, not all patients respond to this modality. With this in mind, several authors have advocated the use of bilateral stimulation. The rationale for this is that each half of the bladder has its own confined innervation. Animal studies in cats have shown that with bilateral stimulation there is a significant increase (33%) in bladder inhibition. In contrast, stimulation of several levels (i.e., S2, S3) does not produce the same effect. Unfortunately, there is very little clinical data to support its use. Scheepens et al performed a randomized prospective crossover trial of unilateral versus bilateral stimulation, but only with the peripheral nerve evaluation (i.e., not with permanent implant) (57). In an effort to minimize poor response due to lead movement, only patients with x-ray confirmation of absence of lead movement were studied. Of the 13 patients with urge incontinence and 13 patients with retention, no significant improvement was noted in bilateral versus unilateral; however, 2 patients who had failed unilateral succeeded with bilateral stimulation. Braun et al published on bilateral stimulation both in the German and the Spanish literature. Patients were implanted after sacral laminectomy (not a technique used here). Their initial work of 20 patients (58) was followed by publication of 30 patients; however, this included the initial 20 patients (59). They reported that at 2 months, bilateral stimulation was successful, but none of these patients had unilateral implants at any stage. Hohenfellner also published on the use of bilateral leads after laminectomy (60). Ten of 11 patients responded, but once again these patients did not have a trial of unilateral lead placement.

Therefore, as the literature stands currently, there is no indication to perform bilateral stimulation as a first-line therapy. Some patients, particularly those with urinary retention, may benefit from bilateral neuromodulation; however, predictive factors for this have not been elucidated. Because of the lack of scientific support and potential expense of bilateral implantation, unilateral stimulation should be the recommended method and bilateral stimulation should be considered only should unilateral fail, particularly in a patient with urinary retention.

Pregnancy

There are a large number of reproductive-age patients who have been implanted. The question arises as to how to manage sacral stimulation once pregnancy is diagnosed. The largest series to date reported on six patients, five who deactivated the stimulator after 7 weeks of pregnancy and one who deactivated it prior to pregnancy (61). One of these patients reactivated the stimulation at 19 weeks. There were no reported teratogenic effects. The only reported complication was a premature delivery in the patient who had neuromodulation during the initial 7 weeks of pregnancy. It is impossible to determine whether this played a role.

The ideal mode for delivery is uncertain. There have been theoretical concerns that the lead may be damaged or displaced during a vaginal delivery. Risks and benefits of elective cesarean section need to be weighed against these potential risks. Current manufacturing guidelines recommend that neuromodulation be discontinued as soon as a diagnosis of pregnancy is made. If the risk of urinary complications from deactivating the device outweighs potential risks to the pregnancy, then reactivation could be considered.

Patient Satisfaction and Quality of Life

Most articles have looked at efficacy, and few have specifically addressed patient satisfaction and quality of life. Four different instruments have been reported in the literature to assess quality of life after implantation: Short Form 36 Health Survey (SF-36), Incontinence Impact Questionnaire (IIQ), Beck Depression Inventory, and a Quality of Life Index Questionnaire. In trials using the SF-36, significant improvement was shown in the emotional raw score, physical functioning score (20), physical health component (28), and change in health perception (31). Using the IIQ, Amundsen et al noted a significantly higher total score in implanted patients compared to baseline (27). Using the Beck inventory, Shaker et al noted a 10% to 40% improvement in scores but did not specify whether these were statistically significant (31). On a 22-item domain-specific quality-of-life questionnaire, Capellano et al showed a significant higher quality-of-life score after implantation (35).

With regards to patient satisfaction, Everaert et al reported that despite the fact that 81% continued to use the device, only 68% of patients were satisfied and only 66% would repeat the procedure (32). They felt the dissatisfaction with long-term success was explained by the occurrence of complications in all patients.

Percutaneous Neuromodulation

One of the challenges of sacral neuromodulation is that between 30% and 50% of candidates will fail their test stimulation stage and therefore not be eligible for permanent implantation. The rate is lower with the new tined lead, but there are still a certain percentage of patients who fail the stage 1. Several authors have described a new technique that directly stimulates the pudendal nerve, the ra-

tionale being that afferent activity is contributed not solely by S3 (35.5%) but also by S1 (4%) and S2 (60.5%) (62). Therefore, for those patients who fail S3 stimulation, direct stimulation of the pudendal nerve, which is innervated by multiple branches, may be a possibility.

In 2005, two research groups simultaneously reported the use of two different leads implanted at the level of the pudendal nerve. Groen et al reported on the use of the Bion (63). This is a self-contained, battery-powered, programmable mini-neurostimulator (size 28 × 3.3 mm, weight 0.7 g) with integrated electrodes that can be implanted adjacent to the pudendal nerve in Alcock's canal. A 3- to 4-mm skin incision is made 1.5 cm medial to the ischial tuberosity, and using a special kit the electrode can be placed. Subjects undergo a test stimulation phase called the percutaneous screening test (PST). The pudendal nerve is stimulated via a needle and an external pulse generator at the same settings as the Bion. Cystometrography is performed prior to stimulation and then after 10 minutes of stimulation. The test stimulation phase is considered positive if stimulation results in a more than 50% increase in bladder volume at the first detrusor contraction or the maximum cystometric capacity. The test is performed on both sides to determine on which side to implant the electrodes. In the operating room, the patient is sedated and local anesthesia used. The electrode is placed using palpation of the ischial spine, fluoroscopy, and electrodiagnosis with surface electrodes perianally.

Simultaneously Spinelli et al described the use of a quadripolar tined lead placed next to the pudendal nerve in Alcock's canal (64). This is also performed with neurophysiological testing. This surgical approach can either be perineal or posterior. With the perineal approach, the patient is given local anesthesia at the level of the ischial tuberosity, 4 cm deep in the direction of the ischial spine. With a finger either in the rectum or the vagina, a 20-gauge insulated needle (Medtronic 041828, 041829) is guided to the ischial spine. It is then directed medially and dorsally to reach the ischiorectal fossa until it is located below and behind the ischial spine in Alcock's canal. The needle is then stimulated, and the external anal sphincter activity is monitored and recorded. The maximum compound muscle action potential (CMAP) is noted and compared to the original test stimulation CMAP, and the position of the needle is adjusted until the tracing reproduces the test stimulation. When correct positioning is confirmed, either a temporary stimulation lead or the definitive quadripolar tined lead can be placed.

This is done in a manner similar to placing the tined lead with the Interstim (i.e., stylet, introducer, feeding of the lead). The introducer is not removed until the lead is confirmed to be in the correct position (i.e., consistent CMAP). The lead is then tunneled and connected to the temporary stimulator. In the posterior approach, the patient is prone and the ischial spine is located by drawing two intersecting lines, one horizontally from the greater trochanter and the second vertically from the tip of the ischial tuberosity. The rest of the procedure is the same. The second stage consists of implanting the IPG (Interstim 3023, Med-tronic). The IPG in this case is then placed in the lower abdomen.

Results

Initial results from pudendal nerve stimulation were described in abstracts in 2003 and 2004. The initial results were published in 2005 (63,64). Using the Bion as described above, Groen et al reported on 14 patients with idiopathic urodynamically demonstrated detrusor instability who had failed previous conservative therapy and neuromodulation (63). Five patients (36%) responded positively to the test phase and received the permanent implant. Six patients were implanted, including one patient who had a significant clinical effect. The number of incontinent episodes, pads used per day, and leakage severity index significantly decreased after 6 months. When the device was deactivated, these values returned to the preoperative ones in a very short period of time. Cystometry showed a significant increase in bladder volume at first detrusor contraction and maximum at cystometric capacity. Side effects included vaginal dryness during intercourse that was resolved by turning the unit off 30 minutes before sexual activity, mechanical irritation during bicycle riding, and altered bowel function (reduced defecatory frequency). It should be noted in this study the patient selection for permanent implantation was based on the result of this so-called PST test, which assesses the response including the use of urodynamic parameters. The authors felt that if urodynamic indices were not included and results were based solely on diaries as used for the other forms of sacral neuromodulation, the rates for a positive test stimulation may be higher. The initial conclusion was that this therapy should be considered in those patients who have failed the current standard sacral neuromodulation.

In the second paper, Spinelli evaluated 15 patients, 6 with the perineal and 9 with the posterior approach (64). Three of these patients had already failed sacral neuromodulation. Patients were screened for 15 to 45 days. The criterion for implantation was greater than an 80% improvement in the number of daily incontinent episodes. Of the 15 patients, 3 had no improvement, 2 had a 50% improvement, 2 had more than an 88% improvement, and 8 were continent. Interestingly, seven patients had associated bowel dysfunction and four reported more normalization of their bowel function. Of the seven patients who had 6 months of follow-up, maximum cystometric capacity significantly increased. Twelve patients had permanent implantation. At 6 months, these patients showed the same efficacy that had been achieved during the screening phase. Interestingly, not all patients used the stimulator in the same way. Five patients used the stimulator "on demand" to increase the time between urgency and voiding, three patients kept the unit on during the day but turned it off at night, and one patient used continuous stimulation. The conclusion of these authors was that implantation of the tined lead into Alcock's canal was feasible using the tools available for sacral nerve stimulation. Neurophysiological guidance is mandatory to verify that the lead is in the correct position and to allow maximal stimulation of the nerve by assessing the CMAP. They felt it offered a therapeutic option to patients who had a poor response to conservative management or the current sacral nerve stimulation.

Obviously, with both of these studies, the results are very preliminary and larger studies are needed to evaluate both the short- and long-term effects, as our knowledge from sacral neuromodulation indicates that efficacy can decrease with time.

PERIPHERAL NEUROMODULATION

Peripheral stimulation (posterior tibial nerve stimulation) is a potential option for patients who are not candidates for sacral or pudendal nerve implantation because of the cost or a desire to avoid an implantable device or those who find the thought of adjusting an implantable device technically overwhelming. From the physician's perspective, placement of a needle in a peripheral nerve is technically less challenging than implantation of a sacral nerve stimulator. The Urgent PC (Uroplasty, Inc, Minneapolis, MN), formerly known as the Stoller afferent nerve stimulator (SANS), provides a means of stimulating S3 via the transcutaneous root at the level of posterior tibial nerve (Fig. 12.8). The posterior tibial nerve is a mixed sensory motor nerve originating from L4 through S3. Stimulation can be obtained by attaching an acupuncture needle (34-gauge) three finger-

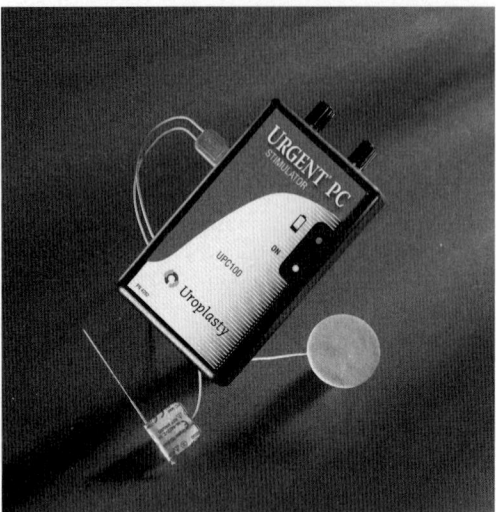

FIGURE 12.8 • The Urgent PC for peripheral modulation.

breadths cephalad to the medial aspect of the medial malleolus (Fig. 12.9). This corresponds to the Spleen-6 acupuncture point. Typically, the stimulator is attached via a connecting lead to the needle and a surface-ground electrode. Stimulation is performed weekly for 20 minutes for an initial 12 sessions. This technique has been studied mostly for irritative voiding syndromes (i.e., overactive bladder), but there is a small amount of data on its use in urinary retention. Table 12.9 details the recent studies. It appears to be effective in decreasing

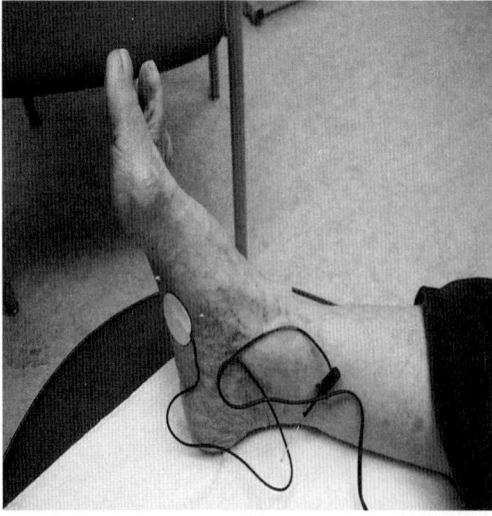

FIGURE 12.9 • Positioning of the needle at the medial malleolus.

both daytime and nighttime frequency and decreasing the number of incontinent episodes. Data on the percentage of patients actually dry is more difficult to obtain, though it does appear that 40% to 50% of patients report a cure. The reader will note, however, that all the studies were performed at 12 weeks, and long-term data on this technique is not available. Herein lies one of the future challenges with this therapy, as we do not know how many total sessions are needed to achieve maximum effect or how often the stimulation needs to be repeated to maintain this effect.

With respect to urinary retention, the two small studies performed show a significant decrease in catheter volume, but it does not appear to abolish the need for catheterization (65–72). Therefore, it does not appear to offer a cure or resolution of retention.

The therapy does appear to alter urodynamic parameters, with an increase in the volume at the first detrusor contraction (73) and an increase in the maximum cystometric capacity (73,74). Vandoninck noted that patients with greater size of their detrusor contractions appeared to have less response to this therapy (68).

There is very little information about its specific use in interstitial cystitis; however, two papers reported pain scores, one in a group of patients with frequency and urgency and the other with chronic pelvic pain. The first paper noted a significant decrease in pain score, from 7.6 to 3.1 (69), and the second paper found a 67% decrease in pain (70).

In summary, the data in the short term looks promising, with improvement rates similar to the standard conservative therapy; however, it must be noted that patients typically in these studies had failed all other means of conservative therapy, so this is obviously a more hardcore group of patients to treat. This appears to be a reasonable alternative to patients who have failed anticholinergic medication and who for financial, cognitive, or other reasons are not candidates for an implantable device. Studies consistently show the lack of any significant side effects for this therapy, so it is very attractive.

BOTULINUM A TOXIN THERAPY

Botulinum toxin (Botox) exerts its effect by inhibiting the release of acetylcholine from the motor nerve. Without the neurotransmitter, the muscles are unable to contract. It has been shown in skeletal muscles that intramuscular injection of the toxin causes temporary chemodenervation and muscle relaxation. It has been hypothesized that

TABLE 12.9

Results with Peripheral Stimulation (SANS)

Author	Study	Diagnosis	n	Voids/Day Voids/Night	Leaks/Day
Van Balken (65)	Multicenter	Overactive bladder, retention	37 & 12	17% decrease 38% decrease	
Govier (66)	Multicenter	Overactive bladder	53	25% decrease 21% decrease	35% decrease
Vandoninck (67)	Multicenter	Overactive bladder	35	12.5/10 (24 h)	5/1
Vandoninck (68)	Multicenter	Overactive bladder	90	13/10 (24 h)	5.2
Klingler (69)	Single-center			16.1/4.4	
		Frequency, urgency	15	8.3/1.4	
		Frequency, urgency,	26	9.2/6.5; 2.9/1.4	
		urge incontinence,	22	8.7/7.1; 2.5/1.3	1.2/0.4
Ruiz (70)	Single-center	interstitial cystitis	3		
Van Balken (71)	Multicenter	Chronic pain	33		
Vandoninck (72)	Multicenter	Retention	39		

Author	Quality of Life	Pain Score	Improvement	Cure	Criteria	Follow-up
Van Balken	Improved		60% want to continue therapy		QOL, diary	12 w
Govier	Significant increase				QOL, diary	12 w
Vandoninck				46%	QOL, diary	12 w
Vandoninck	Significant increase		70%		QOL, diary	12 w
Klinger	Significant increase	7.6/3.1	56%	46.7%	QOL, pain score	12 w
Ruiz		Decrease in 67%			QOL, diary	12 w
Van Balken	Significant increase	Significant decrease	21% >50% improved		QOL	12 w
Vandoninck	Significant increase		41% >50% decrease in no. cath	15%	QOL, diary	12 w

QOL, quality of life.

intradetrusor botulinum toxin may block the presynaptic release of acetylcholine from the parasympathetic nerves, similar to its mechanism with skeletal muscles. Therefore, it has been postulated that it would be an effective treatment for overactive bladder. Currently its use in bladder conditions is not FDA approved.

There appear to be various techniques to inject anywhere from a total of 100 to 300 units of Botox into the bladder mucosa. The technique can be done under local, general, or spinal anesthesia.

Typically, the toxin is diluted in injectable saline. With time, the technique has been redefined, and it appears that lower doses (i.e., 20 units) injected into more sites (i.e., 20 sites) shows significant improvement and lessens the chance of retention. A 1% Xylocaine solution is instilled into the bladder initially to provide some anesthesia. Two hundred or 300 units of Botox are diluted in 20 to 30 mL of saline. Using a rigid cystoscope and a collagen injection needle, 0.5 to 1.0 mL of solution is injected at 20 to 30 sites with a distance of 1 to 1.5 cm between each site. Injections are placed above the trigone in an effort to reduce the theoretical concern of developing ureteral reflux should the Botox diffuse. The patient is continued on antibiotics several days after the procedure. Patients are taught self-catheterization prior to the procedure, as this is a potential risk.

Two studies published in 2005, one in the United States (75) and one in the United Kingdom (76), have shown that it appears effective in patients with idiopathic detrusor instability. Popat reported on 31 patients with detrusor overactivity (76). Maximum cystometric capacity increased from 194 mL to 327 mL in these patients. Frequency decreased from 13.6 to 8.3 per 24 hours, leakage from 3.2 to 0.6. Urgency was also significantly reduced. At 16 weeks, 8 of 14 (57.1% of patients) were continent. Nineteen percent of patients did require intermittent use of self-catheterization. Smith et al reported on one institution's experience using Botox for a variety of voiding dysfunctions (75). One hundred and ten patients were injected either in the bladder (n = 42) or in the urethra (n = 68) for a variety of bladder conditions related to multiple sclerosis, spinal cord injury, interstitial cystitis, stroke, and overactive bladder. Of the 32 patients with pure overactive bladder, there was a 40% decrease in voids per 24-hour period and a decrease in pad use from 93% to 12%. Cystometry showed an increase in capacity from 153 mL to 246 mL. The authors observed that repeated injections appeared to last longer than the initial injection, with some patients maintaining efficacy for more than a year.

Rapp reported the results of Botox for detrusor overactivity in patients who had previously failed anticholinergic therapy (77). Thirty-five patients had a total of 300 units of Botulinum A toxin injected into 30 sites within the bladder. Postinjection efficacy was evaluated using the Incontinence Impact Questionnaire (IIQ-7) and the Urogenital Distress Inventory (UDI-6). Specific information on voiding frequency, pad use, and leakage episodes was not included in the article. The authors reported that 34% of patients had complete resolution of their symptoms, with a further 26% having slight improvement and 40% having no improvement at 3 weeks. At 6 months, the responders noted continued significant improvement; however, it was not as good as the improvement at 3 weeks. Patients noted improvement in their symptoms at a range of 1 to 14 days (mean 5.3) postprocedure and improvement reached maximal effect at 2 to 20 days (mean 8.3). The authors did not report whether any patients required catheterization for retention. A review of early experience from abstract data is available in the *Journal of Urology* (78).

It appears, at least on initial experience, that Botulinum toxin may have a role in patients with overactive bladder that is refractory to other therapies. It should be remembered, however, that this is a nonapproved indication and at this stage is typically not covered by insurance. Long-term effects of repeated Botulinum toxin injections in the bladder are unknown, either locally within the bladder or systemically. Therefore, caution needs to be exercised at embracing this as a first-line therapy for all patients until more long-term data is available.

CONCLUSIONS

Neuromodulation, whether it is sacral, pudendal, or peripheral, is effective therapy for the treatment of frequency, urgency, and urge incontinence in patients with a history of poor response to other therapies. Sacral stimulation is effective for idiopathic retention, with little published data on the other modalities for this condition. Response rates for all of these conditions are remarkable when one considers that studies on neuromodulation are conducted only on patients who have failed conservative therapy and are considered the recalcitrant patients. Unfortunately reoperation rates are high for sacral stimulation and some patients do not maintain efficacy long term. Patients need to be counseled accordingly. The pudendal route is appealing, but there is only a small amount of data to date. Posterior tibial stimulation is more time-consuming for the physician and patient; however, it has a comparable success rate to the other modalities for overactive bladder without the need to permanently implant a device, and it should be considered. Currently Botox is not FDA approved for use in the bladder, but it shows promise.

The other remarkable thing that we need to remember is that prior to these modalities, we had little else to offer a patient who failed conservative therapy, and the existence of these technologies has brought a tremendous improvement in quality of life for those patients who have used them successfully.

REFERENCES

1. Tanagho EA, Schmidt RA. Electrical stimulation in the clinical management of the neurogenic bladder. *J Urol* 1988;140:1331–1339.
2. Wheeler JS, Walter JS, Zaszczurynski PJ. Bladder inhibition by penile nerve stimulation in spinal cord injury patients. *J Urol* 1992;147:100–103.

3. Hassouna MM, Siegel SW, Lycklama À, et al. Sacral neuromodulation in the treatment of urgency-frequency symptoms: A multicenter study on efficacy and safety. *J Urol* 2000;163:1849–1854.

4. Goodwin RJ, Swinn MJ, Fowler CJ. The neurophysiology of urinary retention in young women and its treatment by neuromodulation. *World J Urol* 1998;16:305–307.

5. Fowler CJ, Christmas TJ, Chapple CR, et al. Abnormal electromyographic activity of the urethral sphincter, voiding dysfunction, and polycystic ovaries: a new syndrome? *Br Med J* 1988;297:1436–1438.

6. Swinn MJ, Kitchen ND, Goodwin RJ, et al. Sacral neuromodulation for women with Fowler's syndrome. *Eur Urol* 2000;38:439–443.

7. Fowler CJ, Swinn MJ, Goodwin RJ, et al. Studies of the latency of pelvic floor contraction during peripheral nerve evaluation show that the muscle response is reflexively mediated. *J Urol* 2000;163:881–883.

8. Barbanti G, Maggi CA, Beneforti P, et al. Relief of pain following intravesical capsaicin in patients with hypersensitivity disorders of the lower urinary tract. *Br J Urol* 1993;71:686–691.

9. Long DM. Electrical stimulation for the relief of pain from chronic nerve injury. *J Neurosurg* 1973;39:718–722.

10. Mastropietro M, Fuller E, Benson JT. Electrodiagnostic features of responders and nonresponders to sacral neuromodulation test stimulation. *Int Urogynecol J Pelvic Floor Dysfunct* 2001;12: suppl S1, paper 47.

11. Vaizey CJ, Kamm MA, Turner IC, et al. Effects of short-term sacral stimulation on anal and rectal function in patients with anal incontinence. *Gut* 1999;44:407–412.

12. Carey M, Fynes C, Murray C, et al. Sacral nerve root stimulation for lower urinary tract dysfunction: overcoming the problem of lead migration. *BJU Int* 2001;87:15–18.

13. Dijkema HE, Weil EH, Mijs PT, et al. Neuromodulation of sacral nerves for incontinence and voiding dysfunctions. *Eur Urol* 1993;24:72–76.

14. Koldewijn EL, Rosier PF, Meuleman EJ, et al. Predictors of success with neuromodulation in lower urinary tract dysfunction: Results of trial stimulation in 100 patients. *J Urol* 1994;152:2071–2075.

15. Bosch JL, Groen J. Sacral (S3) segmental nerve stimulation as a treatment for urge incontinence and detrusor instability: results of chronic electrical stimulation using an implantable neural prosthesis. *J Urol* 1995;154:504–507.

16. Weil EH, Ruiz-Cerda JL, Eerdmans PH, et al. Clinical results of sacral stimulation for chronic voiding dysfunction using unilateral sacral foramen electrodes. *World J Urol* 1998;16:313–321.

17. Bosch JL, Groen J. Neuromodulation: urodynamic effects of sacral (S3) spinal nerve stimulation in patients with detrusor instability or detrusor hyperflexia. *Behav Brain Res* 1998;92:141–150.

18. Edlund C, Hellstrom M, Peeker R, et al. First Scandinavian experience of electrical sacral nerve stimulation in the treatment of overactive bladder. *Scand J Urol Nephrol* 2000;34:366–376.

19. Bosch JL, Groen J. Sacral nerve neuromodulation in the treatment of patients with refractory motor urge incontinence: long-term results of a prospective longitudinal study. *J Urol* 2000;163:1219–1222.

20. Weil EH, Ruiz-Cerda JL, Eerdmans PH, et al. Sacral root neuromodulation in the treatment of refractory urinary urge incontinence: a prospective randomized clinical trial. *Eur Urol* 2000;37:161–171.

21. Janknegt RA, Weil EH, Eerdmans PH. Improving neuromodulation technique for refractory voiding dysfunction: two-stage implant. *Urology* 1997;49:358–362.

22. Benson JT. Sacral nerve stimulation results may be improved by electrodiagnostic techniques. *Int Urogynecol J Pelvic Floor Dysfunct* 2000;11:352–357.

23. Spinelli M, Giardiello G, Arduini A, et al. New percutaneous technique of sacral nerve stimulation has high initial success rate: preliminary results. *Eur Urol* 2003;43:70–74.

24. Hijaz A, Vasavada S. Complications and troubleshooting of sacral neuromodulation therapy. *Urol Clin North Am* 2005;32:65–69.

25. Scheepens WA, De Bie RA, Weil EH, et al. Unilateral versus bilateral sacral neuromodulation in patients with chronic voiding dysfunction. *J Urol* 2002;168:2046–2050.

26. Amundsen CL, Romero AA, Jamison MG, et al. Sacral neuromodulation for intractable urge incontinence: are there factors associated with cure? *Urology* 2005;66:746–750.

27. Amundsen CL, Webster GD. Sacral neuromodulation in an older, urge-incontinent population. *Am J Obstet Gynecol* 2002;187:1462–1465.

28. Schmidt RA, Jonas U, Oleson KA, et al. Sacral nerve stimulation for treatment of refractory urinary urge incontinence. *J Urol* 1999;162:352–357,

29. Thon WF, Baskin LS, Jonas U, et al. Neuromodulation of voiding dysfunction and pelvic pain. *World J Urol* 1991;9:138–141.

30. Elabbady AA, Hassouna MM, Elhilali MM. Neural stimulation for chronic voiding dysfunctions. *J Urol* 1994;152:2076–2080.

31. Shaker HS, Hassouna M. Sacral nerve root neuromodulation: an effective treatment for refractory urge incontinence. *J Urol* 1998;159:1516–1519.

32. Everaert K, De Ridder D, Baert L, et al. Patient satisfaction and complications following sacral nerve stimulation for urinary retention, urge incontinence, and perineal pain: a multicenter evaluation. *Int Urogynecol J Pelvic Floor Dysfunct* 2000;11:231–236.

33. Chartier-Kastler EJ, Bosch JL, Perrigot M, et al. Long-term results of sacral nerve stimulation (S3) for the treatment of neurogenic refractory urge incontinence related to detrusor hyperreflexia. *J Urol* 2000;164:1476–1480.

34. Spinelli M, Bertapelle P, Cappellano F, et al. Chronic sacral neuromodulation in patients with lower urinary tract symptoms: results form a national register. *J Urol* 2001;166:541–545.

35. Cappellano F, Ciotti MG, Pizzoccaro M, et al. Sacral root neuromodulation in the treatment of female urge and mixed urinary incontinence. *Urogynaecol Int J* 1998;12(3):111–121.

36. Heesakkers J, Bemelmans BL, Van Kerrebroeck EV, et al. Long-term effects of Interstim in patients suffering from urinary incontinence, urgency/frequency syndrome, and urinary retention: a prospective study. *Eur Urol Suppl* 2003;2(1):143.

37. Janknegt RA, Hassouna MM, Siegel SW, et al. Long-term effectiveness of sacral nerve stimulation for re-

fractory urge incontinence. *Eur Urol* 2001;39(1): 101–106.

38. Spinelli M, Weil E, Ostardo E, et al. New tined lead electrode in sacral neuromodulation: experience from a multicenter European study. *World J Urol* 2005;23:225–229.
39. Elhilali MM, Khaled SM, Kashiwabara T, et al. Sacral neuromodulation: long-term experience of one center. *Urology* 2005;65:1114–1117.
40. Ruiz-Cerda JL, Arlandis S, Gonzalez-Chamorro F, et al. Spanish experience in sacral nerve stimulation: case register of the Spanish Sacral Neuromodulation Group (GENS). *Eur Urol Suppl* 2003;2(1):142.
41. Siegel SW, Catanzaro F, Dijkema HE, et al. Long-term results of a multicenter study on sacral nerve stimulation for treatment of urinary urge incontinence, urgency-frequency, and retention. *Urology* 2000; 56(6:Suppl 1):87–91.
42. Aboseif S, Tamaddon K, Chalfin S, et al. Sacral neuromodulation as an effective treatment for refractory pelvic floor dysfunction. *Urology* 2002;60(1):52–56.
43. Ruffion A, N'Goi C, Dembele D, et al. Sacral root neuromodulation: prospective evaluation in 166 cases. *Eur Urol Suppl* 2003;2(1):143.
44. Koldewijn E, Meuleman EJ, Bemelmans BL, et al. Neuromodulation effective in voiding dysfunction despite high reoperation rate. *J Urol* 1999;161(4 Suppl):255.
45. Dasgupta R, Wiseman OJ, Kitchen N, et al. Long-term results of sacral neuromodulation for women with urinary retention. *BJU Int* 2004;94:335–337.
46. Jonas U, Fowler CJ, Chancellor MB, et al. Efficacy of sacral nerve stimulation for urinary retention: results 18 months after implantation. *J Urol* 2001;165:15–19.
47. Chai TC, Zhang C, Warren JW, et al. Percutaneous sacral third nerve neurostimulation improves symptoms and normalizes urinary BB-EGF levels and antiproliferative activity in patients with interstitial cystitis. *Urology* 2000;55:643–646.
48. Whitmore CE, Payne CK, Diokno AC, et al. Sacral neuromodulation in patients with interstitial cystitis: a multicenter trial. *Int Urogynecol J* 2003;14:305–309.
49. Maher CF, Carey MP, Dwyer PL, et al. Percutaneous sacral nerve root neuromodulation for intractable interstitial cystitis. *J Urol* 2001;165:884–886.
50. Comiter CV. Sacral neuromodulation for the symptomatic treatment of refractory interstitial cystitis: a prospective study. *J Urol* 2003;169:1369–1373.
51. Peters KM, Carey JM, Konstandt DB. Sacral neuromodulation for the treatment of refractory interstitial cystitis: outcomes based on technique. *Int Urogynecol J Pelvic Floor Dysfunct* 2003;14:223–228.
52. Peters KM, Konstandt D. Sacral neuromodulation decreases narcotic requirements in refractory interstitial cystitis. *BJU Int* 2004;93:777–779.
53. Shaker HS, Hassouna M. Sacral root neuromodulation in idiopathic nonobstructive chronic urinary retention. *J Urol* 1998;159:1476–1478.
54. Groen J, van Mastrigt R, Bosch JL. Computerized assessment of detrusor instability in patients treated with sacral neuromodulation. *J Urol* 2001;165:169–173.
55. Walsh IK, Thompson T, Loughridge WG, et al. Non-invasive antidromic neurostimulation: a simple effective method for improving bladder storage. *Neurourol Urodyn* 2001;20:73–84.
56. McLennan MT. The role of electrodiagnostic techniques in the reprogramming of patients with a delayed suboptimal response to sacral nerve stimulation.

Int Urogynecol J Pelvic Floor Dysfunct 2003;14: 98–103.

57. Scheepens WA, De Bie RA, Weil EH, et al. Unilateral versus bilateral sacral neuromodulation in patients with chronic voiding dysfunction. *J Urol* 2002;168: 2046–2050.
58. Braun PM, Seif C, Scheepe JR, et al. Chronic sacral bilateral neuromodulation. Using a minimal invasive implantation technique in patients with disorders of bladder function. *Urologe A* 2002;41:44–47.
59. Braun M, Fernandez MI, Martunez Portillo FJ, et al. Continuous bilateral sacral neuromodulation as a minimally invasive implantation technique with functional bladder changes. *Arch Esp Urol* 2003;56:497–501.
60. Hohenfellner M, Schultz-Lampel D, Dahms S, et al. Bilateral chronic sacral neuromodulation for treatment of lower urinary tract dysfunction. *J Urol* 1998; 160(3:Pt 1):821–824.
61. Wiseman OJ, van der Hombergh U, Koldewijn EL, et al. Sacral neuromodulation and pregnancy. *J Urol* 2002;167:165–168.
62. Huang JC, Deletis V, Vodusek DB, et al. Preservation of pudendal afferents in sacral rhizotomies. *Neurosurgery* 1997;41:411–415.
63. Groen J, Amiel C, Bosch JL. Chronic pudendal nerve neuromodulation in women with idiopathic refractory detrusor overactivity incontinence: results of a pilot study with a novel minimally invasive implantable mini-stimulator. *Neurourol Urodyn* 2005;24:226–230.
64. Spinelli M, Weil E, Ostardo E, et al. New tined lead electrode in sacral neuromodulation: experience from a multicenter European study. *World J Urol* 2005; 23:225–229.
65. Van Balken MR, Vandoninck V, Gisolf KW, et al. Posterior tibial nerve stimulation as neuromodulative treatment of lower urinary tract dysfunction. *J Urol* 2001;166:914–918.
66. Govier FE, Litwiller S, Nitti V, et al. Percutaneous afferent neuromodulation for the refractory overactive bladder: results of a multicenter study. *J Urol* 2001;165:1193–1198.
67. Vandoninck V, Van Balken MR, Finazzi Agro E, et al. Posterior tibial nerve stimulation in the treatment of urge incontinence. *Neurourol Urodyn* 2003;22:17–23.
68. Vandoninck V, Van Balken MR, Finazzi Agro E, et al. Posterior tibial nerve stimulation in the treatment of overactive bladder. *Neurourol Urodyn* 2003;22: 227–232.
69. Klingler HC, Pycha A, Schmidbauer J, et al. Use of peripheral neuromodulation of the S3 region for treatment of detrusor overactivity: a urodynamic-based study. *Urology* 2000;56:766–771.
70. Ruiz BC, Outeirino XMP, Martinez PC, et al. Peripheral afferent nerve stimulation for treatment of lower urinary tract irritative symptoms. *Eur Urol* 2004;45:65–69.
71. van Balken MR, Vandoninck V, Messelink BJ, et al. Percutaneous tibial nerve stimulation as neuromosdulative treatment of chronic pelvic pain. *Eur Urol* 2003;43:158–163.
72. Vandoninck V, Van Balken MR, Finazzi Agr E, et al. Posterior tibial nerve stimulation in the treatment of idiopathic nonobstructive voiding dysfunction. *Urology* 2003;61:567–572.
73. Amarenco G, Ismael SS, Even-Schneider A, et al. Urodynamic effect of acute transcutaneous posterior tibial nerve stimulation in overactive bladder. *J Urol* 2003;169:2210–2215.

74. Walsh IK, Thompson T, Loughridge WG, et al. Non-invasive antidromic neurostimulation: a simple effective method for improving bladder storage. *Neurourol Urodyn* 2001;20:73–84.

75. Smith CP, Nishiguchi J, O'Leary M, et al. Single-institution experience in 110 patients with botulinum toxin A injection into bladder or urethra. *Urology* 2005;65:37–41.

76. Popat R, Apostolidis A, Kalsi V, et al. A comparison between the response of patients with idiopathic detru-sor overactivity and neurogenic detrusor overactivity to the first intradetrusor injection of botulinum A toxin. *J Urol* 2005;174:984–989.

77. Rapp DE, Lucioni A, Katz EE, et al. Use of botulinum A toxin for the treatment of refractory overactive bladder symptoms: an initial experience. *Urology* 2004; 63:1071–1075.

78. Smith CP, Chancellor MB. Emerging role of botulinum toxin in the management of voiding dysfunction. *J Urol* 2004;171:2128–2137.

CHAPTER 13

Conservative Therapy for Stress Incontinence

Laura Scheufele and Karen Abraham

INTRODUCTION

Stress urinary incontinence (SUI) is "the complaint of involuntary leakage on effort or exertion, or on sneezing or coughing," as defined by the International Continence Society (1). Urine leakage from the urethra occurs when the intra-abdominal pressure exceeds the urethral pressure. The reason for the inadequate urethral closure pressure may be multifactorial. Pressure generation is affected by the ability to provide active support (i.e., ability of the smooth and striated muscles of the intrinsic and extrinsic sphincters to generate pressure) and passive support (i.e., nonneuromuscular factors such as the integrity of the connective tissue, vascular plexus, and the urethral lining) to the lower urinary tract. It is the interplay between factors that determines continence.

Interventions for SUI are directed toward improving urethral pressure generation and/or minimizing intra-abdominal pressure. Because of the multifactorial origin of SUI, the best outcomes are often achieved through a combination of interventions. The focus of this chapter is on conservative therapy techniques for SUI. These are nonsurgical techniques that attempt to restore the normal anatomic and mechanical relationships of the lower urinary tract, including pelvic floor muscle exercise, pessary use, lifestyle modifications, and pharmacologic interventions. The Agency for Health Care Policy and Research's Clinical Practice Guidelines on Urinary Incontinence in Adults advise that "the least invasive and least dangerous procedure that is appropriate for the pa-

tient should be the first choice" when treating urinary incontinence (2).

Behavioral management is the treatment of choice for SUI because of the low risk, minimal complications, and noninvasive nature of the techniques. The increased risk and cost of surgical repair make optimizing all nonsurgical therapy a priority. Conservative management should ideally eliminate symptoms and result in long-term improvement in a patient's quality of life. Although incontinence may not be cured, the severity may be lessened such that incontinence no longer has a significant impact upon the patient's lifestyle.

Women with SUI often present with impaired ability to provide both active and passive support to the lower urinary tract. The key component of active support is adequate pelvic floor muscle (PFM) function. The active contraction of the intrinsic and extrinsic sphincters and PFM provide a force that closes the bladder outlet (3). If sudden external pressure is exerted on the bladder, as in coughing, the PFMs respond by quickly contracting to prevent leakage (guarding reflex). An active contraction has been noted to occur 250 msec before the increase in intra-abdominal pressure in asymptomatic individuals (4). This contraction actively closes the bladder outlet, countering the abdominal pressure. Women with SUI have been observed to have significantly lower peak contractions, decreased length of maximal PFM contractions, and a progressive decline by decade in maximal PFM electromyographic activity as compared to continent women (5–7). If PFM function is compromised in any way, such as weakness or impaired innervation, the guarding reflex will be inadequate, resulting in urine leakage.

Women with SUI also have been noted to have impaired passive support of the lower urinary tract. The urothelium and the submucosal vessels of the urethra and bladder neck help to create a "leakproof" mucosal seal (7,8). A urethra that has lost its elasticity and whose submucosal blood supply has been compromised by prior surgery, radiation, obstetric injury, or loss of estrogen may require significantly more force from the active sphincteric mechanism to obtain a urine-tight closure. A hypermobile urethra (i.e., descends with abdominal pressure) allows leakage of urine (9). The slow twitch muscle fibers of the PFMs provide passive support to the urethra and bladder neck at rest, whereas the fast twitch muscle fibers are a part of the active support mechanism (3).

Proper anatomic support of the urethra and its junction with the bladder at the bladder neck is also necessary to resist sudden increases in abdominal pressure. Pressure is transmitted equally to a well-supported urethra and bladder and, therefore, conveys equal force to structures trying to release and to hold urine (3). Tension in the ligaments and fascia supporting the urethra and bladder neck (9) and the suburethral layer of vaginal wall and endopelvic fascia (10) provide a counterforce to the abdominal force that is transmitted to the proximal urethra, thereby closing the bladder outlet. The individual with SUI may have ligaments that are lax and stretched or prolapse of the vaginal walls (11), allowing the bladder neck to descend into a location where increases in intra-abdominal pressure are transmitted only to the bladder and not to the bladder neck and proximal urethra. This produces a significant force for expelling urine.

The magnitude of the pressure exerted on the urethra, which is determined by factors external to the urinary system, such as obesity, chronic lung disease, occupational and recreational stresses, and straining due to constipation, is also crucial in determining the likelihood of SUI (12). These factors not only affect the pressure causing each SUI episode, but may also lead to progressive damage of urethral supports. Numerous other nonmodifiable factors are associated with the onset of SUI, such as genetic factors (13), collagen content (14), race (15), and comorbid disease (16). The remainder of this chapter will discuss management techniques for SUI that affect the modifiable factors related to the onset of SUI. The theoretical rationale and current evidence supporting each intervention will be presented. When applicable, sugges-

tions for improving compliance will also be discussed.

PELVIC FLOOR MUSCLE EXERCISE

PFM exercise, training of the large levator ani and external urethral and anal sphincter muscles, is the most commonly prescribed intervention for the management of SUI (17). The PFM is composed of striated muscle. The levator ani is composed of 70% slow twitch/type I fibers, which use aerobic oxidative metabolism, and 30% fast twitch/type II fibers, which use anaerobic glycolytic metabolism (3,17). Contraction of both muscle types is necessary for normal function. The slow twitch fibers assist in maintaining passive continence, providing pelvic organ support, and are an important part of the postural support system. The fast twitch fibers provide rapid, forceful contractions in response to sudden increases in intra-abdominal pressure, such as with a cough, sneeze, laugh, or lifting maneuver. Interestingly, the slow twitch fibers of the levator ani form are the only weight-bearing muscles in the body whose fibers are oriented transversely.

Individuals with SUI have been shown to have statistically significant differences in PFM function versus continent women (i.e., relative thinning and weakness of the PFM). Continent women were found to have greater PFM thickness than incontinent women as measured by perineal ultrasound (18,19). Mean superficial PFM thickness in healthy women with no history of urinary incontinence or urogynecologic dysfunction was 7.15 mm at rest and 9.41 mm during an active contraction versus 6.34 mm at rest and 8.20 mm during an active contraction in the incontinent women. Greater muscle thickness has been associated with greater strength as measured by vaginal squeeze pressure. Continent women were also found to have a greater squeeze pressure than incontinent women, 39.5 cmH$_2$O versus 32.0 cmH$_2$O, respectively (18,19).

Various factors may affect the strength and thickness of the PFM. When PFM strength was measured in women who had delivered vaginally or via cesarean section and in nulliparous women, PFM strength was significantly lower in the vaginal delivery group compared with the cesarean delivery and nulliparous groups (20). In addition, women who had an episiotomy had significantly weaker pelvic floor muscles at 8 weeks postpartum as compared to women with a spontaneous laceration following vaginal delivery, women who had an elective cesarean, and those with an intact perineum following vaginal delivery (21). The women who had an elective cesarean showed no significant decline in PFM strength from 36 weeks gestation to 8 weeks postpartum. Women in all three vaginal delivery groups had a significant decline in strength as measured by the vaginal cone weight in grams of the heaviest cone able to be retained for 1 minute with the patient in standing and walking.

PFM function can be defined qualitatively by the tone at rest and the strength of a voluntary contraction as strong, weak, or absent or by a validated grading system (e.g., Oxford 1–5) (22). A PFM contraction may be assessed by visual inspection, palpation (external and/or internal), electromyography, real-time ultrasound, or perineometry (23). Factors to be assessed include strength, duration, displacement, and repeatability. These variables will determine the personalized exercise prescription. The PFM does not function in isolation and may have function well beyond our current understanding. Studies have demonstrated that the PFM contracts prior to postural movements along with the transversus abdominis and multifidus to provide important trunk stability to facilitate limb movement. The PFM also cocontracts with the obturator internus, another pelvic muscle, which is an external rotator of the hip joint (24). These relationships may also be utilized when designing exercise protocols to maximize PFM recruitment, facilitate a contraction in those with significant PFM weakness, and identify sources of coexisting dysfunction. Table 13.1 gives tips for identifying an ideal PFM contraction.

PFM exercises may aid in the management of SUI through an increased ability to generate urethral resistance by increasing periurethral muscle tension via a learned program of neuromuscular practice (25). PFM exercises are participatory, proactive, simple, noninvasive, free of side effects, and cost-effective and do not limit more complex options for future treatment. These exercises do, however, require time, effort, and continued practice to produce maximum benefit and continued urinary continence (26). The Cochrane Incontinence Group (27) concluded that PFM training was consistently better than no treatment or placebo treatment for SUI and should be offered as a first-line conservative management to women. This recommendation is based on a number of randomized controlled trials that have examined the effectiveness of PFM exercises in the management of SUI in various populations (28–31).

Participation in a PFM exercise program also results in successful long-term outcomes. With a follow-up of at least 1 year after initiation of PFM

TABLE 13.1

Tips for Identifying an Ideal PFM Contraction

Observation of "puckering" of the anus

Observation of "nodding" of the clitoris

Patient visualization of contraction through use of a handheld mirror

Palpation of superior movement and muscle tension medial to the ischial tuberosity

Palpation of a squeeze around a finger inserted into the vagina

Palpation of a "lift" or anterior movement of the posterior vaginal wall

Negligible visible activity of the gluteals, adductors, and rectus abdominis

Slight inward motion of the abdominal wall (cocontraction of the transversus abdominis)

No visible motion of the spine/pelvis

Maintenance of normal breathing pattern

PFM, pelvic floor muscle.

exercises, 50% of patients previously referred for incontinence surgery avoided the need for surgical intervention (32). A majority of the women (2/3) who chose a PFM exercise program over surgical intervention remained satisfied with their outcome and were not interested in pursuing surgery 5 years later (33).

There has been significant debate, however, as to the most effective way to train the PFM to prevent leakage. Various studies have confirmed that specific exercise instruction is critical to ensure proper performance of a PFM contraction. Performance of a PFM contraction provides little visual or proprioceptive feedback to the person attempting the contraction as there is limited joint motion. Therefore, subjects often report they are unsure if they are performing the PFM contraction correctly. Bump et al showed that more than 50% of stress incontinent women who received verbal instruction alone were performing the PFM contraction incorrectly (34). About half of these women were performing a Valsalva maneuver using contraction of the rectus abdominis muscle, actually promoting versus preventing the loss of urine. These findings were confirmed in a recent study in which perineal ultrasound was used to evaluate the bladder neck during a PFM contraction. During attempts to perform an elevating PFM contraction, 17% of continent and 30% of incontinent women performed an activity that resulted in bladder neck depression (35). This inherent confusion regarding proper performance of a PFM contraction suggests that intervention from a knowledgeable health care professional is needed to ensure proper performance.

A thorough review of the literature reveals numerous different PFM exercise protocols for the management of SUI. However, based on exercise training of skeletal muscles elsewhere in the body, many physical therapists recommend training sessions three or four times per week for at least 15 to 20 weeks, with three repetitions of eight to ten sustained PFM contractions lasting 6 to 8 seconds each time (10). Incorporation of exercises that indirectly recruit the PFM along with the abdominals and the other key muscles of the spinal stabilization system may also be beneficial (36). For many years, women were instructed to palpate their abdomen during performance of PFM exercises and advised to avoid any contraction of the abdominal musculature. Recent studies have demonstrated that contraction of the deepest layer of the abdominals, the transversus abdominis, should occur with a PFM contraction (37) and actually enhances the PFM contraction when patients are instructed to contract both muscles simultaneously.

Another common method of PFM training that has been popularized in the media is instruction to start and stop the stream of urine during normal voiding. This is no longer recommended because of the potential interruption to normal voiding control mechanisms, leading to incomplete bladder emptying and increased risk of bladder infection. This activity should be used only as a method for patients to test their PFM strength and should be limited (once a week maximum).

Numerous devices are available to aid in the instruction and performance of PFM exercises. Clinicians often find other modalities necessary for education, motivation, and compliance. There is limited evidence available to support the addition of biofeedback, intravaginal resistance devices, or electrical or magnetic stimulation of the pelvic floor over PFM training alone (38). These specific modalities will be discussed later in the chapter.

Noncompliance with a PFM exercise program is quite common. The most common reason cited is forgetting to do the exercises (39). Therefore, some sort of reinforcement is important to improve exercise compliance in women with SUI referred for PFM training. In one study, all women received (a) education regarding causes and treatment of SUI, (b) a PFM diagram, (c) detailed verbal instruction about identification and contraction of the PFM, (d) confirmation using biofeedback, (e) a PFM exercise sheet informing patients to exercise 10 minutes twice a day, and (f) verbal encouragement to perform the exercises for 10 minutes twice a day (26). In addition, the experimental group received an audiotape that reinforced the PFM exercise instruction and provided 10 minutes of PFM exercise coaching. At the 4- to 6-week follow-up, only 65% of the control group reported exercise compliance as compared with 100% of the experimental group. Only 12% of the control group performed the exercises twice per day as instructed compared to 71% of the experimental group. The experimental group performed the exercises three times longer than the control group, on average 15.8 minutes per day as compared to 5.4 minutes. A majority of the experimental group (51%) cited the tape as a reminder to do the exercises.

In another study, subjects had weekly visits with a nurse practitioner to answer questions and encourage PFM exercise training. The overall adherence rate in that study to the prescribed home program was 95.4%. Compliance with a PFM exercise program is challenging yet possible. The practicality of compliance measures in clinical practice needs consideration (40).

Who is the ideal candidate for PFM exercises? Studies have shown that PFM exercises are effective in women with complaints of SUI following vaginal delivery (41). A large prospective cohort study attempted to identify the optimal candidate to benefit from PFM exercises to manage SUI symptoms (42). The results of the study suggested that women with more severe SUI (over two pads per day) and longer duration of symptoms (more than 5 years) were more likely to fail conservative management and require surgery. The results of this study raise the question: Would these patients have been able to prevent surgery if PFM exercises had been initiated earlier (before 5 years)? To date, no other consistent variables have been established to identify patients most likely to benefit from PFM exercises.

PFM exercise may also be a strategy to prevent SUI. A Cochrane review performed in 2002 (27) identified 13 randomized trials of PFM training by women specifically to prevent incontinence. However, many of the studies included women with some urinary incontinence symptoms and therefore cannot be considered purely preventative studies. Three of seven trials in childbearing women report less urinary incontinence after pelvic muscle training compared with control subjects 3 months postpartum, whereas four trials found no difference. In one trial, benefits seen at 3 months were no longer present at 12 months.

Therefore, at this time there is not enough evidence to determine whether PFM training can prevent SUI.

BIOFEEDBACK

Biofeedback as applied to the stress urinary population has been defined as "a training technique that aims to reverse urinary incontinence by teaching patients to alter the physiologic responses that mediate urine loss" (43). Biofeedback can be achieved through a variety of methods, ranging from a simple offering of verbal cues during palpation of a PFM contraction to more complex techniques involving equipment such as electromyography (EMG), which monitors electrical activity of muscle during contraction and relaxation (Fig. 13.1), or manometry, which measures pressure generation by a muscle contraction (Fig. 13.2). Biofeedback is not an intervention that is intended to be used in isolation, but is best used in conjunction with other behavioral techniques.

Arnold Kegel was the pioneer in the use of biofeedback as an intervention for the management of SUI (44). In 1956 he reported a 90.56% success rate among 455 women who completed a program of PFM exercise utilizing a vaginal perineometer. He described a number of benefits of the use of the perineometer when performing PFM exercise, which include:

- The ability to correctly identify the pubococcygeus muscle
- The ability to validate that the patient is performing the PFM contraction correctly. This can be reinforced during every exercise session. Kegel believed that a correct contraction with good quality was much more important than a strong contraction.

There are differing opinions and scientific findings reported in the literature as to the benefits of EMG and/or perineometer biofeedback to enhance PFM training. There are a number of reports that describe the benefits of biofeedback training during the initial phase of PFM training (45–47), but there is controversy as to the long-term benefit of a PFM exercise program that is complemented with biofeedback. The Clinical Practice Guidelines published by the Agency for Health Care Policy and Research (2) assigned a strength of evidence rating A to the evidence supporting biofeedback as an intervention for SUI. The intervention was supported by evidence of properly controlled trials.

The reduction in stress incontinence episodes with biofeedback-assisted pelvic floor exercise programs reported in selected studies ranges from 55% to 80% of study participants (47–53). Six of these studies compared groups performing PFM exercises with and without the assistance of biofeedback. In most of the studies, there was no significant difference in the amount of urine leakage between groups. Only one study (50) reported significantly less urine leakage in the group that utilized the biofeedback. A systematic review by Berghmans et al (47) supported the results of the majority of the studies. The authors concluded that PFM exercise with biofeedback is no more effective than PFM exercise alone. Conversely, a meta-analysis of the studies in the systematic review reported a trend in favor of biofeedback-assisted exercise programs.

There may be other benefits to biofeedback-assisted PFM exercise that may influence urine leakage. Aksac et al (53) reported that the biofeedback-assisted group demonstrated a significantly greater improvement in PFM strength as measured with perineometry (a type of manometry), although there was no significant difference in leakage reduction between the biofeedback and nonbiofeedback training groups. Burns et al (49) reported that the biofeedback group had a significantly greater increase in EMG scores with quick contractions than the nonbiofeedback group. These scores were found to negatively correlate with urine loss.

Therefore, biofeedback may be a valuable tool to use as an adjunct to PFM exercise in certain patients, but there is not significant evidence that it is superior to PFM exercise alone. The success of the intervention may also be "highly dependent on the knowledge and skill of the health care provider" who is directing the treatment (2). This may be the rationale behind the 2001 Medicare ruling regarding reimbursement for biofeedback as an intervention for patients with SUI: biofeedback for the treatment of SUI is a covered treatment in cognitively intact patients only if the patient has failed a 4-week trial of pelvic floor exercises. Many clinicians find the addition of biofeedback to be especially helpful when patients are struggling to perform a pelvic floor contraction or if they are particularly weak or kinesthetically challenged. Improved PFM recruitment has been reported following as few as six sessions of biofeedback training (47). Early success with exercise performance may also serve to motivate the patient to comply with the home exercise program.

EMG or manometric training is usually carried out through the use of vaginal or rectal sensors. The use of vaginal and rectal sensors is contraindicated in the presence of an active infection, preg-

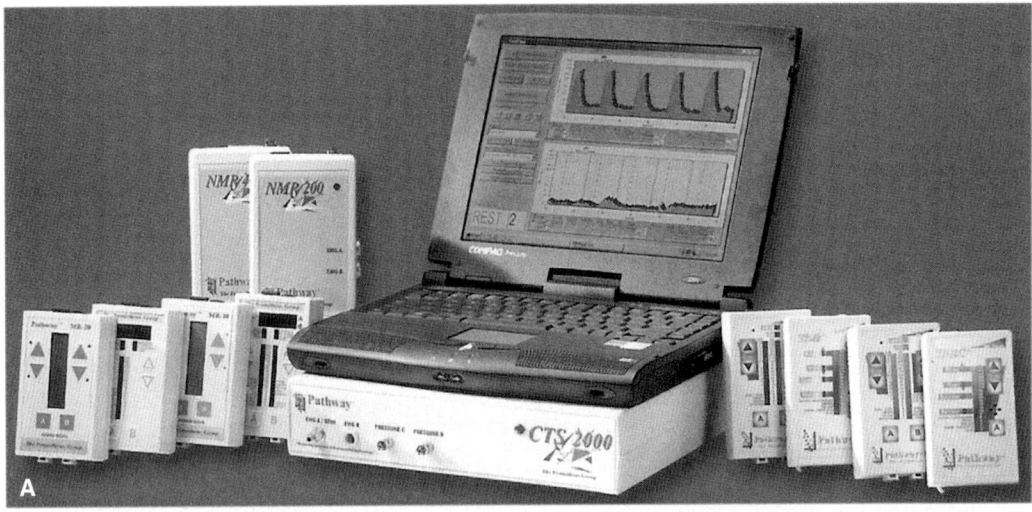

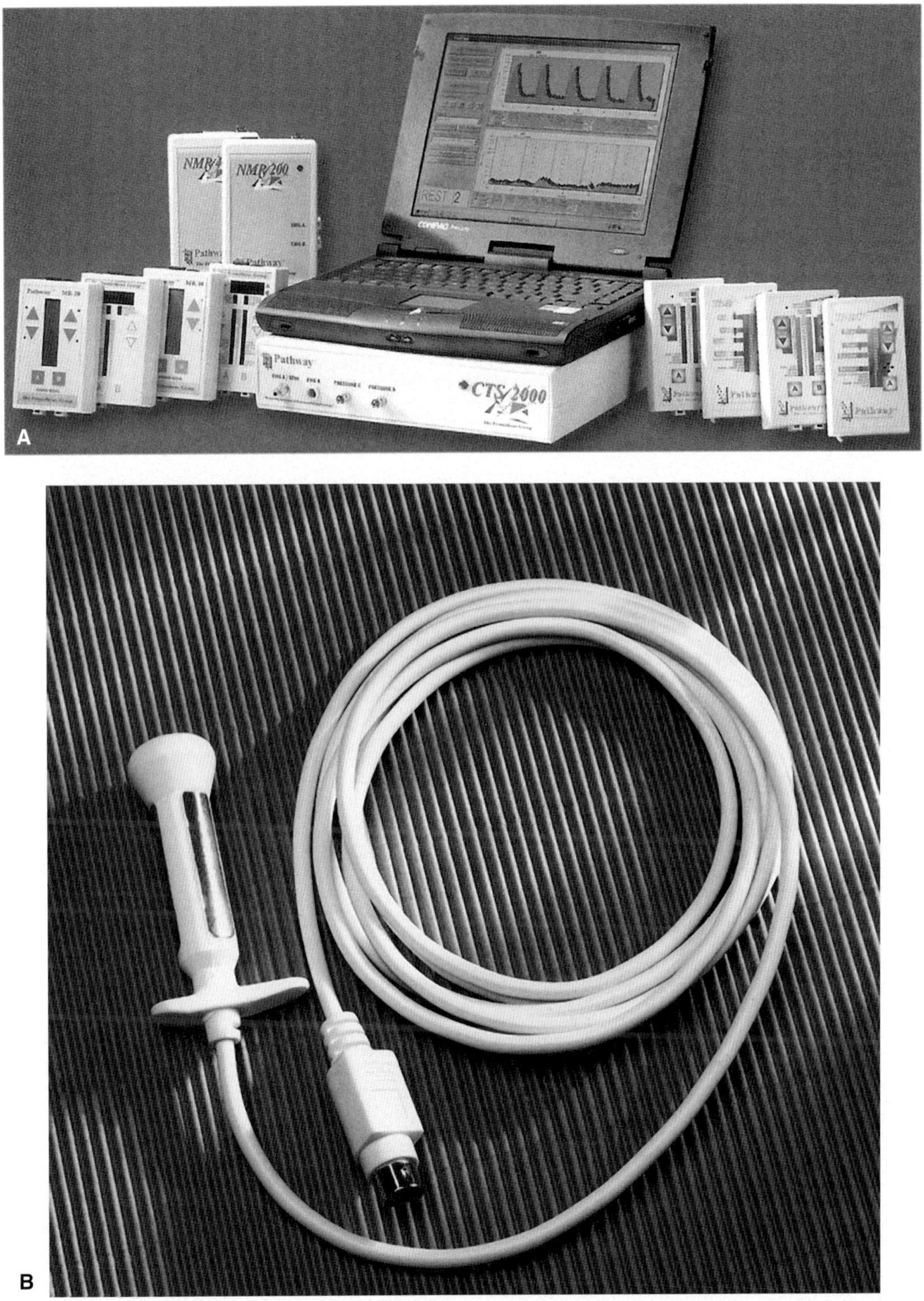

FIGURE 13.1 ● **EMG biofeedback.** A typical EMG biofeedback set-up **(A)** contains the EMG transducer and visual output on a computer screen. PFM activity is generally recorded from a surface electrode, an intravaginal **(B)** or intrarectal sensor. *(continued)*

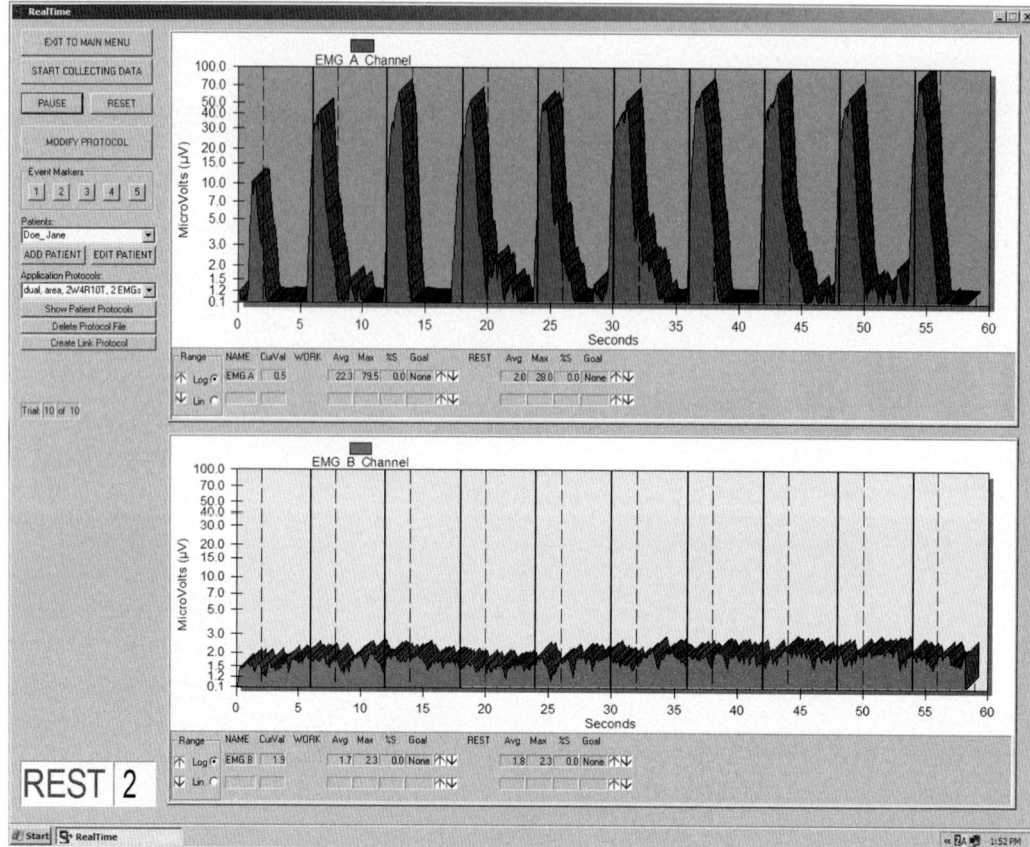

C

FIGURE 13.1 ● *(continued)* The visual display **(C)** allows the patient to see the amount of muscle activity at rest and with muscle activation. In addition, the clinician can assess the quality of the contraction and provide appropriate feedback to the patient during the training session. (Reprinted with permission from the Prometheus Group.)

nancy or less than 6 weeks postpartum, untreated atrophic vaginitis, complaints of pain with insertion of the sensor, recent pelvic or rectal surgical procedure, or if the woman is having her menstrual period (54). Surface electrodes may be an option to replace the internal sensor when contraindications for internal sensor use exist or given personal preference. Optimal monitoring of the PFMs is done with the surface electrodes placed lateral to the anus and medial to the ischial tuberosities.

ELECTRICAL STIMULATION

Electrical stimulation has been proposed as an effective means of activating the PFM in women with SUI (Fig. 13.3). Pelvic floor electrical stimulation can be administered with a single-user vaginal probe or with external surface electrodes, often placed suprapubically and over the sacrum. A high-frequency setting is used (usually between 50 and 100 Hz) to elicit a contraction of the smooth and striated muscles of the pelvic floor (55). Therefore, electrical stimulation may be utilized to provide assistance with active training of the PFM, with the goal of improving the urethral closure mechanism. The use of electrical stimulation may be of greatest value in patients with extreme weakness or those with difficulty eliciting a voluntary contraction of the PFM (29). Although use of electrical stimulation can be limited to clinical use, patients are generally issued a home unit so that training with the stimulator can be completed daily, one or two 20-minute sessions per day.

A number of studies have demonstrated the effectiveness of isolated electrical stimulation in increasing urethral closing pressure and PFM strength and decreasing urine leakage in patients with SUI (56,57). However, the question remains:

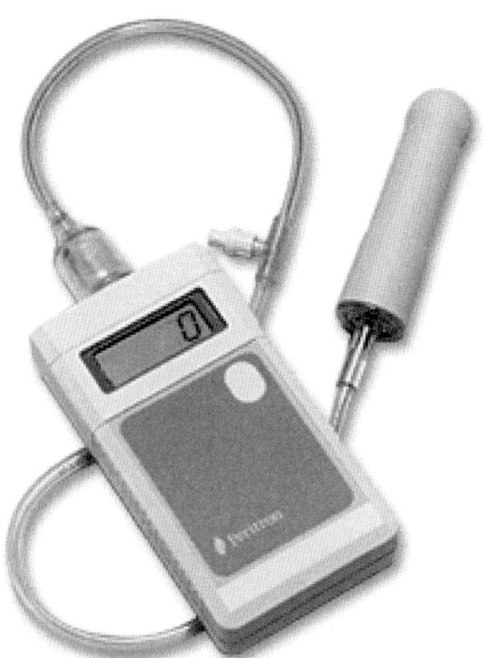

FIGURE 13.2 ● **Perineometer.** The perineometer is used for pressure biofeedback training. The patient inserts the probe into the vagina and performs a PFM contraction. The amount of pressure generated by the contraction is displayed. (Reprinted with permission from Peritron.)

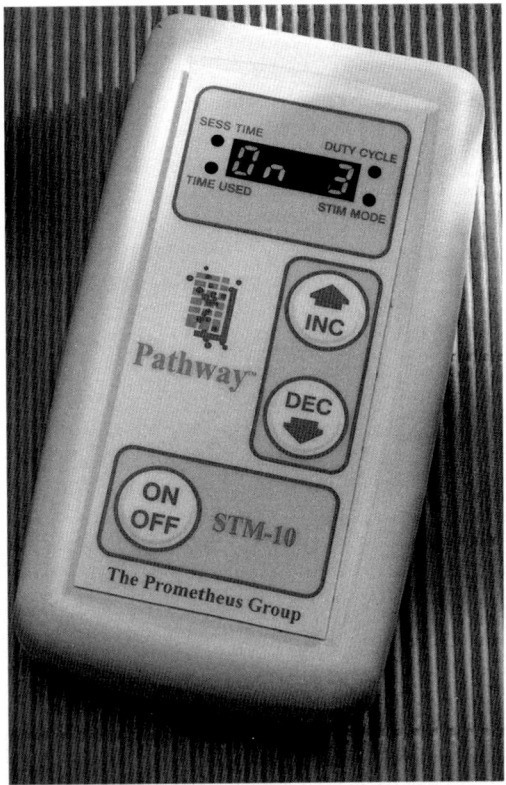

FIGURE 13.3 ● **Electrical stimulation.** Electrical stimulation devices can be utilized for pelvic floor muscle training with surface, intravaginal, or intrarectal electrodes. (Reprinted with permission from the Prometheus Group.)

which is most effective in reducing SUI symptoms: training with electrical stimulation alone, PFM training alone, or the combination of PFM training with electrical stimulation? Several studies have demonstrated that in humans, voluntary muscle contraction is more effective than electrically stimulated muscle contraction for strengthening (58,59). Specifically, voluntary contraction of PFM has been shown to be twice as effective as an electrically stimulated contraction at increasing urethral pressure (60).

In one clinical study, however, PFM exercise augmented with electrical stimulation resulted in the greatest improvement in strength and outcomes as measured with a bladder diary. Greater improvements in symptoms and muscle strength have been noted when comparing the electrical stimulation–augmented exercise group with PFM exercise alone (61). However, a systematic review of the literature performed by Bo in 1998 (62) reviewed nine randomized controlled trials evaluating the effect of electrical stimulation on SUI. Only three studies had a sufficient sample size to enable conclusion on SUI. Of those, only one demonstrated a positive effect of 20% cure and 46% improved as measured by the pad test. Other

prospective randomized controlled trials (29,63) have found that treatment with pelvic floor electrical stimulation did not increase effectiveness of a comprehensive behavioral program for women with stress incontinence.

The clinical usefulness of electrical stimulation may also be limited by the frequent complaint of discomfort during the intervention. Many of the studies cited above report high dropout rates due to discomfort during the stimulation. Use of electrical stimulation is contraindicated in pregnant women, in the presence of an active infection (urinary tract infection/vaginal infection), dementia, complete denervation of the PFM, and/or within 6 weeks of pelvic surgery (64). In addition, current Medicare reimbursement guidelines require a documented failure of a program of PFM exercises for at least 4 weeks prior to reimbursement for the use of electrical stimulation. Electrical stimulation is likely most beneficial in the early stages of rehabilitation when women are weakest and most likely to be struggling to perform a proper PFM contraction.

The results of randomized controlled trials on the effect of electrical stimulation to treat stress incontinence are conflicting. Because of the potential for success, there is a need for more randomized controlled trials with sufficient sample sizes; use of sensitive, reproducible, and valid outcome measures; and optimal stimulation parameters. Based on the information available at this time, PFM should be the first choice of treatment for SUI and electrical stimulation reserved for isolated cases when the patient is unable to perform a correct PFM contraction with visual and/or tactile cues.

VAGINAL CONES

Vaginal cones were introduced as an alternative method for pelvic floor strengthening in 1985 (65) (Fig. 13.4). The original set consisted of nine different cones with increasing weights from 20 to 100 g (66). The cones were presented as an alternative means of biofeedback (sensory) for self-treatment of urinary incontinence (65). The rationale for cone-assisted strengthening is that insertion of a weighted cone into the vagina will result in a reflexive or voluntary PFM contraction to prevent the cone from slipping out (66). Hesse confirmed that insertion of a cone does result in an increase in PFM activity (67). In this study, the pubococcygei muscles were monitored using wire EMG during insertion of a vaginal cone with the subject in a static standing position. A slight increase in muscle activity was detected with insertion of the cone followed by a pattern of variable muscle activity, a waxing and waning pattern, while the subject remained standing (67).

The following is a suggested protocol for training with the cones that has been followed by most clinicians and investigators, with minor modifications (65):

- The patient begins training with the heaviest cone she can retain for 1 minute.
- The patient increases the time she is able to retain the cone up to a maximum of 15 minutes. This process is repeated twice per day.

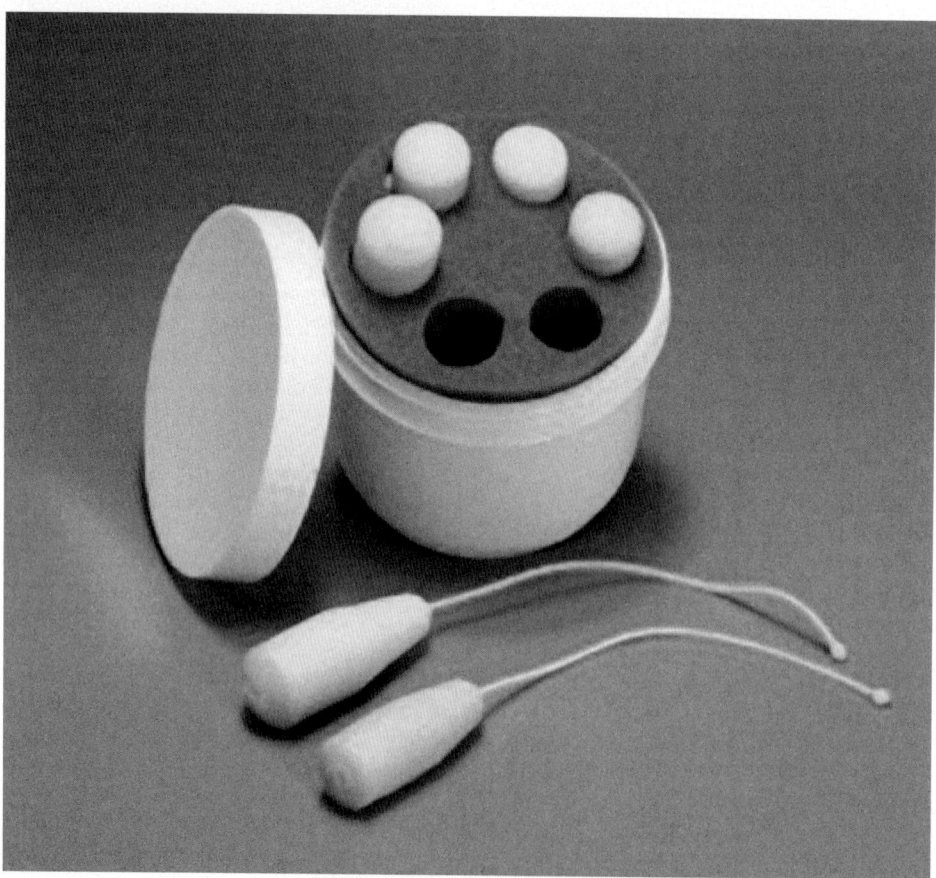

FIGURE 13.4 ● **Vaginal cones.** Weighted vaginal cones used for PFM strengthening.

- Once she has achieved the 15-minute holding time, she is instructed to progress to the next cone weight.

Interestingly, this strengthening program does not follow any other traditional strengthening regimen or follow the basic principles of progressive resistance exercise. In fact, Bo highlights that static muscle contractions are associated with reduced oxygen consumption, muscle pain, and fatigue (66). Despite the apparent contradictions, there are a number of reports of significant reduction of incontinent episodes, ranging between 60% and 90% cure rates, following PFM training using vaginal cones (65,68,69). A systematic review of the literature concluded that cone therapy for the treatment of SUI is of benefit when compared to no treatment and is of equal benefit to PFM exercise and electrical stimulation. The review also found no additional benefit to combining cone therapy with PFM exercise or electrical stimulation (70).

There are several factors that limit the more widespread use of this alternative treatment, despite the apparent benefits from this simple training method. The cones come in standard sizes and are not custom-fit as are other intravaginal devices, such as a pessary or diaphragm. In one study, 17% of the subjects were unable to utilize the cones in a therapeutic way because the cones were either too large or too small in relation to their vagina (68). Also, if improperly placed, very little if any PFM activity may be required to hold the cone in place. In some cases, patients are too weak to even hold the lightest cone, making cone training impossible (65). One must also consider the integrity of the vaginal mucosa before recommending cone therapy. Some clinicians have suggested that elderly women should avoid cone therapy due to the risk of atrophic vaginitis (54). For these and potentially other reasons, there is a dropout rate from studies utilizing vaginal cones ranging from 3% to 27% reported in the literature (65,68,71–73).

Successful intervention with PFM exercise utilizing cone therapy begins with selecting an appropriate candidate. Patients with mild stress incontinence are more likely to respond positively than those with severe incontinence (71). The patient needs the physical ability and willingness to insert the cone vaginally and the motivation to comply with the required cone protocol. Patients may receive the greatest benefit from cone use during the first month of treatment to improve PFM awareness (65). Once the patient is able to perform a PFM contraction independently, she may then transition to a traditional PFM exercise program until a sufficient reduction in urine leakage is achieved.

REAL-TIME ULTRASOUND

The use of real-time ultrasound may also be a valuable form of biofeedback for PFM exercise training. Ultrasound imaging allows for a dynamic study of muscle function as the muscles contract. Ultrasound imaging has been used as an effective form of biofeedback in rehabilitation programs for other areas (74). Of particular value for the patient with urinary incontinence or pelvic organ prolapse is the ability to visualize the "lift" component of the contraction and also the function of the PFMs in resisting rises in intra-abdominal pressure. Because the PFMs are deep and difficult to access and patients receive little proprioceptive feedback from the contraction of the PFM, patients often complain of lack of awareness of muscle contraction. The use of real-time ultrasound allows the patient to visualize the contraction and to observe the functional consequences of the PFM contraction (75). In a study by Dietz et al, of 56 women who were unable to contract the pelvic floor on request, 32 (57%) eventually succeeded with visual ultrasound biofeedback. This may be extremely valuable in assisting and motivating patients to participate in their home exercise program.

Ultrasound imaging has been used experimentally to provide an objective assessment of urethrovesical angle, urethral mobility during a Valsalva maneuver, movement of the anorectal angle, and levator sling angle during contraction of the levator ani (76). At most the specific assessment of muscle function requires 5 additional minutes to the standard ultrasound examination of urogynecologic patients (75). The examination of PFM function can be performed through perineal or abdominal placement of the ultrasound transducer (77).

Assessment using the perineal transducer results in a sagittal view of the lower urinary tract through placement of the transducer just medial to the ischial tuberosities (Fig. 13.5A). Assessment through the abdominal transducer can be achieved with either a perisagittal or transverse abdominal view of the posteroinferior aspect of the bladder wall. With the perisagittal application, the transducer is placed on the abdomen, just superior to the pubic symphysis slightly lateral to midline, and oriented in a superolateral to inferomedial sagittal plane (see Fig. 13.5B). In the transabdominal application the probe is placed transversely in the midline, superior to the pubic symphysis and an-

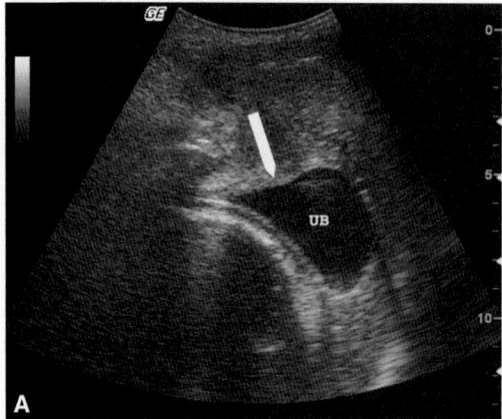

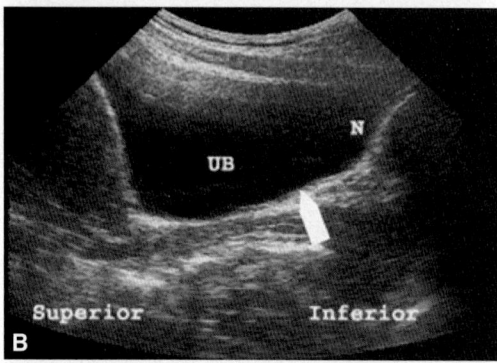

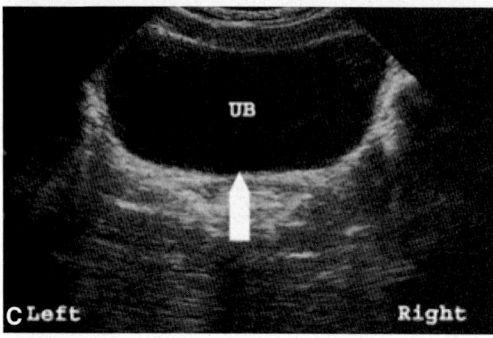

FIGURE 13.5 ● **Real-time ultrasound imaging of pelvic floor muscle contraction.** UB, urinary bladder; N, bladder neck. **(A)** Sagittal view taken with perineal placement of the ultrasound transducer allowing visualization of the urinary bladder, bladder neck, and PFM support. **(B)** Perisagittal view taken with abdominal placement of the ultrasound transducer. *Arrow* represents direction of a PFM contraction that results in encroachment of the posterior/inferior surface of the bladder. (Reprinted with permission from Jackie Whitaker, BScPT, FCAMT, CGIMS, CAFCI.) **(C)** Transverse abdominal placement of the ultrasound transducer. *Arrow* represents direction of a PFM contraction that results in encroachment of the posterior/inferior surface of the bladder.
(Reprinted with permission from Jackie Whitaker, BScPT, FCAMT, CGIMS, CAFCI.)

gled approximately 60 degrees from vertical, aiming towards the posteroinferior aspect of the bladder wall (see Fig. 13.5C). The abdominal placement may be preferred due to the limited difference in image quality while avoiding placement of the transducer in a sensitive area.

An ideal PFM contraction results in an increase in tension in the endopelvic fascia and broadening of the muscle. This results in a slow, isolated indentation of the posteroinferior aspect of the bladder wall accompanied by concurrent cranioventral motion of the bladder (78,79). Christensen et al noted that the bladder wall displacement and cranioventral motion of the bladder is best viewed in the sagittal plane, with the perineal or perisagittal techniques (79). It is this cranioventral motion that is critical for providing pelvic organ support and for maintaining the bladder neck in its optimal position during increases in intra-abdominal pressure such as a cough (80). The transabdominal view allows the examiner to evaluate the left and right sides of the PFMs simultaneously to ensure symmetry between sides. The response is often asymmetrical in patients with dysfunction (81).

Motion of the bladder in a caudodorsal direction and/or lack of an indentation in the posterior wall are considered abnormal. Lack of clear indentation is suggestive of a faulty fascial tensioning mechanism due to changes in the endopelvic fascia (secondary to childbirth, repeated exposure to intra-abdominal pressure, or surgical procedures), recruitment deficits of the PFMs, or impaired innervation to the musculature (77). Motion in the caudodorsal direction is associated with bearing-down or a Valsalva maneuver (78,82).

Although limited evidence exists to substantiate its value versus PFM exercise instruction alone, the use of real-time ultrasound as a visual biofeedback tool during exercise instruction does appear to have potential value. Patients who lack motivation or are struggling to perform a correct PFM contraction are ideal candidates for this type of procedure.

PESSARY

Prescription of a pessary is another way to provide SUI patients the necessary structural support to assist in the maintenance of continence (Fig. 13.6). Pessaries are primarily prescribed for patients with symptomatic pelvic relaxation and organ prolapse (11). However, many patients with pelvic relaxation and/or pelvic organ prolapse also complain of symptoms of SUI. There are no long-term randomized trials comparing the use of pessary devices and other treatments, but devices appear to be an acceptable treatment for some women (10).

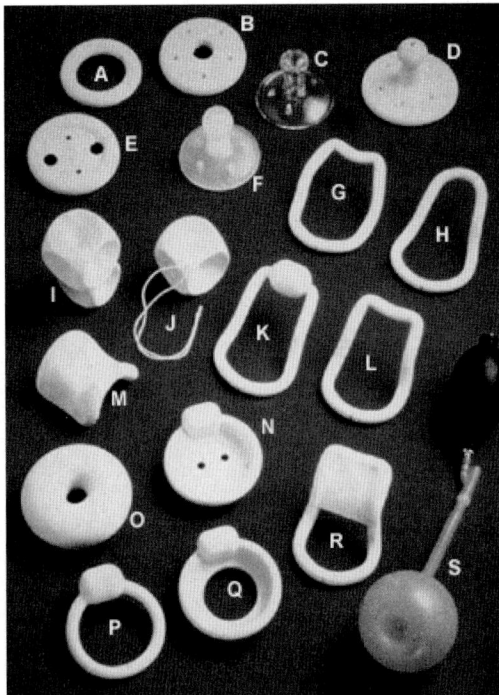

FIGURE 13.6 ● **Pessary.** A variety of different pessary devices are available to provide support to the pelvic organs to minimize pressure on the urethra and prevent urine leakage.

Although the pessary may be an effective tool in managing symptoms, up to 26% of patients cannot be fitted with a pessary and approximately 50% of patients discontinue use after successful fitting (83,84). Predictors of unsuccessful pessary fitting include history of prior vaginal surgery, short vaginal length (less than 6 cm), younger age, and wide vaginal introitus (four fingerbreadths accommodated) (84–86). There may be many reasons why patients choose to discontinue use of the pessary. Severe posterior prolapse is the single predictor reliably identified for pessary discontinuation (86,87). In a study by Robert and Mainprize (88), 38 patients were prescribed a pessary. Of those, at 1-year follow-up only six were still using their pessary. The women who continued use of the pessary were not significantly different from women who discontinued use of the pessary. There was a trend showing that women who continued use were younger (41 versus 52 years old), had less pelvic surgery, and leaked less on semiquantitative pad testing (10.7 g versus 19.2 g). The most frequently cited reasons for discontinuing use of the pessary were complaints of no benefit (69%) and the inability to keep the pessary in place (16%) (88). In a study by Donnelly et al, only 55

of 106 participants fitted for a pessary continued to use the pessary for a median of 13 months. Consistent with other reports, most subjects stopped using the device within the first month following prescription. Reasons cited for discontinuation were consistent with other reports, including persistent urinary incontinence (58%), discomfort (33%), and frequent pessary expulsion (18%) (89).

The best candidates for pessary fitting are those patients with good perineal support so the pessary does not expel spontaneously with bearing-down or active movements (11). Patient motivation and manual dexterity also appear to be significant determinants in successful device use (90). A ring with support is a good first choice because of the ease of insertion and removal. After placement, the patient should be unaware of its presence. If the patient experiences any discomfort, the pessary is likely too large (11).

Most manufacturers of pessaries designed to reduce pelvic organ prolapse also offer modifications specifically for SUI management (12). These devices have additional anterior-to-posterior width near the vaginal introitus. In a study by Nguyen and Jones (91), 82/130 (63%) subjects were successfully fitted with a pessary. Of those, 57 were treated primarily for pelvic relaxation and 25 were treated for both relaxation and SUI. A number of different devices were used: the ring (26%), the ring with incontinence modifications (20%), the ring with support (18%), the gelhorn (14%), continence dish (6%), Gehrung with knot (6%), cube (5%), donut (4%), and regular (1%). The highest success rates for fitting have been reported with prescription of ring pessaries, ring pessaries with support, and gelhorns (85).

Hormone replacement therapy may also influence the success of pessary fitting. In a recent retrospective chart review of 1,216 patients fitted with a pessary, 85% of postmenopausal women were on hormone replacement therapy (HRT) prior to fitting. The highest success rate (78%) occurred in the group of women on both systemic and local HRT (85).

Complications from pessary use are rarely the result of the type of pessary or pessary fit but are more often associated with the inability to perform pessary self-care. In a large study of 76 patients referred for pessary fitting, the following complications were reported: urinary tract infections (13%), bacterial vaginosis (3%), and ulcerations of the vaginal mucosa (24%). The standard protocol for follow-up with the pessary-fitting health care provider is at 7 days and 1 month after successful fitting. Patients able to perform self-care are followed less frequently (every 2 to 6 months) compared to those who are unable or unwilling to perform self-care, who are seen every 4 to 8 weeks (91). The type of pessary may also influence the frequency of follow-up, as there was one published report of an increase in vaginal ulceration rate with the cube type of pessary (84).

Other devices have been introduced for the management of SUI. In 1990, a new conservative treatment for genuine SUI, the urethral plug, was introduced (92). Since then several other mini-devices have been introduced for the conservative management of SUI; however, most of these devices, if not all, have been discontinued. There are two mini-devices available, both intraurethral plugs that occlude the intraluminal space of the urethra. The difference between them is the inclusion of sphincter muscle training. The Danish urethral plug, the VIVA regulator, has had the widest and most reliable evaluation by investigators of the intraurethral plugs. The original reports were promising, with 73% improved continence after 1 week of treatment. The objective success rate at 6 months was 81%. The Reliance urethral plug was similar to the VIVA, but with no spheres on its shaft. Once the device was inserted into the urethra, a small balloon at the tip of the shaft was inflated and stabilized the device in the bladder neck region, thus passively occluding the bladder neck and the urethra. Initial studies were positive (69,93,94), reporting continence rates in 79% to 80% of the patients. However, all groups reported patient difficulty in handling the device. This is believed to be the main reason for the high discontinuation rate, 37% and 31% in the studies noted. This could also be one of the reasons why the urethral plug was withdrawn from the market, as it was no longer profitable. The complication rate was considered "low" despite 25% to 30% of patients developing urinary tract infections.

BEHAVIORAL AND LIFESTYLE INTERVENTIONS

Bladder health education and modification of potentially faulty voiding habits may assist patients in achieving optimal bladder control. This may be achieved by modification of the patient's behavior and/or environment. Typically there are several components to a behavioral management program for the SUI patient, including PFM exercise (with or without the assistance of biofeedback, electrical stimulation, or cone therapy), education, and bladder training. The benefits of PFM training have been discussed previously in this chapter. Although there is evidence to show that bladder training alone can be an effective treatment tool

for SUI, the best results are demonstrated when this technique is combined with PFM exercise and specific lifestyle and bladder education (38).

A bladder training program includes education about the bladder and normal continence mechanisms, positive reinforcement from the health care professional, and development of a timed voiding schedule (2). Active participation from the patient is required to complete a bladder diary before the appropriate recommendation can be made. The diary is a validated record of the total and time of all fluid intake, urine voided, and incontinence episodes that occur over a period of time (95,96) (Fig. 13.7). Though the validation of the instrument suggests that the individual maintain a record for a minimum of 7 days, compliance may be higher and adequate assessment can be made with as little as 1 or 2 days of recording. The bladder diary assists the clinician in establishing a voiding schedule, which the patient is encouraged to follow during waking hours. The goal of the process is to normalize the voiding interval up to a 3- to 4-hour interval, thus improving the bladder capacity and preventing overfilling of the bladder (97). Although bladder training has traditionally been a primary intervention for individuals suffering from urge incontinence, there is evidence to support equal benefit in the stress incontinence population. A reduction in fluid loss and total number of incontinent episodes by greater than 50% has been reported after as little as 6 weeks of a bladder training program in patients with SUI (98).

In addition to a voiding schedule, the clinician may recommend changes in total fluid intake, timing of fluid intake, and the type of fluids consumed. General practice has been to recommend daily fluid intake of between 48 and 64 oz, or a half-ounce of fluid per pound of body weight, including mostly water and/or nonirritating fluids (99,100). Fluid intake should be evenly distributed throughout the day unless the patient suffers from nocturia, in which case patients are instructed to reduce fluids 2 hours before bedtime. However, a recent study of 39 women with SUI reported a significant decrease in wetting episodes when fluid intake was limited to 750 mL (40 oz) of fluid/day (101). Changing from caffeinated to decaffeinated drinks produced no improvement in symptoms (101). Given that 40 oz of fluid is not much less than the recommended minimum of 48 oz of fluid and considerably higher than the average daily fluid intake of many individuals, patients may benefit from counseling to maintain adequate fluid intake but avoid bladder overfilling. Minimizing the intake of caffeine and other potential bladder irritants is likely more important in those suffering

VOIDING DIARY

TIME	FLUID INTAKE (Type/Amount)	FOOD EATEN (Type/ Amount)	URINATED IN TOILET (Ounces)	LEAKAGE (Small, Medium, or Large)	REASON FOR LEAKAGE (Activity)	DID YOU HAVE THE URGE TO GO?

FIGURE 13.7 ● **Voiding diary.** The voiding diary is issued to patients for assessment of voiding and dietary habits that may affect continence. The clinician can make recommendations regarding fluid intake, voiding habits, and activity modification based on the information collected.

from urgency/frequency symptoms and/or urge-associated urine leakage.

The voiding diary provides an opportunity to identify which activities involving an increased intra-abdominal pressure result in incontinent episodes. Once identified, the patient can be counseled to utilize a quick PFM contraction immediately prior to performance of the identified activities. Precontraction of the PFM, also called "the Knack" or stress strategy, limits urine leakage by stabilizing the bladder neck and improving proximal urethral support (4). After instruction in a proper pelvic floor contraction and education to contract just prior to and during a cough, women were able to reduce the amount of urine loss by 98.2% as compared to a cough without pelvic floor precontraction (80). The patients are educated to avoid the Valsalva maneuver during normal activities and to avoid pushing and/or straining with voiding and bowel movements, in the negative effect of excessive abdominal weight on the bladder, and proper weight loss strategies as appropriate. If these behaviors are modified, stress on the bladder, urethra, and PFM will be reduced, thereby limiting urine loss. Women who experience exercise-induced leakage should be instructed to avoid caffeinated beverages 2 to 3 hours prior to exercise to reduce bladder filling and prevent diuresis (102). These women must understand that it is important not to eliminate all fluids prior to exercise because of the possible complication of dehydration.

PHARMACOLOGIC MANAGEMENT

Pharmacologic therapy has not had a significant role in the management of SUI. Pharmacologic management options for SUI have historically been limited to off-label prescription of certain products, particularly estrogens and alpha-adrenergic agonists, and have provided limited improvement in symptoms. On the horizon is a recently released drug called duloxetine. Although initially approved by the Food and Drug Administration (FDA) for the management of major depressive disorder and diabetic peripheral neuropathic pain, initial clinical trials with duloxetine use for the management of SUI are very promising. Pharmacologic therapy will likely gain more attention if duloxetine proves to be successful. Duloxetine inhibits presynaptic serotonin and norepinephrine reuptake in the sacral spinal cord. Administration of duloxetine results in increased urethral closure forces via the stimulation of pudendal motor neuron alpha-1 adrenergic and 5-hydroxytryptamine-2 receptors and thereby reduces episodes of SUI.

Two large multicenter, double-blind, placebo-controlled randomized trials have been performed to assess the efficacy and safety of duloxetine in women with SUI (103,104). In the more recent study, 51% of subjects given duloxetine had a 50% to 100% decrease in frequency of incontinence episodes compared with 34% of those on placebo. These improvements with duloxetine were associated with a significant increase in the voiding interval compared with placebo and they were observed across the spectrum of incontinence severity. Patients reported no serious adverse effects. Nausea was the most common adverse event, reported as mild to moderate in severity and transient in most patients. In both studies, the placebo group demonstrated substantial improvements in frequency of incontinent episodes (34% and 40%). Other studies have also reported high improvement rates in women assigned to placebo

groups. This may be related to the greater awareness of the bladder and bladder habits that occurs with a research protocol and suggests that simply completing a voiding diary may be therapeutic.

The combined therapy of duloxetine and PFM exercise may be the most advantageous treatment. A recent randomized controlled trial compared the benefits of duloxetine alone, PFM training alone, combined treatment, or no active treatment in women with SUI (105). Treatment with duloxetine with or without PFM training was superior to PFM training alone or no active treatment in reducing incontinent episodes. Subjects who received the combined treatment reported a median reduction of 75.8% in the number of incontinent episodes, had the greatest reduction in pad use, and had the highest improvement in quality of life as measured by the Incontinence Quality of Life scale (106).

Estrogens produce some effects on the urethral epithelium, leading to increased blood flow around the bladder neck and midurethra (107), and may be useful in patients with atrophic vaginitis. There is limited evidence supporting its use in women with SUI. In fact, in several large randomized trials women assigned to receive estrogen and progesterone were more likely to experience a worsening of baseline symptoms (108). Alpha-adrenoreceptor agonists have been found to be effective in SUI, but the use of these drugs is limited due to major safety concerns related to cardiovascular side effects (109).

SUMMARY/CONCLUSIONS

The key to resolution of SUI symptoms appears to be restoration of the urethral closure mechanism. This can be accomplished through a variety of methods, including PFM strengthening, use of an orthotic device such as a pessary, or pharmacologic intervention. There is strong evidence to support the value of PFM exercise to improve recruitment and strength of the pelvic floor musculature in order to prevent urine leakage. PFM exercise is the least invasive and best tolerated of all mechanisms. Training programs are likely to be most successful when patients are provided specific instruction and intermittent follow-up. Although no ideal set of exercise parameters has been identified, training of the slow and fast twitch fibers is necessary to optimally train the muscles for their functions. In addition, given the relationship between the PFM and other muscles, such as the transversus abdominis, training programs that involve cocontraction and emphasis on core muscle training may provide optimal training and benefit. Biofeedback, electrical stimulation, ultrasound,

TABLE 13.2

Summary of Recommendations for PFM Training

Confirmation of correct contraction by a knowledge able health professional

Training of both slow and fast twitch muscle fibers

Electrical stimulation may help to "jump start" patients with significant weakness.

Biofeedback training may be appropriate for women with impaired kinesthetic awareness.

Training with vaginal cones is often more successful with younger or more active patients.

Incorporation of PFM contractions into daily activities ("the Knack")

Instruction to start and stop the urine stream as a method of exercise is **not** appropriate.

PFM, pelvic floor muscle.

TABLE 13.3

Keys to Preventing Stress Urine Leakage

Instruct in active contraction of PFM.

Minimize increases in intra-abdominal pressure.

Use PFM contraction to prevent urine leakage.

Void every 2 to 3 hours.

Limit intake of fluids to 5 to 8 cups/day.

Restore anatomic support (i.e., use of pessary or active contraction of PFM).

PFM, pelvic floor muscle.

and vaginal cones may be useful adjuncts to PFM training; however, no evidence suggests that any one of these modalities is superior to PFM training alone (Table 13.2).

It is also important to limit the amount of stress transmitted to the lower urinary tract through rises in intra-abdominal pressure. Pessary use may be beneficial in a certain population of individuals lacking pelvic support to achieve this goal. When properly fit, the success rate of pessary use in controlling symptoms is high. However, patients should be advised that proper fitting may require multiple trials. Given the low compliance rate, this should not be the first treatment option. Education in proper body mechanics and contraction of the PFMs prior to rises in intra-abdominal pressure such as a cough or sneeze are likely the optimal way to prevent excessive force transmission.

Clearly there is evidence to support the value of nonsurgical interventions for the management of SUI (Table 13.3). Given the high success rates, it appears that the majority of patients with SUI will benefit from a trial of conservative therapy prior to referral for a surgical consult. In addition, improved PFM function and anatomic support will likely improve outcomes in patients ultimately referred for surgical intervention. Pharmacologic management has traditionally been a minor consideration in the management of stress incontinence. With the introduction of duloxetine and the success of the early clinical trials, however, pharmacologic intervention may prove to be more

valuable in the future. Care provided by knowledgeable health care professionals is the key to success with any of the conservative methods discussed in this chapter.

REFERENCES

1. Abrams P, Cardozo L, Fall M, et al. The standardisation of terminology in lower urinary tract function: report from the standardization subcommittee of the International Continence Society. *Urology* 2003;61(1): 37–49.
2. *Urinary incontinence in adults: Acute and chronic management.* Rockville, MD: US Department of Health and Human Services, 1996.
3. Ashton-Miller JA, Howard D, DeLancey JO. The functional anatomy of the female pelvic floor and stress continence control system. *Scand J Urol Nephrol Suppl* 2001;(207):1–7, 106–125.
4. Miller JM, Perucchini D, Carchidi LT, et al. Pelvic floor muscle contraction during a cough and decreased vesical neck mobility. *Obstet Gynecol* 2001;97(2):255–260.
5. Gunnarsson M, Mattiasson A. Female stress, urge, and mixed urinary incontinence are associated with a chronic and progressive pelvic floor/vaginal neuromuscular disorder: An investigation of 317 healthy and incontinent women using vaginal surface electromyography. *Neurourol Urodyn* 1999;18(6):613–621.
6. Gunnarsson M, Teleman P, Mattiason A, et al. Effects of pelvic floor exercises in middle-aged women with a history of naive urinary incontinence: a population-based study. *Eur Urol* 2002;41(5):556–561.
7. Zhang Q, Wang L, Zheng W. Surface electromyography of pelvic floor muscles in stress urinary incontinence. *Int J Gynaecol Obstet* 2006(Aug 18).
8. Robinson D, Cardozo LD. The role of estrogens in female lower urinary tract dysfunction. *Urology* 2003; 62(4 Suppl 1):45–51.
9. Kim KJ, Ashton-Miller JA, Strohbehn K, et al. The vesico-urethral pressuregram analysis of urethral function under stress. *J Biomech* 1997;30(1):19–25.
10. Nygaard IE, Heit M. Stress urinary incontinence. *Obstet Gynecol* 2004;104(3):607–620.
11. Rush CB, Entman SS. Pelvic organ prolapse and stress urinary incontinence. *Med Clin North Am* 1995;79(6): 1473–1479.

12. Miller K. Stress urinary incontinence in women: review and update on neurological control. *J Womens Health* 2005;14(7):595–608.

13. Chen B, Wen Y, Zhang Z, et al. Microarray analysis of differentially expressed genes in vaginal tissues from women with stress urinary incontinence compared with asymptomatic women. *Hum Reprod* 2006;21(1):22–29.

14. Radziszewski P, Borkowski A, Torz C, et al. Distribution of collagen type VII in connective tissues of postmenopausal stress-incontinent women. *Gynecol Endocrinol* 2005;20(3):121–126.

15. Sampselle CM, Harlow SD, Skumick J, et al. Urinary incontinence predictors and life impact in ethnically diverse perimenopausal women. *Obstet Gynecol* 2002;100(6):1230–1238.

16. McGrother CW, Donaldson MM, Hayward T, et al. Urinary storage symptoms and comorbidities: a prospective population cohort study in middle-aged and older women. *Age Ageing* 2006;35(1):16–24.

17. Freeman RM. Initial management of stress urinary incontinence: pelvic floor muscle training and duloxetine. *Br J Obstet Gynaecol* 2006;113(Suppl 1):10–16.

18. Morkved S, Salvesen KA, Bo K, et al. Pelvic floor muscle strength and thickness in continent and incontinent nulliparous pregnant women. *Int Urogynecol J Pelvic Floor Dysfunct* 2004;15(6):384–390.

19. Bernstein IT. The pelvic floor muscles: muscle thickness in healthy and urinary-incontinent women measured by perineal ultrasonography with reference to the effect of pelvic floor training. Estrogen receptor studies. *Neurourol Urodyn* 1997;16(4):237–275.

20. Baytur YB, Deveci A, Uyar Y, et al. Mode of delivery and pelvic floor muscle strength and sexual function after childbirth. *Int J Gynaecol Obstet* 2005;88(3):276–280.

21. Rockner G, Jonasson A, Olund A. The effect of mediolateral episiotomy at delivery on pelvic floor muscle strength evaluated with vaginal cones. *Acta Obstet Gynecol Scand* 1991;70(1):51–54.

22. Bo K, Finckenhagen HB. Vaginal palpation of pelvic floor muscle strength: intertest reproducibility and comparison between palpation and vaginal squeeze pressure. *Acta Obstet Gynecol Scand* 2001;80(10):883–887.

23. Bo K, Sherburn M. Evaluation of female pelvic-floor muscle function and strength. *Phys Ther* 2005;85(3):269–282.

24. Bo K, Stien R. Needle EMG registration of striated urethral wall and pelvic floor muscle activity patterns during cough, Valsalva, abdominal, hip adductor, and gluteal muscle contractions in nulliparous healthy females. *Neurourol Urodyn* 1994;13(1):35–41.

25. Wells TJ. Pelvic (floor) muscle exercise. *J Am Geriatr Soc* 1990;38(3):333–337.

26. Gallo ML, Staskin DR. Cues to action: pelvic floor muscle exercise compliance in women with stress urinary incontinence. *Neurourol Urodyn* 1997;16(3):167–177.

27. Hay-Smith J, Herbison P, Morkved S. Physical therapies for prevention of urinary and fecal incontinence in adults. *Cochrane Database Syst Rev* 2002(2):CD003191.

28. Turkan A, Inci Y, Fazli D. The short-term effects of physical therapy in different intensities of urodynamic stress incontinence. *Gynecol Obstet Invest* 2005;59(1):43–48.

29. Goode PS, Burgio KL, Locher JL, et al. Effect of behavioral training with or without pelvic floor electrical stimulation on stress incontinence in women: a randomized controlled trial. *JAMA* 2003;290(3):345–352.

30. Theofrastous JP, Wyman JF, Bump RC, et al. Effects of pelvic floor muscle training on strength and predictors of response in the treatment of urinary incontinence. *Neurourol Urodyn* 2002;21(5):486–490.

31. Laycock J, Brown J, Cusack C, et al. Pelvic floor reeducation for stress incontinence: comparing three methods. *Br J Community Nurs* 2001;6(5):230–237.

32. Mouritsen L, Frimodt-Moller C, Moller M. Long-term effect of pelvic floor exercises on female urinary incontinence. *Br J Urol* 1991;68(1):32–37.

33. Lagro-Janssen T, van Weel C. Long-term effect of treatment of female incontinence in general practice. *Br J Gen Pract* 1998;48(436):1735–1738.

34. Bump RC, Hurt WG, Fantl JA, et al. Assessment of Kegel pelvic muscle exercise performance after brief verbal instruction. *Am J Obstet Gynecol* 1991;165(2):322–329.

35. Thompson JA, O'Sullivan PB, Briffa NK, et al. Assessment of voluntary pelvic floor muscle contraction in continent and incontinent women using transperineal ultrasound, manual muscle testing, and vaginal squeeze pressure measurements. *Int Urogynecol J Pelvic Floor Dysfunct* 2006;17:624–630.

36. Morkved S, Bo K, Schei B, et al. Pelvic floor muscle training during pregnancy to prevent urinary incontinence: a single-blind randomized controlled trial. *Obstet Gynecol* 2003;101(2):313–319.

37. Sapsford RR, Hodges PW, Richardson CA, et al. Coactivation of the abdominal and pelvic floor muscles during voluntary exercises. *Neurourol Urodyn* 2001;20(1):31–42.

38. Wyman JF, Fantl JA, McClish DK, et al. Comparative efficacy of behavioral interventions in the management of female urinary incontinence. Continence Program for Women Research Group. *Am J Obstet Gynecol* 1998;179(4):999–1007.

39. Dolman M, Chase J. Comparison between the Health Belief Model and Subjective Expected Utility Theory: predicting incontinence prevention behaviour in postpartum women. *J Eval Clin Pract* 1996;2(3):217–222.

40. Mooney RA, Dougherty MC. Adherence in clinical nursing research. *West J Nurs Res* 1989;11(5):533–547.

41. Meyer S, Hohlfeld P, Achtari C, et al. Pelvic floor education after vaginal delivery. *Obstet Gynecol* 2001;97(5 Pt 1):673–677.

42. Cammu H, Van Nylen M. Pelvic floor exercises versus vaginal weight cones in genuine stress incontinence. *Eur J Obstet Gynecol Reprod Biol* 1998;77(1):89–93.

43. Burgio KL, Engel BT. Biofeedback-assisted behavioral training for elderly men and women. *J Am Geriatr Soc* 1990;38(3):338–340.

44. Kegel AH. Stress incontinence of urine in women; physiologic treatment. *J Int Coll Surg* 1956;25(4 Part 1):487–499.

45. Glavind K, Nohr SB, Walter S. Biofeedback and physiotherapy versus physiotherapy alone in the treatment of genuine stress urinary incontinence. *Int Urogynecol J Pelvic Floor Dysfunct* 1996;7(6):339–343.

46. Castleden CM, Duffin HM, Mitchell EP. The effect of physiotherapy on stress incontinence. *Age Ageing* 1984;13(4):235–237.

47. Berghmans LC, Frederiks CM, de Bie RA, et al. Efficacy of biofeedback, when included with pelvic floor muscle exercise treatment, for genuine stress incontinence. *Neurourol Urodyn* 1996;15(1):37–52.

48. Morkved S, Bo K, Fjortoft T. Effect of adding biofeedback to pelvic floor muscle training to treat urodynamic stress incontinence. *Obstet Gynecol* 2002;100(4):730–739.

49. Burns PA, Pranioff K, Nochajski T, et al. Treatment of stress incontinence with pelvic floor exercises and biofeedback. *J Am Geriatr Soc* 1990;38(3):341–344.

50. Burgio KL, Robinson JC, Engel BT. The role of biofeedback in Kegel exercise training for stress urinary incontinence. *Am J Obstet Gynecol* 1986;154(1):58–64.

51. Burton JR, Pearce KL, Burgio KL, et al. Behavioral training for urinary incontinence in elderly ambulatory patients. *J Am Geriatr Soc* 1988;36(8):693–698.

52. Henderson JS, Taylor KH. Age as a variable in an exercise program for the treatment of simple urinary stress incontinence. *J Obstet Gynecol Neonatal Nurs* 1987;16(4):266–272.

53. Aksac B, Aki S, Karan A, et al. Biofeedback and pelvic floor exercises for the rehabilitation of urinary stress incontinence. *Gynecol Obstet Invest* 2003;56(1):23–27.

54. Newman DK, Smith DA. Pelvic muscle reeducation as a nursing treatment for incontinence. *Urol Nurs* 1992;12(1):9–15.

55. Bo K, Maanum M. Does vaginal electrical stimulation cause pelvic floor muscle contraction? A pilot study. *Scand J Urol Nephrol Suppl* 1996;179:39–45.

56. Yamanishi T, Yasuda K. Electrical stimulation for stress incontinence. *Int Urogynecol J Pelvic Floor Dysfunct* 1998;9(5):281–290.

57. Amaro JL, Gameiro MO, Padovani CR. Effect of intravaginal electrical stimulation on pelvic floor muscle strength. *Int Urogynecol J Pelvic Floor Dysfunct* 2005;16(5):355–358.

58. Use of electrical stimulation in strength and power training. In Dudley G, Harris R, Komi P, eds. *Strength and power in sport.* Oxford: Blackwell Scientific Publications, 1992:329–337.

59. Physical activity, fitness, and health. Consensus statement. In Bouchard C, Shephard R, Stephens T, eds. *Physical activity, fitness, and health: status and determinants. Adjuvants to physical activity.* Champaign, IL: Human Kinetics Publishers, 1993:33–40.

60. Bo K, Talseth T. Change in urethral pressure during voluntary pelvic floor muscle contraction and vaginal electrical stimulation. *Int Urogynecol J Pelvic Floor Dysfunct* 1997;8(1):3–7.

61. Sung MS, Hong JY, Choi YH, et al. FES-biofeedback versus intensive pelvic floor muscle exercise for the prevention and treatment of genuine stress incontinence. *J Korean Med Sci* 2000;15(3):303–308.

62. Bo K. Effect of electrical stimulation on stress and urge urinary incontinence. Clinical outcome and practical recommendations based on randomized controlled trials. *Acta Obstet Gynecol Scand Suppl* 1998;168:3–11.

63. Parkkinen A, Karjalainen E, Vartianen M, et al. Physiotherapy for female stress urinary incontinence: individual therapy at the outpatient clinic versus home-based pelvic floor training: a 5-year follow-up study. *Neurourol Urodyn* 2004;23(7):643–648.

64. Lee JY, Chancellor MB. Using electrical stimulation for urinary incontinence. *Rev Urol* 2002;4(1):49–50.

65. Peattie AB, Plevnik S, Stanton SL. Vaginal cones: a conservative method of treating genuine stress incontinence. *Br J Obstet Gynaecol* 1988;95(10):1049–1053.

66. Bo K. Vaginal weight cones. Theoretical framework, effect on pelvic floor muscle strength, and female stress urinary incontinence. *Acta Obstet Gynecol Scand* 1995;74(2):87–92.

67. Hesse U, Vodusek DB, Deindl FM, et al. Neurophysiological assessment of treatment with vaginal cones. *Neurourol Urodyn* 1991;10:394–395.

68. Olah KS, Bridges N, Denning J, et al. The conservative management of patients with symptoms of stress incontinence: a randomized, prospective study comparing weighted vaginal cones and interferential therapy. *Am J Obstet Gynecol* 1990;162(1):87–92.

69. Sand PK, Staskin D, Miller J, et al. Effect of a urinary control insert on quality of life in incontinent women. *Int Urogynecol J Pelvic Floor Dysfunct* 1999;10(2):100–105.

70. Herbison P, Plevnik S, Mantle J. Weighted vaginal cones for urinary incontinence. *Cochrane Database Syst Rev* 2002(1):CD002114.

71. Kato K, Kondo A. Clinical value of vaginal cones for the management of female stress incontinence. *Int Urogynecol J Pelvic Floor Dysfunct* 1997;8(5):314–317.

72. Bo K, Talseth T, Holme I. Single-blind, randomized controlled trial of pelvic floor exercises, electrical stimulation, vaginal cones, and no treatment in management of genuine stress incontinence in women. *Br Med J* 1999;318(7182):487–493.

73. Kondo A, Yamada Y, Niijima R. Treatment of stress incontinence by vaginal cones: short- and long-term results and predictive parameters. *Br J Urol* 1995;76(4):464–466.

74. Hides JA, Richardson CA, Jull GA. Use of real-time ultrasound imaging for feedback in rehabilitation. *Manual Ther* 1998;3(3):125–131.

75. Dietz HP, Wilson PD, Clarke B. The use of perineal ultrasound to quantify levator activity and teach pelvic floor muscle exercises. *Int Urogynecol J Pelvic Floor Dysfunct* 2001;12(3):166–169.

76. Costantini S, Esposito C, Nadalini D, et al. Ultrasound imaging of the female perineum: the effect of vaginal delivery on pelvic floor dynamics. *Ultrasound Obstet Gynecol* 2006;27(2):183–187.

77. Whittaker J. Abdominal ultrasound imaging of pelvic floor muscle function in individuals with low back pain. *J Manual Manip Ther* 2004;12(1):44–49.

78. Bo K, Lilleas F, Talseth T, et al. Dynamic MRI of the pelvic floor muscles in an upright sitting position. *Neurourol Urodyn* 2001;20(2):167–174.

79. Christensen LL, Djurhuus JC, Constantinou CE. Imaging of pelvic floor contractions using MRI. *Neurourol Urodyn* 1995;14(3):209–216.

80. Miller JM, Ashton-Miller JA, DeLancey JO. A pelvic muscle precontraction can reduce cough-related urine loss in selected women with mild SUI. *J Am Geriatr Soc* 1998;46(7):870–874.

81. Lee LJ, Lee DG. Treating the lumbo-pelvic-hip dysfunction. In Lee DG, ed. *The pelvic girdle.* New York: Elsevier Science, 2005.

82. Fielding JR, Griffiths D, Versi E, et al. MR imaging of pelvic floor continence mechanisms in the supine and sitting positions. *AJR Am J Roentgenol* 1998;171(6):1607–1610.

83. Sulak PJ, Kuehl TJ, Shull BL. Vaginal pessaries and their use in pelvic relaxation. *J Reprod Med* 1993;38(12):919–923.

84. Wu V, Farrell SA, Baskett TF, et al. A simplified protocol for pessary management. *Obstet Gynecol* 1997;90(6):990–994.

85. Hanson LA, Schuly JA, Flood CG, et al. Vaginal pessaries in managing women with pelvic organ prolapse and urinary incontinence: patient characteristics and factors contributing to success. *Int Urogynecol J Pelvic Floor Dysfunct* 2006;17(2):155–159.

86. Clemons JL, Aguilar VC, Tillinghast TA, et al. Risk factors associated with an unsuccessful pessary fitting trial in women with pelvic organ prolapse. *Am J Obstet Gynecol* 2004;190(2):345–350.

87. Maito JM, Quam ZA, Craig E, et al. Predictors of successful pessary fitting and continued use in a nurse-midwifery pessary clinic. *J Midwifery Womens Health* 2006;51(2):78–84.

88. Robert M, Mainprize TC. Long-term assessment of the incontinence ring pessary for the treatment of stress incontinence. *Int Urogynecol J Pelvic Floor Dysfunct* 2002;13(5):326–329.

89. Donnelly MJ, Powell-Morgan S, Olsen AL, et al. Vaginal pessaries for the management of stress and mixed urinary incontinence. *Int Urogynecol J Pelvic Floor Dysfunct* 2004;15(5):302–307.

90. Wilson TS, Zimmern PE. Tailor-made incontinence care. Match type of incontinence to resident assessment for optimal treatment. Part 2. *Contemp Longterm Care* 2002;25(9):18–20.

91. Nguyen JN, Jones CR. Pessary treatment of pelvic relaxation: factors affecting successful fitting and continued use. *J Wound Ostomy Continence Nurs* 2005; 32(4):255–261.

92. Nielsen KK, Kromann-Andersen B, Jacobsen H, et al. The urethral plug: a new treatment modality for genuine urinary stress incontinence in women. *J Urol* 1990; 144(5):1199–1202.

93. Staskin D, Bavendam T, Miller J, et al. Effectiveness of a urinary control insert in the management of stress urinary incontinence: early results of a multicenter study. *Urology* 1996;47(5):629–636.

94. Miller JL, Bavendam T. Treatment with the Reliance urinary control insert: one-year experience. *J Endourol* 1996;10(3):287–292.

95. Wyman JF, Choi SC, Harkins SW, et al. The urinary diary in evaluation of incontinent women: a test-retest analysis. *Obstet Gynecol* 1988;71(6 Pt 1):812–817.

96. Locher JL, Goode PS, Roth DL, et al. Reliability assessment of the bladder diary for urinary incontinence in older women. *J Gerontol A Biol Sci Med Sci* 2001;56(1):M32–35.

97. Wallace SA, Roe B, Williams K, et al. Bladder training for urinary incontinence in adults. *Cochrane Database Syst Rev* 2004(1):CD001308.

98. Fantl JA, Wyman JF, McClish DK, et al. Efficacy of bladder training in older women with urinary incontinence. *JAMA* 1991;265(5):609–613.

99. Gormley EA. Biofeedback and behavioral therapy for the management of female urinary incontinence. *Urol Clin North Am* 2002;29:551–557.

100. Iselin CE, Webster GD. Office management of female urinary incontinence. *Urol Clin North Am* 1998; 25(4):625–645.

101. Swithinbank L, Hashim H, Abrams P. The effect of fluid intake on urinary symptoms in women. *J Urol* 2005;174(1):187–189.

102. Sherman RA, Davis GD, Wong MF. Behavioral treatment of exercise-induced urinary incontinence among female soldiers. *Mil Med* 1997;162(10):690–694.

103. Dmochowski RR, Miklos JR, Norton PA, et al. Duloxetine versus placebo for the treatment of North American women with stress urinary incontinence. *J Urol* 2003;170(4 Pt 1):1259–1263.

104. Norton PA, Zinner NR, Yalcin I, et al. Duloxetine versus placebo in the treatment of stress urinary incontinence. *Am J Obstet Gynecol* 2002;187(1): 40–48.

105. Ghoniem GM, Van Leeuwen JS, Elser DM, et al. A randomized controlled trial of duloxetine alone, pelvic floor muscle training alone, combined treatment and no active treatment in women with stress urinary incontinence. *J Urol* 2005;173(5):1647–1653.

106. Wagner TH, Patrick DL, Bavendam TG, et al. Quality of life of persons with urinary incontinence: development of a new measure. *Urology* 1996;47(1): 67–72.

107. Long CY, Liu CM, Hsu SC, et al. A randomized comparative study of the effects of oral and topical estrogen therapy on the lower urinary tract of hysterectomized postmenopausal women. *Fertil Steril* 2006;85(1):155–160.

108. Goldstein SR, Johnson S, Watts NB, et al. Incidence of urinary incontinence in postmenopausal women treated with raloxifene or estrogen. *Menopause* 2005;12(2):160–164.

109. Castro-Diaz D, Amoros MA. Pharmacotherapy for stress urinary incontinence. *Curr Opin Urol* 2005; 15(4):227–230.

Surgical Treatment of Stress Urinary Incontinence

Matthew D. Barber

Surgery for stress urinary incontinence (SUI) represents one of the most common indications for surgery in women. Approximately 4% of women will undergo surgery for SUI during their lifetime (1). An estimated 119,663 inpatient surgical procedures for SUI were performed in the United States in 2003, with the majority being performed for women age 45 to 64 (58,660) (2). The number of ambulatory procedures performed for SUI approximated 15,900 in 1996 and is certainly much higher today given the recent widespread adoption of minimally invasive sling procedures such as the tension-free vaginal tape (3).

HISTORICAL PERSPECTIVE

Over 1,000 surgical procedures for treating SUI have been described; however, only a small number have both withstood the test of time and held up to scientific scrutiny (Table 14.1). As of the writing of this chapter, only three techniques have consistently demonstrated superior efficacy for the treatment of SUI and are supported by level 1 evidence:

1. Retropubic colposuspensions, including the Burch colposuspension and the Marshall-Marchetti-Krantz procedure (MMK)
2. The traditional bladder-neck sling
3. The tension-free vaginal tape procedure

Several newer techniques show promise, such as the transobturator sling, but clinical trials evaluating their efficacy either have yet to be performed or are still ongoing.

The evolution of the surgical treatment of SUI largely occurred in the last century. In 1913, Howard Kelly first described his anterior plication stitch—a horizontal mattress stitch placed at the urethrovesical junction (UVJ) designed to narrow the patulous urethra and provide elevation of the bladder neck (4). The Kelly plication, along with later modifications by Kennedy (5), evolved into the modern-day anterior colporrhaphy. Because of its relative simplicity, low morbidity, and transvaginal approach, the anterior colporrhaphy became the primary treatment of SUI among gynecologists for much of the 20th century. After a number of studies demonstrated that the success rate for anterior colporrhaphy with Kelly plication was significantly less than that of retropubic colposuspensions or traditional slings, it fell out of favor for the treatment of SUI. While no longer an acceptable treatment for SUI, anterior colporrhaphy still remains an acceptable and commonly used technique for transvaginal correction of anterior vaginal prolapse.

The first suburethral sling procedure was described in 1907 by von Giordano using a gracilis muscle flap. In 1910, Goebel described detaching the pyramidalis muscle and suturing it beneath the urethra (6). Frangenheim modified the technique in 1914 by attaching a vertical strip of rectus fascia to the pyramidalis muscle (7). The final alteration of the initial Goebel-Frangenheim-Stoekel procedure included securing the pyramidalis muscle and the rectus fascia beneath the urethra after plication of the periurethral fascia (8). Later, in 1933, Price described the first sling constructed from fascia lata (9). In 1942, Aldridge described the rectus fascia

TABLE 14.1

Surgical Procedures for Stress Urinary Incontinence

Superior efficacy, recommended—Level 1 evidence
    Retropubic colposuspension (Burch colposuspension, Marshall-Marchetti-Krantz procedure)
    Traditional sling procedures
    Tension-free vaginal tape (TVT)
Inferior efficacy, not recommended—Level 1 evidence
    Anterior colporrhaphy
    Needle suspension procedures (e.g., Pereyra, Raz, Stamey, Gittes)
    Paravaginal repair
Unknown efficacy—no Level 1 evidence available
    Tension-free midurethral slings other than TVT (e.g., SPARC [American Medical Systems, Minnetonka, MN],
        anterior intravaginal slingplasty)
    Transobturator tape procedures (TOT)
    Radiofrequency ablation techniques

---

sling (10). He used two strips of rectus fascia sutured in the midline below the urethra via a separate vaginal incision. The fascial strips were brought down through the rectus muscle, behind the symphysis pubis, and united as a sling beneath the urethra at the UVJ. This provided a reliable cure for recurrent cases of SUI and served as the foundation for modern-day sling techniques. For most of the 20th century, sling procedures were used to treat patients with the most severe disease, those with recurrent incontinence and/or intrinsic sphincter deficiency, and were not used in the treatment of primary SUI. This is largely because sling procedures, as they were traditionally performed, were associated with an increased rate of voiding dysfunction and morbidity when compared to other prevailing techniques. It was not until the 1990s, after surgeons recognized the importance of "loosely tensioning" slings to minimize voiding dysfunction, that traditional sling procedures gained popularity as a first-line treatment for SUI.

The first retropubic operation for the treatment of SUI was described in 1949 by Marshall et al (11). In the mid-1940s, Victor Marshall, a urologist, began to develop an operation for treating voiding dysfunction that developed after rectal resection in men as a result of pronounced urethral hypermobility. He employed a suprapubic approach to suspend the bladder and bladder neck by placement of interrupted chromic catgut sutures to the periostium of the symphysis and posterior rectus sheath. Thereafter he collaborated with two gynecologists, Andrew Marchetti and Kermit Krantz, refining and modifying the procedure to treat urinary incontinence in women. Over the next several decades the MMK procedure became a standard for the treatment of SUI in women and is still used by some today.

John Burch described his retropubic colposuspension technique in 1961 after noting that when performing a MMK procedure the sutures in the periosteum of the pubic symphysis often pulled out (12). Burch identified Cooper's ligament, the thick band of fibrous tissue running along the superior surface of the superior ramus of the pubic bone, as a more consistent point of attachment for the suspension sutures. In Burch's original description of his operation, three sutures were placed in the periurethral tissues on either side and sutured to Cooper's ligament. In 1976, Tanagho described his modification of the Burch procedure in which two sutures are placed in the anterior vaginal wall on each side, one at the midurethra and one at the UVJ, lateral enough to avoid damaging the urethral sphincteric mechanism (13). The sutures are passed through Cooper's ligament and tied so that the urethra is preferentially elevated, but not compressed. He emphasized that the presence of a "suture gap" between the vaginal attachment and Cooper's ligament was of no disadvantage and perhaps desirable. It is Tanagho's modification of the Burch colposuspension that is most commonly performed today. While the available evidence suggests that the MMK procedure and the Burch colposuspension have similar efficacy, the Burch procedure is often preferred because it avoids the risk of osteitis pubis that is associated with the MMK.

The transvaginal needle suspension procedure was first described by Pereyra in 1959 (14). The needle urethropexy underwent more than 20 modifications in an attempt to improve the cure rates and minimize complications, including the Raz, Gittes, and Stamey procedures (15). Modifications involved various amounts of dissection and different anchoring tissue and materials. Although extremely popular in the 1980s and early 1990s, particularly among urologists, these procedures were largely abandoned after several comprehensive reviews and randomized trials demonstrated that they were significantly less effective than retropubic colposuspensions and traditional sling procedures (15).

The tension-free vaginal tape (TVT) procedure was introduced Ulmsten et al in 1996 and over the subsequent decade gained world-wide popularity (16). This operation introduced two new concepts to the mechanism of cure for slings: placement at the midurethra, and placement without tension ("tension-free"). The primary advantage that TVT offered over other surgical treatments for SUI, however, is that it could be performed on an outpatient basis. Often patients can void the day of surgery and be discharged home without a catheter. Several randomized trials and numerous cohort studies suggest that the TVT procedure has similar cure rates to the Burch colposuspension, with a quicker return to normal voiding and fewer postoperative complications (17–19). The success of the TVT has prompted the development of a number of similar minimally invasive midurethral slings with varying differences in sling material and surgical approach. To date, these "TVT-like" devices are largely unstudied.

The most recent innovation in the surgical management of SUI is the transobturator tape (TOT), which was first described by Delorme in 2001 (20). Like the TVT, this is a minimally invasive midurethral sling using a synthetic tape; however, it is placed using a transobturator approach rather than a retropubic one. The impetus for the development of this technique was to reduce the risk of bladder perforation and eliminate the rare but life-threatening complications of bowel perforation and major vascular injury that have been reported with TVT. Published data are limited regarding the relative efficacy and risk of complications with this new approach.

INDICATIONS FOR SURGERY

Surgery is indicated for the treatment of SUI when conservative treatments have failed to satisfactorily relieve the symptoms and the patient wishes further treatment in an effort to achieve continence (21). Prevailing opinion suggests that surgery should be delayed until childbearing is complete because the effect of subsequent pregnancy on continence surgery is unknown; however, the desire for future childbearing should not be considered an absolute contraindication (21,22).

Prior to surgery, the minimum evaluation should include a comprehensive history, physical examination, urinalysis, and measurement of postvoid residual volume. Stress incontinence should be objectively documented, with direct visualization of urine loss from the urethra with stress. Urethral hypermobility should be demonstrated with Q-tip testing or some similar method.

Urodynamics should be performed prior to surgery when the diagnosis is unclear or the patient is at high risk for treatment failure or complications. Not all patients with urinary incontinence require urodynamic testing prior to surgery, however. According to the AHCPR Urinary Incontinence Clinical Practice Guidelines, patients who lose urine only with physical exertion; have normal voiding habits (eight or fewer voiding episodes per day, two or fewer per night); have a normal neurologic examination and have no history of previous continence surgery or radical pelvic surgery; possess a hypermobile urethra and pliable vaginal wall on physical examination; have a normal postvoid residual volume and are not pregnant do not require urodynamics prior to continence surgery (23). These guidelines are based largely on expert opinion, however, and a considerable amount of research is required before evidence-based guidelines can be developed. Preoperative urodynamics should be strongly considered in patients with advanced age, a history of previous continence surgery, symptoms suggestive of detrusor overactivity or voiding dysfunction, an abnormal sacral neurologic examination, an elevated postvoid residual, or whenever the diagnosis of SUI is otherwise in question (21,23).

Factors that may negatively influence the results of SUI surgery include advancing age, obesity, a history of previous incontinence surgery, a nonmobile urethra, and preoperative detrusor overactivity (24). The evidence supporting these negative predictors is generally weak, however. As such, they should not be considered contraindications to continence surgery, but instead be used for patient counseling. Contraindications to SUI surgery include the presence of pure detrusor overactivity, an atonic bladder, or a neurogenic bladder. Also, patients who are otherwise at high risk for postoperative urinary retention who are unable or unwilling to perform self-catheterization may not be good candidates for SUI surgery.

Intrinsic Sphincter Deficiency

Subjects with severe urinary incontinence and urodynamic evidence of poor urethral sphincter function are said to have intrinsic sphincter deficiency (ISD), sometimes called type III incontinence or "low-pressure urethra." Some authors have suggested that subjects with ISD are at risk for poor results after continence surgery, particularly after a retropubic colposuspension (24–26). They suggest that patients who demonstrate a low leak point pressure (less than 60 cm H_2O) or low maximum urethral closure pressure (less than 20 cm H_2O) are best served by a procedure such as a sling that is more obstructive. These findings are not consistent, however, with some authors finding no association between commonly used measures of urethral function and continence surgery success (27–29). Additionally, systematic reviews of the two most common measures of urethral sphincteric function, urethral pressure profilometry and leak point pressure measurement, have concluded that these tests are not well standardized and have poor reproducibility (30,31). In 2005, the World Health Organization's Third International Consultation on Incontinence concluded that there is no consensus definition for ISD and there is currently no evidence that such a diagnosis influences the outcome of SUI surgery or should be used to choose the type of surgical treatment (24). In spite of this, many surgeons continue to use the results of urethral function testing in an attempt to provide prognostic information about the success of certain surgical procedures and to triage patients accordingly. A recent example is the suggestion by some that patients with ISD have a high failure rate after TOT procedures (32). Clearly, high-quality studies are needed to clarify the role of urethral function testing and the ISD diagnosis in the management of patients with SUI.

Mixed Urinary Incontinence

Approximately one third of patients with urodynamic stress incontinence have coexisting detrusor overactivity. These patients are said to have mixed urinary incontinence. There is some controversy about the best management for these patients. Studies have shown that patients with mixed urinary incontinence may have lower cure rates after surgery than those with pure SUI (33–35). Generally, 30% to 60% of women with mixed incontinence will have resolution of their urge incontinence after SUI surgery, with 5% to 10% developing worse urge incontinence and the remainder not changing (19,36,37). Unfortunately,

attempts to use clinical or urodynamic data to predict who will improve and who will worsen have been unsuccessful (38). Most authors recommend that patients with mixed urinary incontinence undergo a trial of medical and behavioral therapy prior to considering surgery. Approximately one third of patients with mixed incontinence can be expected to become dry with conservative therapy alone (39). In those who have persistent bothersome incontinence after a trial of conservative therapy, surgery can be considered after appropriate patient counseling.

RETROPUBIC COLPOSUSPENSIONS

Retropubic colposuspensions are indicated for women with a diagnosis of urodynamic stress incontinence and a hypermobile urethra. They can be performed through an abdominal incision or laparoscopically. The Third International Consultation on Incontinence concluded that based on the currently available evidence, retropubic colposuspensions, particularly the open Burch colposuspension, "can be recommended as a procedure which is as effective as any other procedure for primary or secondary surgery with proven long-term success" in the treatment of SUI (24). The Burch colposuspension has historically been one of the most commonly performed operations for SUI, particularly among gynecologists. With the recent widespread adoption of minimally invasive slings, the popularity of the retropubic colposuspension has waned somewhat, with many surgeons reserving this procedure for instances where a laparotomy (or laparoscopy) is being performed for another indication (e.g., abdominal sacral colpopexy). No other continence operation has demonstrated greater efficacy or longer durability than the Burch colposuspension, however. As such, it should remain an important option in the surgical management of SUI.

Mechanism

SUI occurs when there is an unequal transmission of pressure between the bladder and urethra during stress such that the bladder pressure exceeds maximal urethral closure pressure (unaccompanied by a detrusor contraction), resulting in urine leakage. One commonly proposed theory holds that loss of urethrovesical support contributes to inefficient pressure transmission of the urethra because the urethra is displaced out of the abdominal cavity (40). Retropubic colposuspensions are designed to provide preferential elevation and support of the bladder neck by the placement of sutures in the vagina near the urethra. This results in elevation of the hypermobile urethra back into an intra-abdominal position. Perhaps more importantly, it provides mechanical compression of the urethra against the stable, elevated anterior vaginal wall and/or the posterior-superior aspect of the symphysis pubis during episodes of increased abdominal pressure. The principal urodynamic change after these procedures is increased pressure transmission to the urethra, relative to the bladder, during elevations in intra-abdominal pressure (41,42). Resting urethral pressure and functional urethral length are unchanged, suggesting that the intrinsic function of the urethra is not altered appreciably by this type of surgery. Appropriate elevation of the bladder neck and urethra, accompanied by pressure transmission ratios near 100%, results in continence in most patients (42). Penttinen et al demonstrated a significant negative correlation between postoperative bladder neck mobility and pressure transmission ratios, suggesting that correction of the urethrovesical anatomic disorder eliminates the functional disorder and restores continence (43). Retropubic procedures, particularly the MMK, probably tend to overelevate and fix the urethra in a retropubic position. Hilton and Stanton found that pressure transmission profiles after successful Burch colposuspensions differed from those of continent control subjects, with pressure transmission ratios in the proximal half of the urethra significantly higher than 100% (44). This observation suggests that an additional mechanism that likely contributes to the success of these operations is partial outflow obstruction. Bump et al determined that patients with postoperative voiding abnormalities and detrusor instability after Burch colposuspensions had pressure transmission ratios significantly greater than 100%, supporting the hypothesis that obstruction, when excessive, also plays a role in postoperative voiding dysfunction and detrusor instability after these operations (41,42).

Access to the Retropubic Space

The patient is placed in modified lithotomy position using low leg holders such as Allen stirrups and is draped to allow both abdominal and vaginal access. The bladder is drained with a Foley catheter with a 10 cc or larger balloon. One perioperative intravenous dose of an appropriate antibiotic should be given as prophylaxis against infection. The abdomen may be entered through a transverse or vertical abdominal incision or laparoscopically. The laparoscopic approach will be discussed later in the chapter. While retropubic col-

posuspensions can be performed entirely retroperitoneally, some find that entering the peritoneal cavity and packing the bowel out of the pelvis often provides better visualization of the retropubic space. Entering the peritoneal cavity also allows for concurrent hysterectomy or additional abdominal prolapse repairs that may be necessary.

To access the retropubic space, the rectus abdominis muscles are separated in the midline and the underlying transversalis fascia is bluntly separated off the pubic symphysis. The retropubic space is developed using blunt dissection. The surgeon's hand is placed along the underside of the pubic bone and the underlying bladder is displaced posteriorly. Sharp dissection is typically unnecessary in primary cases. Cooper's ligament, the obturator neurovascular bundle, any accessory obturator vessels, and the lateral attachments of the vagina (arcus tendineus fascia pelvis) are identified. A fluffed-up gauze and a medium malleable retractor can be useful to retract the bladder medially to expose these lateral structures. The surgeon's nondominant hand is placed into the vagina to elevate the paravaginal tissues and identify the urethra and bladder neck. Identification of the UVJ can be facilitated by gently placing traction on the Foley catheter and palpating the lower edge of the balloon. Adipose tissue is dissected off the anterior vaginal wall lateral to the urethra and UVJ using forceps, a peanut dissector, or some similar device. This dissection is facilitated by forcefully elevating the surgeon's vaginal fingers until glistening white periurethral fascia and vaginal wall are seen. Dissection in the midline over the urethra and UVJ should be avoided to avoid trauma to the urethral sphincter mechanism. The retropubic space and paravaginal tissues are highly vascular, and careful attention and gentle dissection are required to avoid excessive bleeding. Hemostasis is achieved with hemoclips, cautery, or sutures.

If previous retropubic surgery has been performed, dense adhesions from the anterior bladder wall and urethra to the pubic symphysis are often present. These adhesions should be dissected sharply from the pubic bone until the anterior bladder wall, urethra, and vagina are free of adhesions and are mobile. If identification of the urethra or lower border of the bladder is difficult, one may perform a cystotomy, which, with a finger inside the bladder, helps to define the bladder's lower limits for easier dissection, mobilization, and elevation.

Marshall-Marchetti-Krantz Procedure

The retropubic space is entered and the urethra and UVJ are exposed as described above. The surgeon's nondominant hand is placed in the vagina with the index and middle fingers placed on either side of the urethra to facilitate elevation of the urethra and UVJ. Permanent sutures are placed with the needle initially entering closest to the urethra and then coursing lateral perpendicular to the urethra to include almost the full thickness of the anterior vaginal wall. One to three pairs of sutures are placed on either side of the urethra, with the most proximal pair at the UVJ (Fig. 14.1). Sutures are generally placed much closer to the urethra during an MMK than is typical with a Burch colposuspension. All sutures are passed through the midline cartilage of the symphysis and tied. Hyperelevation of the urethra is avoided by tying the sutures so that there is sufficient space for the operator to easily place a finger between the pubic symphysis and urethra. Symmonds recommended performing a dome cystotomy when performing an MMK in order to allow directive visualization of the UVJ to facilitate appropriate placement of the proximal sutures (45). This is probably unnecessary with the use of routine intraoperative cystoscopy, however. Postoperatively, the bladder is drained with either a transurethral or suprapubic catheter until normal voiding occurs.

Burch Colposuspension

The retropubic space is entered, the urethra and UVJ are identified, and the periurethral anterior vaginal wall is cleared of all fat as described above. Two permanent sutures are placed on each side of the urethra through the anterior vaginal wall using double bites for each suture. Sutures should be placed almost full thickness through the anterior vaginal wall with the needle parallel to the urethra. The proximal suture is placed approximately 2 cm lateral to the UVJ. The distal suture is placed 2 cm lateral to the mid-urethra. The index and middle fingers of the vaginal hand are used to elevate the anterior vaginal wall on either side of

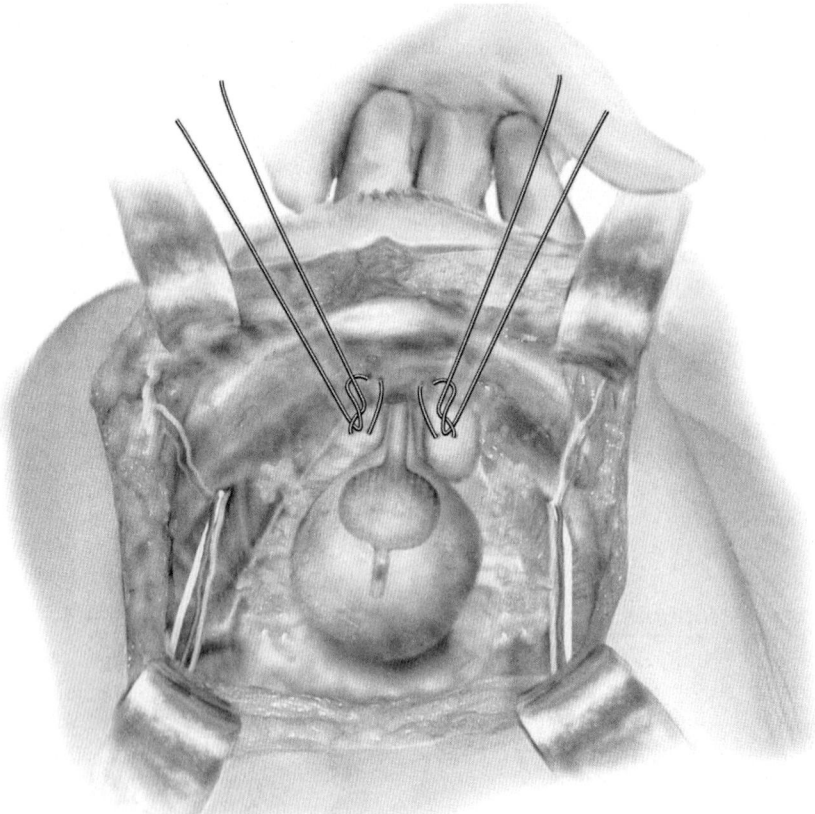

FIGURE 14.1 ● The Marshall-Marchetti-Krantz procedure. One to three sutures are placed on either side of the urethra and sutured to the midline cartilage of the pubic symphysis. (Reproduced with permission from Baggish M, Karram M, eds. *Atlas of pelvic anatomy and gynecologic surgery.* Philadelphia: WB Saunders, 2001.)

the urethra during placement of the sutures. Alternatively, Allis clamps can be used to grasp and elevate the periurethral tissue at the proximal and distal suture sites and the sutures can be placed underneath the clamp in order to avoid an inadvertent needle injury of the vaginal fingers. On each side, after the two sutures are placed, they are passed through Cooper's (pectineal) ligament so that all four suture ends exit above the ligament (Fig. 14.2). The sutures are tied so that there is a small amount of preferential elevation to the ure-

thra while allowing two fingers to easily fit between the pubic bone and the urethra. A suture bridging between anterior vaginal wall and Cooper's ligament is desired in order to prevent compression or hyperelevation of the urethra. As noted previously, this area is extremely vascular, and visible vessels should be avoided if possible. When excessive bleeding occurs, it can be controlled by direct pressure, sutures, cautery, or hemoclips. Less severe bleeding usually stops with direct pressure and after tying the Burch sutures.

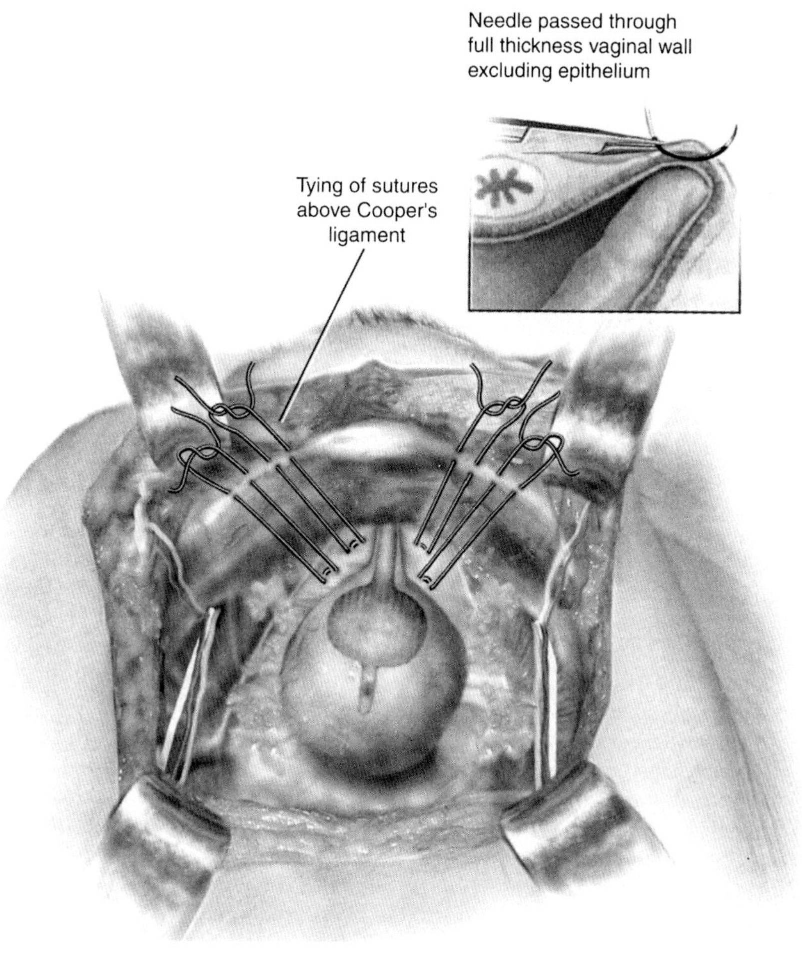

Needle passed through full thickness vaginal wall excluding epithelium

Tying of sutures above Cooper's ligament

FIGURE 14.2 ● Burch colposuspension. Two sutures are placed on each side of the urethra. The proximal suture is placed approximately 2 cm lateral to the urethrovesical junction and the distal suture is placed 2 cm lateral to the mid-urethra. Each is passed through Cooper's (pectineal) ligament so that all four suture ends exit above the ligament. The sutures are tied so that there is a small amount of preferential elevation to the urethra while allowing two fingers to easily fit between the pubic bone and the urethra. *Inset:* The index and middle finger of the vaginal hand are used to elevate the anterior vaginal wall on either side of the urethra during placement of the sutures. The needle should be passed through the full thickness of the vaginal wall, excluding the epithelium. (Reproduced with permission from Baggish M, Karram M, eds. *Atlas of pelvic anatomy and gynecologic surgery.* Philadelphia: WB Saunders, 2001.)

At the end of the procedure, cystoscopy should be performed to document the absence of intravesical sutures. Closed-suction drainage of the retropubic space is rarely indicated. Postoperatively, the bladder is drained with either a transurethral or suprapubic catheter until normal voiding occurs.

Laparoscopic Burch Colposuspension

Advances in minimally invasive techniques in the 1990s allowed for the development of the laparoscopic retropubic colposuspension. The potential advantages of the laparoscopic approach over the open approach include improved visualization of the retropubic space, shortened hospital stay, decreased postoperative pain, faster recovery, and improved cosmesis. Disadvantages of the laparoscopic approach include a steep learning curve in acquiring suturing skills, technical difficulty of retroperitoneal dissection, increased operating time early in the surgeon's experience, and potentially greater costs related to longer operating time and use of disposable surgical instruments. Although various modifications have been described in an attempt to overcome the technical difficulty associated with laparoscopic suturing, many experts agree that laparoscopic retropubic colposuspensions should be performed in a manner identical to that of the open procedure, with the only difference being that of access to the retropubic space (46–48). The use of mesh, staples, bone anchors, or similar devices cannot be recommended.

As with the open procedure, the patient is placed in modified lithotomy position using low leg holders such as Allen stirrups and is draped to allow both abdominal and vaginal access. A three-way Foley catheter with a 20- to 30-mL balloon is attached to continuous drainage, and the irrigation port is connected to sterile water or saline. For the transperitoneal approach, a 5- or 10-mm trocar and laparoscope are placed through a standard infraumbilical incision. Two additional lateral trocars are placed: a 5/12-mm disposable trocar with reducer in the right lower quadrant (if knot-tying from the right) lateral to the right inferior epigastric vessels and a reusable 5-mm port or an additional 5/12-mm disposable trocar with reducer in the left lower quadrant lateral to the left inferior epigastric vessels. Trocars are placed lateral to the rectus muscle, approximately 3 cm medial to and above the anterior superior iliac spine. The retropubic space is developed by first identifying the two medial umbilical folds (the peritoneum overlying the obliterated umbilical arteries). These serve as lateral landmarks of dissection for transperitoneal entry into the retropubic space. The upper margin of the dome of the bladder is located several centimeters above the pubic symphysis. This can be easily visualized by filling the bladder with 300 cc of fluid via the three-way Foley. After emptying the bladder, the peritoneum is incised 2 cm above the bladder dome in between the medial umbilical folds. The retropubic space is developed with blunt dissection and important landmarks are identified as described earlier for the open procedure.

Although used less commonly, some prefer to access the retropubic space using an extraperitoneal approach. For this approach an infraumbilical incision is made with dissection to the preperitoneal space. The dissection is carried caudal into the retropubic space using a balloon dilator or similar technique. Once the retropubic space is entered, CO_2 is insufflated to develop a "pneumo-Retzius," additional trocars are placed, and the remainder of the procedure is performed similar to the transperitoneal approach.

Using laparoscopic needle drivers, 0- or 2-0 permanent sutures with an SH or CT-2 needle are placed at the bladder neck and midurethra on each side and then brought through Cooper's ligaments, similar to the open procedure. Extracorporeal knot-tying is preferred because of technical facility and the ability to hold more tension on the suture. Thirty-six-inch or 48-inch sutures are necessary to facilitate extracorporeal knot-tying. At the completion of the procedure, cystoscopy is performed to assess the integrity of the bladder. Postoperatively, the bladder is drained with either a transurethral or suprapubic catheter until normal voiding occurs. Peritoneum of the retropubic space may be left open or closed according to surgeon preference. Generally patients can be discharged on the day of surgery after this procedure.

Adjuvant Procedures

Although hysterectomy is frequently performed at the time of SUI surgery, prospective studies, including clinical trials, demonstrate that the addition of a hysterectomy at the time of retropubic colposuspension does not improve SUI cure rates. Langer et al randomized 45 subjects to Burch colposuspension alone or colposuspension plus abdominal hysterectomy and cul-de-sac obliteration (49). Six months after surgery the objective (urodynamic) cure rates were not significantly different between groups (95.5% vs. 95.7% respectively). In 2001, Meltomaa et al reported their results from a prospective study evaluating morbidity and long-term subjective outcomes between Burch colposuspension alone and Burch with abdominal hysterectomy (50). There was no difference in subjective outcomes up to 5 years after surgery. Complications were higher in the Burch-plus-hysterectomy group (46.2%) than in the group who received a Burch alone (29.2%). These studies support the conclusion that hysterectomy should not be routinely performed at the time of a retropubic colposuspension unless there is a clear indication for the hysterectomy other than SUI.

Pelvic organ prolapse, particularly apical and posterior vaginal wall prolapse, has been reported to occur in 22.1% of women (range 9.5% to 38.2%) after a Burch colposuspension (24). Most are asymptomatic, however, and less than 5% request subsequent reconstructive surgery (24). Whether these findings are the result of an increased propensity for patients with SUI to develop future prolapse or are a direct result of the Burch procedure itself is largely unknown; however, pelvic organ prolapse appears to be more common after Burch colposuspension than after anterior colporrhaphy and sling procedures (19). In a randomized trial comparing the open Burch colposuspension to the TVT, anterior vaginal wall prolapse was more common in the TVT group but enterocele and apical prolapse were more common in the Burch group 2 years after surgery (17). In order to reduce the risk of subsequent prolapse, many authors suggest that a prophylactic cul-de-sac obliteration procedure such as a uterosacral plication, Moschcowitz procedure, or Halban's culdoplasty be performed at the time of retropubic colposuspension whenever possible. Although frequently advocated, the efficacy of this prophylactic maneuver is unstudied. At a minimum, patients who receive a retropubic colposuspension should be assessed for concurrent vaginal support defects at the time of their surgery and, when present, these should be corrected.

Outcome

A Cochrane Collaboration review of retropubic colposuspensions in 2005 identified 39 randomized clinical trials involving a total of 3,301 women, making retropubic colposuspension the most studied surgery for SUI in terms of level 1 evidence (19). The available evidence indicates that open retropubic colposuspension is an effective treatment for SUI, especially in the long term (19). Within the first year of treatment, the overall continence rate is approximately 85% to 90%. After 5 years, approximately 70% of patients can expect to be dry.

Both the Burch colposuspension and the MMK procedure appear to be durable, with only modest declines in efficacy over 10 to 20 years. Langer et al followed 127 women who received a Burch colposuspension for an average of 12.4 years and reported an objective cure rate of 93.7% (51). All failures in this study occurred within 1 year of the operation. Alcalay et al followed a cohort of 109 women after a Burch colposuspension for 10 to 20 years and found that the cure rate was time-dependent, with an initial decline for 10 to 12 years and a plateau of 69% thereafter (52). McDuffie et al found that the efficacy of the MMK procedure declined from 90% at 1 year to 75% at 15 years (53).

Retropubic colposuspensions have demonstrated a lower subjective failure rate than anterior colporrhaphy in six randomized trials with a relative risk (RR) of failure of 0.43 (95% CI 0.32 to 0.57) at 1 to 5 years after surgery and a RR of 0.49 (95% CI 0.32 to 0.75) at greater than 5 years (19). Similarly, retropubic procedures have demonstrated a lower failure rate than needle procedures in seven clinical trials, particularly after the first year postsurgery (RR 0.48; 95% CI 0.33 to 0.71) (19). The retropubic colposuspension has been compared to the paravaginal defect repair in a single randomized trial. Colombo et al found that after 6 months of follow-up, the objective cure rate of the Burch procedure was 100% compared to only 72% for those undergoing a paravaginal repair (54).

Retropubic colposuspensions have been compared to traditional sling procedures in five trials, and in each there was no significant difference between the two techniques, regardless of whether the procedure was a primary or secondary operation (55). However, these five trials all had small sample sizes ($n = 22$ to 72), limiting their ability to detect even large differences between the two treatments. The NIH-sponsored Urinary Incontinence Treatment Group (UITN) has recently completed the Stress Incontinence Surgical Treatment Efficacy Results (SISTEr) Trial, a randomized trial of autologous rectus fascia sling versus Burch colposuspension for the treatment of SUI with urethral hypermobility (56). This trial enrolled over 650 subjects from nine centers and followed them for a minimum of 2 years. As of the writing of this chapter, the results of this trial have not been reported. The size, quality, and scope of this trial should provide significant insight into the relative efficacy of these two "gold standard" operations.

Ward et al performed a large multicenter randomized trial comparing open Burch colposuspension to TVT for urodynamic SUI (17,57). They found no significant difference in objective or subjective cure rates of these two procedures. Six months after surgery the objective cure rate, defined as a negative 1-hour pad test and negative stress test on urodynamics, was 57% for the Burch group and 66% for the TVT group ($p = 0.10$) when the authors considered those subjects who withdrew or were lost to follow-up as treatment failures (57). When the authors analyzed their data at 2 years and ignored subject withdrawals, the objective cure rate (negative 1-hour pad test) was 80% for colposuspension and 81% for TVT (17).

Most studies comparing the Burch procedure to the MMK are retrospective and demonstrate similar cure rates for the two procedures. Only two randomized trials have compared these two procedures directly. Colombo et al randomized 80 women to either Burch colposuspension or MMK and followed them for 2 to 7 years (58). Differences in cure rates were not statistically significant between the two groups, with a subjective cure rate of 92% in those who received a Burch and 85% for those who received an MMK and objective cure rates of 80% and 60%, respectively (58). Burch colposuspension was associated with shorter hospital stay (mean difference of 1 day) and later resumption of voiding than the MMK (mean difference of 8 days) in this trial, however. Liapas et al randomized 170 women with SUI to receive a Burch colposuspension, a MMK procedure, or an anterior colporrhaphy and followed them for up to 5 years. The Burch procedure had a significantly greater subjective cure rate (88%) than the MMK (67%) or the anterior colporrhaphy (52%) (59). The results of these two trials and the risk of osteitis pubis that is uniquely associated with the MMK suggest that the Burch colposuspension should be the retropubic procedure of choice for SUI.

In 2003, the Cochrane Incontinence Group published a systematic review on laparoscopic retropubic colposuspension (60). They identified five randomized trials comparing laparoscopic to open colposuspension. A meta-analysis of these trials found similar subjective cure rates between the two approaches, ranging from 85% to 96% in the laparoscopic group and 85% to 100% in the open group 6 to 18 months after surgery (60). In contrast, objective cure (stress test at urodynamics) favored open colposuspension over the laparoscopic approach (RR 2.30, 95% CI 1.06 to 4.99) (60). One trial of subjects undergoing laparoscopic colposuspension demonstrated that two sutures on each side of the urethra resulted in a significantly higher cure rate than one suture (48). Notably, the trials included in this review have small sample sizes and short follow-up and are of relatively poor quality. Three of the five studies have only been published as abstracts. These weaknesses limit the strength of the review's conclusions.

Since the publication of the Cochrane review, Smith et al presented the results of a large multicenter trial comparing open to laparoscopic Burch colposuspension (61). Two hundred ninety-one subjects were randomized from one of six centers in the United Kingdom and followed for 2 years. Two years after surgery, the objective cure rate (negative pad test) was similar for the two procedures (79% for the laparoscopic colposuspension vs. 70% for the open procedure) (61). The proportion of subjects reporting that they have "never leaked" since their procedure was 55% in the laparoscopic group and 53% for the open group. Laparoscopic Burch colposuspension was associated with decreased postoperative pain, decreased infectious morbidity, and greater cost than open Burch colposuspension.

In 2004, Paraiso et al randomized 72 women with SUI to receive a laparoscopic Burch colposuspension or a TVT (62). One year after surgery there was a greater rate of urodynamic stress incontinence in the laparoscopic Burch colposuspension group than the TVT group: 18.8% versus 3.2% (RR 1.19, 95% CI 1.00 to 1.42). Additionally, the time to development of recurrent urinary incontinence symptoms was earlier after laparoscopic Burch than with TVT.

Thus, while laparoscopic Burch colposuspension provides a minimally invasive alternative to its open counterpart, its role in the current environment of minimally invasive slings is unclear.

Complications

In general, the rate of perioperative complications associated with retropubic colposuspensions is low. In a review of 2,712 MMK procedures, Mainprize and Drutz noted a lower urinary tract injury rate of 1.6%, a wound complication rate of 5.5%, and a fistula rate of 0.3% (63). Similarly, Kenton et al noted that after Burch colposuspension lower urinary tract injuries were uncommon (less than 1%), while incisional complications were the most frequent perioperative complication (3%) (64). While laparoscopic colposuspension is associated with a shorter hospital stay and less blood loss than open colposuspension, the Cochrane review noted a longer operating time and a trend toward higher complication rates with the laparoscopic approach (60). Smith et al noted that laparoscopic colposuspension was associated with a lower infectious morbidity rate than open colposuspension, but otherwise there was no difference in complications between the two approaches (61). While nerve injury appears to be uncommon after retropubic colposuspension, Galloway et al have described the "post-colposuspension syndrome" in which women develop pain in one or both ilioinguinal regions following colposuspension (65). Demirci reported the occurrence of groin or suprapubic pain in 15 of 200 women (6.8%) after Burch colposuspension (66).

The most common long-term complication after retropubic colposuspension is de novo urge incontinence, which occurs in 5% to 27% of cases (19,24). Transient voiding dysfunction occurs in 6% to 37% of subjects after a Burch colposuspension, depending upon how it is defined (24). Voiding dysfunction that persists beyond 6 weeks after surgery is uncommon, however. Viereck et al reported persistent voiding difficulties in 3.5% of 310 women who underwent a Burch colposuspension with a mean follow-up of 36 months (67). Risk factors for prolonged voiding after a Burch colposuspension include advanced age, previous incontinence surgery, increased first sensation to void on preoperative urodynamics, high postvoid residual volume preoperatively, and postoperative cystitis (68).

Generally, overactive bladder symptoms and voiding dysfunction that occur after a retropubic colposuspension can be managed conservatively or are self-limiting. When these symptoms are refractory to behavioral or medical management, a urethrolysis performed either retropubically or vaginally may provide relief.

Osteitis pubis occurs after 0.74% to 2.5% of MMK procedures but is rare after Burch colposuspension (24). Patients with osteitis pubis typically present 2 to 12 weeks after surgery with suprapubic pain radiating to the thighs that is exacerbated by walking or abduction of the thighs, along with marked tenderness of the pubic symphysis. Radiologic investigation may demonstrate evidence of bone destruction and symphysis separation. The etiology of this condition is unclear, but most cases are noninfectious. Suggested therapy includes rest, physical therapy, and nonsteroidal anti-inflammatory agents and, if necessary, steroids. The clinical course may be prolonged but is typically self-limiting. When conservative therapy fails to result in symptom relief, pubic osteomyelitis should be considered and a biopsy with bacterial culture performed. Kammerer-Doak et al found positive cultures in 71% of patients with clinical osteitis pubis who failed to respond to conservative therapy (69). Pubic osteomyelitis is treated with antibiotics and if necessary débridement and/or symphyseal wedge resection.

TRADITIONAL SLING PROCEDURES

Traditional sling procedures, sometimes referred to as pubovaginal slings or bladder neck slings,

have undergone a considerable number of modifications since their earliest description in beginning of the 20th century. The fundamentals of the procedure have changed little, however: a strap of material, whether biologic or synthetic, is placed suburethrally at the level of the bladder neck, and the arms are passed behind the symphysis pubis and fixed to the rectus fascia or pubic bone using a combined abdominal–vaginal approach. The newer minimally invasive midurethral slings such as the TVT represent a significant evolution from the traditional sling procedures and are described later in the chapter. As noted previously, traditional sling procedures were classically reserved for use as salvage operations in patients who had failed previous continence surgery or for patients with significant sphincter deficiency. More recently, traditional sling procedures have been advocated for the primary treatment of SUI with urethral hypermobility. A survey of practice patterns in 2000 found that sling procedures were the most common SUI surgery performed by urologists in the United States (70). In 1997, the American Urological Association (AUA)-sponsored Female Stress Urinary Incontinence Clinical Guidelines Panel evaluated the published outcomes data on surgical procedures to treat female SUI (71). The panel concluded, based on the available evidence at the time, that sling procedures, along with retropubic colposuspensions, are the most efficacious procedures for long-term success (71). More recently, the Third International Consultation on Incontinence concluded that "autologous slings provide effective long-term cure for stress incontinence" (24). They were more hesitant in their conclusions regarding slings that use allograft or xenografts, however, because they "have yet to show long-term cure rates equivalent to those reported for autologous fascia" (24).

Mechanism

Although there is some debate regarding the mechanism of action of traditional sling procedures, they are generally thought to restore continence through two mechanisms: (a) re-establishing UVJ position and support and (b) providing a stable suburethral base that results in mechanical compression of the proximal urethra during stress. In patients with SUI and urethral hypermobility, bladder neck slings reposition the UVJ into its normal position and prevent proximal urethral descent during stress (72). As with retropubic colposuspensions, this results in increased pressure transmission to the urethra, relative to the bladder, during elevations in intra-abdominal pressure, thereby promoting continence (73,74). Consistent with this, Summit et al noted that the success rate of traditional sling procedures is compromised in patients without urethral hypermobility (75). Unlike retropubic operations, sling procedures also create a hammock underneath the proximal urethra that allows mechanical compression of the urethra during stress. When the tightness or anterior elevation of a sling is increased, it results in increased mechanical compression of the urethra and greater urethral resistance. While this promotes continence, it is also can result in voiding dysfunction, the most common complication of sling procedures. Because of this, it is generally recommended that slings be placed loosely so that there is no tension on the urethra at rest. In rare instances where urethral function is completely compromised, resulting in continuous incontinence at rest, it may be desirable to provide greater urethral compression or even complete obstruction as long as the patient is willing to permanently self-catheterize.

The importance of the suburethral portion of the sling for promoting continence was recently questioned in an interesting animal experiment. Using a rat sling model, Hijaz et al performed slings on 40 animals with SUI (76). Half of the rats received intact slings and the other half received slings in which the suburethral portion was cut at the time of the initial operation. Six weeks after surgery, there was a significant improvement in leak point pressures in both groups compared to animals who received sham operations, and there was no difference between the intact or cut sling groups (76). This implies that, in rats, the lateral arms of the sling are more important for restoring urethral function than the suburethral portion of the sling. Whether these findings translate to humans is currently unknown.

Technique

Although a myriad of different sling techniques have been described, they all follow the same fundamental principles, with the critical variables being: (a) the length of the sling (full-length versus a smaller sling or "patch" that is placed suburethrally and fixed via suspending sutures); (b) the type of sling material (autograft, allograft, xenografts, or synthetic); and (c) the point of fixation (rectus fascia, pubic bone, or Cooper's ligament). Additionally, some surgeons feel that it is important that the sling arms penetrate the periurethral tissues to enter the retropubic space, while others feel this is not necessary (Fig. 14.3). To date, there have been no randomized trials comparing

the various sling alternatives, and with few exceptions the existing evidence does not favor one technique over another. As such, the sling technique and choice of material can be left to the discretion of the individual surgeon. A discussion of the advantages and disadvantages of the different sling materials can be found later in the chapter.

The most common autologous tissues used for traditional sling procedures are fascia lata and rectus fascia. If a surgeon chooses to perform an autologous sling, the tissue is typically harvested at the beginning of the procedure, prior to any vaginal dissection. To harvest fascia lata, the patient is placed in the lateral decubitus position with the hip and knee flexed, each at approximately 45 degrees. The leg is prepped from above the hip to below the knee. A 3- to 4-cm incision is made either horizontally or vertically just above the lateral femoral condyle. Dissection is carried down to the underlying fascia lata and the fat is cleaned off with blunt dissection. For a full-length sling, a fascial stripper is used. Typically a 2-cm × 20- to 25-cm strip of fascia lata can be obtained. For a patch sling, the desired graft size, usually 2 cm × 6 to 8 cm, can easily be harvested through the small leg incision. There is no need to reapproximate the fascial defect. After obtaining hemostasis, the subcutaneous tissues are reapproximated, the skin is closed, and a pressure dressing is applied. If a full-length sling has been harvested, it is prudent to apply a pressure dressing to the entire thigh to prevent hematoma formation. To harvest rectus fascia, a low transverse abdominal incision is made two fingerbreadths above the pubic symphysis. Using blunt dissection the fat is dissected off underlying rectus fascia to provide exposure to the harvest site. A strip of rectus fascia of the desired size is harvested in a transverse direction using sharp dissection. Published reports describe harvesting grafts ranging in size from full-length strips of 20 cm in length (77) to patch slings as small as 4 cm in length (78). The typical width is 1 to 3 cm. The fascial incision is closed with No. 0 delayed absorbable suture and the abdominal incision is packed until the vaginal portion of the procedure is completed.

After a decision is made about the type of sling material to be used and, in the case of autologous graft, the material has been harvested, the patient is placed in dorsal lithotomy position in high stirrups and the vagina and lower abdomen are prepped and draped. A Foley catheter is inserted and placed to dependent drainage. Preoperative antibiotics should be administered on-call to the operating room and antithrombotic compression devices applied. If rectus fascia has not been pre-

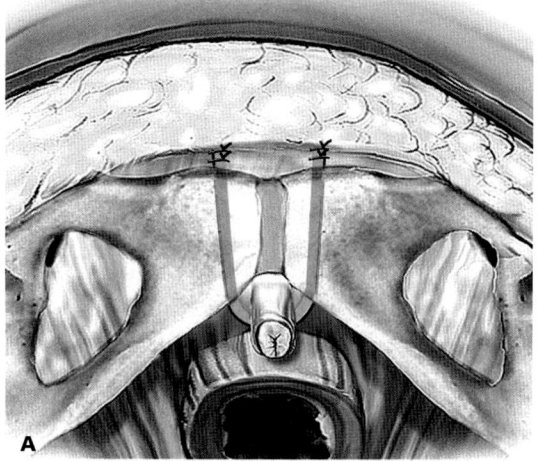

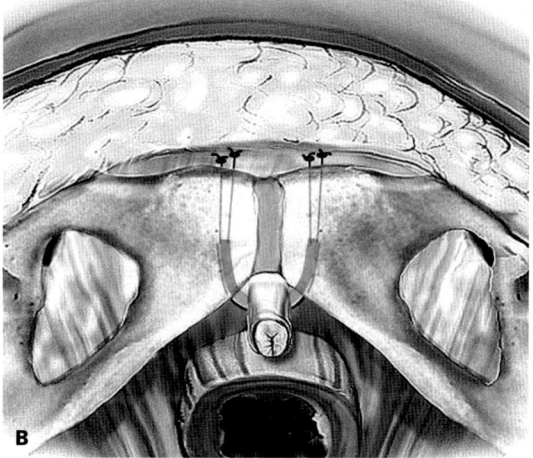

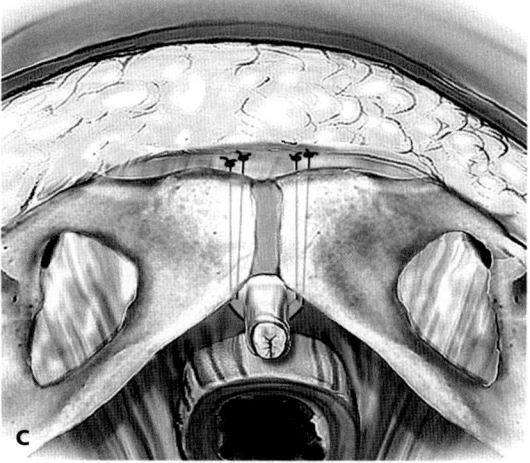

FIGURE 14.3 ● Traditional sling procedure modifications. **(A)** Full-length traditional pubo-vaginal sling. **(B)** Patch sling with the sling arms entering the retropubic space and a "suture bridge" fixing the sling to the rectus fascia. **(C)** Small patch sling with arms that do not enter the retropubic space. (Modified from Walters MD, Karram MM, eds. *Urogynecology and reconstructive pelvic surgery*, 3rd ed. St. Louis: Mosby, 2006.)

viously harvested, a 4-cm low transverse abdominal incision is made just above the pubic bone, carried down to the rectus fascia, and then packed. Attention is turned to the vagina, where a midline incision or an inverted-U incision is made in the vaginal epithelium from the distal urethra to just beyond the UVJ. The vaginal epithelium is dissected from the underlying tissues laterally to the inferior lateral aspect of the pubic rami. Transvaginal perforation of the endopelvic fascia along the posterior surface of the inferior pubic ramus to enter the retropubic space is accomplished using blunt or sharp dissection on each side of the urethra. Once accomplished, the surgeon should be able to easily pass a finger along the back side of the pubic bone to the inferior aspect of the rectus muscle. During this dissection, care should be taken to remain lateral to the urethra and medial to the pubic tubercle to avoid injury to adjacent structures.

Two small stab incisions are made in the rectus fascia just above the pubic symphysis on either side of the midline. Uterine dressing forceps or a needle ligature carrier is passed through the stab incision, behind the pubic bone, and into the vaginal field on each side of the urethra under the guidance of the surgeon's vaginal finger. For a full-length sling, the arms of the sling are grasped by the forceps or attached to the ligature carrier and pulled into the abdominal field. For a patch sling, permanent sutures are fixed to each end of the graft and it is the sutures that are grasped and pulled through to the abdominal field. These permanent sutures will act as a "suture bridge" between the sling and the fixation point at the rectus fascia. The midportion of the sling is placed under the proximal urethra at the level of the UVJ. Some surgeons secure the sling in this location with two to four sutures, while others leave the suburethral portion of the sling unattached. The sling is placed at the desired tension and the arms or suture bridges are secured to the rectus fascia. Cystoscopy is performed to ensure that no bladder or urethral injury has occurred. The abdominal and vaginal incisions are closed. The bladder is drained transurethrally or suprapubically until normal voiding resumes.

Some surgeons prefer to fix the sling arms to the pubic bone or Cooper's ligament rather than the rectus fascia. This can be accomplished using bone anchoring devices or, for fixation to Cooper's ligament, a curved Capio needle driver (Boston Scientific, Natick, MA) The use of these alternative fixation points allows the sling to be placed entirely through the vaginal incision while avoiding the need for the abdominal incision. The potential advantages and disadvantages of using bone anchors have been reviewed by several authors (79–81).

Perhaps the most important step when performing a traditional sling procedure is determining how much tension to apply to the sling when securing the sling arms. Numerous techniques have been described to determine optimal sling tension, including measuring the degree of urethral deflection with a Q-tip, placing a spacer such as a right-angle clamp, Hegar dilator, or cystoscope sheath between the sling and the urethra, and even intraoperative urodynamic assessment of urethral function (82–85). Unfortunately, there is no standardized technique that can be applied to all patients. Generally, slings should be placed loosely so that there is no compression of the urethra at rest. As mentioned previously, in a patient with severe incontinence and compromise to urethral function, it may be desirable to tension the sling tighter so that it is purposefully obstructive. However, these instances are rare and the patient must be willing to accept the possibility of voiding dysfunction requiring regular self-catheterization.

Outcomes

Although one of the most popular procedures for the treatment for SUI, the quality of the evidence regarding the efficacy of traditional sling procedures is, somewhat surprisingly, considerably less than that of retropubic colposuspensions. The Cochrane Collaboration review of traditional sling procedures in 2005 identified 13 randomized trials involving a total of 760 women evaluating this procedure (55). Most of the studies were of small size ($n = 20$ to 165) and poor quality (55). That being said, the level 1 evidence that does exist, along with a large volume of retrospective and prospective cohort studies, do support the conclusion that traditional sling procedures are effective in the management of SUI. Five randomized trials have compared the traditional sling to the retropubic colposuspension, and in each there was no difference in efficacy between the two procedures (86–90). In the majority of the nonrandomized studies in the literature, traditional sling procedures were used as salvage surgery in women who had failed previous continence surgery. In this capacity, the objective cure rates reported in the literature range from 61% to 100%, with a mean cure rate of 85% (91%). While there are fewer studies evaluating traditional slings as first-line therapy for SUI, the reported cure rates as a first operation are 87% to 94% (24,91). As mentioned, the UITN's SISTEr trial, which has randomized 650 women with SUI to either rectus fascia sling or Burch colposuspension, should provide valuable information about the relative merits of these two procedures (56).

Autologous Slings

Autologous rectus fascia and fascia lata are historically the most common materials used for traditional sling procedures. Based on the available evidence, slings using these materials should be considered the "gold standard" to which other slings are compared (24). The primary advantage of using these autologous tissues, as opposed to other sling materials, is that there is a large body of literature supporting their long-term efficacy, there is an exceedingly low risk of graft complications or erosions, and there is no risk of viral transmission, as might be seen from allograft or xenograft. The primary disadvantage of autologous grafts is the increased operating time required to harvest the tissue and the risk of donor site complications. While the objective and subjective cure rates of autologous fascial slings vary in the literature from 50% to 100%, the mean cure rate is approximately 87% (24). Long-term follow-up for as long as 10 years demonstrates minimal decline in continence rates (92–94).

Both rectus fascia and fascia lata appear to have similar tissue properties, although tissue quality may vary from patient to patient. Generally, the tissues remain viable, undergo neovascularization and fibroblastic proliferation with some remodeling, and do not degenerate (95). The degree of fibrosis varies between patients, with some women replacing the fascia with dense fibrosis and others producing only minimal fibrosis (24). Harvesting fascia lata avoids a large abdominal incision but requires a change in patient position and can be associated with incisional leg pain and formation of thigh hematomas and seromas. Rectus fascia harvest is generally easier than harvesting fascia lata, but larger strips for full-length slings are harder to obtain and there may be an increased risk for abdominal wall hernia. Other autologous materials have been used for sling construction, including skin, rectus abdominis muscle flap, aponeurosis of the external oblique muscle, and vaginal wall free graft (55). While some of these alternative materials have been associated with acceptable short-term results, long-term results are unavailable.

Allograft Slings

The motivation for the development of alternative sling materials has been the desire to reduce operative time and eliminate the morbidity associated with autograft harvest. Cadaveric allografts have been used successfully in orthopaedics for over 20 years, and in the past decade they have been adopted for sling procedures. Allograft materials that have been used for slings include cadaveric fascia lata, lyophilized human dura mater, and human acellular dermis. The main advantage of allografts is the elimination of the time and morbidity associated with harvesting autologous fascia.

Allografts also appear to have a very low risk of graft complications, infections, or erosions. The disadvantages of allografts include the potential for tissue antigenicity and rejection, the risk of disease transmission, and the potential for loss of tissue integrity over time. Additionally, there is considerable variation in tissue processing from tissue bank to tissue bank, which may influence allograft quality and strength.

To minimize the risk of disease transmission, allografts are frozen or freeze-dried after harvest, making them essentially acellular. Additionally, serologic screening for human immunodeficiency virus (HIV) and hepatitis B is routinely performed on all cadaveric tissue. To date, there have been no reported cases of disease transmission from an allograft sling (24). False-negative results from viral serologic screens are possible, however. Additionally, cellular DNA has been detected in cadaveric fascia lata and acellular dermis, raising the possibility that disease transmission could occur (96). The risk of HIV transmission from human allografts is estimated at 1 in 8 million (97). The risk of developing Creutzfeldt-Jakob disease (CJD) is approximately 1 in 3.5 million (98).

Cadaveric fascia lata is the most common allograft material used in sling surgery. There are two main techniques of processing this tissue: solvent dehydration with gamma irradiation (Tutoplast [Mentor, Santa Barbara, CA]) and freeze drying (local tissue banks and FasLata [Bard, Covington, GA]) (24). For both preparations, tissue rehydration for 15 to 30 minutes is recommended prior to implantation. Studies by Lemer et al and Hinton et al suggest that the biomechanical properties of solvent-dehydrated fascia lata are superior to those of freeze-dried tissue in terms of maximum load to failure, stiffness, and load/graft width (99–101). Others have found no difference in graft strength between the two methods of processing, however (102).

While most authors report cure rates similar to those of autologous slings, some have reported a high early failure rate, with as many as 20% of subjects developing recurrent incontinence with 3 months of surgery (24). This risk of early failure seems to be primarily associated with freeze-dried preparations (102,103). Fitzgerald et al reported early sling failure in 6 of 35 women who underwent an allograft sling with irradiated freeze-dried cadaveric fascia lata. The mean time to failure was 11.5 weeks (range 1 to 20 weeks). At reoperation, four grafts appeared to have been reabsorbed and two were significantly fragmented (102). Several mechanisms of allograft loss have been proposed, including host-versus-graft reaction, potential accelerated immunity, and autolysis (24). Currently, the processing of cadaveric tissue is not standardized and varies considerably between different companies and tissue banks. It is likely that differences in processing explain, at least in part, the wide differences in success rates experienced with cadaveric fascia lata slings.

Currently, there are no clinical trials comparing cadaveric fascia lata slings to autologous slings. McBride et al retrospectively compared the results of 39 women who underwent an autologous fascia lata sling to 31 women who underwent a sling with solvent-dehydrated cadaveric fascia lata sling (104). Two or more years after surgery, none of the subjects who had an autologous fascia lata sling developed recurrence, compared to 41% who received an allograft sling ($p = 0.007$).

Lyophilized dura mater has been used as a sling material by several authors. With follow-up ranging from 6 to 150 months, the cure rates of lyophilized dura mater slings range from 86% to 94% (24). A small clinical trial ($n = 72$) comparing lyophilized dura sling to the Burch colposuspension found no difference in cure rates between the two procedures at 32 to 48 months; however, those who received a sling had a significantly higher rate of postoperative irritative voiding symptoms (10% vs. 29%) (86). To date, there have been no cases of viral or prion transmission from a urologic procedure using lyophilized dura mater. However, a case of CJD being transmitted to a male who received a dura mater implant 12 years earlier has been reported (105). Acellular cadaveric dermal allografts have also been used for traditional sling procedures. Biomechanical testing demonstrates that dermal allografts are strong, demonstrating similar load-to-failure characteristics as autologous tissues. Dermal grafts appear to maintain their integrity and strength after implantation through neovascularization and host incorporation (24). The short-term success with dermal allografts appears promising (80% to 95% cure); however, no long-term data is available (106–108).

In summary, the use of cadaveric allograft material for traditional slings has the potential to decrease operative time and eliminate the morbidity associated with autograft harvest. However, there is considerable variation in tissue processing, which may affect the integrity and long-term durability of the sling. This appears to be particularly true for cadaveric fascia lata that is freeze-dried. For slings made with other allograft material, the short-term success rates approach that of autologous slings; however, studies of long-term success (beyond 2 years) are generally lacking. Disease transmission with cadaveric tissues appears to be exceedingly rare but can occur.

Xenograft Slings

As with allografts, animal tissues have become widely available and are being increasingly adapted to pelvic reconstructive surgery. Xenograft materials that have been used for traditional slings include porcine dermis, porcine small intestinal submucosa (SIS), and bovine pericardium. Slings using xenograft material have many of the same advantages and disadvantages that are associated with slings using allograft materials. The manufacturers claim that each of these tissues is biocompatible, has excellent tensile strength, is nonimmunogenic, and is devoid of viruses or prions. The published evidence supporting these claims is limited, however (24).

At present, the only tissue with long-term follow-up data available is porcine dermis. Nicholson et al followed 24 women who underwent a traditional sling procedure with porcine dermis for a mean of 49 months (range 12 to 132 months) and reported a 79.2% cure rate (109). Interestingly, they also noted the development of delayed urinary retention developing 1 or more years after surgery in 13%, suggesting there may be some tissue shrinkage associated with this material. Abdel-Fattah et al randomized 142 women with SUI to receive a sling with porcine dermis (Pelvicol [Bard, Covington, GA]) or a TVT (110). After a median follow-up of 36 months, the cure rates were 82% and 88%, respectively ($p = $ NS). Delayed retention was not observed in this study and the rate of voiding dysfunction was similar between the two groups.

Porcine SIS has more recently been marketed for use in sling surgery. After the intestinal submucosa is harvested, the tissue is processed so that the cellular material is removed and only the extracellular matrix remains, along with associated growth factors. SIS is somewhat unusual among biologic grafts in that it acts as a tissue scaffold that over time is completely degraded and replaced by the host's connective tissue. How this affects the strength and long-term durability of the graft is largely unknown. Kubricht et al found that the mean pullout load for SIS was less than freeze-dried cadaveric fascia lata (111).

There are currently two retrospective case series of slings using SIS for the treatment of SUI in the literature (112,113). These studies report a success rate of 79.2% to 94% 2 to 3 years after surgery. Given the relative paucity of long-term data (4 years or longer) on slings using xenograft materials, the Third Consultation on Incontinence has recommended that they not be used outside of a well-constructed research trial until high-level evidence comparing the different types of biological materials is available (24).

Synthetic Slings

The use of permanent synthetic materials for traditional sling procedures has several potential advantages over autologous slings and slings using biologic grafts. Synthetic materials are readily available, have consistent and durable strength, have no potential for infectious disease transmission, avoid the time and potential morbidity of tissue harvest, and are relatively inexpensive. The primary disadvantage of synthetic slings, however, is the potential for mesh complications such as erosion, infections, sinus tract formation, and fistulas. Historically, these types of complications have been seen in as many as 14% to 23% of patients, causing many surgeons to abandon the use of permanent synthetic materials for sling procedures (114–116). More recently, however, there has been a considerable improvement in our understanding of mesh properties that encourage biocompatibility and minimize the risk of mesh complications. With the adoption of newer materials, particularly loosely knitted, macroporous monofilament polypropylene mesh, the rate of erosions and mesh complications has decreased to 1% to 2% (117).

In addition to the biochemical makeup of a synthetic material, the properties that appear to be important for predicting biocompatibility and potential complications include type of pore size and filamentous structure (monofilament vs. multifilament). A classification scheme based on these properties has been developed (118). Pore sizes larger than 75 microns are considered "macroporous." This pore size is thought to be clinically significant because it is the size required for the admission of macrophages, fibroblasts, blood vessels, and collagen fibrils (118). Thus, pore sizes smaller than this may inhibit tissue ingrowth and decrease the host immune response to infections. Multifilament meshes typically have interstices within the filamentous fibers that can be smaller than 10 microns. As with microporous materials, these small interstices allow entry of bacteria (as small as 1 micron) and prevent access of host immune cells. Type I meshes are macroporous and monofilament. It is type I mesh materials that are preferred for vaginal placement because they are thought to have the lowest risk of erosion and infection. Type II mesh is microporous, with pore sizes less than 10 microns. Type III meshes are multifilament materials. Type IV meshes are

"coated" biomaterials that contain submicronic (less than 1 pore size). A more detailed discussion of synthetic mesh properties can be found in Chapter 32, Sutures and Grafts in Pelvic Reconstructive Surgery.

In the 1980s and early 1990s, the use of type II and III synthetic meshes such as Dacron, Mersilene, and Gore-tex was common and associated with significant mesh complications. Largely with the introduction of the TVT procedure in 1997, loosely knitted monofilament polypropylene meshes have gained popularity. The large worldwide experience with this procedure has confirmed a low erosion rate with this material, with more serious mesh complications being exceedingly rare. The size of the mesh and the location where the mesh is placed almost certainly play a role in the risk of mesh complications, however. Unlike the smaller pieces of mesh (1 to 2 cm in width) placed under the urethra for slings, which have erosion rates of less than 2%, large sheets of polypropylene mesh placed in the anterior and posterior vaginal wall at the time of prolapse surgery are associated with mesh erosion rates of 6% to 12% (119).

Complications

Generally, the rate of surgical complications associated with traditional sling procedures is no higher than that of other continence operations (24,120). In fact, the wound complication rate associated with slings is lower than that of open retropubic colpsuspensions (55). Although some early series suggested a greater complication rate with sling procedures than retropubic colposuspensions, this is most likely due to a difference in surgical indications for the two procedures. Many patients in the early sling series had prior failed procedures, which can be associated with periurethral and retropubic scarring and an increased complication rate. More recent series in which traditional sling procedures were used as primary operations demonstrate a lower complication rate similar to that of other procedures (24,55). The bladder injury rate is approximately 2% after traditional sling procedures, making routine intraoperative cystoscopy essential for this procedure.

As with the Burch colposuspension, the most common chronic complications after traditional sling procedures are voiding dysfunction and de novo irritative voiding symptoms. In his 1994 systematic review, Jarvis found a mean incidence of voiding disorders of 12.8% (range 2% to 37%) (91). Such symptoms may include positional voiding, a feeling of incomplete emptying, hesitancy, intermittent urinary stream, the need to use the Credé maneuver to void, or even complete retention. The recent emphasis on avoiding excess sling tension has likely lowered the voiding dysfunction rate after sling procedures substantially, however. In fact, more recent series report chronic voiding dysfunction rates between 2% and 10% (24). Preoperative factors that have been associated with delayed postoperative voiding after traditional sling procedures include advanced age, low flow rates (less than 20 mL/sec), and concomitant prolapse surgery (121). Patients with elevated postvoid residual volumes, weak detrusor contractions, and low flow rates preoperatively are likely to be at increased risk of postoperative urinary retention; however, this has not been consistently demonstrated in the literature. Urinary retention or bothersome voiding symptoms that persist beyond 6 weeks postoperatively are unlikely to resolve spontaneously and usually require management with intermittent self-catheterization or urethrolysis. Urethrolysis after a traditional sling procedure is most easily accomplished transvaginally and usually results in resolution of voiding symptoms. The rate of recurrent stress incontinence after a sling release is approximately 15% (122–125).

Irritative voiding symptoms such as urgency, frequency, nocturia, dysuria, and urge incontinence have been report to occur in 3% to 30% of patients after a traditional sling procedure (24,55,120). Urodynamic evaluation may or may not demonstrate de novo detrusor instability. A systematic review performed by the American Urological Association found the incidence of de novo detrusor instability to be 7% (95% CI 3% to 11%) (71%). Several hypotheses exist to explain these new irritative symptoms, including an unmasking of pre-existing detrusor overactivity, local irritation, foreign body reaction, denervation, and partial urethral obstruction. After ruling out an infection, first-line therapy for these de novo symptoms includes standard medical and behavioral treatment. Some patients will not respond to conservative therapy, however. Cystoscopy is often warranted in these patients to rule out an erosion of the sling material into the bladder or urethra. Refractory urge incontinence has been reported to occur in as many as 6% to 24% of patients after a sling procedure, although most authors report a lower incidence than this (24). In patients with persistent bothersome irritative bladder symptoms that are refractory to conservative therapy, a urethrolysis should be considered. As with urethrolysis for urinary retention, patients should be counseled about the possibility of recurrent stress incontinence.

TENSION-FREE VAGINAL TAPE

Since its introduction in 1996 by Ulmsten et al, the TVT procedure has gained worldwide popularity and may be the continence operation most commonly performed today (16). The popularity of this minimally invasive sling procedure is largely due to its ability to be performed in an ambulatory setting without the delayed voiding seen in many other procedures. Cure rates for the TVT appear to be similar to that of the Burch colposuspension and traditional sling procedures (17,18,24,126). While based on the traditional sling technique, TVT has several characteristics that make it unique, including placement of the sling at the midurethra, sling arms that are "self-fixing" and do not require suturing of fixation to the rectus fascia, the use of trocars that pass the sling from the urethra to the abdomen ("down-to-up" trocar passage), the use of loosely knitted polypropylene mesh for the sling material, and "tension-free" placement (Table 14.2). TVT is indicated for the primary treatment of SUI with urethral hypermobility. There is some evidence that it may also have a role as a salvage operation in subjects who have failed previous SUI surgery and in the treatment of ISD. TVT is not recommended in women without urethral hypermobility, however.

Mechanism

Petros and Ulmsten developed the TVT procedure based a theory of pathophysiology of SUI that they termed the "integral theory" (127). In their integral theory, SUI is the result of impairment of the pubourethral ligament supporting the urethra to the pubic bone. The goal of the TVT is "correction of inadequate urethral support from the pubourethral vesical ligaments" (16,127). The TVT is placed under the midurethra where, based on urethral pressure profilometry, the pubourethral ligaments are assumed to have their functional attachment. Recent anatomic and radiologic studies have questioned the importance of the pubourethral ligaments in maintaining continence. A recent anatomic study by Fritsh et al concluded that the female urethra has no direct ligamentous fixation to the pubic bone (128). They did identify "delicate cords" of smooth muscle running from the pubic bone to the bladder neck, which they proposed should be called the "pubovesical muscles" rather than pubourethral ligaments. They concluded that because of the low content of connective tissue and small dimensions of these structures, they cannot be considered a supportive structure of the urethra

TABLE 14.2

Comparison of the Tension-Free Vaginal Tape (TVT) to Traditional Sling Procedures

	Traditional Sling	Tension-free Vaginal Tape (TVT)
Sling placement (urethra)	Bladder neck	Midurethra
Sling arms	Fixed to rectus fascia or pubic bone	Self-fixing
Sling material	Variable	1 cm × 40 cm polypropylene mesh
Instrument passage through retropubic space	Abdomen to vagina ("up to down") with guidance from the surgeon's fingers	Vagina to abdomen ("down to up"); passed blindly
Sling tension	Variable	Tension-free
Mechanism of Cure:		
Repositions bladder neck?	Yes	No
Urethral compression?	Variable	No
Urethral kinking with stress?	??	Yes

(128). Similarly, magnetic resonance imaging and sonographic data demonstrate that the urethra is a mobile structure that can be moved up and down and is not fixed to the pubic bone (129,130). These findings suggest that the "integral theory" may not provide the best explanation for the efficacy of the TVT procedure.

A more plausible mechanism of action is that of transient urethral kinking during stress. Unlike traditional sling procedures or retropubic colposuspensions, the efficacy of the TVT does not appear to be related to correction of urethral hypermobility. Most patients with urethral hypermobility preoperatively will continue to have urethral hypermobility postoperatively while still achieving high cure rates (131). Ultrasound studies demonstrate that during Valsalva or a cough, dynamic urethral kinking occurs after a TVT, with the suburethral portion of the TVT serving as the fulcrum (132,133). At rest, there is no compression or kinking of the urethra. This suggests that urethral mobility may be important in the mechanism of action of the TVT. Urodynamic studies demonstrate an increase in pressure transmission ratios after a TVT with no change in maximum urethral closure pressure (134). Although midurethral placement is often emphasized, postoperative ultrasonography demonstrates marked variation of sling placement relative to the urethra, with little apparent effect on symptoms or continence rates (135,136). Dietz et al noted a weak association between irritative voiding symptoms and proximal urethral placement, however (135).

Technique

In their original description of the TVT technique, Ulmsten et al used local anesthesia with intravenous sedation (16). General or regional anesthesia is also acceptable. After anesthesia is satisfactorily obtained, the patient is placed in the dorsal lithotomy position in high stirrups and the vagina and lower abdomen are prepped and draped. An 18-French Foley catheter is inserted and placed to dependent drainage. Preoperative antibiotics should be administered on-call to the operating room and antithrombotic compression devices applied.

Using a marking pen, the sites for the two 1-cm suprapubic stab incisions are marked just superior to the pubic symphysis two fingerbreadths lateral to the midline on each side. Local anesthetic such as 1% lidocaine is injected at the two suprapubic sites, 10 mL on each side. Using a spinal needle, the injection is carried down behind the pubic bone and should include the rectus muscle, fascia, and skin. Attention is then turned to the vagina, where a weighted speculum is placed for exposure. The site for the 1.5-cm midurethral incision is marked vertically beginning 1 cm from the external urethral meatus. Local anesthetic (10 mL) with dilute epinephrine (1:200,000) is infiltrated in the anterior vaginal wall at the location of the urethral incision site and laterally to the inferior pubic rami for hydrodissection and hemostasis. Provided the maximum dose of lidocaine is not exceeded, a large-volume infiltration of a dilute mixture (1/4% with 1/200,000 to 1/400,000 epinephrine) retropubically and vaginally (100 mL in all) may provide improved hydrodissection to help prevent bladder perforation. The urethral incision is made and dissection is carried laterally with Metzenbaum scissors to create a tunnel to the inferior pubic ramus on each side of the urethra.

The TVT kit (Ethicon Inc., Somerville, NJ) includes two curved stainless steel trocars connected by a 1-cm × 40-cm piece of polypropylene mesh encased in a plastic sheath as well as a nondisposable handle that attaches to the trocars (Fig. 14.4). The plastic sheath covering the mesh consists of two pieces that overlap in the midline, allowing for easy removal after the sling is placed. A hemostat placed in the middle of the sling in the area of overlap is useful for marking the midline and preventing sheath slippage during placement. One of the two trocars is attached to the trocar handle. Prior to each trocar passage, the bladder is drained and a rigid catheter guide is placed in the Foley catheter and directed to the ipsilateral side of trocar placement to displace the UVJ away from the path of the trocar.

The trocar handle is held in the hand contralateral to the side of trocar placement while the thumb of the ipsilateral hand stabilizes the trocar as it curves into the vagina and the index finger maintains proper alignment of the tip. The tip of the trocar is placed in the periurethral tunnel and directed toward the patient's ipsilateral shoulder and the marked suprapubic exit site. The endopelvic fascia is perforated and the trocar is directed along the back of the pubic symphysis to exit at the previously marked abdominal incision sites (Fig. 14.5). After each trocar is placed, the urethral catheter is removed and the bladder is inspected with a 70-degree cystoscope. It is important that the bladder is filled to capacity during cystoscopic inspection so that a bladder perforation is not missed behind a mucosal fold. The area at highest risk for bladder perforation is the anterolateral portion of the bladder dome.

After bladder integrity is confirmed, the handle is detached from the trocar and the trocar is pulled through the abdominal incision. The encased mesh is clamped just below the trocar and cut so that the trocar can be removed from the operative field. The second trocar is then placed on the opposite side using the same technique. Should bladder perforation occur, the trocar is withdrawn, the bladder is

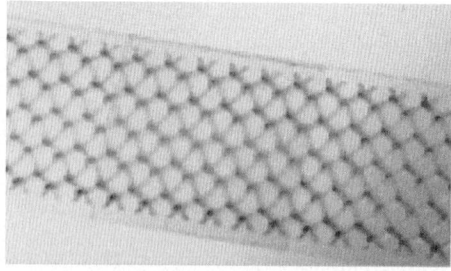

A

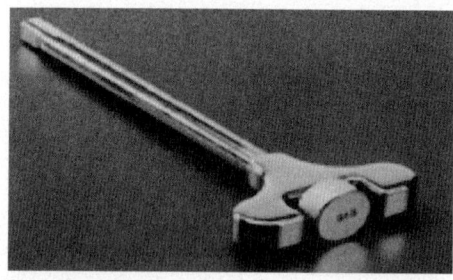

B

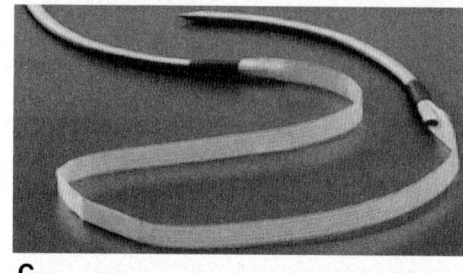

C

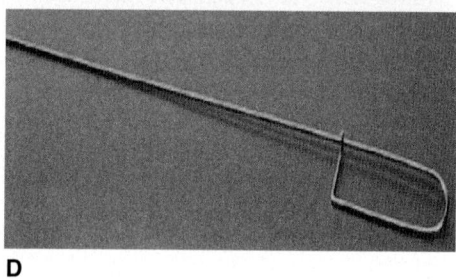

D

FIGURE 14.4 ● The tension-free vaginal tape (TVT) device. **(A)** Loosely knitted polypropylene mesh tape. **(B)** Introducer. **(C)** TVT needles with attached mesh encased in a plastic sheath. **(D)** Rigid catheter guide. (Reproduced with permission from Ethicon Inc., Somerville, NJ.)

drained, the appropriate landmarks are reviewed, and a second attempt at trocar placement is made, taking care to stay as close as possible to the back of the pubic bone. As the typical TVT bladder injury is small (1 cm), extraperitoneal, and in the bladder dome, it is usually unnecessary to perform any type of repair. Some surgeons prefer to drain the bladder for 24 to 48 hours after such an injury, but it is not clear if even this is necessary.

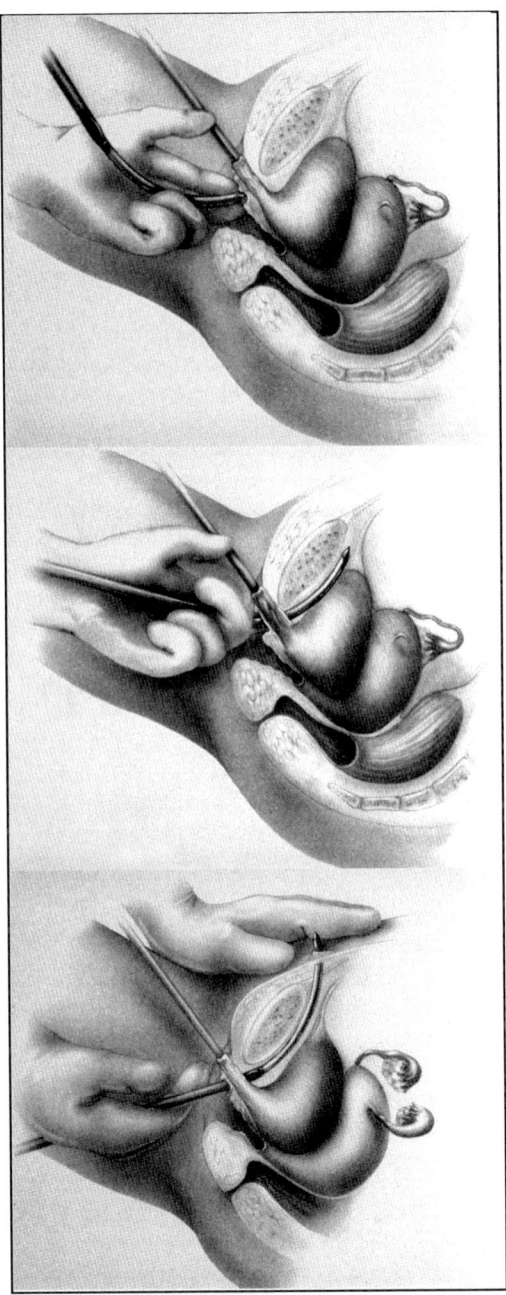

FIGURE 14.5 ● TVT trocar introduced into the periurethral incision (*top*), passing through the retropubic space along the inside of the pubic symphysis (*middle*) to exit at the previously marked abdominal incision sites (*bottom*). (Reproduced with permission from Ethicon Inc., Somerville, NJ.)

The tension of the TVT sling is adjusted so that it allows for dynamic urethral kinking while avoiding any compression of the urethra at rest. If the procedure is performed using local anesthesia, the patient is asked to cough repeatedly with a bladder volume of 250 to 300 mL. The sling is tightened so that a few drops of urine are present at the external meatus during coughing. This ensures that the sling is not too tight and minimizes the risk of urinary retention. If general anesthesia is used, the sling is tightened empirically without the benefit of the cough test. Some surgeons use a spacer such as a Mayo scissor, a size 10 Hegar dilator, or their index finger between the urethra and the sling to adjust the TVT to the appropriate tension. Others use a Credé maneuver with a full bladder to simulate a Valsalva maneuver. In patients who receive regional anesthesia, any of the above techniques may be used, depending upon the patient's level of consciousness and ability to perform forceful cough or Valsalva. The use of the cough test to guide TVT tensioning was originally thought to be an important component of the TVT procedure; however, numerous authors have reported high cure rates with a low incidence of voiding dysfunction in patients who received general anesthesia or when the cough test was otherwise omitted (62,110,137–139). Some authors have found that when compared with general anesthesia, the use of local anesthesia with a cough test improved continence rates, while others have found no relationship between anesthesia type and TVT efficacy (140,141). Adamiak et al randomized 103 women with SUI to undergo a TVT with either local anesthetic or spinal anesthesia and found no difference in efficacy or safety between the two types of anesthesia (137). No randomized trials have compared different methods of TVT tensioning.

Once the desired tension is achieved, the sheath encasing the sling is removed while stabilizing the sling below the urethra. The abdominal ends of the sling are cut below the skin surface and the incisions are closed with 4-0 absorbable suture, Steristrips, or skin adhesive. The vaginal incision is closed with 2-0 or 3-0 absorbable suture in a running fashion. If the TVT is performed in isolation, the patient can attempt to void in the recovery room. If she voids successfully, she can be discharged home without bladder drainage. It is prudent to check at least one postvoid residual prior to discharging the patient home. If the TVT is performed in conjunction with other pelvic reconstructive surgery, effective voiding in the immediate postoperative period is unlikely and postoperative bladder drainage with a transurethral or suprapubic catheter or intermittent self-catheterization is usually necessary for a few days.

Outcomes

More than 300 articles have been published on the TVT procedure, including 14 randomized trials, making it one of the most studied surgical procedures for the treatment of SUI. The currently available data suggests that TVT has short- and medium-term efficacy similar to that of the open Burch colposuspension but is associated with shorter operating times, less delayed voiding, and quicker recovery (24). The reported cure rates range from 63% to 97% depending upon the outcome measured and the length of follow-up (17,24,62). A prospective study of 129 women treated with TVT noted a negative pad test in 81% and negative cough stress test in 74% of subjects 6 years after surgery (142). Efficacy data with follow-up of 10 years or more, such as is available for the Burch colposuspension and the autologous sling, is not yet available for the TVT.

Four clinical trials have compared TVT to open Burch colposuspension with follow-up ranging from 6 months to 2 years. Each found no significant difference in efficacy rates between the two procedures (17,18,126,138). The UK TVT Trial randomized 344 women with urodynamic SUI to receive either a TVT or open Burch colposuspension, making it one of the largest trials for the surgical management of SUI. Six months after surgery, objective and subjective outcomes were not significantly different between the two procedures (57). At the 2-year follow-up, 81% of the Burch group and 80% of the TVT group who were available for follow-up were objectively cured (negative 1-hour pad test) (17). Only 20% of subjects in the Burch group and 25% of subjects in the TVT group reported no leakage under any circumstance 2 years after surgery, however. Bladder injury was more common in the TVT group (9% vs. 3%). However, TVT was associated with less blood loss, shorter operating time, shorter hospital stay, quicker return to normal activities, and less delayed voiding (57). Additionally, an economic analysis of this trial found TVT to be cost-saving when compared to the Burch colposuspension (143).

Three trials have compared the TVT to the laparoscopic Burch colposuspension (62,144,145). A multicenter study performed by Paraiso et al randomized 72 women to one of these two procedures and followed them for an average of 21 months (range 6 to 43) (62). TVT was associated with a lower rate of urodynamic SUI than the la-

paroscopic Burch colposuspension 1 year after surgery (3.2% vs. 18%). Similarly, those who received a TVT were less likely to develop subjective incontinence (stress and urge) than those who received a laparoscopic Burch procedure. The operating time was shorter for the TVT group; however, the hospital stay, duration of catheter use, blood loss, and procedure cost were similar. Valpas et al also found a higher objective and subjective cure rate after TVT than with laparoscopic Burch colposuspension (145).

Thus far, TVT has been compared to sling procedures in only two trials. Abdel-Fattah et al randomized 142 women with urodynamic stress incontinence to either a TVT or a Pelvicol pubovaginal sling (110). Three years after surgery, the subjective continence rate and patient satisfaction were similar between the two procedures. Similarly, Wadie et al found no difference in incontinence cure between rectus fascia sling and TVT; however, subjects were followed for only 6 months (146).

Factors that may negatively influence the success of the TVT procedure include increasing body mass index (BMI), preoperative overactive bladder symptoms, and presence of a nonmobile urethra. A prospective nonrandomized comparison of TVT and a traditional sling procedure with polypropylene mesh found that TVT performed better in patients with lower BMI (less than 27 kg/m^2), while the sling procedure had greater efficacy in patients with higher BMIs (147). Rafii et al prospectively compared the success of TVT in 149 normal and overweight women to 30 obese (BMI more than 30 kg/m^2) women and found that obese women had a higher rate of postoperative urge incontinence (18% vs. 5%, $p = 0.02$), with no effect on objective or subjective cure of SUI (148). In contrast, retrospective studies have demonstrated satisfactory efficacy for TVT in obese women comparable to that of nonobese women (149).

Davis et al evaluated predictors of patient satisfaction after TVT in a prospective cohort of 97 women (150). They found that the only preoperative predictors of decreased satisfaction 1 year after surgery were symptoms of overactive bladder or voiding difficulty before surgery. While several studies have demonstrated similar cure rates in women with mixed urinary incontinence symptoms preoperatively to those with pure stress incontinence symptoms (35,151,152), a recent study suggests that those with mixed incontinence symptoms have a higher failure rate in the long term. Holgrom et al surveyed 760 women 2 to 8 years after their TVT procedure. Those with pure stress incontinence had a persistent cure rate of

85% during the follow-up period. Women with mixed incontinence had persistent cure rates of 60% up to 4 years postoperatively, which declined to 30% 4 to 8 years after surgery (36). Most of the recurrence appeared to be related to urge incontinence symptoms.

Preoperative urethral immobility (urethral straining angle less than 30 degrees) is associated with TVT success rates of less than 50% and should probably be considered a contraindication for this procedure (131,132,153). The results of TVT in women with ISD and urethral hypermobility vary considerably in the literature. Some studies have found similar cure rates in women with low-pressure urethra compared to women with normal urethral closure pressures (154,155), while others have found low maximum urethral closure pressures to be an independent risk factor for treatment failure (156). This is likely due to differences in definitions of ISD and the difficulties in making measurements of urethral insufficiency, as was discussed earlier in the chapter.

Several studies suggest that TVT is effective as a salvage surgery in women who have failed previous surgical treatment, at least in the short term. A retrospective multicenter study of 245 consecutive women with urodynamic stress incontinence treated with TVT found that cure rates in women with recurrent SUI after previous surgical treatment were similar to those with primary SUI (85% vs. 87%) after a mean follow-up of 38 weeks

(157). Similarly, two prospective studies of women with recurrent SUI treated with TVT with mean follow-ups beyond 4 years found success rates of 82% and 84.7% (158,159). It is worth noting that in these studies the previously failed surgery was always something other than TVT. The use of TVT as a salvage surgery for someone who has failed a previous TVT has not been studied.

Complications

One of the aspects of the TVT procedure that differentiates it from more traditional continence procedures is the blind trocar passage through the retropubic space. This blind trocar passage has been the source of some concern, particularly with regard to perioperative complications. Generally, the complication rate with the TVT procedure is low, however, perhaps even lower than the Burch colposuspension or traditional sling procedures. The complication rates noted in nationwide registries from Finland and Austria are shown in Table 14.3. The one complication that occurs more frequently with TVT than with other procedures is bladder injury, the rate of which ranges from 2.9% to 9% in the literature (57,160,161). Fortunately, the long-term sequelae from these bladder perforations appear to be minimal, assuming they are identified intraoperatively. Trocar injuries to the bladder are typically small and extraperitoneal, requiring no intervention other than replacement of

TABLE 14.3

Complications of the Tension-Free Vaginal Tape Procedure (TVT) in Two Nationwide Registries

	Austrian TVT Registry (161)	Finnish nationwide TVT study (160)
n	5,578	1,455
Bladder perforation	2.7%	3.8%
Urethral injury	0 %	0.1%
Bowel perforation	0.02%	0%
Increased blood loss	1.9%	1.9%
Retropubic hematoma	1.1%	1.9%
Reoperation for hematoma	0.8%	0.5%
Blood transfusion	0.3%	0.3%
Mesh erosion	0.7%	0.1%
Reoperation for voiding dysfunction	1.3%	2.3%
Urinary tract infection	4.1%	17%
Vesicovaginal fistula	0%	0.1%

the trocar in the proper location. Trocar injuries of the bowel and major blood vessels have been reported but are exceedingly rare (160,161).

On average, the intraoperative blood loss from a TVT is less than that from an open or laparoscopic Burch colposuspension (57,62). The rate of postoperative bleeding and retropubic hematomas appears to be higher with the TVT, however (57). The blood transfusion rate after a TVT ranges from 0.3% to 0.6% in large series (162). Postoperative hematomas develop in up to 4.1% of patients; however, the majority can be managed expectantly (162,163). Correct orientation of the TVT trocar during placement is critical for avoiding cystotomy and damage to major blood vessels. The orientation of the trocar and handle is best kept slightly lateral to the midline sagittal plane, directed to the ipsilateral shoulder during retropubic passage (164). Care must be taken to minimize external or internal rotation of the device, as the average distance to major vascular structures ranges from 3.2 to 4.9 cm away from the proper trocar path (164) (Fig. 14.6).

Generally, return to normal voiding occurs quicker with the TVT than with more traditional continence procedures (24,57). Short-term voiding dysfunction has been reported in 4% to 17% of women (24). Over 80% of women with short-term voiding dysfunction will have resolution of their symptoms by 6 weeks after surgery (165). Urinary retention requiring transection of the tape occurs in 1% to 5% of subjects (160,161,165,166). The risk of urinary retention is greater in women who have had a previous incontinence procedure (odds ratio 2.9) than in women treated for primary SUI (165). In women with prolonged urinary retention, transvaginal transection of the TVT tape almost universally resolves the voiding dysfunction, with only a small proportion developing recurrent SUI. De novo urinary urgency after TVT has been reported at rates similar to or lower than that of other continence operations (24,57).

The rate of vaginal mesh erosion or exposure after TVT is 1% or less (17,160,161). This rate is lower than that typically reported for traditional slings using synthetic materials and is likely the result of a combination of factors, including the use of monofilament, loosely knitted polypropylene mesh, and a small vaginal incision with minimal dissection. In patients who are asymptomatic and have small (less than 1 cm) erosions, topical estrogen therapy and observation may result in re-epithelialization. In symptomatic patients and those with larger erosions, a reoperation to excise the ex-

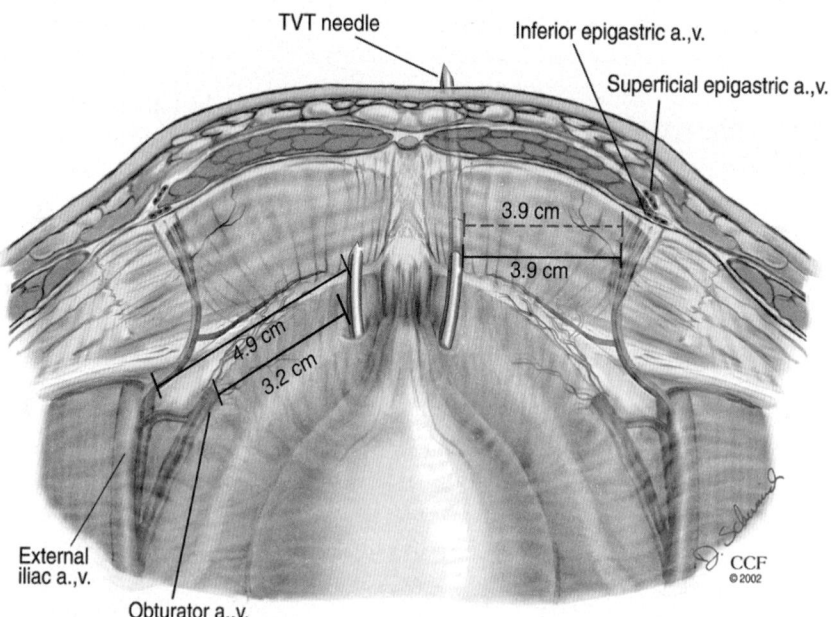

FIGURE 14.6 ● The relationship of the tension-free vaginal tape (TVT) needle to the vascular anatomy of the anterior abdominal wall and retropubic space. Numbers represent the mean distance from the lateral aspect of the TVT needle to the medial edge of the vessels. a = artery; v = vein. (From Muir TW, Tulikangas PK, Fidela Paraiso M, et al. The relationship of tension-free vaginal tape insertion and the vascular anatomy. *Obstet Gynecol* 2003;101:933–936.)

posed mesh and reapproximate the vaginal epithelium is required. Excision of a larger portion of the mesh or the entire sling is necessary only in cases of severe infection or intractable pain. Mesh erosions into the bladder and urethra have occurred but are very rare. The presence of the TVT mesh in the bladder or urethra in the postoperative period is more likely the result of intraoperative perforation that was missed during cystoscopy than a postoperative erosion.

Other Midurethral Slings

The popularity and commercial success of the TVT has led a number of companies to develop their own midurethral slings. All are minimally invasive, intended to be performed as ambulatory procedures, are placed at the midurethra, and have self-fixing arms. Each has modifications that differentiate it from the TVT. In some, the trocars are passed from the abdomen to the vagina ("up to down" trocar passage; SPARC [American Medical Systems, Minnetonka, MN]) rather than the "down to up" passage used in the TVT. Others allow trocar passage in either direction (Uretex [Bard Urological, Covington, GA]). Some use a multifilament, more tightly woven polypropylene (anterior intravaginal slingplasty [anterior IVS; US Surgical, Chicago, IL]) and others a biological graft (Sabre [Mentor, Santa Barbara, CA; PelviLace [Bard Urological, Covington, GA]). In general, there are very few studies evaluating the safety and efficacy of these non-TVT midurethral slings. Thus, it is unclear if these procedures offer any advantages or disadvantages over the TVT for the surgical management of SUI.

The majority of the studies investigating the alternative midurethral slings evaluated the SPARC procedure and anterior IVS procedure. Dietz et al retrospectively compared 37 women who underwent a SPARC procedure to 63 who received a TVT (167). The subjective cure rate of the two procedures was similar, but the objective cure rate was higher in those who received a TVT. Translabial ultrasound demonstrated that the SPARC tape was situated more cranially at rest and was more mobile than the TVT (167). Three small randomized trials with short-term follow-up have compared the SPARC to the TVT, and each has demonstrated no significant differences in cure rates (139,168,169). However, Tseng et al reported a higher bladder injury rate with SPARC than with the TVT (12.9% vs. 0%) (169). The SUSPEND trial randomized 195 women with urodynamic stress incontinence to receive a SPARC, TVT, or anterior IVS (139). There was a trend for a lower objective cure rate with the SPARC procedure

at short-term (6 to 12 weeks) follow-up (cure rates: 72.4%, 87.9%, and 81.5%, respectively, $p = 0.11$), and SPARC was associated with a significantly greater mesh erosion rate that the other two procedures (13.1% vs. 3.3% and 1.7%, $p = 0.04$) (139). The bladder injury rate for the three procedures was similar. Rechberger et al performed a clinical trial comparing TVT to the anterior IVS and found similar cure rates (170). Subjects who received an anterior IVS were more likely to void on the day of surgery than those who received a TVT. Several retrospective studies have demonstrated a higher mesh erosion rate with anterior IVS than with TVT, with one study demonstrating an erosion rate of 14.2% with the IVS (171,172). This is thought to be due to the multifilament nature of the IVS mesh. Properly designed clinical trials with larger sample sizes and longer follow-up are necessary to accurately compare the relative merits of these alternative midurethral slings to the TVT procedure.

TRANSOBTURATOR SLINGS

In 2001, Delorme described the transobturator suburethral sling (20). Like the TVT, this is a minimally invasive midurethral sling using a synthetic tape; however, it is placed using a transobturator approach rather than a retropubic one. Placement of the transobturator tape (TOT) involves the blind passage of a curved trocar from just lateral to the labia majora, around the ischiopubic ramus, and through the obturator foramen to pass into the anterior vaginal wall at the level of the midurethra (20,173). This is the so-called outside-in approach. Techniques using a inside-out approach in which the trocar is passed from the periurethral incision around the ischiopubic ramus to an incision on the inner thigh have also been described (174). The anatomic approach of the TOT differs from other sling procedures because the retropubic space is not entered. Additionally, the relationship between the sling and the urethra is different for the TOT than for other slings. In other sling techniques, including the TVT, the sling axis is roughly vertical in relation to the urethral axis (173). In contrast, the axis of the TOT is more horizontal in relation to the urethral axis. As such, the TOT provides less circumferential compression of the urethra than do traditional slings and the TVT.

Potential advantages of the TOT include a reduction in the incidence of bladder, bowel, and major vascular injuries compared to TVT. There is also some data to suggest that the TOT results in less voiding dysfunction and postoperative irritative bladder symptoms than the TVT and traditional sling procedures (175). Potential disadvantages include the risk of leg or obturator compartment injuries, including hematomas and abscesses. Additionally it is possible that the decreased urethral compression noted with the TOT may translate into lower cure rates for SUI. Initial studies of this approach have been promising (176–178), but there is very little data yet available comparing the efficacy of the TOT to other standard procedures. Some authors have suggested the TOT may have inferior efficacy in patients with ISD (32). Large properly designed clinical trials are necessary to determine the role of TOT in the treatment of SUI.

Obturator Anatomy

Because of the increased popularity of the TOT technique, pelvic surgeons should develop an intimate knowledge of obturator compartment anatomy in order to properly perform this procedure

and/or manage its complications (Fig. 14.7). The obturator membrane is a fibrous sheath that spans the obturator foramen, through which the obturator neurovascular bundle penetrates via the obturator canal. The obturator internus muscle lies on the superior (intrapelvic) side of the obturator membrane. The obturator internus origin is on the inferior margin of the superior pubic ramus and the pelvic surface of the obturator membrane. Its tendon passes through the lesser sciatic foramen to insert onto the greater trochanter of the femur to laterally rotate the thigh. The obturator artery and vein originate as branches of the internal iliac vessels. As they emerge from the cranial side of the obturator membrane via the obturator canal and enter the obturator space, they divide into many small branches supplying the muscles of the adductor compartment of the thigh (Fig. 14.8). Recent cadaver work by Whiteside et al has con-

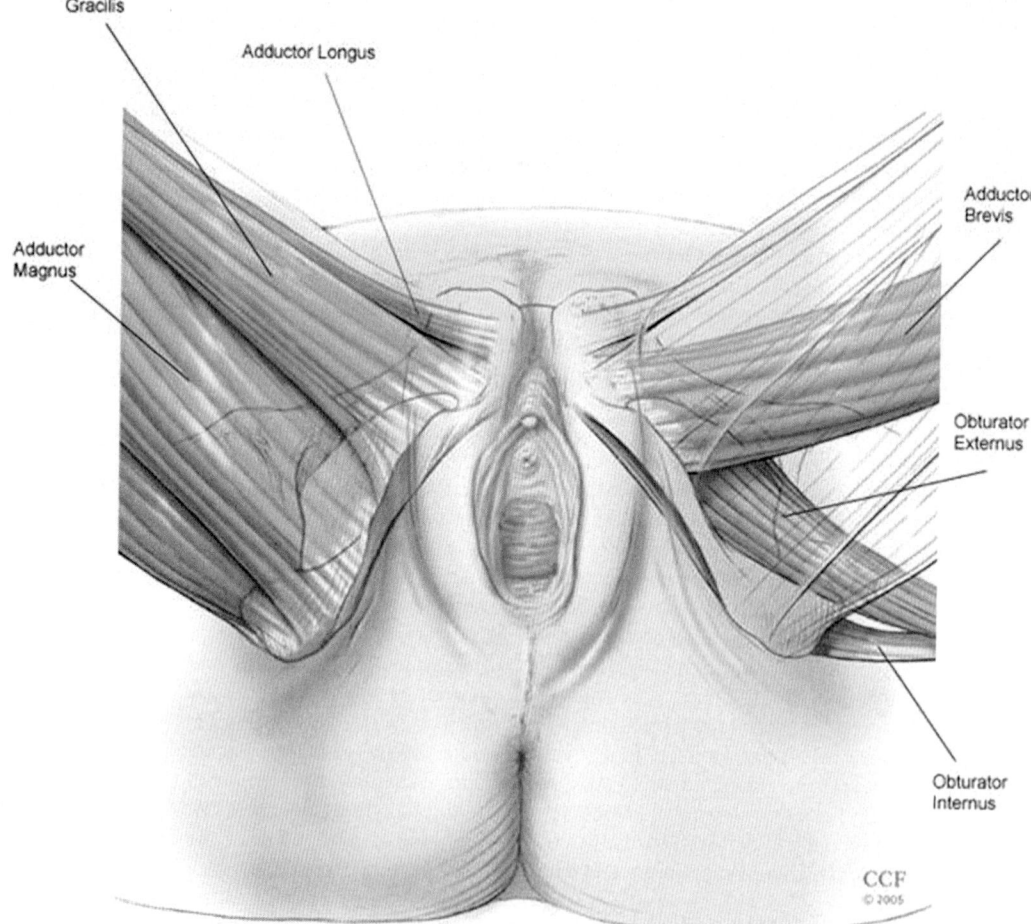

FIGURE 14.7 ● Muscles of the obturator compartment. The superficial muscles are illustrated on the *left*. On the *right*, the superficial muscles have been made transparent to illustrate the deeper muscles. (Reproduced with permission from Cleveland Clinic Foundation.)

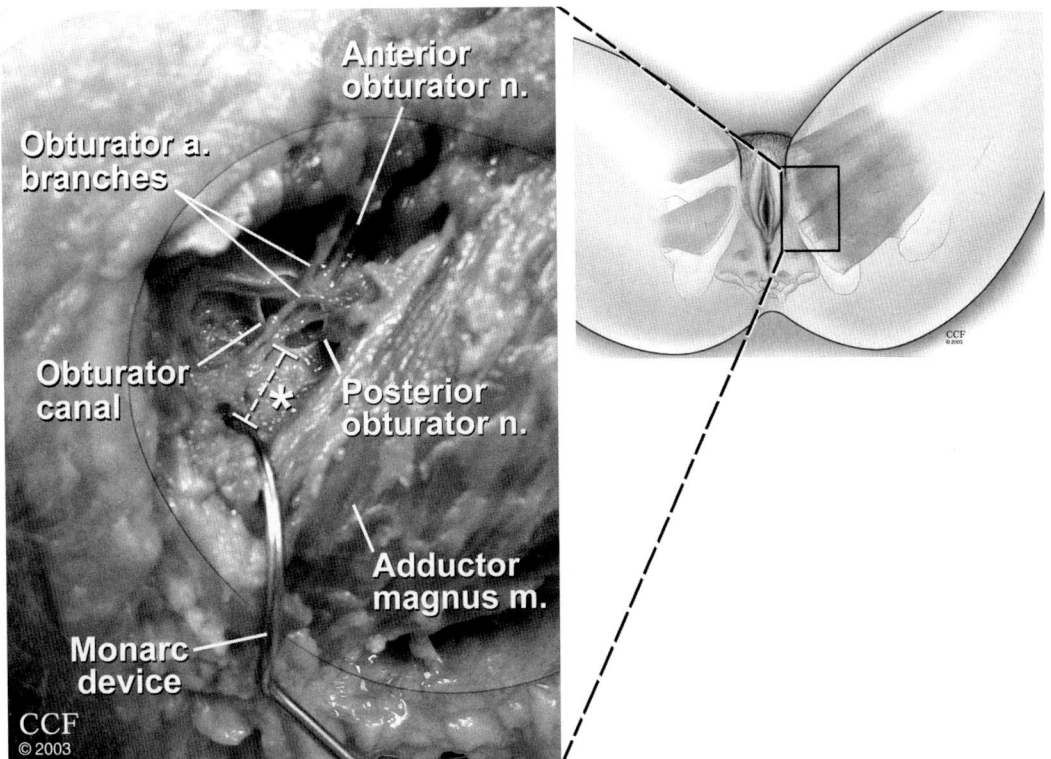

FIGURE 14.8 • Photograph and drawing of dissected left external obturator region. Margins of the obturator foramen are highlighted in the photograph. Displayed are the anterior and posterior obturator nerves as they emerge from the obturator canal (ghosted). Multiple obturator artery branches are displayed after emergence from the canal along with adductor magnus muscle. The TOT device is shown passing around the left ischiopubic ramus. The distance from the device to the canal (*) is on average 2.3 cm. (From Whiteside JL, Walters MD. Anatomy of the obturator region: relations to a transobturator sling. *Int Urogynecol J Pelvic Floor Dysfunct* 2004;15:223–226.)

tradicted previous reports of the obturator vessels bifurcating into medial and lateral branches (173). Rather, the vessels are predominantly small (less than 5 mm in diameter) and splinter into variable courses. The muscles of the medial thigh and adductor compartment are, from superficial to deep, the gracilis, adductor longus, adductor brevis, adductor magnus, and obturator externus muscles.

In contrast to the vessels, the obturator nerve emerges from the obturator membrane and bifurcates into anterior and posterior divisions traveling distally down the thigh to supply the muscles of the adductor compartment. With the patient in the dorsal lithotomy position, the nerves and vessels follow the thigh and course laterally away from the ischiopubic ramus.

Technique

General, regional, or local anesthesia with sedation is appropriate. The patient is placed in dorsal litho-

tomy position in high stirrups with the buttocks at the end of the table. The vagina, lower abdomen, and inner thighs are prepped and draped and a Foley catheter is inserted and placed to dependent drainage. Preoperative antibiotics should be administered on-call to the operating room and antithrombotic compression devices applied. Important landmarks in the obturator compartment are identified, including the ischiopubic ramus and the adductor longus tendon. When using an outside-in approach, the location of the inner thigh incisions is identified by palpating the notch below the adductor longus tendon and just lateral to the labia majora. A marking pen is used to mark the location of the incisions on each side within this notch at the level of the clitoris. The location of these incisions sites is approximately 2.5 cm medial to the obturator neurovascular bundle as it exits the obturator canal (173). If the procedure is being performed using local anesthetic, 10 to 60 mL of local anesthetic with dilute epinephrine is injected into the incision site and carried down to the underlying muscle, to the level of the obturator membrane just lateral to the ischiopubic ramus on each side. A 1-cm stab incision is then made at the marked sites.

Attention is then turned to the vagina, where a weighted speculum is placed for exposure. Using the marking pen, the site for the 2-cm midurethral incision is marked vertically beginning 1 cm from the external urethral meatus. Local anesthetic (10 to 40 mL) with dilute epinephrine (1:200,000) is infiltrated in the anterior vaginal wall at the location of the urethral incision site and laterally to the inferior pubic rami for hydrodissection and hemostasis. The urethral incision is made and dissection is carried laterally with Metzenbaum scissors to create a tunnel to the inferior pubic ramus on each side of the urethra large enough to insert an index finger.

Several different transobturator sling kits have been marketed (Monarc [American Medical Systems, Minnetonka, MN]; Obtryx [Boston Scientific, Natick, MA]; ObTape [Mentor, Santa Barbara, CA]), with some using helical trocars and others using curved trocars. The surgeon should follow the manufacturer's recommendations for each kit. The angle of trocar passage from the thigh incision to the periurethral incision is approximately 30 to 40 degrees. The trocar is oriented appropriately and held with the ipsilateral hand. The surgeon's contralateral index finger is inserted into the periurethral tunnel to the medial edge of the ramus. The trocar passes through the following layers as it is passed around the ischiopubic ramus: the skin, subcutaneous fat, gracilis muscle, adductor brevis, obturator externus muscle, obturator membrane, obturator internus muscle, and periurethral endopelvic fascia (173) (Fig. 14.9). If passed properly, the trocar tip will meet the surgeon's finger as passes around the ramus so that it can be guided out the periurethral tunnel lateral to the urethra. The sling is connected to the trocar and pulled through the periurethral tunnel, around the ischiopubic ramus and out the inner thigh incision (Fig. 14.10). The sling is clamped and cut just below the trocar and the trocar is removed from the operative field. This procedure is repeated on the opposite side (Fig. 14.11).

Although some have suggested that intraoperative cystoscopy may be unnecessary with the TOT, bladder injuries have been reported (179,180). We recommend routine cystoscopy when performing

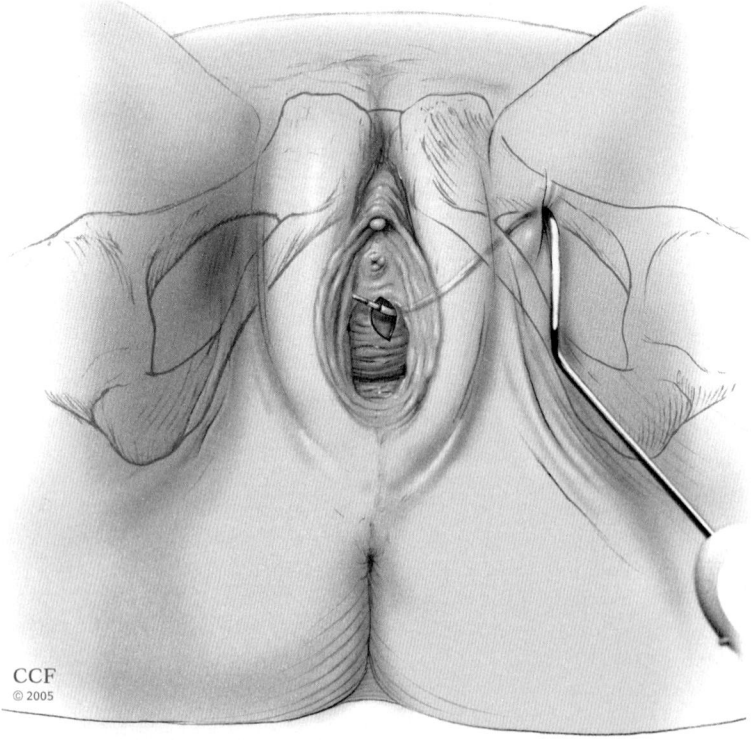

CCF
© 2005

FIGURE 14.9 ● Transobturator sling placed using outside-in technique. (Reproduced with permission from Cleveland Clinic Foundation.)

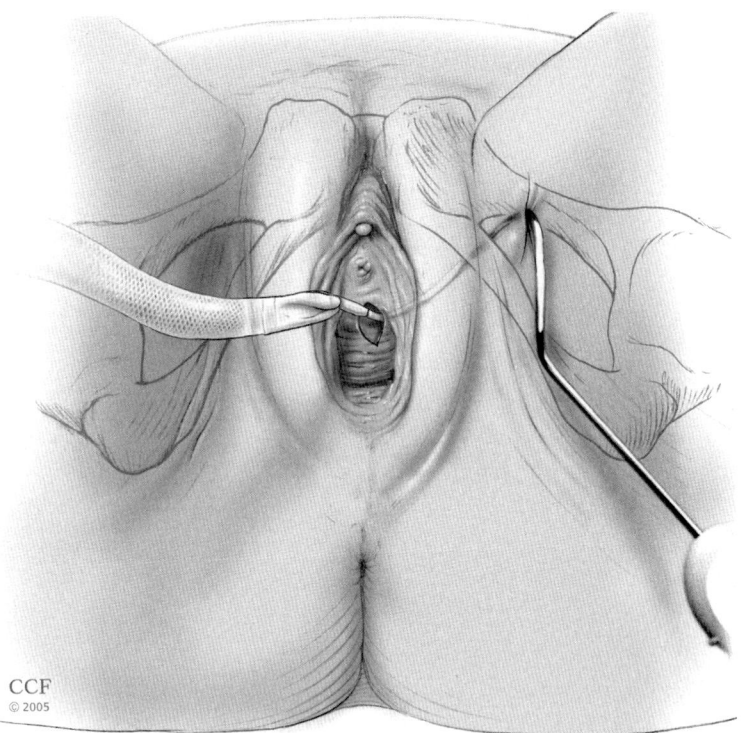

FIGURE 14.10 ● Transobturator sling is connected to the trocar and pulled through the periurethral tunnel, around the ischiopubic ramus and out the inner thigh incision. (Reproduced with permission from Cleveland Clinic Foundation.)

TOT because of the significant adverse consequences that can occur with an unrecognized bladder injury involving an exposed foreign body within the bladder.

The sling should be adjusted so that is tension-free beneath the midurethra. Tensioning techniques similar to those described for TVT can be used. Some authors have suggested that TOT slings should be tensioned somewhat tighter than would be typical for a TVT; however, there no randomized trials evaluating different TOT tensioning techniques. Once the desired tension is achieved, the sheath encasing the sling is removed while stabilizing the sling below the urethra. The outer ends of the sling are cut below the skin surface and the incisions are closed with 4-0 absorbable suture. The vaginal incision is closed with 2-0 or 3-0 absorbable suture in a running fashion. Most patients will be able to void in the recovery room, making postoperative bladder drainage unnecessary. At least one postvoid residual should be obtained in the recovery room. If the patient is unable to void postoperatively, either the patient can be taught self-catheterization or a Foley catheter can be inserted and the patient

asked to return to the clinic in several days for a voiding trial. Most patients will be able to void in 1 or 2 days.

Unlike other TOT kits, the TVT Obturator (TVT-O) System (Ethicon, Inc., Somerville, NJ) uses an "inside-out" out approach. The patient is prepared as above. Similar to the TOT procedure, a 2-cm midurethral incision is made and periurethral tunnels are developed bilaterally. Unlike the TOT, where the dissection stops at the ischiopubic ramus, with the TVT-O the obturator membrane is perforated with the tip of the scissors. Included within the TVT-O kit is a winged metal trocar guide whose purpose is to help guide the helical TVT-O trocars around the ischiopubic ramus. The winged guide is inserted into the periurethral tunnels and its tip is pushed just beyond the perforated obturator membrane. The tip of the helical trocar is passed into the periurethral tunnel just inside the metal guide (Fig. 14.12). The trocar is then rotated around the ischiopubic ramus to exit out the skin through stab incisions (Fig. 14.13). The inner thigh incisions of the TVT-O are somewhat lateral to those of the outside-in technique, located 2 cm above a horizontal line at the level of

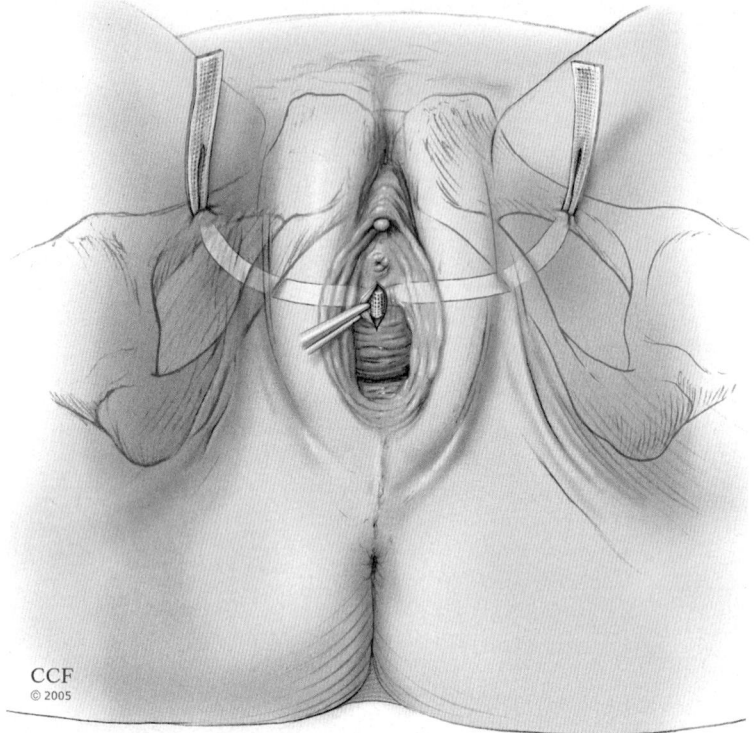

FIGURE 14.11 ● Transobturator sling. (Reproduced with permission from Cleveland Clinic Foundation.)

the urethral meatus and 2 cm outside the thigh folds. The sling is then pulled through the thigh incision and held. The same procedure is repeated on the opposite side. The sling is tensioned and the procedure completed similar to technique described above.

Outcomes

There is relatively little outcome data currently published for the TOT. As of the writing of this chapter, less than 30 original research articles have been published on this approach, with the majority being case reports and observational studies. The cure rates in published case series range from 59% to 97%, with few studies reporting results beyond 1 year of follow-up (32,177,178). Two randomized trials have been published that evaluate the TOT. Unfortunately, one of the studies was retracted because of ethical concerns (181,182) and the other only reports short-term data (less than 6 weeks) (176).

David-Montefiore et al randomized 88 women to undergo a suburethral sling by either the retropubic or the transobturator approach (176). The I-STOP device (CL Medical, Lyon, France), a sling

made of macroporous, nonelastic monofilament polypropylene, was used for both approaches. In their initial report, the authors presented data on perioperative complications and postoperative pain. There was no difference in overall morbidity or hospital stay between the two approaches (176). Bladder injuries were more common in the retropubic sling group (9% vs. 0%), while vaginal lacerations were more common in the transobturator group (0% vs. 11%). Pain scores were lower in those patients who received a transobturator sling. Over 90% of subjects in both groups were dry 6 weeks after surgery. Efficacy data from this trial with longer follow-up is anticipated in the future.

Fischer et al retrospectively compared the first 220 TOT procedures to the first 220 TVT procedures performed at their institution (183). One year after surgery, a negative 1-hour pad test was noted in 81% of the TOT group and in 76% of those who received TVT (183). De novo urge incontinence occurred more frequently in the TVT group (4% vs. 0%). Bladder injuries were also more common in the TVT group (4.5% vs. 0.5%); however, this did not reach statistical significance. Roumeguere followed 120 women after TOT for a minimum of 1 year (range 12 to 30 months) and

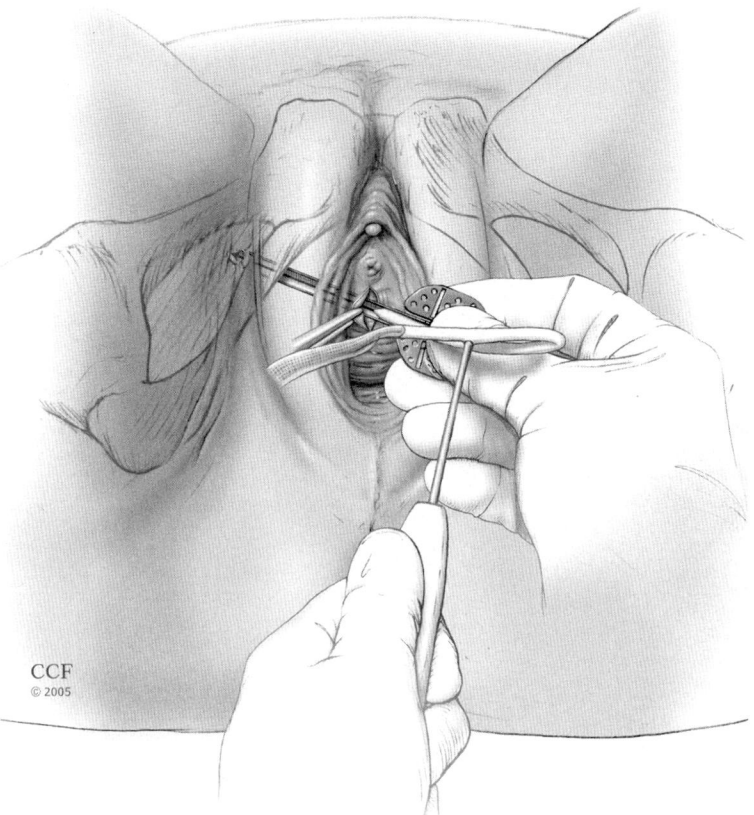

FIGURE 14.12 ● The trocar of the TVT-O procedure is passed using an inside-out technique. The tip of the helical trocar is passed into the peri-urethral tunnel just inside the winged metal guide. (Reproduced with permission from Cleveland Clinic Foundation.)

found that 80% of subjects were dry at 1 year, with an additional 12% greatly improved (32). The cure rate for subjects with a maximum urethral closure pressure below 20 was 70% compared to 85% for those with higher maximum urethral closure pressures, suggesting that TOT may not be the ideal procedure for patients with ISD. Few studies have evaluated the efficacy of the TVT-O procedure and none have compared the relative merits of the outside-in and inside-out approaches.

Complications

TOT has been advocated because it avoids the retropubic space and, at least in theory, should reduce the risk of bladder, bowel, and iliac vessel injury compared to TVT. Several comparative studies have confirmed a lower rate of bladder injury for TOT than TVT (175,176,183). Some authors have suggested that the rate of bladder injury with TOT is low enough that routine cystoscopy is not necessary (20,183). However, while uncommon,

lower urinary tract injuries can occur with TOT, with bladder injuries reported in up to 0.5% of cases, and urethral injuries occur in up to 1.1% of cases (20,179,180). Minaglia et al reported three bladder injuries in their first 61 cases of TOT, two of which would not have been identified without routine intraoperative cystoscopy (180). Given the adverse consequences of an unrecognized bladder injury, intraoperative cystoscopy at the time of TOT seems prudent.

The novel anatomic approach of the TOT, while avoiding the space of Retzius and thereby reducing the risk of bladder injury, does allow for the potential for other complications, including obturator neurovascular injury and lower extremity complications not seen with other approaches. Hematomas and abscesses of the obturator compartment have been reported after procedures using the transobturator approach. In a study comparing the perioperative complications of 205 consecutive patients undergoing a TOT to 213 women receiving a TVT, no obturator nerve injuries, thigh

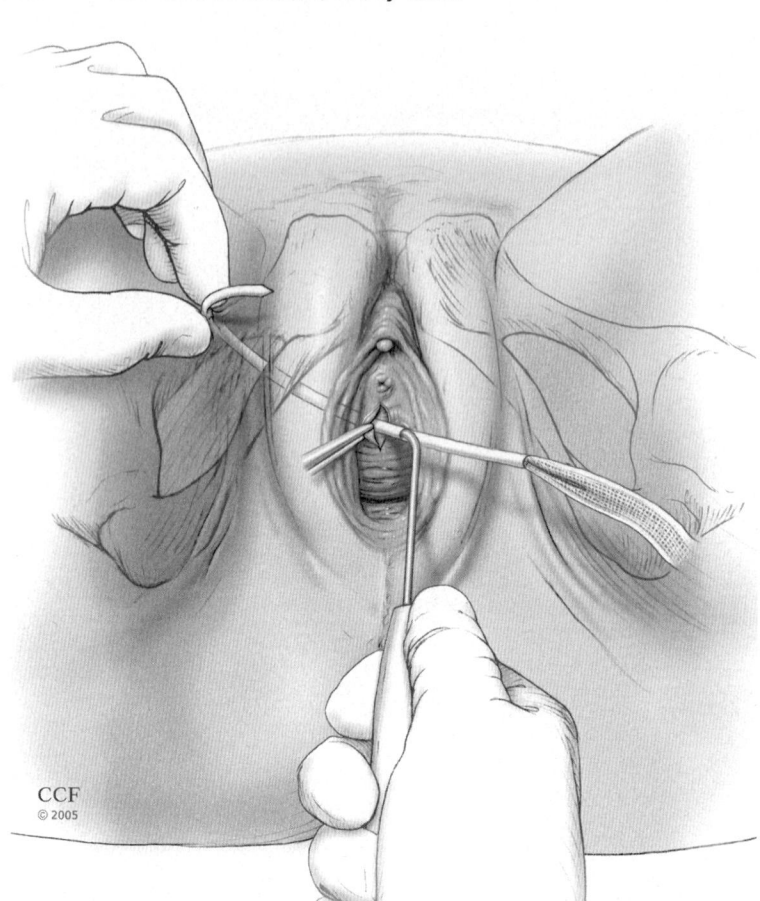

FIGURE 14.13 ● TVT-O trocar rotating around the ischiopubic ramus to exit out the skin through stab incisions on inner thigh. (Reproduced with permission from Cleveland Clinic Foundation.)

hematomas, or infections were seen in the TOT group (175). The rate of postoperative leg pain was low (0.5%) and similar to that of subjects receiving a TVT. Similarly, Davila et al reported only two minor lower extremity complications after 200 MONARC TOT placements: leg numbness in one patient, which resolved spontaneously, and a small abscess of a groin incision (suture removed, resolved) (177). Thus, while obturator and other leg complications are possible with TOT, they appear to be rare. Nonetheless, surgeons should be aware of these unique adverse events and counsel patients accordingly. Whether the TVT-O offers any advantages or disadvantages in terms of bladder injuries or obturator compartment complications is currently unknown. The relative

location of vascular structures to the TOT trocar is somewhat different when using an outside-in approach compared to an inside-out approach (173,184). One might expect a different rate of bleeding complications with these two different techniques, but this has yet to be determined, as no comparative studies currently exist.

The less compressive nature of the TOT sling appears to translate into a lower rate of voiding dysfunction and irritative bladder symptoms than the TVT procedure. In a retrospective comparison of the Monarc TOT to TVT, Barber et al noted that subjects who received TVT were significantly more likely to require urethrolysis for voiding dysfunction or urinary urgency (adjusted odds ratio 3.2 [95% CI 1.2 to 10.1], $p = 0.026$) and more likely to use anticholinergic medications postoperatively (adjusted odds ratio 2.1 [1.02 to 4.70], $p = 0.046$) than those who received a TOT (175). These results are similar to those of Fisher et al described previously (183). Whether the less obstructive nature of the TOT results in lower cure rates for subjects with ISD or lower cure rates for SUI in general has yet to be determined, however.

As with other slings using synthetic mesh, the risk of mesh complications after TOT appears to be largely dependent upon the type of mesh used. For instance, Domingo et al noted a 13.8% erosion rate after TOT procedures that used a fusion-welded, nonwoven, nonknitted polypropylene mesh with and without silicone coating (Uratape/Obtape, Mentor-Porges, Le Plessis-Ronbinson, France) (185). In contrast, the mesh erosion rate seen in studies of TOT devices that use loosely knitted polypropylene is low (less than 1%) (175,176).

SUMMARY

The Burch colposuspension, the traditional sling procedure using autologous or synthetic graft, and the TVT are the most effective and durable procedures currently available for the surgical management of SUI. As such they should be considered the "gold standards" to which newer operations should be compared. Objective cure can be expected in approximately 85% of patients after each of these operations. In many circumstances, the choice of procedure will be dictated by the need for (or lack of) concurrent surgery. Because it can be performed in an ambulatory setting and is associated with less pain, quicker recovery, and quicker return to normal voiding, TVT is probably the optimal choice for the management of isolated primary SUI. The principal caveat is that the durability of TVT beyond 10 years has not yet been demonstrated, while it has for the Burch colposuspension and autologous fascial sling. Each of the three "gold standard" operations has demonstrated success in the treatment of recurrent SUI; however, the traditional sling procedure has the longest history in this regard, often being reserved for the most difficult cases. Thus, in today's era of minimally invasive midurethral slings, the traditional sling may have a special role in the management of patients with multiple previous recurrences, severely impaired urethral sphincter function, and other challenging cases. The transobturator slings offer the promise of increased safety and decreased voiding dysfunction; however, their long-term efficacy is currently unknown. The results of several ongoing clinical trials should prove valuable in determining the role of this newer approach.

REFERENCES

1. Olsen AL, Smith VJ, Bergstrom JO, et al. Epidemiology of surgically managed pelvic organ prolapse and urinary incontinence. *Obstet Gynecol* 1997;89:501–506.
2. http://hcup.ahrq.gov/HCUPnet.asp.
3. Boyles SH, Weber AM, Meyn L. Ambulatory procedures for urinary incontinence in the United States, 1994–1996. *Am J Obstet Gynecol* 2004;190:33–36.
4. Kelly HA. Incontinence of urine in women. *Urol Cutan Rev* 1913;17:291–293.
5. Kennedy WT. Incontinence of urine in the female, the urethral sphincter mechanism, damage of function and restoration of control. *Am J Obstet Gynecol* 1937;34:576–586.
6. Goebel R. Zur operitaven beseitigung der angebornen incontinentia vesicae. *Zeitscher Gynakol* 1910;2: 187–191.
7. Frangenheim P. Zu operativen behandlung der inkontinenz der mannlichen harnohre. *Ver Dtsch Ges Chir* 1914;43:149–154.
8. Ridley JG. Appraisal of the Goebell-Stoekel-Frankenheim sling procedure. *Am J Obstet Gynecol* 1966;95:714.
9. Price PB. Plastic operations for incontinence of urine and feces. *Arch Surg* 1933;26:1043–1048.
10. Aldridge AH. Transplanation of fascia for relief of urinary stress incontinence. *Am J Obstet Gynecol* 1942;44:398–411.
11. Marshall VF, Marchetti AA, Krantz KE. The correction of stress incontinence by simple vesicourethral suspension. *Surg Gynecol Obstet* 1949;88:509–518.
12. Burch JC. Urethrovaginal fixation to Cooper's ligament for correction of stress incontinence, cystocele, and prolapse. *Am J Obstet Gynecol* 1961;81:281–290.
13. Tanagho EA. Colpocystourethropexy: the way we do it. *J Urol* 1976;116:751–753.
14. Pereyra AJ. A simplified surgical procedure for the correction of stress incontinence in women. *West J Surg* 1959;67:223–228.
15. Glazener CM, Cooper K. Bladder neck needle suspension for urinary incontinence in women. *Cochrane Database Syst Rev* 2002:CD003636.
16. Ulmsten U, Henriksson L, Johnson P, et al. An ambulatory surgical procedure under local anesthesia for treatment of female urinary incontinence. *Int Urogynecol J Pelvic Floor Dysfunct* 1996;7:81–85.
17. Ward KL, Hilton P. A prospective multicenter randomized trial of tension-free vaginal tape and colposuspension for primary urodynamic stress incontinence: two-year follow-up. *Am J Obstet Gynecol* 2004;190:324–331.
18. Liapis A, Bakas P, Creatsas G. Burch colposuspension and tension-free vaginal tape in the management of stress urinary incontinence in women. *Eur Urol* 2002;41:469–473.
19. Lapitan MC, Cody DJ, Grant AM. Open retropubic colposuspension for urinary incontinence in women. *Cochrane Database Syst Rev* 2005:CD002912.
20. Delorme E. [Transobturator urethral suspension: mini-invasive procedure in the treatment of stress urinary

incontinence in women]. *Prog Urol* 2001;11: 1306–1313.

21. ACOG Practice Bulletin No. 63. Urinary incontinence in women. *Obstet Gynecol* 2006;105:1533–1545.

22. Brubaker L. Surgical treatment of urinary incontinence in women. *Gastroenterology* 2004;126:S71–76.

23. AHCPR. *Clinical Practice Guidelines: urinary incontinence in adults*: Washington: Dept. of Health and Human Services (US), Agency for Health Care Policy and Research, 1992.

24. Smith ARB, Daneshgari F, Dmochowski R, et al. Surgery for urinary incontinence in women. In: Abrahms P, Cordozo L, Koury S, et al, eds. *Third Consultation on Incontinence.* Paris: Health Publication Ltd., 2005.

25. Sand PK, Bowen LW, Panganiban R, et al. The low pressure urethra as a factor in failed retropubic urethropexy. *Obstet Gynecol* 1987;69:399–402.

26. McGuire EJ. Urodynamic findings in patients after failure of stress incontinence operations. *Prog Clin Biol Res* 1981;78:351–360.

27. Bergman A, Koonings PP, Ballard CA. The Ball-Burch procedure for stress incontinence with low urethral pressure. *J Reprod Med* 1991;36:137–140.

28. Meschia M. Unsuccessful Burch colposuspension: analysis of risk factors. *Int Urogynecol J Pelvic Floor Dysfunct* 1991;2:19–21.

29. Monga A, Stanton SL. Predicting outcome of colposuspension. A prospective evaluation. *Neurourol Urodyn* 1997;16:354–355.

30. Weber AM. Leak point pressure measurement and stress urinary incontinence. *Curr Womens Health Rep* 2001;1:45–52.

31. Weber AM. Is urethral pressure profilometry a useful diagnostic test for stress urinary incontinence? *Obstet Gynecol Surv* 2001;56:720–735.

32. Roumeguere T, Quackels T, Bollens R, et al. Transobturator vaginal tape (TOT) for female stress incontinence: one year follow-up in 120 patients. *Eur Urol* 2005;48:805–809.

33. Colombo M, Zanetta G, Vitobello D, et al. The Burch colposuspension for women with and without detrusor overactivity. *Br J Obstet Gynaecol* 1996;103: 255–260.

34. Scotti RJ, Angell G, Flora R, Greston WM. Antecedent history as a predictor of surgical cure of urgency symptoms in mixed incontinence. *Obstet Gynecol* 1998;91:51–54.

35. Laurikainen E, Kiilholma P. The tension-free vaginal tape procedure for female urinary incontinence without preoperative urodynamic evaluation. *J Am Coll Surg* 2003;196:579–583.

36. Holmgren C, Nilsson S, Lanner L, et al. Long-term results with tension-free vaginal tape on mixed and stress urinary incontinence. *Obstet Gynecol* 2005; 106:38–43.

37. Segal JL, Vassallo B, Kleeman S, et al. Prevalence of persistent and de novo overactive bladder symptoms after the tension-free vaginal tape. *Obstet Gynecol* 2004;104:1263–1269.

38. Brown K, Hilton P. The incidence of detrusor instability before and after colposuspension: a study using conventional and ambulatory urodynamic monitoring. *BJU Int* 1999;84:961–965.

39. Karram MM, Bhatia NN. Management of coexistent stress and urge urinary incontinence. *Obstet Gynecol* 1989;73:4–7.

40. Enhorning G. Simultaneous recording of intraurethral and intravesical pressure: a study of urethral closure pressure and stress incontinence in women. *Acta Chir Scand* 1961;276, Suppl 1.

41. Bump RC, Fantl JA, Hurt WG. Dynamic urethral pressure profilometry pressure transmission ratio determinations after continence surgery: understanding the mechanism of success, failure, and complications. *Obstet Gynecol* 1988;72:870–874.

42. Bump RC, Hurt WG, Elser DM, et al. Understanding lower urinary tract function in women soon after bladder neck surgery. Continence Program for Women Research Group. *Neurourol Urodyn* 1999;18: 629–637.

43. Penttinen J, Lindholm EL, Kaar K, et al. Successful colposuspension in stress urinary incontinence reduces bladder neck mobility and increases pressure transmission to the urethra. *Arch Gynecol Obstet* 1989;244: 233–238.

44. Hilton P, Stanton SL. A clinical and urodynamic assessment of the Burch colposuspension for genuine stress incontinence. *Br J Obstet Gynaecol* 1983;90: 934–939.

45. Symmonds RE. The suprapubic approach to anterior vaginal relaxation and urinary stress incontinence. *Clin Obstet Gynecol* 1972;15:1107–1121.

46. Miklos JR, Kohli N. Laparoscopic paravaginal repair plus Burch colposuspension: review and descriptive technique. *Urology* 2000;56:64–69.

47. Paraiso MF, Falcone T, Walters MD. Laparoscopic surgery for genuine stress incontinence. *Int Urogynecol J Pelvic Floor Dysfunct* 1999;10:237–247.

48. Persson J, Wolner-Hanssen P. Laparoscopic Burch colposuspension for stress urinary incontinence: a randomized comparison of one or two sutures on each side of the urethra. *Obstet Gynecol* 2000;95:151–155.

49. Langer R, Ron-El R, Neuman M, et al. The value of simultaneous hysterectomy during Burch colposuspension for urinary stress incontinence. *Obstet Gynecol* 1988;72:866–869.

50. Meltomaa SS, Haarala MA, Taalikka MO, et al. Outcome of Burch retropubic urethropexy and the effect of concomitant abdominal hysterectomy: a prospective long-term follow-up study. *Int Urogynecol J Pelvic Floor Dysfunct* 2001;12:3–8.

51. Langer R, Lipshitz Y, Halperin R, et al. Long-term (10–15 years) follow-up after Burch colposuspension for urinary stress incontinence. *Int Urogynecol J Pelvic Floor Dysfunct* 2001;12:323–327.

52. Alcalay M, Monga A, Stanton SL. Burch colposuspension: a 10- to 20-year follow up. *Br J Obstet Gynaecol* 1995;102:740–745.

53. McDuffie RW, Jr., Litin RB, Blundon KE. Urethrovesical suspension (Marshall-Marchetti-Krantz). Experience with 204 cases. *Am J Surg* 1981;141:297–298.

54. Colombo M, Milani R, Vitobello D, et al. A randomized comparison of Burch colposuspension and abdominal paravaginal defect repair for female stress urinary incontinence. *Am J Obstet Gynecol* 1996;175:78–84.

55. Bezerra CA, Bruschini H, Cody DJ. Traditional suburethral sling operations for urinary incontinence in women. *Cochrane Database Syst Rev* 2005:CD001754.

56. Tennstedt S. Design of the Stress Incontinence Surgical Treatment Efficacy Trial (SISTEr). *Urology* 2005;66:1213–1217.

57. Ward K, Hilton P. Prospective multicenter randomized trial of tension-free vaginal tape and colposuspension as primary treatment for stress incontinence. *Br Med J* 2002;325:67.

58. Colombo M, Scalambrino S, Maggioni A, et al. Burch colposuspension versus modified Marshall-Marchetti-Krantz urethropexy for primary genuine stress urinary incontinence: a prospective, randomized clinical trial. *Am J Obstet Gynecol* 1994;171:1573–1579.

59. Liapis AE, Asimidis V, Loghis CD, et al. A randomized prospective study of three operative methods for genuine stress incontinence. *J Gynecol Surg* 1996;12:7–14.

60. Moehrer B, Ellis G, Carey M, et al. Laparoscopic colposuspension for urinary incontinence in women. *Cochrane Database Syst Rev* 2002:CD002239.

61. Smith A, Kitchener H, Dunne G, et al. *A prospective randomized controlled trial of open and laparoscopic Burch colposuspension.* [Abstract] Presented at International Continence Society's 35th annual meeting, Montreal, Canada, 2005.

62. Paraiso MF, Walters MD, Karram MM, et al. Laparoscopic Burch colposuspension versus tension-free vaginal tape: a randomized trial. *Obstet Gynecol* 2004;104:1249–1258.

63. Mainprize TC, Drutz HP. The Marshall-Marchetti-Krantz procedure: a critical review. *Obstet Gynecol Surv* 1988;43:724–729.

64. Kenton K, Oldham L, Brubaker L. Open Burch urethropexy has a low rate of perioperative complications. *Am J Obstet Gynecol* 2002;187:107–110.

65. Galloway NT, Davies N, Stephenson TP. The complications of colposuspension. *Br J Urol* 1987;60:122–124.

66. Demirci F, Yucel O, Eren S, et al. Long-term results of Burch colposuspension. *Gynecol Obstet Invest* 2001;51:243–247.

67. Viereck V, Pauer HU, Bader W, et al. Introital ultrasound of the lower genital tract before and after colposuspension: a 4-year objective follow-up. *Ultrasound Obstet Gynecol* 2004;23:277–283.

68. Kobak WH, Walters MD, Piedmonte MR. Determinants of voiding after three types of incontinence surgery: a multivariable analysis. *Obstet Gynecol* 2001;97:86–91.

69. Kammerer-Doak DN, Cornella JL, Magrina JF, et al. Osteitis pubis after Marshall-Marchetti-Krantz urethropexy: a pubic osteomyelitis. *Am J Obstet Gynecol* 1998;179:586–590.

70. Kim HL, Gerber GS, Patel RV, et al. Practice patterns in the treatment of female urinary incontinence: a postal and internet survey. *Urology* 2001;57:45–48.

71. Leach GE, Dmochowski RR, Appell RA, et al. Female Stress Urinary Incontinence Clinical Guidelines Panel summary report on surgical management of female stress urinary incontinence. The American Urological Association. *J Urol* 1997;158:875–880.

72. Kuo HC. Videourodynamic results after pubovaginal sling procedure for stress urinary incontinence. *Urology* 1999;54:802–807.

73. Hilton P. A clinical and urodynamic study comparing the Stamey bladder neck suspension and suburethral sling procedures in the treatment of genuine stress incontinence. *Br J Obstet Gynaecol* 1989;96:213–220.

74. Rottenberg RD, Weil A, Brioschi PA, et al. Urodynamic and clinical assessment of the Lyodura sling operation for urinary stress incontinence. *Br J Obstet Gynaecol* 1985;92:829–834.

75. Summitt RL, Jr., Bent AE, Ostergard DR, et al. Stress incontinence and low urethral closure pressure. Correlation of preoperative urethral hypermobility with successful suburethral sling procedures. *J Reprod Med* 1990;35:877–880.

76. Hijaz A, Daneshgari F, Huang X, et al. Role of sling integrity in the restoration of leak point pressure in the rat vaginal sling model. *J Urol* 2005;174:771–775.

77. Kuo HC. Comparison of video urodynamic results after the pubovaginal sling procedure using rectus fascia and polypropylene mesh for stress urinary incontinence. *J Urol* 2001;165:163–168.

78. Mason RC, Roach M. Modified pubovaginal sling for treatment of intrinsic sphincteric deficiency. *J Urol* 1996;156:1991–1994.

79. Heit M. What is the scientific evidence for bone anchor use during bladder neck suspension? *Int Urogynecol J Pelvic Floor Dysfunct* 2002;13:143–144.

80. Schultheiss D, Jonas U. Do we need bone anchors in urogynecology? *Int Urogynecol J Pelvic Floor Dysfunct* 1999;10:153–154.

81. Winters JC, Scarpero HM, Appell RA. Use of bone anchors in female urology. *Urology* 2000;56:15–22.

82. Beck RP, Grove D, Arnusch D, et al. Recurrent urinary stress incontinence treated by the fascia lata sling procedure. *Am J Obstet Gynecol* 1974;120:613–621.

83. Govier FE, Gibbons RP, Correa RJ, et al. Pubovaginal slings using fascia lata for the treatment of intrinsic sphincter deficiency. *J Urol* 1997;157:117–121.

84. McGuire EJ, Bennett CJ, Konnak JA, et al. Experience with pubovaginal slings for urinary incontinence at the University of Michigan. *J Urol* 1987;138:525–526.

85. Rovner ES, Ginsberg DA, Raz S. A method for intraoperative adjustment of sling tension: prevention of outlet obstruction during vaginal wall sling. *Urology* 1997;50:273–276.

86. Enzelsberger H, Helmer H, Schatten C. Comparison of Burch and Iyodura sling procedures for repair of unsuccessful incontinence surgery. *Obstet Gynecol* 1996;88:251–256.

87. Sand PK, Winkler H, Blackhurst DW, et al. A prospective randomized study comparing modified Burch retropubic urethropexy and suburethral sling for treatment of genuine stress incontinence with low-pressure urethra. *Am J Obstet Gynecol* 2000;182:30–34.

88. Demirci F, Yucel O. Comparison of pubovaginal sling and Burch colposuspension procedures in type I/II genuine stress incontinence. *Arch Gynecol Obstet* 2001;265:190–194.

89. Henriksson L, Ulmsten U. A urodynamic evaluation of the effects of abdominal urethrocystopexy and vaginal sling urethroplasty in women with stress incontinence. *Am J Obstet Gynecol* 1978;131:77–82.

90. Fischer JR, Hale DS, McClellan E, et al. The use of urethral electrodiagnosis to select the method of surgery in women with intrinsic sphincter deficiency (Abstract). *Int Urogynecol J Pelvic Floor Dysfunct* 2001;12 (Supp 1):S33.

91. Jarvis GJ. Surgery for genuine stress incontinence. *Br J Obstet Gynaecol* 1994;101:371–374.

92. Beck RP, McCormick S, Nordstrom L. The fascia lata sling procedure for treating recurrent genuine stress incontinence of urine. *Obstet Gynecol* 1988;72:699–703.

93. Chaikin DC, Rosenthal J, Blaivas JG. Pubovaginal fascial sling for all types of stress urinary inconti-

nence: long-term analysis. *J Urol* 1998;160: 1312–1316.

94. Richter HE, Varner RE, Sanders E, et al. Effects of pubovaginal sling procedure on patients with urethral hypermobility and intrinsic sphincteric deficiency: would they do it again? *Am J Obstet Gynecol* 2001;184:14–19.

95. FitzGerald MP, Mollenhauer J, Brubaker L. The fate of rectus fascia suburethral slings. *Am J Obstet Gynecol* 2000;183:964–966.

96. Choe JM, Bell T. Genetic material is present in cadaveric dermis and cadaveric fascia lata. *J Urol* 2001;166:122–124.

97. Liscic RM, Brinar V, Miklic P, et al. Creutzfeldt-Jakob disease in a patient with a lyophilized dura mater graft. *Acta Med Croatica* 1999;53:93–96.

98. Handa VL, Jensen JK, Germain MM, et al. Banked human fascia lata for the suburethral sling procedure: a preliminary report. *Obstet Gynecol* 1996;88: 1045–1049.

99. Hinton R, Jinnah RH, Johnson C, et al. A biomechanical analysis of solvent-dehydrated and freeze-dried human fascia lata allografts. A preliminary report. *Am J Sports Med* 1992;20:607–612.

100. Lemer ML, Chaikin DC, Blaivas JG. Tissue strength analysis of autologous and cadaveric allografts for the pubovaginal sling. *Neurourol Urodyn* 1999;18: 497–503.

101. Sutaria P, Staskin D. A comparison of fascial "pull-through" strength using four different suture fixation techniques. *J Urol* 1999;161:79–80.

102. Fitzgerald MP, Mollenhauer J, Brubaker L. Failure of allograft suburethral slings. *BJU Int* 1999;84:785–788.

103. FitzGerald MP, Edwards SR, Fenner D. Medium-term follow-up on use of freeze-dried, irradiated donor fascia for sacrocolpopexy and sling procedures. *Int Urogynecol J Pelvic Floor Dysfunct* 2004;15:238–242.

104. McBride AW, Ellerkmann RM, Bent AE, et al. Comparison of long-term outcomes of autologous fascia lata slings with Suspend Tutoplast fascia lata allograft slings for stress incontinence. *Am J Obstet Gynecol* 2005;192:1677–1681.

105. Mochizuki Y, Mizutani T, Tajiri N, et al. Creutzfeldt-Jakob disease with florid plaques after cadaveric dura mater graft. *Neuropathology* 2003;23:136–140.

106. Chung SY, Franks M, Smith CP, et al. Technique of combined pubovaginal sling and cystocele repair using a single piece of cadaveric dermal graft. *Urology* 2002;59:538–541.

107. Onur R, Singla A. Solvent-dehydrated cadaveric dermis: a new allograft for pubovaginal sling surgery. *Int J Urol* 2005;12:801–805.

108. Owens DC, Winters JC. Pubovaginal sling using Duraderm graft: intermediate follow-up and patient satisfaction. *Neurourol Urodyn* 2004;23:115–118.

109. Nicholson SC, Brown AD. The long-term success of abdominovaginal sling operations for genuine stress incontinence and a cystocoele: a questionnaire-based study. *J Obstet Gynaecol* 2001;21:162–165.

110. Abdel-Fattah M, Barrington JW, Arunkalaivanan AS. Pelvicol pubovaginal sling versus tension-free vaginal tape for treatment of urodynamic stress incontinence: a prospective randomized three-year follow-up study. *Eur Urol* 2004;46:629–635.

111. Kubricht WS, 3rd, Williams BJ, Eastham JA, et al. Tensile strength of cadaveric fascia lata compared to small intestinal submucosa using suture pull through analysis. *J Urol* 2001;165:486–490.

112. Jones JS, Rackley RR, Berglund R, et al. Porcine small intestinal submucosa as a percutaneous midurethral sling: 2-year results. *BJU Int* 2005;96:103–106.

113. Rutner AB, Levine SR, Schmaelzle JF. Processed porcine small intestine submucosa as a graft material for pubovaginal slings: durability and results. *Urology* 2003;62:805–809.

114. Bent AE, Ostergard DR, Zwick-Zaffuto M. Tissue reaction to expanded polytetrafluoroethylene suburethral sling for urinary incontinence: clinical and histologic study. *Am J Obstet Gynecol* 1993;169: 1198–204.

115. Ghoniem GM, Shaaban A. Suburethral slings for the treatment of stress urinary incontinence. *Int Urogynecol J Pelvic Floor Dysfunct* 1994;5:228–239.

116. Weinberger MW, Ostergard DR. Long-term clinical and urodynamic evaluation of the polytetrafluoroethylene suburethral sling for treatment of genuine stress incontinence. *Obstet Gynecol* 1995;86:92–96.

117. Bukkapatnam R, Rodriguez LV. Synthetic sling options for stress urinary incontinence. *Curr Urol Rep* 2004;5:374–580.

118. Cosson M, Debodinance P, Boukerrou M, et al. Mechanical properties of synthetic implants used in the repair of prolapse and urinary incontinence in women: which is the ideal material? *Int Urogynecol J Pelvic Floor Dysfunct* 2003;14:169–178.

119. Winters JC, Fitzgerald MP, Barber MD. The use of synthetic mesh in female pelvic reconstructive surgery. *BJU Int* 2006;98(Suppl 1):70–77.

120. Bidmead J, Cardozo L. Sling techniques in the treatment of genuine stress incontinence. *Br J Obstet Gynaecol* 2000;107:147–156.

121. McLennan MT, Melick CF, Bent AE. Clinical and urodynamic predictors of delayed voiding after fascia lata suburethral sling. *Obstet Gynecol* 1998;92:608–612.

122. Amundsen CL, Guralnick ML, Webster GD. Variations in strategy for the treatment of urethral obstruction after a pubovaginal sling procedure. *J Urol* 2000;164:434–437.

123. Ghoniem GM, Elgamasy AN. Simplified surgical approach to bladder outlet obstruction following pubovaginal sling. *J Urol* 1995;154:181–183.

124. Goldman HB, Rackley RR, Appell RA. The efficacy of urethrolysis without resuspension for iatrogenic urethral obstruction. *J Urol* 1999;161:196–199.

125. McLennan MT, Bent AE. Sling incision with associated vaginal wall interposition for obstructed voiding secondary to suburethral sling procedure. *Int Urogynecol J Pelvic Floor Dysfunct* 1997;8:168–172.

126. Wang AC, Chen MC. Comparison of tension-free vaginal taping versus modified Burch colposuspension on urethral obstruction: a randomized controlled trial. *Neurourol Urodyn* 2003;22:185–190.

127. Petros PE, Ulmsten UI. An integral theory of female urinary incontinence. Experimental and clinical considerations. *Acta Obstet Gynecol Scand Suppl* 1990;153:7–31.

128. Fritsch H, Pinggera GM, Lienemann A, et al. What are the supportive structures of the female urethra? *Neurourol Urodyn* 2006;25:128–134.

129. Brandt FT, Albuquerque CDC, Lorenzato FR, et al. Perineal assessment of urethrovesical junction mobility in young continent females. *Int Urogynecol J Pelvic Floor Dysfunct* 2000;11:18–22.

130. Fielding JR, Griffiths DJ, Versi E, et al. MR imaging of pelvic floor continence mechanisms in the supine and sitting positions. *AJR Am J Roentgenol* 1998;171:1607–1610.

131. Klutke JJ, Carlin BI, Klutke CG. The tension-free vaginal tape procedure: correction of stress incontinence with minimal alteration in proximal urethral mobility. *Urology* 2000;55:512–514.

132. Lo TS, Horng SG, Liang CC, et al. Ultrasound assessment of midurethra tape at three-year follow-up after tension-free vaginal tape procedure. *Urology* 2004;63:671–675.

133. Sarlos D, Kuronen M, Schaer GN. How does tension-free vaginal tape correct stress incontinence? Investigation by perineal ultrasound. *Int Urogynecol J Pelvic Floor Dysfunct* 2003;14:395–398.

134. Mutone N, Mastropietro M, Brizendine E, et al. Effect of tension-free vaginal tape procedure on urodynamic continence indices. *Obstet Gynecol* 2001;98:638–645.

135. Dietz HP, Mouritsen L, Ellis G, et al. How important is TVT location? *Acta Obstet Gynecol Scand* 2004;83:904–908.

136. Ng CC, Lee LC, Han WH. Use of three-dimensional ultrasound scan to assess the clinical importance of midurethral placement of the tension-free vaginal tape (TVT) for treatment of incontinence. *Int Urogynecol J Pelvic Floor Dysfunct* 2005;16:220–225.

137. Adamiak A, Milart P, Skorupski P, et al. The efficacy and safety of the tension-free vaginal tape procedure do not depend on the method of analgesia. *Eur Urol* 2002;42:29–33.

138. El-Barky E, El-Shazly A, El-Wahab OA, et al. Tension-free vaginal tape versus Burch colposuspension for treatment of female stress urinary incontinence. *Int Urol Nephrol* 2005;37:277–281.

139. Lim YN, Muller R, Corstiaans A, et al. Suburethral slingplasty evaluation study in North Queensland, Australia: the SUSPEND trial. *Aust N Z J Obstet Gynaecol* 2005;45:52–59.

140. Ghezzi F, Cromi A, Raio L, et al. Influence of the type of anesthesia and hydrodissection on the complication rate after tension-free vaginal tape procedure. *Eur J Obstet Gynecol Reprod Biol* 2005;118:96–100.

141. Murphy M, Culligan PJ, Arce CM, et al. Is the cough-stress test necessary when placing the tension-free vaginal tape? *Obstet Gynecol* 2005;105:319–324.

142. Kuuva N, Nilsson CG. Long-term results of the tension-free vaginal tape operation in an unselected group of 129 stress incontinent women. *Acta Obstet Gynecol Scand* 2006;85:482–487.

143. Manca A, Sculpher MJ, Ward K, et al. A cost-utility analysis of tension-free vaginal tape versus colposuspension for primary urodynamic stress incontinence. *Br J Obstet Gynaecol* 2003;110:255–262.

144. Ustun Y, Engin-Ustun Y, Gungor M, et al. Tension-free vaginal tape compared with laparoscopic Burch urethropexy. *J Am Assoc Gynecol Laparosc* 2003;10:386–389.

145. Valpas A, Kivela A, Penttinen J, et al. Tension-free vaginal tape and laparoscopic mesh colposuspension for stress urinary incontinence. *Obstet Gynecol* 2004;104:42–49.

146. Wadie BS, Edwan A, Nabeeh AM. Autologous fascial sling vs polypropylene tape at short-term follow-up: a prospective randomized study. *J Urol* 2005;174:990–993.

147. Hung MJ, Liu FS, Shen PS, et al. Analysis of two sling procedures using polypropylene mesh for treatment of stress urinary incontinence. *Int J Gynaecol Obstet* 2004;84:133–141.

148. Rafii A, Darai E, Haab F, et al. Body mass index and outcome of tension-free vaginal tape. *Eur Urol* 2003;43:288–292.

149. Mukherjee K, Constantine G. Urinary stress incontinence in obese women: tension-free vaginal tape is the answer. *BJU Int* 2001;88:881–883.

150. Davis TL, Lukacz ES, Luber KM, et al. Determinants of patient satisfaction after the tension-free vaginal tape procedure. *Am J Obstet Gynecol* 2004;191:176–181.

151. Debodinance P, Delporte P, Engrand JB, et al. Tension-free vaginal tape (TVT) in the treatment of urinary stress incontinence: 3 years experience involving 256 operations. *Eur J Obstet Gynecol Reprod Biol* 2002;105:49–58.

152. Rezapour M, Ulmsten U. Tension-free vaginal tape (TVT) in women with mixed urinary incontinence—a long-term follow-up. *Int Urogynecol J Pelvic Floor Dysfunct* 2001;12 Suppl 2:S15–18.

153. Liapis A, Bakas P, Lazaris D, et al. Tension-free vaginal tape in the management of recurrent stress incontinence. *Arch Gynecol Obstet* 2004;269:205–207.

154. Meschia M, Pifarotti P, Buonaguidi A, et al. Tension-free vaginal tape (TVT) for treatment of stress urinary incontinence in women with low-pressure urethra. *Eur J Obstet Gynecol Reprod Biol* 2005;122:118–121.

155. Rezapour M, Falconer C, Ulmsten U. Tension-free vaginal tape (TVT) in stress incontinent women with intrinsic sphincter deficiency (ISD)—a long-term follow-up. *Int Urogynecol J Pelvic Floor Dysfunct* 2001;12 Suppl 2:S12–14.

156. Paick JS, Ku JH, Shin JW, et al. Tension-free vaginal tape procedure for urinary incontinence with low Valsalva leak point pressure. *J Urol* 2004;172:1370–1373.

157. Rardin CR, Kohli N, Rosenblatt PL, et al. Tension-free vaginal tape: outcomes among women with primary versus recurrent stress urinary incontinence. *Obstet Gynecol* 2002;100:893–897.

158. Nilsson CG, Kuuva N, Falconer C, et al. Long-term results of the tension-free vaginal tape (TVT) procedure for surgical treatment of female stress urinary incontinence. *Int Urogynecol J Pelvic Floor Dysfunct* 2001;12 Suppl 2:S5–8.

159. Rezapour M, Ulmsten U. Tension-free vaginal tape (TVT) in women with recurrent stress urinary incontinence—a long-term follow up. *Int Urogynecol J Pelvic Floor Dysfunct* 2001;12 Suppl 2:S9–11.

160. Kuuva N, Nilsson CG. A nationwide analysis of complications associated with the tension-free vaginal tape (TVT) procedure. *Acta Obstet Gynecol Scand* 2002;81:72–77.

161. Tamussino K, Hanzal E, Kolle D, et al. The Austrian tension-free vaginal tape registry. *Int Urogynecol J Pelvic Floor Dysfunct* 2001;12 Suppl 2:S28–29.

162. Kolle D, Tamussino K, Hanzal E, et al. Bleeding complications with the tension-free vaginal tape operation. *Am J Obstet Gynecol* 2005;193:2045–2049.

163. Flock F, Reich A, Muche R, et al. Hemorrhagic complications associated with tension-free vaginal tape procedure. *Obstet Gynecol* 2004;104:989–994.

164. Muir TW, Tulikangas PK, Fidela Paraiso M, et al. The relationship of tension-free vaginal tape insertion and the vascular anatomy. *Obstet Gynecol* 2003;101:933–936.

165. Sokol AI, Jelovsek JE, Walters MD, et al. Incidence and predictors of prolonged urinary retention after TVT with and without concurrent prolapse surgery. *Am J Obstet Gynecol* 2005;192:1537–1543.

166. Meschia M, Pifarotti P, Bernasconi F, et al. Tension-free vaginal tape: analysis of outcomes and complica-

tions in 404 stress incontinent women. *Int Urogynecol J Pelvic Floor Dysfunct* 2001;12 Suppl 2:S24–27.

167. Dietz HP, Foote AJ, Mak HL, et al. TVT and SPARC suburethral slings: a case-control series. *Int Urogynecol J Pelvic Floor Dysfunct* 2004;15: 129–131.

168. Andonian S, Chen T, St-Denis B, et al. Randomized clinical trial comparing suprapubic arch sling (SPARC) and tension-free vaginal tape (TVT): one-year results. *Eur Urol* 2005;47:537–541.

169. Tseng LH, Wang AC, Lin YH, et al. Randomized comparison of the suprapubic arc sling procedure vs tension-free vaginal taping for stress incontinent women. *Int Urogynecol J Pelvic Floor Dysfunct* 2005;16:230–235.

170. Rechberger T, Rzezniczuk K, Skorupski P, et al. A randomized comparison between monofilament and multifilament tapes for stress incontinence surgery. *Int Urogynecol J Pelvic Floor Dysfunct* 2003;14: 432–436.

171. Bafghi A, Valerio L, Benizri EI, et al. Comparison between monofilament and multifilament polypropylene tapes in urinary incontinence. *Eur J Obstet Gynecol Reprod Biol* 2005;122:232–236.

172. Glavind K, Sander P. Erosion, defective healing, and extrusion after tension-free urethropexy for the treatment of stress urinary incontinence. *Int Urogynecol J Pelvic Floor Dysfunct* 2004;15:179–182.

173. Whiteside JL, Walters MD. Anatomy of the obturator region: relations to a transobturator sling. *Int Urogynecol J Pelvic Floor Dysfunct* 2004;15: 223–226.

174. de Leval J. Novel surgical technique for the treatment of female stress urinary incontinence: transobturator vaginal tape inside-out. *Eur Urol* 2003;44:724–730.

175. Barber MD, Gustilo-Ashby AM, Chen CCG, et al. Perioperative complications and adverse events of the MONARC™ transobturator tape compared to the tension-free vaginal tape. *Am J Obstet Gynecol* 2006;195: 1820–1825.

176. David-Montefiore E, Frobert JL, Grisard-Anaf M, et al. Perioperative complications and pain after the suburethral sling procedure for urinary stress incontinence: a French prospective randomized multicenter study comparing the retropubic and transobturator routes. *Eur Urol* 2006;49:133–138.

177. Davila GW, Johnson JD, Serels S. Multicenter experience with the Monarc transobturator sling system to treat stress urinary incontinence. *Int Urogynecol J Pelvic Floor Dysfunct* 2006;17:460–465.

178. Naidu A, Lim YN, Barry C, et al. Transobturator tape for stress incontinence: the North Queensland experience. *Aust N Z J Obstet Gynaecol* 2005;45:446–449.

179. Mellier G, Benayed B, Bretones S, et al. Suburethral tape via the obturator route: is the TOT a simplification of the TVT? *Int Urogynecol J Pelvic Floor Dysfunct* 2004;15:227–232.

180. Minaglia S, Ozel B, Klutke C, et al. Bladder injury during transobturator sling. *Urology* 2004;64: 376–377.

181. deTayrac R, Deffieux X, Droupy S, et al. A prospective randomized trial comparing tension-free vaginal tape and transobturator suburethral tape for surgical treatment of stress urinary incontinence. *Am J Obstet Gynecol* 2004;190:602–608.

182. Editors. Comment on notice of retraction. *Am J Obstet Gynecol* 2005;192:339.

183. Fischer A, Fink T, Zachmann S, et al. Comparison of retropubic and outside-in transoburator sling systems for the cure of female genuine stress urinary incontinence. *Eur Urol* 2005;48:799–804.

184. Costa P, Delmas V. Transobturator-tape procedure—"inside out or outside in": current concepts and evidence base. *Curr Opin Urol* 2004;14:313–315.

185. Domingo S, Alama P, Ruiz N, et al. Diagnosis, management, and prognosis of vaginal erosion after transobturator suburethral tape procedure using a nonwoven thermally bonded polypropylene mesh. *J Urol* 2005;173:1627–1630.

CHAPTER 15

Periurethral Bulking

Alfred E. Bent

The injection treatment of stress incontinence using sodium morrhuate was reported in 1938 (1). Injectable polytetrafluoroethylene (PTFE) was developed in the 1970s (2). The major breakthrough in modern bulking techniques came in 1989 with the development of a new product, glutaraldehyde cross-linked collagen (3). The approval of Contigen® (C.R. Bard, Inc., Covington, GA) in the United States (4) was followed in 1994 by Medicare approval for funding of treatment (5). Treatment was expanded in a second Medicare publication in 1996 (6). The ideal material is biocompatible, nonimmunologic, and hypoallergenic. It retains its bulking characteristics for a prolonged interval and therefore should not biodegrade, nor should it migrate (particle size over 80 μm). The material should be easy to prepare and easy to inject. The ideal material is safe, readily obtainable, inexpensive, efficacious, and durable and induces minimal tissue reaction. The theory on how injectable materials treat incontinence is by mucosal coaptation with subsequent increased urethral resistance to outflow of urine.

INDICATIONS AND CONTRAINDICATIONS

There is controversy regarding the characteristics of patients best treated with bulking agents. In 1992 the term "intrinsic sphincter deficiency" (ISD) was coined to describe patients with a damaged urethral sphincteric mechanism (Fig. 15.1), regardless of cause (7). While many, including the author of this chapter, believe the ideal patient for urethral bulking has both limited mobility of the bladder neck and a poorly functioning sphincteric mechanism, others consider that any patient desiring conservative treatment of stress urinary incontinence is a candidate. One of the aspects against use in young patients is that repeat injections of current agents are usually required to maintain effect, and this could mean many injections for such a patient. While some reports indicate equal effectiveness in patients with hypermobility of the bladder neck (8–10), others have noted impaired effect in these patients (11). Medicare guidelines for reimbursement require immobility of the bladder neck (5). It was not specified as to how immobility was to be determined, but most physicians use a Q-tip test with a straining value of less than 30 to 40 degrees as the cut-off value for hypermobility. Hypermobility has also been determined radiologically by a standing stress test with 2 cm or greater descent of the bladder neck, but there is no indication that imaging provides any more information than the standard Q-tip test. Other techniques include ultrasound and voiding cystourethrography (12). Medicare still requires a leak point pressure of 100 cm of water or less for reimbursement (6). The guidelines for this measurement require at least 150 mL of bladder filling, but there is no requirement regarding maximum bladder volume, position of the patient, size of urethral catheter, or kind of effort used to increase the intra-abdominal pressure. Without study confirmation, it is the author's opinion that the most important pretreatment indication is impaired mobility of the bladder neck. If an anti-incontinence procedure or other

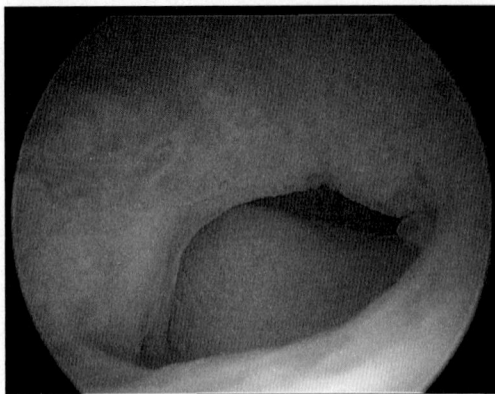

FIGURE 15.1 ● Urethroscopic appearance of damaged urethral sphincter. The bladder neck is open at rest and there is minimal mobility of the tissues during hold or strain maneuvers. The urethral lining is often pale or white rather than the usual pink appearance.

pelvic floor surgery has been performed, and stress incontinence persists or occurs, there is no contraindication to using a bulking agent, and often it is effective. This may be done as early as 6 weeks after surgery.

Generally, bulking agents are not indicated for patients with urethral hypermobility, especially now where there are minimally invasive tension-free slings that have excellent cure rates (see Chapter 14, Surgical Treatment of Stress Urinary Incontinence). There are situations in high-risk patients where a pessary has provided excellent control of pelvic organ prolapse, and there has been some temporary stabilization of bladder neck mobility. Periurethral bulking has been considered in this patient since when the prolapse is reduced by the pessary, the masking effect of the prolapse on the urethra is removed, and stress incontinence can result. This has not been studied definitively. The result of periurethral bulking after radiation therapy has not been encouraging. Contraindications include active urinary tract infection, high residual urine, severe detrusor overactivity, and reduced bladder capacity (less than 250 mL).

The ideal candidate for bulking therapy may be the patient with an immobile urethra and symptomatic stress incontinence, although there are other patients who could benefit from this approach (Table 15.1).

EVALUATION

Evaluation prior to therapy includes the basic evaluation consisting of history, physical examination, neurological screening examination, 24-hour void-

TABLE 15.1

Patients with Stress Urinary Incontinence Who Are Candidates for Periurethral Bulking Therapy

Intrinsic sphincter deficiency and hypomobility of the bladder neck

Intrinsic sphincter deficiency without hypomobility of the bladder neck

Medically compromised patient

Recent unsuccessful surgery

Childbearing age and wishes to have more children

Patient preference for most conservative approach

ing diary, residual urine determination, Q-tip test, and urinalysis and/or culture (see Chapter 5, Basic Evaluation of the Incontinent Female Patient). This is complemented by a cystometrogram (CMG) with leak point pressure determination and urethrocystoscopy. The procedure needs to be fully explained to the patient, including the need for repeat injections.

MATERIALS (Table 15.2)

Bulking agents should be of uniform spheroidal particle size over 110 microns in order to avoid phagocytization by macrophages and possible migration to distant locations. The injection performed under a low-pressure technique may prevent introduction into the vascular system.

Contigen® was approved by the Food and Drug Administration (FDA) in 1993. The material is prepared by glutaraldehyde cross-linking of bovine dermal collagen that is dispersed in phosphate-buffered physiologic saline, which may represent up to 65% of the total volume. The material contains 95% type I collagen and 1% to 5% type III collagen. It requires a skin test to be placed 30 days prior to injection to ensure absence of an allergic response, which occurs in 2% to 5% of women. The material biodegrades in 3 to 19 months and repeat injections may be required to re-establish efficacy. However, patients have been satisfactorily managed by one injection for as long as 6 years. The material is readily available and up to 1999 was the only injectable agent approved in the United States. The material comes in 2.5-mL syringes, injects through a 22-gauge needle, and requires one to three syringes injected transurethrally, and more as a periurethral injection. The contraindications to therapy include positive

TABLE 15.2

Periurethral Bulking Agents in North America

Trade Name	Company	Approval
Contigen®	C.R. Bard, Inc., Covington, GA	1993
Durasphere® EXP	Boston Scientific, Boston, MA Carbon Medical Technologies Inc., St. Paul, MN	1999
Tegress™	C.R. Bard, Inc., Covington, GA	2004
Macroplastique®	Uroplasty, Inc., Minneapolis, MN	FDA trials ongoing; approved in Canada, Europe
Zuidex™	Q-Med AB, Uppsala, Sweden	FDA trial ongoing; approved in Europe
Coaptite®	BioForm Medical, Inc., San Mateo, CA	2006
Permacol™	TSL, Aldershot, Hampshire, UK	FDA trials starting; approved in Europe

skin test for Contigen® implant, history of allergy to any bovine collagen products, patients undergoing desensitization to meat products, or in patients with a history of severe allergies.

Durasphere® (Boston Scientific, Natick, MA) was approved by the FDA in 1999. It consists of pyrolytic carbon-coated zirconium oxide beads suspended in a water-based carrier gel containing beta-glucan. The newer preparation (Durasphere EXP) has a particle size of 95 to 200 μm compared to the older material, which had particle size of 251 to 300 μm. The material is nonbiodegradable and is radiopaque but requires injection with an 18-gauge needle. The material comes in 1-mL syringes and requires two to four syringes for injection. The initial evaluation showed efficacy equal to Contigen® (13).

Tegress® (C.R. Bard, Inc., Covington, GA) is an ethylene vinyl copolymer dissolved in dimethyl sulfoxide (DMSO), approved in the United States in the fall of 2004. Upon contact with a liquid medium, diffusion of DMSO occurs, and a solid polymer precipitates. It comes in a 2.8-mL vial and is injected through a 25-gauge needle at a total of three sites, with no more than 1 mL at any one site and the total injection not to exceed 2.5 mL (14).

Macroplastique® (Uroplasty, Inc., Minneapolis, MN) is approved for use in Europe and in Canada but remains in study protocols in the United States. It is made from highly textured polydimethyl-siloxane macroparticles suspended in a bioexcretable carrier hydrogel of polyvinyl-pyrrolidone. It consists of silicone microimplants of size 73 to 100 μm and is prepared in 2.5-mL syringes. It requires a special injection apparatus for

transurethral injection, but recently it has been applied periurethrally using the Macroplastique Implantation System (15). The silicone name will most likely inhibit ease of approval in the United States.

Calcium hydroxylapatite (Coaptite®; BioForm Medical, Inc., San Mateo, CA) consists of 100-μm hydroxylapatite spheres suspended in an aqueous gel of sodium carboxylmethylcellulose. The material is a natural constituent of bones and teeth and has been used in dental and orthopaedic applications for a number of years. It was approved by the FDA in the spring of 2006 for use in the United States. It is injected via a 21-gauge needle, requires only 2.5 mL on initial injection, and can be visualized radiographically or by ultrasound (16).

Permacol™ (Tissue Science Laboratories plc [TSL], Aldershot, Hampshire, UK) is approved for use in Europe and is under study protocol in the Unites States. It is a sterile injectable suspension of acellular cross-linked porcine collagen matrix. It is a 60% suspension in saline of cryogenically milled Permacol® surgical implant. Its safety has largely been assumed through thousands of implants of porcine collagen sheets in pelvic reconstructive surgery. No skin test is required prior to use and comparative studies are favorable (17).

Zuidex™ gel (Q-Med AB, Uppsala, Sweden) is a combination of dextranomer (cross-linked polysaccharides) and hyaluronic acid. Dextranomer has been used in wound treatment for a number of years. Nonanimal stabilized hyaluronic acid (NASHA) is similar to natural hyaluronic acid found in the body. The material is prepared in 0.7-mL syringes and is used periurethrally with an implantation device (Implacer™) and the injection of four syringes of material (18,19). The material is in current use in the United States for ureterovesical reflux and is marketed as Deflux™. While marketed in Europe and Canada as a bulking agent, it is currently under study in the United States.

The best materials will probably come from tissue engineering and autologous cell bioimplants. This was briefly studied in the past by the use of autologous ear cartilage and in vitro expansion of cells for implant (20). The technology was not advanced because of cost and use of other readily available and cheaper products. The other material of interest in this area is human bladder muscle cells (21).

TECHNIQUES

The methods of injection described relate to use of current bulking materials (22). In some cases (Macroplastique®) there is need for a special delivery device, but in most cases, the materials are injected through spinal needles, specially made needles for injection directly in the periurethral tissue or by an implacement device, disposable injection needles that fit the operating channel of a cystoscope sheath, or with a reusable needle adapted to an operating sheath and bridge set. The amount of

material injected is usually greater for periurethral techniques, though the efficacy of periurethral versus transurethral is the same. There is a limit to the amount of some materials injected, such as Tegress™, which is restricted to 2.5 mL per session. Transurethral injection sites include the 3 and 9 o'clock positions, the 4, 8, and 12 o'clock positions, or the circumferential techniques using material at 3, 6, 9, and 12 o'clock. The material is intended for injection into the submucosa of the urethra.

Periurethral

Lidocaine 2% gel or a mixture of lidocaine 2% and benzocaine 20% may be placed in the urethra at the start of the procedure. The injection materials are assembled. (Fig. 15.2). The sites for injection of local anesthesia are selected at the level of the Skene duct openings on either side of the urethra, and using a 27- to 30-gauge needle, 0.5 to 1.0 mL of Xylocaine solution is injected 0.5 to 1.0 cm lateral to the urethral meatus (Fig. 15.3). The scope with zero-degree lens is inserted to the urethrovesical junction and then withdrawn to observe the proximal urethra. A syringe with lidocaine 1% solution and an attached 22-gauge spinal needle, with or without a small amount of indigo carmine to stain the tissues, is inserted and guided parallel to the urethra, directing the needle bevel

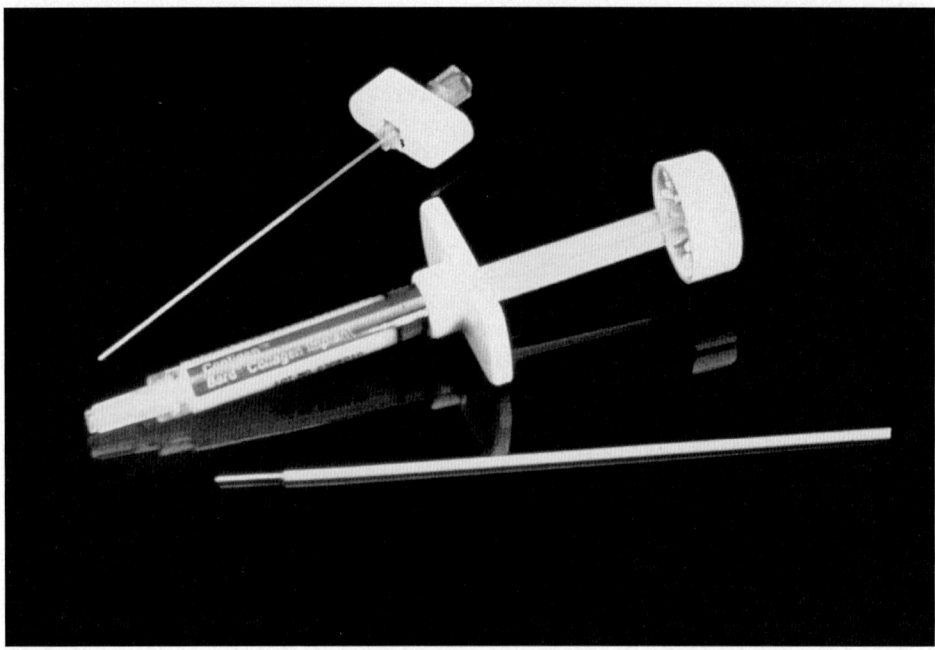

FIGURE 15.2 ● Contigen® injection syringe and needles. (Bard Urological Division, Covington, GA.)

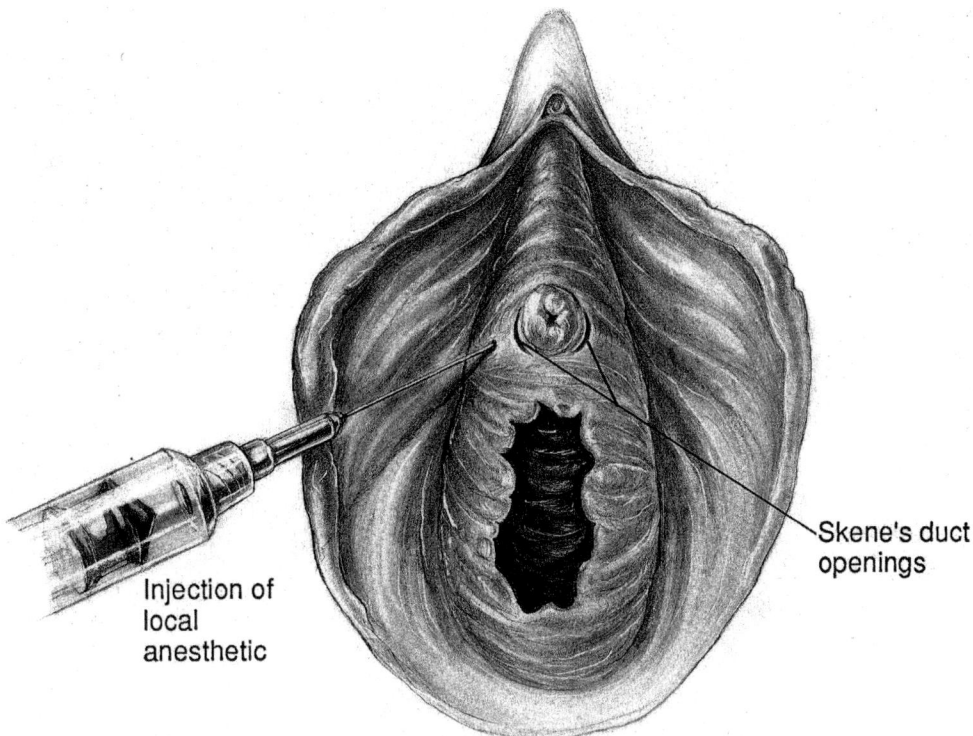

FIGURE 15.3 ● Periurethral bulking technique. Injection of local anesthetic at Skene duct openings. (From Bent AE. Periurethral collagen injections. *Oper Tech Gynecol Surg* 1997;2:54, with permission.)

medially toward the urethral lumen. This allows the injecting material to be viewed more easily as the position of the needle is determined (Fig. 15.4). The scope is used to observe the advancing needle and the syringe is moved in short strokes to allow the needle tip to be seen under the tissue at the proximal urethra. Once the correct location has been determined the syringe is replaced with a syringe of bulking agent, and the material is injected until the entire syringe has been injected or there has been adequate effect noted with urethral bulking (Fig. 15.5). The process is repeated on the opposite site, though the second side is always more difficult due to the distortion of the proximal urethra caused by the initial injection. The amount of Contigen® averages 3.75 mL for each of two sites, which is 7.5 mL of product. Durasphere® EXP comes with its own injection needle, which is 18 gauge in size and angled so as to aid the submucosal placement of the needle.

Alternatively, the periurethral anesthesia can be applied using a small injection needle (e.g., 25 gauge 1.5 inch) and left for 5 to 10 minutes. The bulking agent can then be placed by an appropriate delivery method without using the urethroscope.

Both Macroplastique® and Zuidex™ have a delivery apparatus that is placed into the urethra without urethroscopic or cystoscopic guidance. A marker on the apparatus allows location of the urethrovesical junction, the delivery needles are inserted into the device, and then the material is injected without visual control of the injection (Fig. 15.6).

Transurethral

The transurethral method normally has required the use of a cystoscope with a 12- or 25-degree lens with the appropriate sheath (20 or 21 French with no fenestration) and operating channel to allow the passage of a 5-French thermoplastic injection catheter and beveled 22-gauge disposable injection needle (Fig. 15.7). Alternatively, some physicians use a zero- or 30-degree lens, but this makes simultaneous viewing of the needle puncture site and impact of the injection difficult. A built-in needle delivery system is found in some systems, and the delivery mechanism is spring-loaded to allow advancement of the needle into the urethral submucosa for shallow or deep injection,

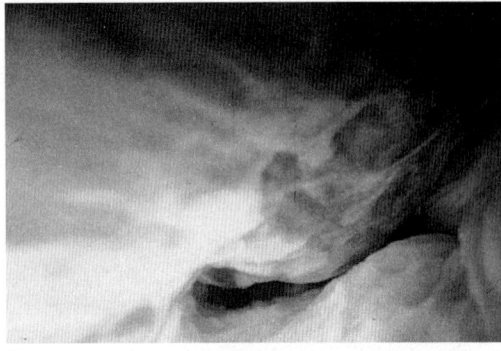
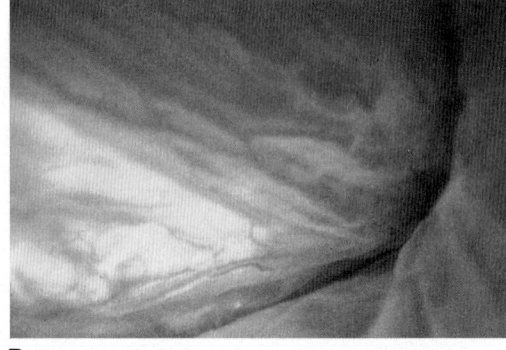

A   **B**

FIGURE 15.4 ● **(A)** Periurethral injection of indigo carmine has stained the urethral submucosa. **(B)** Bulking in place at the proximal urethra after periurethral injection completed.

and then removal of the needle just by releasing the thumb-operated mechanism (Karl Storz, Tuttlingen, Germany; Richard Wolf Medical Instruments Corporation, Vernon Hills, IL). The various materials for injection may dictate injection systems, such as the pressure gun required for injection of Macroplastique®. On the other hand, material like Tegress™ can be injected through a 25-gauge needle.

The procedure begins with optional placement of 2% lidocaine gel (or a mixture of 2% lidocaine and 20% benzocaine) in the urethra for 5 to 10 minutes. The injection needle may be preloaded with Xylocaine 1% solution (0.4 mL fills the 22-gauge disposable injection needle [C.R. Bard, Inc., Covington, GA), and this is injected into the selected site. The selected site may be as much as 2 cm distal to the bladder neck, but the needle bevel extends 1 cm from the hub, and the site of injection ends up 1 cm distal to the bladder neck. The injection should gradually cause distention of the urethral mucosa, and this is observed by appropriate angling of the cystoscope lens during the injection (Fig. 15.8). Should the injection be too superficial, there will be blanching or superficial appearance of the injection material under the urethral mucosa, and the needle must be repositioned. There is always discussion as to whether the needle bevel should turn toward the urethral lumen or away from it. The needle inserts better into the tissue if the bevel is turned away from the lumen during insertion, and then it can be rotated according to visualized effect. After injecting the first side, Xylocaine is flushed through the injecting needle to clear the remaining collagen. The second syringe of bulking agent is attached and the injection at the second site commences as the lidocaine solution is first delivered to provide anesthesia, fol-

lowed by the bulking material. The urethral mucosa should swell with the injection and gradually the injection sites meet in the midline as the bladder neck is occluded.

The injection of Tegress™ may be completed with a 25-gauge needle, and any local anesthetic has to be injected through a different needle than the one carrying the bulking agent. Also, the material is seldom seen occluding the bladder neck, and the injected volume is limited to 2.5 mL.

Durasphere® requires an 18-gauge needle for injection. A modified injection technique has been described for Durasphere® that consists of a single needlestick at 4 o'clock, hydrodissection with 1.5 mL of 1% lidocaine, gradual withdrawal, advancement, or rotation of the needle tip after resistance is noted, and holding the needle in position 10 seconds after coaptation is achieved to prevent leakage of material from the injection site. Recently the description has changed and is posted on the website. Insert the transurethral injection needle at 45 degrees to the tissue with the bevel facing the urethral lumen until the bevel is just under the mucosal surface. Reangle the scope parallel to the urethra and guide the needle tip toward the bladder neck until it is approximately 1 cm distal to the bladder neck. Inject slowly. The objective is to obtain closure from the bladder neck to the midurethra.

POSTINJECTION FOLLOW-UP

Patients may have urethral burning with urination that lasts for only part of a day and can be controlled with phenazopyridine (Pyridium). Antibiotics are not mandatory but may be given immediately before and/or 1 or 2 days after injection, since the rate of urinary tract infection is 10%. The patient is allowed to void after the injection, and

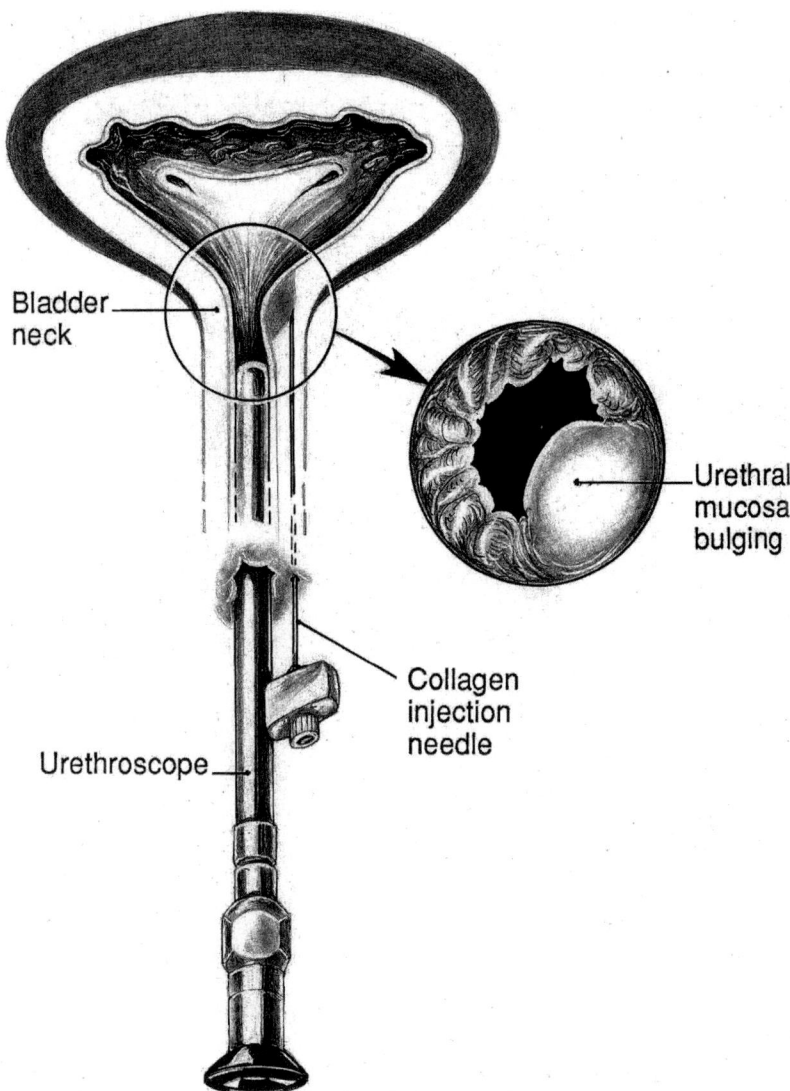

Bladder neck

Urethral mucosa bulging

Collagen injection needle

Urethroscope

FIGURE 15.5 ● Urethroscopic guidance of periurethral injection. *Circled insert* shows effect at proximal urethral location. (From Bent AE. Periurethral collagen injections. *Oper Tech Gynecol Surg* 1997;2:54, with permission.)

she should be prepared to stay in the clinic area for 1 to 2 hours to allow the initial swelling from the injection to diminish enough to allow voiding. If voiding does not occur or is associated with high residual urine (over 200 mL as determined by bladder scan, ultrasound, or straight catheter), then the patient needs to either be instructed in self-catheterization, or have an 8 to 10 French Foley catheter placed, using no more than 5 mL in the balloon. One technique is to teach patients self-catheterization prior to the injection, but this means that as many as 70% to 80% of patients are taught unnecessarily. One can resort to teaching

those who need it after the injection. If a Foley catheter is placed, it is left for 24 to 48 hours, and then the patient returns for voiding assessment. Those who utilize self-catheterization should do so after attempts at voiding, four or five times a day. There is no longer a need to perform self-catheterization after voiding commences, and residual urine amounts are less than 100 mL, or less than 25% of the voided volume, which must exceed 100 mL. Voiding dysfunction usually resolves in 12 to 24 hours. Patients should be called the day following the injection to be sure there is no continuing problem. A follow-up appointment is made

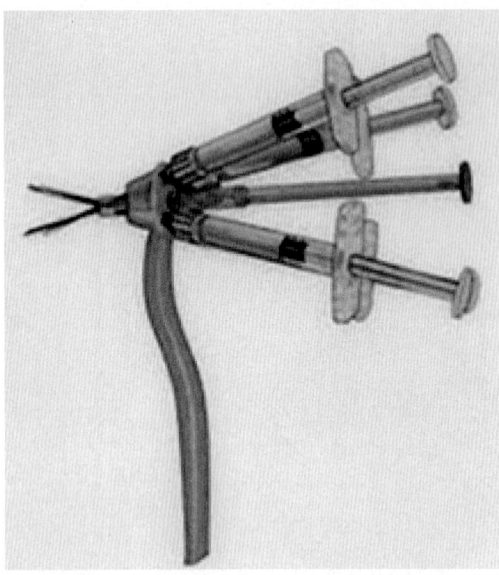

FIGURE 15.6 ● Zuidex™ implacer. (Q-Med Scandinavia, Inc, Princeton, NJ, and AB, Seminariegatan 21, SE-752 28 Uppsala, Sweden.)

for 4 weeks, and at that time, in addition to patient history, assessment is made for voiding function, urinary tract infection, and swelling at the suburethral injection site. Additionally, the effectiveness of the injection and need for further injection are assessed, and overactive bladder symptoms are addressed if appropriate.

COMPLICATIONS

The most common complication during the procedure is pain. For those having treatment in a clinic or office setting, this can be minimized with intraurethral topical anesthetic gel, and/or injection of local anesthetic into the submucosal injection site. Most patients are able to tolerate the procedure without any difficulty and usually observe on the monitor. Extrusion of material may be avoided by submucosal placement of the needle approximately 1 cm into the tissue, and then observing the injection effect on the urethral lining. If the injection is too superficial, and the lining distends rapidly, then an alternative site should be selected. A small amount of bleeding may occur from the injection site, or the material may start to extrude from the puncture site. In this case, when using a disposable needle, the hub should be pressed against the lining of the urethra, and this will usually control the situation. After injection, a small amount of material may leak from the site, but this is seldom a problem unless the material used is Tegress™. In this situation, the extruded material needs to be removed since it is permanent and can lead to recurrent irritative voiding symptoms and infections.

The most common complications in the immediate period are urinary retention and voiding dysfunction. Most patients void within 1 to 2 hours, and a few may need catheter management. Voiding discomfort occurs in some patients and the incidence of urinary tract infection is as high as 10% to 15%. Since antibiotic treatment immediately before or after the injection may not prevent an infection, the urine should be checked at the initial postoperative visit.

Delayed complications are rare. Suburethral abscess is associated with increasing voiding dysfunction with or without pain. A more common problem is recurrent urinary tract infections requiring prophylactic antibiotics. Cystoscopy may be required to be certain there is no bulking material resting in the urethra. Occasionally patients have a problem with overactive bladder. Macroplastique® was associated with a high incidence of dysuria for 48 hours.

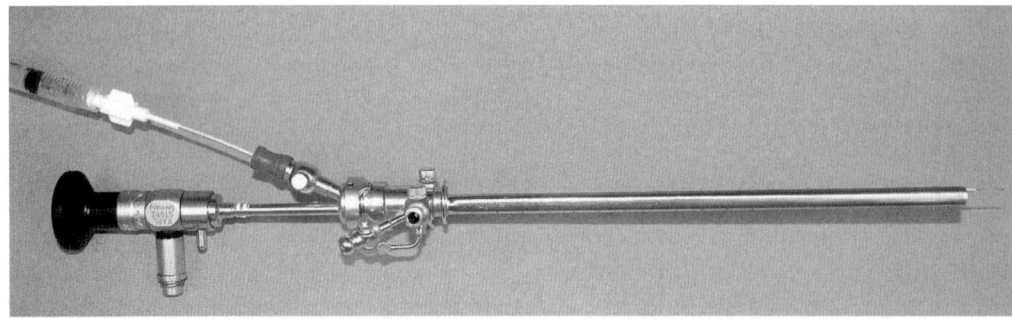

FIGURE 15.7 ● Cystoscope with straight bevel at end, 12-degree lens, and disposable injection needle in operating channel.

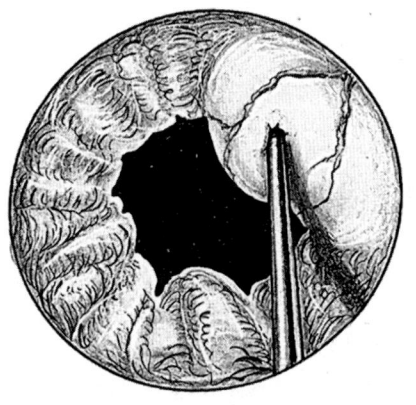

A

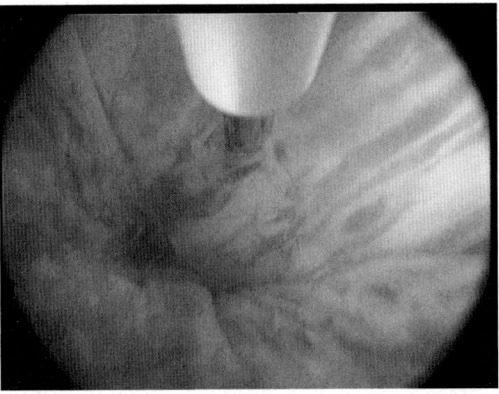

B

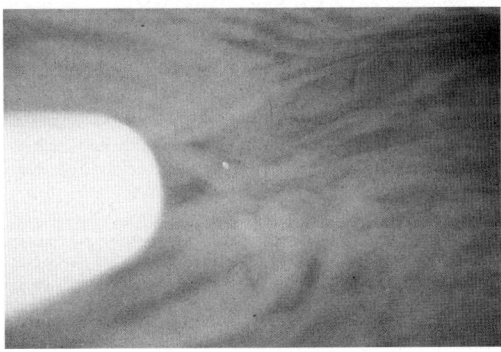

C

FIGURE 15.8 ● Transurethral collagen injection. **(A)** Transurethral needle placement in urethral submucosa. (From Bent AE. Periurethral collagen injections. *Oper Tech Gynecol Surg* 1997;2:54, with permission.) Transurethral needle **(B)** partially advanced and **(C)** advanced to hub for transurethral bulking.

EFFECTIVENESS

There is no standardized manner in which to evaluate effectiveness of therapy. Most of the FDA-approved trials utilize voiding diaries, pad tests, and subjective data such as the Stamey scoring system. Urodynamic testing and leak point pressures have not proven useful. Definitions of cure, improvement, and failure can vary. It may require two injections to provide continence or significant improvement, and these can be performed as close together as 1 month. If there is no improvement after two injections, then there is unlikely to be a response. Cure or improvement will occur in 60% to 80% of patients, with cure around 40%. Repeat injections are required at varying intervals to maintain the effect (Table 15.3).

The review in the Cochrane Database (28) indicates that randomized trials suggest, but do not prove, that periurethral injection of established bulking agents results in objective and subjective short-term improvement of symptomatic stress incontinence in females. Many of the study papers on Contigen® included patients with severe incontinence (leak point pressures less than 65 cm H_2O) and minimal urethral mobility, precluding operative intervention other than obstructive slings. A number of these patients were significantly improved, and while injection therapy may only last 12 months, repeat injections are generally helpful again.

The statement from the Third International Consultation on Incontinence quoted a success rate of approximately 70%, based on level IV evidence (29). The 30 studies reviewed showed small numbers (only 13 with follow-up over 1 year) and with many variables related to techniques. There were not enough patients or studies to comment on any bulking agent except collagen. However, these finding are almost the same as those published after the 2002 meeting. All studies on new injectable agents in the United States and Canada go through a rigorous randomized comparison, usually to Contigen®. The main problem with these studies is that patients tend to drop out and disappear when they are not better. Hopefully there will be enough published studies to accurately represent the 70% improvement that many quote. While the International Consultation suggests comparative studies to conservative therapies, most of the current trials have already had conservative therapy failures. There is no point in comparing injectable therapy to surgical procedures, since the injections are not permanent. However, many patients have significant improvement from periurethral bulking and are able to carry on activities without invasive surgery. They gladly accept another clinic visit in a year or so to redo their bulking. The ACOG Practice Bulletin (30) stresses the limitations of bulking agents: durability and long-

TABLE 15.3

Results of Injectable Urethral Bulking Agents in Women (Minimum 60 Patients)

Investigator	Agent	Number of patients	Follow-up, months (range)	Mean number/volume of injections (mL)	Dry/improved/ failed (%)
Cross (23)	Collagen	139	18 (6–36)	NR	74/20/6
Groutz (24)	Collagen	63	12 (1–32)	2.08/3.1	13/27/60
Herschorn (25)	Collagen	187	22 (4–69)	2.5/9.65	23/52/25
Monga (9)	Collagen	60	24	1.6/19	48/20/32
Smith (26)	Collagen	96	14 (6–21)	2.1/11.9	38/28/34
Swami (27)	Collagen	111	40	NR	25/40/35
Lightner (13)	Durasphere®	61	12	1/4.3	na/80/20

term results. However, for women with extensive comorbidity, injection of bulking agents could provide useful relief. Taking it a step further, most of these patients would gladly come into the clinic each year for their annual "top up" in order to avoid surgical risks and other inconveniences.

FUTURE CONSIDERATIONS

Contigen® remains the bulking agent of choice in the United States. This is because of a good safety profile for the 13 years of use, ease of injection, and its effectiveness in providing relief of symptoms in a large proportion of patients. Tegress™ is being promoted for ease of injection, but effectiveness has not been shown to be better than Contigen®. It may have some irritative effects due to the leakage of material into the urethra after injection. Durasphere® may increase in popularity as long as the injection technique is made user-friendly. There is very poor data on any large number of patients receiving Macroplastique®. The newer products approaching FDA approval may be equally effective, but long-term data is required to determine durability. Only autologous injection of either muscle cells or collagen may prove to be better, and this remains a long way off. Studies have illustrated that skeletal muscle proliferates and appears to persist favorably following injection into the bladder and urethral smooth muscle (21). These preliminary studies indicate that autologous skeletal muscle injection may come to represent a viable alternative to other injectable agents currently available.

REFERENCES

1. Murless BC. The injection treatment of stress incontinence. *J Obstet Gynaecol Br Emp* 1938;45:67–73.
2. Shortliffe LM, Freiha FS, Kessler R, et al. Treatment of urinary incontinence by the periurethral implantation of glutaraldehyde cross-linked collagen. *J Urol* 1989;141:538–541.
3. Berg S. Polytef augmentation urethroplasty. Correction of surgically incurable urinary incontinence by injection technique. *Arch Surg* 1973;107:379–381.
4. Appell RA, McGuire EJ, DeRidder PA, et al. Summary of effectiveness and safety in the prospective, open, multicenter investigation of collagen implant for incontinence due to intrinsic sphincteric deficiency in females [abstract]. *J Urol* 1994;151:418.
5. *Medicare Coverage Issues Manual: Incontinence Control Devices.* Department of Health and Human Services, Health Care Financing Administration, June 1994, Transmittal No. 70. Section 65–69.
6. *Medicare Coverage Issues Manual: Incontinence Control Devices.* Department of Health and Human Services, Health Care Financing Administration, September 1996, Transmittal No. 89. Section 65–69.
7. Agency for Health Care Policy and Research. *Urinary Incontinence in Adults: Clinical Practice Guidelines.* US Department of Health Care and Human Resources Publication 92-0038. Rockville, MD: Agency for Health Care Policy and Research, 1996.
8. Herschorn S, Radomski SB, Steele DJ. Early experience with intraurethral collagen injections for urinary incontinence. *J Urol* 1992;148:1797–1800.
9. Monga AK, Robinson D, Stanton SL. Periurethral collagen injections for genuine stress incontinence: a two-year follow-up. *Br J Urol* 1995;76:156–160.
10. Herschorn S, Radomski SB. Collagen injections for genuine stress urinary incontinence: patient selection and durability. *Int Urogynecol J* 1997;8:18–24.
11. Bent AE, Foote J, Siegel S, et al. Collagen implant for treating stress urinary incontinence in women with urethral hypermobility. *J Urol* 2001;166:1354–1357.

12. Kelvin FM, Maglinte DD, Hale D, et al. Voiding cystourethrography in female stress incontinence. *AJR Am J Roentgenol* 1996;167:1065–1066.

13. Lightner D, Calvosa C, Anderson R et al. A new injectable bulking agent for treatment of stress urinary incontinence: results of a multicenter, randomized, controlled, double-blind study of Durasphere®. *Urology* 2001;58:12–15.

14. URYX® Urethral Bulking Agent. FDA summary of safety and effectiveness. www.fda.gov/cdrh/PDF3/p030030b.pdf.

15. Taminini JT, D'Ancona CA, Tadini V, et al. Macroplastique® implantation system for the treatment of female stress urinary incontinence. *J Urol* 2003;169: 2229–2233.

16. Mayer R, Lightfoot M, Jung I. Preliminary evaluation of calcium hydroxylapatite as a transurethral bulking agent for stress urinary incontinence. *Urology* 2001;57: 434–438.

17. Bano F, Barrington JW, Dyer R. Comparison between porcine dermal implant (Permacol®) and silicone injection (Macroplastique™) for urodynamic stress incontinence. *Int Urogynecol J* 2005;16:147–150.

18. van Kerrebroeck P, ter Meulen F, Larsson G, et al. Efficacy and safety of a novel system (NASHA/Dx copolymer via the Implacer™ device) for the treatment of stress urinary incontinence. *Urology* 2004;64:276–281.

19. Chapple CR, Haab F, Cervigni M, et al. An open, multicentre study of NASHA/Dx gel (Zuidex™) for the treatment of stress urinary incontinence. *Eur Urol* 2005;48:488–494.

20. Bent AE, Tutrone RT, McLennan MT, et al. Treatment of intrinsic sphincter deficiency using autologous ear chondrocytes as a bulking agent. *Neurourol Urodyn* 2001;20:157–165.

21. Yokoyama T, Yoshimura N, Dhir R, et al. Persistence and survival of autologous muscle derived cells versus bovine collagen as potential treatment of stress urinary incontinence. *J Urol* 2001;165:271–276.

22. Bent AE. Periurethral collagen injections. *Oper Tech Gynecol Surg* 1997;2:51–55.

23. Cross CA, English SF, Cespedes RD, et al. A follow-up on transurethral collagen injection therapy for urinary incontinence. *J Urol* 1998;159:106–108.

24. Groutz A, Blaivas JG, Kesler SS, et al. Outcome results of transurethral collagen injection for female stress incontinence: assessment by urinary incontinence score. *J Urol* 2000;164:2006–2009.

25. Herschorn S, Steele DJ, Radomski SB. Follow-up of intraurethral collagen for female stress urinary incontinence. *J Urol* 1996;156:1305–1309.

26. Smith DN, Appell RA, Winters JC, et al. Collagen injection therapy for female intrinsic sphincteric deficiency. *J Urol* 1997;157:1275–1278.

27. Swami S, Batista JE, Abrams P. Collagen for female genuine stress incontinence after a minimum 2-year follow-up. *Br J Urol* 1997;80:757–761.

28. Pickard R, Reaper J, Wyness L, et al. Periurethral injection therapy for urinary incontinence in women. *The Cochrane Library*, 2003, Volume 3.

29. Smith T, Daneshgari F, Dmochowski R, et al. Surgery for urinary incontinence in women. In Abrams P, Cardozo L, Khoury S, et al, eds. *Incontinence*. Third International Consultation on Incontinence, June 26–29, 2004. Health Publications Ltd, Paris, 2005, pp. 1297–1370.

30. ACOG Practice Bulletin. *Urinary incontinence in women.* Clinical management guidelines for Obstetricians-Gynecologists. Number 63, June 2005.

CHAPTER 16

Mixed Urinary Incontinence

Patrick J. Woodman

DEFINITION

Mixed urinary incontinence (MUI) is the complaint of involuntary leakage associated with urgency and also with exertion, effort, sneezing, or coughing (1). Thus, it is a complex clinical condition of the leakage of urine with acute rises in abdominal pressure (stress urinary incontinence) *and* leakage that occurs as a result of spontaneous or triggered rises in bladder pressure (urge urinary incontinence). The rises in abdominal pressure that typically occur with exertion, cough, laugh, or sneeze result in transient spikes in bladder pressure. More persistent rises in bladder pressure are commonly associated with urgency. Urgency can be spontaneous, as a result of a detrusor contraction, or can occur as a result of socialized and environmental cues, such as being startled, passing a restroom, acute drops in outside temperature, and hearing or feeling water run. On occasion, detrusor contractility and urinary leakage may be insensible.

A distinction should be made between the symptom, sign, urodynamic observation, and condition of urinary incontinence. For the purposes of this chapter, the definitions as specified by the International Continence Society (1,2) will be used unless otherwise specified. Overactive bladder (OAB) is a symptomatic diagnosis whereby a patient has urgency and frequency with or without urge incontinence. Detrusor overactivity is a urodynamic diagnosis of OAB associated with urodynamic evidence of detrusor contractions. Urge incontinence is the actual leakage of urine with urge, either reported by the patient (symptom) or observed during bladder filling (sign). Since stress

incontinence also has its own nuances, even well-done research studies are sometimes difficult to interpret due to confusion over the definition of MUI. For instance, a woman with urodynamic stress incontinence and urodynamically recorded urge incontinence has mixed incontinence. This situation happens only 27% of the time (3). The sensitivity (specificity) of urodynamics in women with a history of mixed incontinence is only 0.51 (0.66) (4). Those patients with MUI symptoms show only urodynamic stress incontinence on urodynamics 55% of the time and detrusor overactivity incontinence in 38% (5). Since detrusor overactivity can be missing on as many as 46% of urodynamics in those with OAB (6), it seems prudent to use a combination of symptomatic and objective evidence in the definition of MUI. The woman who has observed stress leakage in the office but also reports symptoms of OAB would also qualify as having MUI. This dichotomy affects the diagnosis, decision to treat, and eventual treatment outcomes of MUI.

INCIDENCE

MUI is one of the most common types of urinary incontinence in patients presenting to their physicians with complaints of urinary loss. It has been estimated that 29% to 62% of women with urinary incontinence have MUI (7–13). MUI is associated with an increasing number of vaginal deliveries, a history of operative vaginal delivery, and a history of chronic obstructive pulmonary disease and neurologic disease (12). Women with MUI tend to have a more severe degree of incontinence symptoms than do women with pure stress or urge incontinence (10,13) and have greater degrees of bother (13). Patients who undergo surgical procedures for the stress component of their condition and have urgency or urge incontinence have a reduced patient satisfaction, and in many series the urge component reduces the overall continence rates (14). Although the weekly MUI rate is as low as 3% in young, pregnant patients primiparas who had vaginal deliveries were found to have a higher risk of stress or MUI than their nulliparous counterparts (odds ratio 5.7) (15). The incidence of MUI is known to rise in women after the sixth decade.

Incontinence has been shown to have a detrimental effect on health-related quality of life (HRQL), and those with urge incontinence or MUI may be more greatly affected (16). Women with MUI have more reported incontinent episodes when compared with stress incontinence. Indeed, the stress and urge components have a synergistically negative effect on patient symptomatology, distress (17), and quality of life (18). Nocturia can lead to sleep deprivation and either worsen or trigger depression, resulting in even further functional and quality-of-life deficits. Women with MUI are 13.5 times more likely to have major depression than women with stress incontinence (11).

ETIOLOGY

There are several theories of the etiology of mixed incontinence, one of which is iatrogenic. The first, and most commonly held, is that MUI is merely a combination of stress incontinence and urge incontinence, with their individual respective etiologies. In this scenario, correcting the stress component would be expected not to change the urge component. However, in a significant number of cases of surgical correction of the stress component of MUI, the urge component is cured or improved.

Another theory is that MUI is due to a urethral event. By forcing urine (or passive urine leakage) into the bladder neck, the patient is set up for the normal neurologic response of voiding: triggering a conscious urgency and/or bladder contractions that are initially suppressed. Eventually, however, neuropathic or myopathic changes may occur that make the spread of contractile signals more effective, resulting in the unconscious let-down of urethral and sometimes pelvic floor tone. McLennan et al describe a shorter functional urethral length in women with urethral instability (19). This shortening is a physiologic event coordinated with detrusor contraction and posterior slackening of the endopelvic fascial hammock that occurs during normal voiding. Bump et al have supported this theory: they found that the main determining factor as to whether urge incontinence symptoms were present in their MUI subjects seemed to be incontinence severity (8). Others have not found this to be the case (20).

It also has been suggested that there is a myogenic (21–24) and/or neurologic (9,25) basis for the development of urge incontinence. Myocytes have stretch-sensitive cation channels that can depolarize and trigger action potentials, and this can result from stretching part of the bladder wall (22). Unlike skeletal muscle, denervated smooth muscle becomes hypersensitive to acetylcholine and small rises can trigger a large reaction. If the stimulus for the action potential is persistent, electrically coupling can happen, leading to a spreading of the muscular action potential (23). Vaginal electromyographic changes are seen in urge, stress, and mixed incontinence and successively decrease with age (9). Others have proposed that the pelvic nerves stretch as a result of increased abdominal pressure and that this stimulates a bladder contraction (26).

However, there is an important subgroup of mixed incontinence that deserves particular attention: those who present with MUI after a stress incontinence surgical procedure (27). Worsening or de novo urge symptoms after surgery may indicate bladder outlet obstruction, a vesical or urethral foreign body (such as a stitch or sling material), or a urinary tract fistula or diverticulum (28). Cystourethroscopy and interval urodynamics with pressure-flow studies should be entertained for this subset of patients.

EVALUATION

The evaluation of urinary incontinence is covered in Chapters 5 through 7.

TREATMENT

Although the true etiology may be in question, most experts agree that MUI is a difficult problem to treat. The expectations of the patient are that whatever treatment the physician recommends will stop the leakage, when in fact a total cure may not be attainable. Treating the urge component of MUI alone may not change the stress component. Treating the stress component may not only result in an unchanged urge component (18) but in 10% to 15% can exacerbate urge symptoms (29).

The most common recommendation is to treat the predominant symptom first. If the patient suffers from stress-predominant MUI, surgical repair of the stress component can cure or improve the urge component in 25% to 75% of cases. Since surgery for SUI can cause bladder outlet obstruction, the worsening of urge incontinence symptoms after surgery should trigger investigation (28). Lower urinary tract symptoms such as urge incontinence have been shown to be more bothersome and more distressing than the occasional leakage of urine with a cough or sneeze (27). If the predominant symptom is urge incontinence, the prudent choice would be to aggressively treat the urge component until stable, then address any residual stress incontinence. This achieves two things: it identifies a therapy already proven to control the patient's urge, and it establishes a baseline (on treatment) that can be used to determine if the patient's urge symptoms change or worsen after surgical correction of stress incontinence.

Since most MUI treatment approaches hinge on addressing the individual symptom components, various therapies have been employed to treat MUI over the years. Many of these are addressed, at length, in previous chapters (Chapters 11 through 15). A summary of treatment options is listed in Table 16.1. The evidence-based literature available about MUI-specific treatments and outcomes will be discussed.

Behavioral Therapy

Behavioral therapy is a broad category of interventions designed to "unlearn" negative behaviors and learn or relearn good behaviors. They can be as simple as adjusting the time and amount of fluid intake and avoiding certain foods or drinks, or as complex as preferential contraction of the levator ani or pelvic floor muscles. As a treatment option group, behavioral therapies have minimal side effects or risks but help a large number of patients. These therapies should be considered as first-line empiric therapy for MUI.

Bladder training or "bladder drill" is a behavioral therapy focused on changing bladder habits

TABLE 16.1

Treatments for Mixed Urinary Incontinence

Treatment	Usefulness
Behavioral Therapy	
Dietary changes/water restriction	UUI, SUI
Bladder training	UUI, SUI
Kegel exercises	UUI, SUI
Prompted voiding	UUI, (SUI)
Drug Therapy	
Serotonin & noradrenaline reuptake inhibitors	SUI
Alpha-adrenergic agents	SUI
Estrogen	UUI, (SUI)
Anticholinergic agents	UUI
Barriers	
Pessaries	SUI, HM
Urethral inserts/patches	SUI
Surgical Therapy	
Bladder neck suspension	SUI, HM
Suburethral sling procedures	SUI, ISD
Bulking agents	SUI, ISD

UUI, urge component; SUI, stress component; HM, hypermobility of bladder neck; ISD, intrinsic sphincteric deficiency.

to reduce urinary incontinence by increasing bladder capacity and restoring normal bladder function (30). One starts with an attainable goal, based on the patient's voiding diary. Slowly, over the course of 6 to 12 weeks, the patient is encouraged to delay micturition 15 minutes longer than she would normally wait to empty. After 1 to 2 weeks of stability with no leakage episodes, then the time goal is increased another 15 to 30 minutes, until a goal of voiding every 2 to 3 hours is reached. Cure rates range from 44% to 90% in urge incontinence, although one randomized controlled trial (RCT) of bladder training in older women (with a 57% reduction in incontinence episodes) revealed that similar results could be seen in stress incontinence (31). The mechanisms of improvement in bladder training are still unexplained.

Most people are unaware of exactly the type and quantity of the fluid they drink, or how often they actually void. Fluid management is done by initially recording this information in a voiding diary so estimates of the amount of each void and the frequency of incontinent episodes can be made. Using this information, the physician may make recommendations for the patient to drink more water, for instance, or to restrict fluids before bedtime. Although a desired fluid intake has not been substantiated by clinical studies, many experts recommend six to eight 8-ounce glasses of water per day, or 15 cc per pound of body weight (32). These recommendations can lead to adequate quantities of dilute, nonirritating urine and provide the body with plenty of fluid to perform functional tasks, such as optimizing stool consistency. A randomized trial of fluid management found that 33% of incontinent patients benefited by increasing fluids by 500 cc (not to exceed 2,400 cc/day) (33).

Timed voiding is a way to prevent the distention triggering of a detrusor contraction that may be uncontrolled by emptying *earlier* than the patient would normally do so. If waiting 4 hours between voids reliably results in a severe urge to void and an urge incontinent episode, then the patient is encouraged to void every 3 hours. If the interval necessary for timed voiding is too close together, then timed voiding can be combined with bladder training over time to increase bladder capacity. If the stress component of MUI is worse when the bladder is full, then emptying earlier would decrease potential incontinence. No quality-controlled studies have been done with timed voiding for MUI (32).

Reducing caffeine ingestion is another commonly recommended item, since caffeine acts as a natural diuretic and bladder irritant in susceptible individuals. Although there is some evidence to support this recommendation (33), restriction of other dietary substances thought to irritate the bladder, such as artificial sweeteners, spicy food, and citrus foods, is not yet supported by the data.

Weight reduction after bariatric surgery has been associated with improvement in both stress and urge incontinence (34). However, no studies have suggested that nonsurgical weight loss in mild to moderately overweight individuals had any benefit (33).

Constipation has been cited as a factor that makes urge incontinence worse, especially when coexisting with a large rectocele. However, no data exist to support this recommendation (33). Smoking has been cited as a risk factor for both stress and urge incontinence, as well as other lower urinary tract symptoms, but evidence of a link is also inconclusive (33). Recreational, daily, and occupational activity has been linked to pelvic organ prolapse (35) but not definitively to incontinence.

Pelvic Floor Muscle Exercises (Kegel Exercises)

Pelvic floor muscle training (PFMT) is considered a first-line therapy for MUI. The three-layer muscular plate of the levator ani spanning the pelvic outlet is known to contract together to cause an inward lift and squeeze around the urethra, vagina, and rectum (36). Strength training and timing are two ways that the pelvic floor muscle can be trained to effect an improvement in continence. Costs for behavioral therapy for MUI are approximately $2,500 per patient, which is comparable to the approximately $2,100 per year for medical interventions, and much less than the average direct costs for surgical intervention of $20,000 (37). Women who are not wearing protective pads prior to starting therapy, women with fewer incontinent episodes, and women who had previous surgery for incontinence seem to have more success with PFMT for their urge symptoms (37). For primarily stress symptoms, women with fewer leakage episodes on bladder diary and who have *never* been treated for stress incontinence seem to have more success with PFMT (37). The optimal number of pelvic floor muscle exercises has not been determined (38), but 24 to 160 contractions per day, in divided sets, are usually recommended.

Although studies on women with stress incontinence or urge incontinence alone are fairly numerous, most studies of PFMT exercises on women with MUI are post hoc analyses of the MUI patients. For instance, Dattilo demonstrated a greater than 50% improvement in 18 MUI subjects (81.6%)

doing 50 to 60 exercises per day for 5 to 6 weeks, and 45% had maintained that benefit at a mean of 16.6 months after treatment (37). Nygaard et al performed an intent-to-treat analysis of women with urinary incontinence treated by a 3-month course of PFMT as first-line therapy (39). Subjects were instructed to perform 36 to 75 exercises per day in divided sessions. Forty-four percent of all enrollees had at least 50% improvement in the number of incontinent episodes per day, and this increased to 55% for those who completed the course of therapy. All subjects with MUI ($n = 17$) decreased their incontinence frequency from 3.9 incontinent episodes to 3.2 episodes per day. Of those MUI subjects who completed their course of therapy ($n = 10$), the incontinence frequency decreased from 3.0 to 1.7 episodes per day. Six months later, one third of all enrollees reported that they continued to have good or excellent results and desired no further treatment.

The timing of pelvic floor muscle contraction can also influence leakage parameters. Miller et al have described what they call "the Knack," which involves timing a pelvic floor contraction just before an impending cough or sneeze (40). Subjects able to demonstrate "the Knack" showed 98.1% less urine leakage during a medium cough test compared with subjects who were not taught "the Knack." Timing a pelvic floor contraction can help with the urge component of MUI as well by sustaining a contraction of the pelvic floor muscles or quickly "flicking" the pelvic floor muscles continually when a seemingly irrepressible urge is felt. In this way, the subject can competitively inhibit the detrusor contraction and then calmly make her way to the restroom.

In some studies, when compared to oxybutynin and placebo, PFMT has performed better than medical therapy. PFMT was significantly more effective in the treatment of urge ($n = 90$) or MUI ($n = 107$), and both PFMT and oxybutynin were better than placebo (41). The subjects in this group received an 8-week course of 45 exercises in divided sets. Attrition was 6.2% in the behavioral group, 17.9% in the drug group, and 18.5% in the placebo group. Behavioral therapy resulted in a mean 80.7% improvement in incontinent episodes, the best patient-perceived improvement (74.1% "much better" compared to 50.9% in drug group and 26.9% for placebo), and the lowest percent of subjects wanting to change therapies (14.0% vs. 75.5% in each of the other groups). Although this was a large group of subjects with MUI, the authors did not break out the MUI-specific outcomes compared to urge incontinence subjects.

Biofeedback is a form of operant learning or re-education with auditory, visual, or tactile feedback. Biofeedback is most commonly added to PFMT in order to teach a patient to selectively contract the pelvic floor muscles. Bump et al found that although 49% of women given brief instructions on PFMT could mount an "ideal" contraction, 25% would trigger a Valsalva maneuver, which was counterproductive (42). Cure or improvement rates ranged from 68% to 92%. In studies that measured incontinent episode frequency, typical reductions ranged between 61% and 85% (30). Biofeedback can be a simple verbal instruction or encouragement, a simple vaginal balloon device, or a complicated computer-based urethral catheter or anal manometer. Electromyographic monitoring of the buttocks or rectus muscles can also be provided to determine whether the pelvic floor is being isolated during PFMT. Biofeedback seems to be more effective in cases of moderate to severe incontinence. When biofeedback is added to behavioral treatment, it has been shown to be more effective than either oxybutynin or placebo in another treatment study of MUI (5).

One type of biofeedback device is done with a set of six vaginal cones of graded size and weight. By inserting the largest and lightest cone, the patient is asked to try to maintain the cone above the pelvic floor twice a day for 15-minute sessions. Once the first cone can be maintained, then the patient moves up to the next smallest (and heaviest) cone, until the smallest and heaviest cone can be maintained. A Cochrane database systematic review determined that vaginal cones worked better than no intervention but, when used in conjunction with PFMT or electrical stimulation, did not work any better than those interventions alone (43). Improvement in continence with vaginal cones is reported to be 60% to 90%; however, the discontinuation rate is as high as 20% to 40% (32).

Electrical stimulation is another conservative measure, usually reserved for those patients having difficulty locating or isolating the pelvic floor muscles. Barroso et al performed a double-blind RCT of transvaginal electrical stimulation using a battery-powered, portable electrical stimulator at 20 to 50 Hz with 5 seconds of stimulation and 5-second rests. The subjects used the stimulation twice a day for 20-minute sessions over a 12-week period. Most patients had MUI or urge incontinence (71%), and they found a significant reduction in total voids, urgent voids, nocturia episodes, and number of incontinent episodes (44). There were also significant increases in cystometric bladder capacity. Siegel et al found similar benefits by stimulating every other day compared to a daily treatment group (45). Electrical stimulation is limited by discomfort and normal mechanical wear-and-tear.

Functional magnetic stimulation (FMS) has been investigated as a treatment modality for urge-predominant MUI (46). But et al randomly assigned 39 women to a portable FMS device that generated a percutaneous electromagnetic field at 18.5 Hz per minute or a placebo device. The pulsating field could not be felt or heard, effectively blinding subjects to group assignment. The devices were worn continuously for 2 months. The FMS group had significant decreases in daytime frequency and nocturia and significant increases in first sensation to void and maximum cystometric capacity. A subjective "success rate" was reported by subjects as being 42%, and 74% wanted to continue therapy. FMS can also be delivered while the patient sits in an office-based chair (Neotonus Inc., Marietta, GA).

Barrier Devices

Barrier devices, such as pessaries, have commonly been used for stress incontinence, but their use in women with urge has been somewhat limited since pressure at the bladder or trigone sometimes stimulates a detrusor contraction. However, unlike PFMT or electrical stimulation, results can be quick and dramatic. Donnelly et al reported on 31 women with urodynamic criteria for MUI who were fitted with a variety of "incontinence" pessaries or ones with "support" (47). Fifty-five percent of subjects ($n = 16$) wore the pessary beyond the 6-month study period, which the investigators equated with control of urinary leakage ($n = 16$).

Another form of barrier device is the urethral insert. Robinson et al compared two different balloon-tip urethral inserts in women with MUI or stress incontinence (48). Although the sample size was not large enough to show a difference between the two devices, each group had a 59% to 68% reduction in urine loss and a 62.5% to 75% reduction in pad-weight measurements. These devices demand some manual dexterity, and the most common side effects are awareness of the device (62.5%), urgency (29.2%), urethral discomfort (20.8%), and hematuria (15.8%). When examined alone, 79% of patients were completely dry at 12 months with the Reliance™ device in situ and 16% were significantly better using patient diaries and pad-weight tests (49). This study showed much better rates of awareness (7%) and urethral discomfort (9%) at 12 months, but the longer study period resulted in higher numbers of hematuria (24%) and symptomatic bacteriuria (30%). There are no data available on urethral patches and MUI.

Medications

Numerous medications have been used to treat the urge component of MUI, with several new anti-incontinence medications now on the market (50). Medications have not been specifically designed to treat MUI, although several studies have recently been published investigating the use of these anti-incontinence medications in MUI. Unfortunately, the pharmacologic activities of these agents are not entirely selective for the urinary tract, and multiple systemic side effects are common.

A Cochrane database systematic review of the use of alpha-adrenergic medications such as phenylpropanolamine (which has been removed from the American market) and pseudoephedrine for incontinence suggested weak evidence for improving stress incontinence symptoms and almost no mention of MUI (51). Imipramine (Tofranil) and desipramine are tricyclic antidepressants that have been shown to have some anticholinergic properties on bladder muscle and alpha-adrenergic properties on the urethra (50). Long used in children to treat enuresis, imipramine has been shown to decrease urge incontinent episodes in women with mixed incontinence and has been shown to improve the HRQL in treated women (52). Combined therapy with estrogen and/or oxybutynin demonstrates a 32% cure rate and an improvement rate (more than 50%) of 28% (53). Lin et al reported similar findings with imipramine monotherapy (54).

Estrogen has been recommended for years as a treatment for stress, urge, and MUI. However, some recent epidemiologic studies have cast doubt on its usefulness as a treatment modality for urinary incontinence (7,55). One such study showed an increase in the incidence of both urge incontinence and stress incontinence in women taking estrogen and progesterone supplementation compared to those taking placebo (7). However, other studies still show a protective effect against MUI and urinary incontinence in general (12). A Cochrane database systematic review and meta-analysis on estrogen for urinary incontinence looked at 28 trials investigating the relationship of estrogen and incontinence. Taken together, 50% of women treated with estrogen were cured or improved of their incontinence, compared with 25% with placebo. This translated to one or two fewer voids per day, although the effect appeared to be better in women with urge-predominant incontinence (56). There were no statistically significant differences in frequency, nocturia, or urgency. When subjective cure and improvement were considered together, statistically higher cure and improvement rates were shown for both urge (57% vs. 28% on placebo) and stress (43% vs. 27%) incontinence. The conclusion of the authors of this meta-analysis was that there were not enough data to make recommendations about estrogen in combination with progesterone.

Duloxetine hydrochloride (Yentreve, Cymbalta) is a selective serotonin and norepinephrine reuptake inhibitor that inhibits parasympathetic activity and enhances sympathetic and somatic activity in the lower urinary tract. Although not approved for the treatment of MUI in the United States, this medication is available for treatment of depression. Duloxetine promotes urine storage and decreases bladder contractility by its noradrenergic effect enhancing sympathetic stimulation (57). A double-blind, placebo-controlled RCT of duloxetine was performed on 553 women with stress or MUI (n = 171) (8). Women with MUI were more likely to have a significantly shorter voiding interval, more likely to have voiding frequency (at least 9 voids/day) and urgent urination, and more likely to show detrusor overactivity on urodynamics, when compared to those subjects with stress incontinence. At the end of the 12-week treatment period, 34% of subjects with MUI had persistent mixed symptoms, but subjects taking 40 mg (80 mg) of duloxetine had an average of 62% (63%) fewer incontinent episodes compared to pretreatment (8). A Cochrane database systematic review showed that there was good evidence that duloxetine improved the quality of life in women with stress and mixed incontinence and perception of improvement. Although individual studies demonstrated a 50% reduction in incontinent episodes, a meta-analysis of stress-pad test and 24-hour pad-weight change failed to show an objective benefit to duloxetine therapy (58).

Oxybutynin hydrochloride (Ditropan) is a nonselective M2 and M3 receptor anticholinergic and antispasmodic agent. It is available in injectable, oral immediate-release, oral extended-release, an impregnated vaginal ring, and transdermal delivery. It is known that oxybutynin antagonizes acetylcholine-induced stimulation of postganglionic parasympathetic receptors, although this is comparatively weak. However, oxybutynin is also a musculotropic agent with a weak direct relaxant effect on the bladder smooth muscle (59).

The use of immediate-release oxybutynin is useful in the treatment of MUI; however, its side effect profile is considered by many to limit its use. Extended-release oxybutynin has the benefit of avoiding the peak and trough drug levels that occur with immediate-release administration (50). In a placebo-controlled RCT of extended-release and immediate-release oxybutynin, mean reductions in the weekly number of incontinence episodes of 92% and 72% were achieved, respectively, compared with 45% for placebo (60). Significantly more subjects on extended-release oxybutynin achieved continence (51%) compared to the immediate-release form (28%) and placebo (13%). The extended-release formula achieves significantly less dry mouth and other side effects. There are no data available regarding the use of the oxybutynin ring for MUI.

Transdermal oxybutynin as been reported to limit the first-pass effect and effectively decrease anticholinergic side effects. A double-blind, double-dummy RCT study comparing transdermal oxybutynin (3.9 mg) to extended-release tolterodine (4 mg) and placebo found that oxybutynin significantly reduced the number of incontinence episodes per day, increased the average voided volume, and led to significant increases in HRQL (61). The most common side effect was application site pruritus (14% vs. 4% for placebo) and dry mouth (4.1% vs. 1.7% for placebo). There were no differences in the outcome parameters comparing transdermal oxybutynin and extended-release tolterodine.

Tolterodine tartrate (Detrol) is a competitive M2 receptor muscarinic receptor antagonist (M2 receptors predominate in smooth muscle), with a greater affinity for the bladder than the salivary glands (50). Extended-release tolterodine has been shown to statistically decrease urge-related urine loss in a placebo-controlled RCT of women with MUI (62). The Mixed Incontinence Effectiveness Research Investigating Tolterodine (MERIT) study found a 90% improvement in HRQL compared to placebo, and reported more treatment benefit and bladder improvement over the 8-week treatment period. There were no differences in women whose first symptom of MUI was urge, compared with stress (63).

Solifenacin succinate (Vesicare) is a non (receptor)-selective antimuscarinic agent that has some target-organ selectivity for the bladder. Its half-life is 52 hours. Metabolism is in the liver, and the majority is excreted in the urine and the gastrointestinal tract. Solifenacin was examined with four 12-week, placebo-controlled RCTs with urge-predominant MUI or urge incontinence (64). The mean reduction in urge incontinent episodes was 2.7 per 24 hours using the typical dose of 10 mg qd, compared to placebo. There was also a significant increase in average bladder volume voided per micturition of 42.5 cc. Specific investigations of MUI have not been performed.

Trospium chloride (Sanctura) is an antimuscarinic, antispasmodic agent that can be used for MUI. Darifenacin hydrobromide (Enablex) is a selective M3 receptor antagonist with a higher affinity for the bladder, but less dry mouth has not been definitively proven. There are no data available on the use of trospium or darifenacin for MUI.

Surgical Therapy for Mixed Incontinence

Surgical correction of urethral hypermobility is thought to increase pressure transmission to the urethra (as related to the bladder) during periods of elevated abdominal pressure (29). Many authors have noted that correcting the stress component of MUI can have a positive effect on the urge component. For instance, Schrepferman et al examined 69 women with MUI and noted complete resolution of motor urgency (urge incontinence) in 58.5% and improvement in an additional 17.1% (65). For subjects with sensory urgency (urge with no urine loss), 39.3% were cured and 32.1% were improved. If the subjects with urge incontinence were subdivided by low bladder pressures (detrusor rises of 25 cm H_2O pressure or less), the low-pressure group had a cure rate of 91.3% and an improvement of an additional 8.7%. Of those with high-pressure motor urgency (detrusor rises of more than 25 cm H_2O), only 27.8% were cured and 27.8% improved.

The difficulty with looking at any surgical studies investigating MUI is that very few look at pure mixed incontinence. More commonly, these studies tend to look at the results of surgery done for stress urinary incontinence and mixed incontinence

Surgical correction of significant pelvic organ prolapse itself has also been proposed as a way to cure the urge component of mixed incontinence (66). Nguyen and Bhatia have suggested that low-amplitude (less than 25 cm H_2O) detrusor contractions on urodynamic study or bladder trabeculations on cystoscopy were independent predictors of urge resolution after pelvic organ prolapse surgery.

A long-term follow-up of Pereyra bladder neck suspension showed that 67% of patients undergoing needle suspension for stress incontinence had preoperative MUI symptoms (only 13% had urodynamic mixed urinary incontinence) (67). Although 29.6% were lost to follow-up, nearly as many subjects (65%) had postoperative urgency an average of 10 years later. Only 20% claimed no incontinence of any type, although 71% reported improvement compared to their preoperative state. Only 24% reported they were completely satisfied and 62% now wore protection from incontinence. A Cochrane database systematic review on the ef-

fects of needle suspension on stress or mixed incontinence suggested that there were no significant differences between needle suspensions and anterior colporrhaphy (36% failed after needle suspension, 39% failed after anterior colporrhaphy). However, needle suspensions were more likely to fail than Burch colposuspension (68).

The anterior colporrhaphy was once the standard vaginal repair for stress urinary incontinence, but it has been shown to have poor long-term success rates (69). One RCT between anterior repair and Burch colposuspension in 103 women with MUI was done (70). At 3 months, 31% of anterior colporrhaphy subjects and 33% of Burch subjects were still incontinent. However, at 12 months, 3 years, and 5 years, the proportion of subjects who remained incontinent continued to drop, so that only 16% of anterior colporrhaphy subjects and 8% of Burch subjects remained incontinent at 5 years. However, a Cochrane database systematic review of anterior colporrhaphy showed the opposite: that the anterior colporrhaphy was less effective than the Burch procedure (41% failed vs. 17%) at 5 years, irrespective of the coexistence of prolapse (71).

Burch retropubic urethropexy has been a mainstay of surgical treatment for stress incontinence. It has comparable long-term results to suburethral sling procedures. In one study, the Burch procedure was shown to have a 59% cure rate, with an additional 22% improved, in women with MUI (53). All "failures" ($n = 5$) after Burch urethropexy were due to urge persistence after surgery. Karram and Bhatia found no specific preoperative urodynamic parameters that predicted success or failure of Burch for MUI. The Burch procedure may also relieve the urge component in a number of cases. Langer et al reported the results of a study of 30 women with MUI symptoms who underwent Burch colposuspension (72). Prior to the procedure, 73.3% had urodynamic evidence of detrusor instability, and this proportion dropped to 33.3% after surgery. A Cochrane database systematic review comparing Burch and slings showed comparable rates, but long-term results of four RCTs were not extensive enough to make recommendations (73).

Traditional pubovaginal slings placed at the urethrovesical junction have been used effectively in women with MUI. Chou et al evaluated 52 women with MUI who underwent a pubovaginal sling a median of 3 years previously (74). Cure rate was 93% in the MUI group, slightly less than the 97% cure rate for stress incontinence ($p = $ NS). An increased number of total voids did not affect the sling results. However, those who failed or were only improved had more episodes of sensory urgency and more episodes of urge incontinence than those whose procedures were successful. A Cochrane database systematic review comparing traditional sling results showed comparable rates between different types of traditional slings, as well as comparable results to other types of continence surgery. Confidence intervals in these studies were wide, so clinically important differences could not be ruled out (75).

The tension-free vaginal tape (TVT; Gynecare, Somerville, NJ) suburethral sling has shown excellent short-term and long-term efficacy for MUI. After 6 months, one group described a cure rate of 89% in 128 women with MUI (76). Concentrating on the urge component of MUI, Segal et al found a 63.1% resolution of urge in 65 women with preoperative MUI symptoms (26). However, they also reported de novo detrusor overactivity in as many as 13.4% of subjects who had an isolated TVT. A review of 80 women who had TVT procedures 3 to 5 years previously showed an 85% cure rate (negative cough stress test, a 90% quality-of-life improvement, and 10 g pad weight or less on a 24-hour pad test) and an additional 4% improved (77). Twenty-five percent retained sensory urgency (75% resolution) without incontinence, and there was no worsening of the urge component. In all three studies, cure or improvement was accompanied by HRQL improvements and decreases in leakage episodes and patient-evaluated subjective assessments.

The TVT procedure can also be done with ancillary surgery, such as for pelvic organ prolapse (78). Women with MUI had a 91% cure rate at a mean follow-up of 11 months; however, only 21.6% had a vaginal vault suspension as one of the ancillary procedures. Meltomaa et al compared the results of 75 women with stress or MUI (41%) who underwent a TVT with ancillary surgery (group 1) with 75 women who had a TVT alone (group 2), and found the 3-year success rates to be 87% for group 1 and 92% for group 2 ($p = NS$) (79). Postoperatively, there was a 50% resolution of urge symptoms in both groups and a de novo urge incontinence rate of 6%.

A recent Cochrane database systematic review of the use of bulking agents for the treatment of incontinence did not suggest a benefit in the use of these agents for the treatment of MUI (80).

SUMMARY

MUI is a multifactorial and complex clinical challenge for the physician who deals with incontinence. Symptomatic control is paramount and often requires treatment of both components (urge and stress) of leakage. Many conservative measures can be used. If surgery is chosen, most professionals recommend control of the urge component prior to surgical repair if the patient has urge-predominant or urge-equal mixed incontinence. If the patient has stress-predominant mixed incontinence or a mild urge component, then surgical correction can improve or cure the urge component in a majority of cases. Worsening of the urge component immediately after surgical repair can be the first clinical clue of partial bladder outlet obstruction and requires further work-up.

ACKNOWLEDGMENTS

I'd like to thank my wife, Nora, for her unwavering support and patience during the development of this chapter. My parents and kids were a constant source of inspiration. I'd also like to thank my colleagues, Drs. Hale, Benson, and Bump, for their contributions. The Methodist Hospital (Indianapolis) library staff was invaluable in the researching of this topic. No supporting research grant funds were used.

REFERENCES

1. Abrams P, Cardozo L, Fall M, et al. The standardization of terminology of lower urinary tract function: report from the Standardization Subcommittee of the International Continence Society. *Neurourol Urodynam* 2002;21:167–178.
2. Weber AM, Abrams P, Brubaker L, et al. The standardization of terminology for researchers in female pelvic floor disorders. *Int Urogynecol J Pelvic Floor Dysfunct* 2001;12:178–186.
3. Weidner AC, Myers ER, Visco AG, et al. Which women with stress incontinence require urodynamics? *Am J Obstet Gynecol* 2001;184:20–27.
4. Colli E, Artibani W, Goka J, et al. Are urodynamic tests useful tools for the initial conservative management of nonneurogenic urinary incontinence? A review of the literature. *Eur Urol* 2003;43:63–69.
5. Cardozo LD. Biofeedback in overactive bladder. *Urology* 2000;55(5A):24–28.
6. Digesu GA, Khullar V, Cardozo L, et al. Overactive bladder symptoms: do we need urodynamics? *Neurourol Urodynam* 2003;22:105–108.
7. Brown JS, Grady D, Ouslander JG, et al, for the Heart & Estrogen/Progestin Replacement Study (HERS) Research Group. Prevalence of urinary incontinence and associated risk factors in postmenopausal women. *Obstet Gynecol* 1999;94:66–70.
8. Bump RC, Norton PA, Zinner NR, et al, for the Duloxetine Urinary Incontinence Study Group. Mixed urinary incontinence symptoms: urodynamic findings, incontinence severity, and treatment response. *Obstet Gynecol* 2003;102:76–83.
9. Gunnarsson M, Mattiasson A. Female stress, urge, and mixed urinary incontinence are associated with a chronic and progressive pelvic floor/vaginal neuromuscular disorder: an investigation of 317 healthy and in-

continent women using vaginal surface electromyography. *Neurourol Urodynam* 1999;18:613–621.

10. Sandvik H, Hunskaar S, Vanvik A, et al. Diagnostic classification of female urinary incontinence: an epidemiological survey corrected for validity. *J Clin Epidemiol* 1995;48:339–343.

11. Melville JL, Walker E, Katon W, et al. Prevalence of comorbid psychiatric illness and its impact on symptom perception, quality of life, and functional status in women with urinary incontinence. *Am J Obstet Gynecol* 2002;187:80–87.

12. Parazzini F, Chiaffarino F, Lavezzari M, et al, on behalf of the VIVA Study Group. Risk factors for stress, urge, or mixed urinary incontinence in Italy. *Int J Obstet Gynaecol* 2003;110:927–933.

13. Hannestad YS, Rortveit G, Sandvik H, et al. A community-based epidemiological survey of female urinary incontinence: the Norwegian EPINCONT study. *J Clin Epidemiol* 2000;53:1150–1157.

14. Anger JT, Rodriguez LV. Mixed incontinence: stressing about urge. *Curr Urol Rep* 2004;5:427–431.

15. Hojberg KE, Salvig JD, Winslow NA, et al. Urinary incontinence: prevalence and risk factors at 16 weeks of gestation. *Br J Obstet Gynaecol* 1999;106:842–850.

16. Coyne KS, Zhou Z, Thompson C, et al. The impact on health-related quality of life of stress, urge, and mixed urinary incontinence. *BJU Intl* 2003;92:731–735.

17. Valerius AJ. The psychosocial impact of urinary incontinence on women aged 25 to 45 years. *Urol Nurs* 1997;17:96–103.

18. O'Donnell PD. Mixed urinary incontinence. In: O'Donnell PD, ed. *Urinary incontinence*. Mosby: St. Louis, 1997:202–206.

19. McLennan MT, Melick C, Bent AE. Urethral instability: clinical and urodynamic characteristics. *Neurourol Urodynam* 2001;20:653–660.

20. Paick JS, Ku JH, Shin JW, et al. Significance of pad test loss for the evaluation of women with urinary incontinence. *Neurourol Urodynam* 2005;24:39–43.

21. Rovner ES, Gomes CM, Banner MP, et al. Ventral hernia of the urinary bladder with mixed urinary incontinence: treatment with herniorrhaphy and allograft fascial sling. *Urology* 2000;55:145vii–145ix.

22. Coolsaet BLRA, van Duyl WA, van Os-Bossagh P, et al. New concepts in relation to urge and detrusor activity. *Neurourol Urodynam* 1993;12:463–471.

23. Brading AF. A myogenic basis for the overactive bladder. *Urology* 1997;50(Supp 6A):57–67.

24. Elbadawi A, Yalla SV, Resnick NM. Structural basis of geriatric voiding dysfunction. III. Detrusor overactivity. *J Urol* 1993;150:1668–1680.

25. Gunnarsson M, Mattiasson A. Circumvaginal surface electromyography in women with urinary incontinence and in healthy volunteers. *Scand J Urol Nephrol* 1994;157:89–95.

26. Segal JL, Vassallo B, Kleeman S, et al. Prevalence of persistent and de novo overactive bladder symptoms after the tension-free vaginal tape. *Obstet Gynecol* 2004;104:1263–1269.

27. Brubaker L. Mixed urinary incontinence. In: Weber AM, Brubaker L, Schaffer J, et al, eds. *Office urogynecology*. New York: McGraw-Hill, 2004:89–98.

28. Carr LK, Webster GD. Voiding dysfunction following incontinence surgery: diagnosis and treatment with retropubic or vaginal urethrolysis. *J Urol* 1997;157:821–823.

29. Karram MM. Detrusor instability and hyperreflexia. In: Walters MD, Karram MM, eds. *Urogynecology and re-*constructive pelvic surgery, 2nd ed. St. Louis: Mosby, 1999:297–314.

30. Burgio KL, Goode PS. Behavioral interventions for incontinence in ambulatory geriatric patients. *Am J Med Sci* 1997;314:257–261.

31. Fantl JA, Wyman JF, McClish DK, et al. Efficacy of bladder training in older women with urinary incontinence. *JAMA* 1991;265:609–613.

32. Gormley EA. Biofeedback and behavioral therapy for the management of female urinary incontinence. *Urol Clin North Am* 2002;29:551–557.

33. Wyman JF. Management of urinary incontinence in adult ambulatory care populations. *Ann Rev Nurs Res* 2000;18:171–194.

34. Bump RC, Sugerman HJ, Fantl JA, et al. Obesity and lower urinary tract function in women: effect of surgically induced weight loss. *Am J Obstet Gynecol* 1992;167:392–397.

35. Woodman P, Swift S, O'Boyle A, et al. Prevalence of severe pelvic organ prolapse in relation to job-description and socioeconomic status: a multicenter, cross-sectional study. *Int Urogynecol J Pelvic Floor Dysfunct* 2006;17:340–345.

36. Bo K. Pelvic floor muscle training is effective in treatment of female stress urinary incontinence, but how does it work? *Int Urogynecol J Pelvic Floor Dysfunct* 2004;15:76–84.

37. Datillo J. A long-term study of patient outcomes with pelvic muscle re-education for urinary in continence. *J Wound Ostomy Cont Nurs* 2001;28:199–205.

38. Burgio KL, Goode PS, Locher JL, et al. Predictors of outcome in the behavioral treatment of urinary incontinence in women. *Obstet Gynecol* 2003;102:940–947.

39. Nygaard IE, Kreder KJ, Lepic MM, et al. Efficacy of pelvic floor muscle exercises in women with stress, urge, and mixed urinary incontinence. *Am J Obstet Gynecol* 1996;174:120–125.

40. Miller JM, Ashton-Miller JA, DeLancey JOL. The Knack: Use of precisely timed pelvic muscle exercise contraction can reduce leakage in SUI. *Neurourol Urodynam* 1996;15:302–393.

41. Burgio KL, Locher JL, Goode PS, et al. Behavioral vs. drug treatment for urge urinary incontinence in older women: a randomized controlled trial. *JAMA* 1998;280:1995–2000.

42. Bump RC, Hurt WG, Fantl JA, et al. Assessment of Kegel pelvic muscle exercise performance after brief verbal instruction. *Am J Obstet Gynecol* 1991;165:322–329.

43. Herbison P, Plevnik S, Mantle J. Weighted vaginal cones for urinary incontinence (Cochrane Review). In: *The Cochrane Library*. Chichester, UK: John Wiley & Sons, Ltd., 2004;(2).

44. Barroso JCV, Ramos JGL, Martins-Costa S, et al. Transvaginal electrical stimulation in the treatment of urinary incontinence. *BJU Intl* 2004;93:319–323.

45. Siegel SW, Richardson DA, Miller KL, et al. Pelvic floor electrical stimulation for the treatment of urge and mixed urinary incontinence in women. *Urology* 1997;50:934–940.

46. But I, Faganelj M, Sostaric A. Functional magnetic stimulation for mixed urinary incontinence. *J Urol* 2005;173:1644–1646.

47. Donnelly MJ, Powell-Morgan S, Olsen AL, et al. Vaginal pessary for the management of stress and mixed urinary incontinence. *Int Urogynecol J Pelvic Floor Dysfunct* 2004;15:302–307.

48. Robinson H, Schulz J, Flood C, Hansen L. A randomized controlled trial of the NEAT expandable tip conti-

nence device. *Int Urogynecol J Pelvic Floor Dysfunct* 2003;14:199–203.

49. Miller JL, Bavendam T. Treatment with Reliance urinary control insert: one-year experience. *J Endourol* 1996;10:287–292.

50. Guay DR. Clinical pharmacokinetics of drugs used to treat urge incontinence. *Clin Pharmacokinetics* 2003;42:1243–1285.

51. Alhasso A, Glazener CMA, Pickard R, et al. Adrenergic drugs for urinary incontinence in adults. (Cochrane Review). In: *The Cochrane Library*. Chichester, UK: John Wiley & Sons, Ltd., 2004;(2).

52. Woodman P, Misko C, Fisher J. The use of short-form quality-of-life questionnaires to measure the impact of imipramine on women with urge incontinence. *Int Urogynecol J Pelvic Floor Dysfunct* 2001;12:312–316.

53. Karram MM, Bhatia NN. Management of coexistent stress and urge urinary incontinence. *Obstet Gynecol* 1989;73:4–7.

54. Lin HH, Sheu BC, Lo MC, et al. Comparison of treatment outcomes for imipramine for female genuine stress incontinence. *Br J Obstet Gynaecol* 1999;106: 1089–1092.

55. Hendrix SL, Cochrane BB, Nygaard IE, et al. Effects of estrogen with and without progestin on urinary incontinence. *JAMA* 2005;293:935–948.

56. Moehrer B, Hextall A, Jackson S. Oestrogens for urinary incontinence in women (Cochrane Review). In: *The Cochrane Library*. Chichester, UK: John Wiley & Sons, Ltd., 2004;(2).

57. Norton PA, Zinner NR, Yalcin I, et al, for the Duloxetine Urinary Incontinence Study Group. Duloxetine versus placebo in the treatment of stress urinary incontinence. *Am J Obstet Gynecol* 2002;187: 40–48.

58. Mariappan P, Ballantyne Z, N'Dow JM, et al. Serotonin and noradrenaline reuptake inhibitors (SNRI) for stress urinary incontinence in adults. (Cochrane Review). In: *The Cochrane Library*. Chichester, UK: John Wiley & Sons, Ltd., 2005;(3).

59. Goldenberg MM. An extended-release formulation of oxybutynin chloride for the treatment of overactive urinary bladder. *Clin Therapeutics* 1999;21:634–642.

60. Anderson RU, Mobley D, Blank B, et al. Once-daily controlled versus immediate-release oxybutynin chloride for urge urinary incontinence. OROS Oxybutynin Study Group. *J Urol* 1999;161(6):1809–1812.

61. Dmochowski RR, Sand PK, Zinner NR, et al, for the Transdermal Oxybutynin Study Group. Comparative efficacy and safety of transdermal oxybutynin and oral tolterodine versus placebo in previously treated patients with urge and mixed urinary incontinence. *Urology* 2003;62:237–242.

62. Khullar V, Hill S, Laval KU, et al. Treatment of urge-predominant mixed urinary incontinence with tolterodine extended release: a randomized, placebo-controlled trial. *Urology* 2004;64:269–275.

63. Khullar V, Digesu A, Chaliha C, et al. Mixed incontinence: how should it be treated? *Neurourol Urodynam* 2002;21:378–379 [abstract 73].

64. Chapple CR, Rechberger T, Al-Shukri S, et al, on behalf of the YM-905 Study Group. Randomized, double-blind placebo- and tolterodine-controlled trial of the once-daily antimuscarinic agent solifenacin in patients with symptomatic overactive bladder. *BJU Intl* 2004;93:303–310.

65. Schrepferman CG, Griebling TL, Nygaard IE, et al. Resolution of urge symptoms following sling cystourethropexy. *J Urol* 2000;164:1628–1631.

66. Nguyen JK, Bhattia NN. Resolution of motor urge incontinence after surgical repair of pelvic organ prolapse. *J Urol* 2001;166:2263–2266.

67. Trockman BA, Leach GE, Hamilton J, et al. Modified Pereyra bladder neck suspension: a 10-year mean follow-up using outcomes analysis in 125 patients. *J Urol* 1995;154:1841–1847.

68. Glazener CM, Cooper K. Bladder neck needle suspension for urinary incontinence in women. (Cochrane Review). In: *The Cochrane Library*. Chichester, UK: John Wiley & Sons, Ltd., 2002;(2).

69. Bergman A, Elia G. Three surgical procedures for genuine stress incontinence: Five-year follow-up of a prospective randomized study. *Am J Obstet Gynecol* 1995;173:66–71.

70. Quadri G, Scalambrino S, Boisio N, et al. Randomized surgery for incontinence and prolapse: retropubic colposuspension vs. anterior repair [abstract]. *Arch Gynecol* 1985;237(Suppl):402.

71. Glazener CM, Cooper K. Anterior vaginal repair for urinary incontinence in women. (Cochrane Review). In: *The Cochrane Library*. Chichester, UK: John Wiley & Sons, Ltd., 2001;(1).

72. Langer R, Ron-El R, Bukovsky I, et al. Colposuspension in patients with combined stress incontinence and detrusor instability. *Eur Urol* 1988;14: 437–439.

73. Bezerra CA, Bruschini H. Suburethral sling for urinary incontinence in women. (Cochrane Review). In: *The Cochrane Library*. Chichester, UK: John Wiley & Sons, Ltd., 2001;(3).

74. Chou ECL, Flisser AJ, Panagopoulos G, et al. Effective treatment for mixed urinary incontinence with a pubovaginal sling. *J Urol* 2003;170:494–497.

75. Bezerra CA, Bruschini H, Cody DJ. Traditional suburethral sling operations for urinary incontinence in women. (Cochrane Review). In: *The Cochrane Library*. Chichester, UK: John Wiley & Sons, Ltd., 2005;(3).

76. Abdel-Hady ES, Constantine G. Outcome of the use of tension-free vaginal tape in women with mixed urinary incontinence, previous failed surgery, or low Valsalva pressure. *J Obstet Gynaecol Res* 2005;31:38–42.

77. Rezapour M, Ulmsten U. Tension-free vaginal tape (TVT) in women with mixed urinary incontinence—a long term follow-up. *Int Urogynecol J Pelvic Floor Dysfunct* 2001;12(S2):S15–S18.

78. Partoll LM. Efficacy of tension-free vaginal tape with other pelvic reconstructive surgery. *Am J Obstet Gynecol* 2002;186:1292–1298.

79. Meltomaa S, Backman T, Haarala M. Concomitant vaginal surgery did not affect outcome of the tension-free vaginal tape operation during a prospective 3-year follow-up study. *J Urol* 2004;172:222–226.

80. Pickard R, Reaper J, Wyness L, et al. Periurethral injection therapy for urinary incontinence in women (Cochrane Review). In: *The Cochrane Library*. Chichester, UK: John Wiley & Sons, Ltd., 2004;(2).

CHAPTER 17

Fistula and Urethral Diverticulum

Ralph R. Chesson, Jr., and Okechukwu A. Ibeanu

INTRODUCTION

Vesicovaginal fistulas are a most distressing condition for women. Their constant drainage of urine creates emotional and physical distress affecting their everyday life. In developing countries they are social outcasts because of the constant smell of urine. They withdraw from society. In the United States postoperative fistulas are becoming a more common cause of malpractice cases because of the long social isolation these patients endure.

Luiz de Mercado in Valladolid, Spain, first used the term *fistula* instead of *rupture* (1). Although John Peter Mettauer, a rural Virginia surgeon, reported the first successful cure of a fistula in the United States (2), James Marion Sims, a rural Alabama surgeon, is recognized as the father of American gynecology and is most associated with the repair of vesicovaginal fistula (3).

Neglected obstetric labor and gynecologic surgical complications are the main etiologic factors for the formation of vesicovaginal fistulas. Worldwide, most vesicovaginal fistulas are from neglected obstetrics, especially in sub-Saharan Africa, where the true incidence is unknown. Some report an incidence of 1 or 2 per 1,000 deliveries (4), but recent presentations and discussions at an international fistula conference at Johns Hopkins, Baltimore, Maryland, in August 2005 suggest that all estimates are inaccurate (5).

The problem of obstetric fistula has been eradicated in the United States, Scandinavia, and Western Europe, with the exception of vesicouterine/vesicocervical fistulas. Today most fistulas seen in the United States are from gynecologic surgery, in particular abdominal hysterectomy (6). Fistulas from gynecologic malignancy and/or radiation therapy are quite rare. The high prevalence of obstetric fistulas still remains a problem in Africa and less developed regions of Asia and Oceania (7). Until there are improvements in obstetric care, especially the elimination of prolonged obstructed labor, the problem of obstetric fistula will persist in these areas.

We will discuss the gynecologic and obstetric fistulas separately as their cause and cure are different. Obstetric injuries are a "field" injury with ischemic changes to the bladder and vagina from the prolonged pressure of an impacted fetal head against the tissues (7). Most gynecologic injuries, with the exception of radiation injuries, are a local injury with minimal changes in the adjacent tissues.

GYNECOLOGIC FISTULA

Etiology

In gynecologic practice in the United States, vesicovaginal fistulas most commonly follow hysterectomies. Specifically, 88% of the vesicovaginal fistula cases are complications of gynecologic and obstetric surgery (1) and 82% are from hysterectomy (6). Urologic procedures account for 6% of cases, while radiation treatment, trauma, and malignant disease account for approximately 4% of cases (8). Vesicovaginal fistulas result from "faulty" dissection of the bladder from the cervix and lower uterine segment. Distortion of tissues is caused by uterine leiomyomata, previous cesareans, and other pelvic conditions such as endometriosis and pelvic inflammatory disease that lead to loss of surgical planes. Tissue trauma, electrocautery, infection, smoking, radiation, and diabetes contribute to local tissue breakdown and poor wound healing. Wound healing has four phases: coagulation, inflammation, fibroplasia, and remodeling. During the fibroplasia phase the rate of formation of fibroplastic collagen peaks at day 7 and formation continues for 2 to 3 weeks. It is this time period during which tissue breakdown is most likely to occur. Inadvertent suture in the bladder may contribute to poor healing, but Meeks (9) suggests that a suture in the bladder is not associated with fistula formation. Seventy percent to 80% of bladder injuries during gynecologic surgery go unrecognized (10). Radiation fistulas occur with endarteritis and tissue ischemia with necrosis and fibrosis. These radiation-induced lesions may present months to years after treatment (11). Minimizing the risk of injury at the time of surgery is the goal of the surgeon (Table 17.1).

Presentation

Patients may complain of urine loss immediately following the procedure once the urethral catheter is removed if there is a gross bladder defect. This would entail a combined vaginal opening as well as a laceration or other direct injury to the bladder, allowing the urine to escape from the vagina and resulting in symptomatic urinary leakage. More commonly the leakage starts in 2 to 4 weeks after surgery, once the sutures placed through the vagina and the bladder have started to dissolve. Other symptoms include hematuria at the time of surgery and in the first few days after surgery. Fever and chills may precede loss of urine, followed by defervescence. Abdominal flank pain may also be present, but this association is more common for ureterovaginal fistula. This latter case is accompanied by a transient serum creatinine elevation lasting 1 or 2 days. In most cases of posthysterectomy vesicovaginal fistula, however, patients remain relatively symptom-free and complain of only occasional abnormal vaginal discharge until there is sudden urinary leakage soaking through pads and clothing. It has been estimated that 50% of postsurgical fistulas present after 10 days (8). Signs of peritonitis and ileus frequently accompany intraperitoneal leakage of urine, which occurs when there has been direct bladder injury and the site remains open to the peritoneal cavity, while the vagina is tightly closed. The serum creatinine will be elevated as long as there is peritoneal urine leakage.

TABLE 17.1

Surgical Techniques for Minimizing Lower Urinary Tract Injuries During Gynecologic Surgery

1. Proper positioning of the patient to allow abdominal and vaginal access
2. Adequate exposure and lighting of the surgical field
3. Surgeon familiarity with the anatomy of the space being entered
4. Performance of blunt and sharp dissection where appropriate. Blunt dissection is appropriate along certain established spaces in the pelvis (i.e., pubocervical space), but sharp dissection is needed to enter the space. When unsure, always use sharp dissection.
5. Be aware of the course of the ureter and protect it from injury.
6. Control bleeding with pressure, suction, identification of source, and correction.
7. Avoid large pedicles.
8. Continuous bladder drainage for abdominal cases
9. Intraoperative cystoscopy for all hysterectomy and pelvic reconstructive surgery to ensure the integrity of the lower urinary tract system (10)
10. Minimize use of electrocautery in the area of the bladder in proximity to the vaginal cuff.

Diagnosis

The initial management of leakage of urine from the vagina should be prompted by a high index of suspicion for a vesicovaginal fistula. Unless very small, the fistula may be visualized with a vaginal speculum. Diagnosis is aided by instilling methylene blue dye into the bladder. If the blue is not seen vaginally, a tampon is placed in the vagina and the patient is asked to walk for a few minutes. Blue coloration of the tampon at the vaginal vault location indicates loss from a fistula. Blue color on the end closest to the vaginal entry indicates urethral loss. If no blue is seen, then an ureterovaginal fistula must be considered. Either indigo carmine intravenously or phenazopyridine (Pyridium) orally may be given to stain the urine as it exits the kidney. Again, placing a tampon in the vagina will help to determine if the leakage is from an ureterovaginal fistula. If still unclear, intravenous pyelography should be performed, but especially if there is a suspicion of a compound fistula including the bladder and ureter. Cystoscopy is indicated to view the bladder site of a vesicovaginal fistula and proximity to the ureters. If there has been ureteral compromise, cystoscopy with intravenous indigo carmine and retrograde studies may also be performed. Contrast cystography can also be used as a diagnostic test; however, it is not as sensitive and has a higher false-negative rate than other tests.

Urinalysis with culture and sensitivity should be performed. At the time of cystoscopy suture material should be removed from the area of the fistula to facilitate resolution of inflammation prior to repair.

Treatment

Nonsurgical

Five percent to 10% of small vesicovaginal fistulas may heal spontaneously with prolonged bladder drainage using a suprapubic or urethral catheter. Bladder drainage and the use of a Foley catheter connected to a birth control diaphragm may lessen perineal irritation by diverting the urine flow. Four weeks of drainage should allow time for healing if the defect is going to close. Otherwise, surgical intervention is required.

Surgical

Traditionally, an interval of at least 3 to 6 months was advised before the surgical repair of a vesicovaginal fistula. Once the inflammation has resolved, it is considered appropriate to proceed with repair, and this has not led to failures of the Latzko colpocleisis procedure in uncomplicated unradiated patients (12). Fistula associated with radiation therapy should not be immediately repaired, as the radiation scarring will continue to affect tissues for a much longer time.

Several surgical techniques have been described for closure of vesicovaginal fistula. Regardless of the technique used, any repair must be performed with strict adherence to basic surgical principles in order to maximize the chances of a successful repair. Meticulous tissue dissection should be performed in order to adequately expose the fistula site, and all layers of closure should be tension-free, watertight, and nonopposing. If deemed necessary, a tissue interposition flap (Martius) should be employed in order to enhance blood supply and healing.

The surgical repair may be approached transvaginally or transabdominally. Most urogyneco-logic surgeons favor the transvaginal route, with the transabdominal route reserved for fistulas involving the ureter or other organs, including bowel. The use of specialty vaginal retractors such as those made by Lone Star Medical Products (www.lsmp.com) and/or the use of a generous episiotomy will allow adequate access to most fistulas, including most "high" fistulas.

Techniques

Latzko Partial Colpocleisis

Latzko's method of partial colpocleisis (13) has the advantage of minimal tissue dissection as well as avoiding incision of the bladder (Fig. 17.1). After patient positioning and exposure of the operative site with proper retractors, the fistula is again visualized using methylene blue dye if necessary. Repeat cystoscopy is performed if necessary. After locating the fistula, stay sutures are placed between 3 and 4 cm from the fistula at four quadrants (2, 5, 8, and 11 o'clock) to delineate the area of epithelium to remove. The principle of the Latzko repair is a partial colpocleisis of the upper vagina to close the fistula tract without actually excising it. All vaginal epithelium must be removed to prevent epithelial inclusion cyst formation or failure of the fibromuscularis tissues to scar together. A generous amount of epithelium removal will increase the success rate of this procedure. Generally, a 1.5- to 2-cm border around the fistula margin is sufficient. The incision is closed in two or three layers with interrupted 3-0 or 4-0 polyglactin sutures anterior to posterior.

If the procedure is a repeat procedure or vascularity is compromised, a Martius flap is placed (Figs. 17.2). The Martius flap utilizes the fat pad overlying the bulbocavernosus muscle. The fat pad is mobilized, usually leaving the posterior pedicle attached. It is brought into the vaginal incision though a subepithelial tunnel and is sutured to the fibromuscularis prior to closing the vaginal epithelium.

Postoperative drainage should be from 10 to 14 days either by indwelling Foley or suprapubic catheter. The method of drainage and length should be individualized to the surgeon's comfort with his or her estimation of the quality of the closure and the vascularity of the tissues.

Excisional Transvaginal Repair of Vesicovaginal Fistula

Sometimes the amount of scarring precludes a standard Latzko approach, and the fistula tract must be excised (Fig. 17.3). This procedure is also utilized in most obstetric fistulas to be discussed later. The fistula is exposed as in the Latzko repair and the fistula tract is excised. If significant scarring is encountered, Potts scissors (sharp-pointed

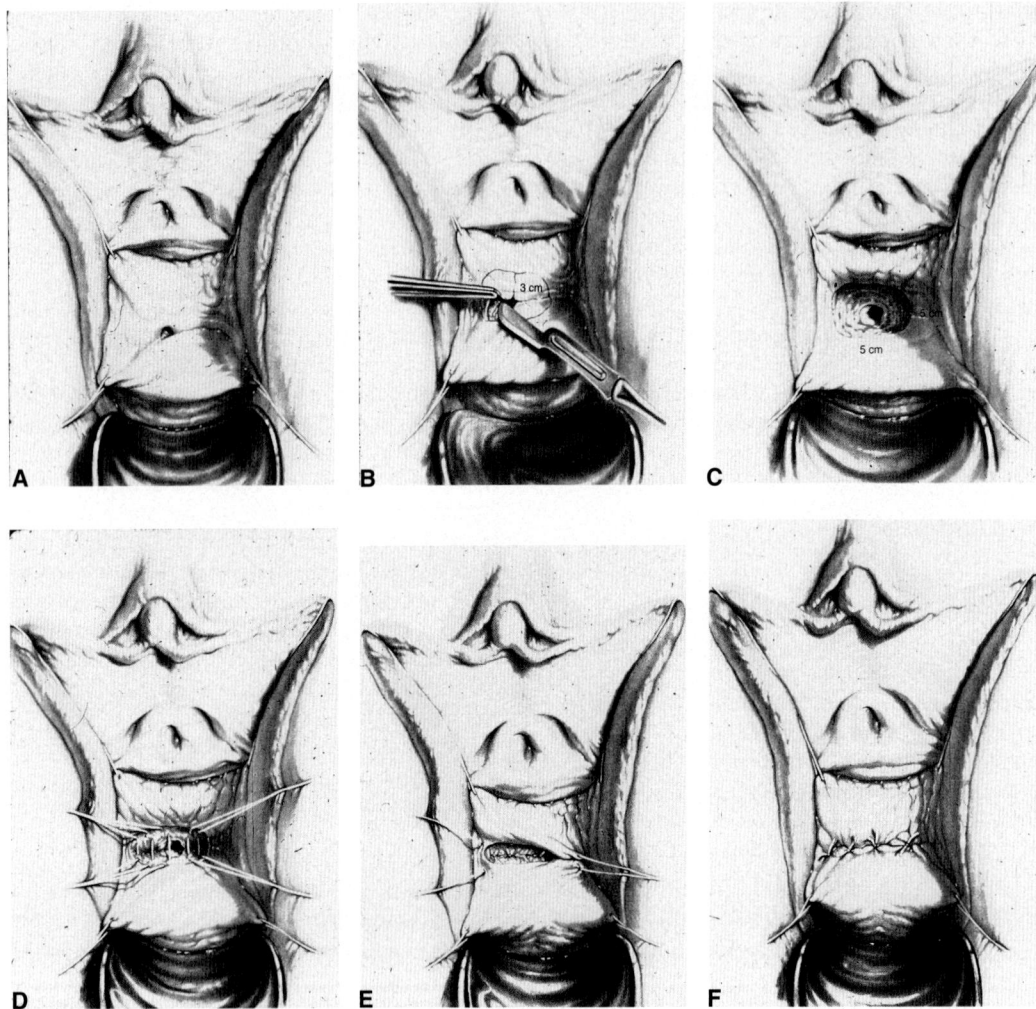

FIGURE 17.1   ●   Latzko procedure. **(A)** Stay sutures or Lone Star hooks are placed at 10, 2, 4, and 8 o'clock. **(B)** A rectangular excision of epithelial tissue at least 3 cm from the fistula tract is excised from the underlying fibromuscularis. **(C)** The epithelium has been excised from the underlying fibromuscularis with at least a 5 × 5-cm defect. **(D)** The first layer is closed with interrupted delayed absorbable 3-0 sutures on an RB or SH needle. **(E)** After two layers of suture, watertight integrity has been checked and the epithelium is being closed. **(F)** The epithelium has been closed with interrupted sutures.

scissors) are helpful in the dissection. The vaginal epithelium is mobilized from the underlying fibromuscularis, and the fistula is excised. The margins of the defect in the bladder mucosa and muscularis are identified and closed without tension. The bladder is closed with 3-0 or 4-0 polyglactin sutures in two layers. Pubocervical fibromuscularis is then used to interpose between the bladder and vaginal mucosa. The vaginal mucosa is closed in similar fashion with the same suture. A Martius flap should be considered in cases where the risk of breakdown is relatively high. Bladder drainage postoperatively is as described above.

Transabdominal Repair

While some urologists favor this approach (Figs. 17.4, 17.5, 17.6), more surgeons reserve the transabdominal route for cases of vesicovaginal fistula complicated by ureteral injury, radiated fistula, or cases with bowel involvement. This route may also be used for vesicouterine fistula when uterine preservation is desired.

Transvesical Approach

The incision is usually made at the dome of the bladder, exposing and identifying the fistula location. Indigo carmine may be given intravenously to help in identification of the ureteric orifices.

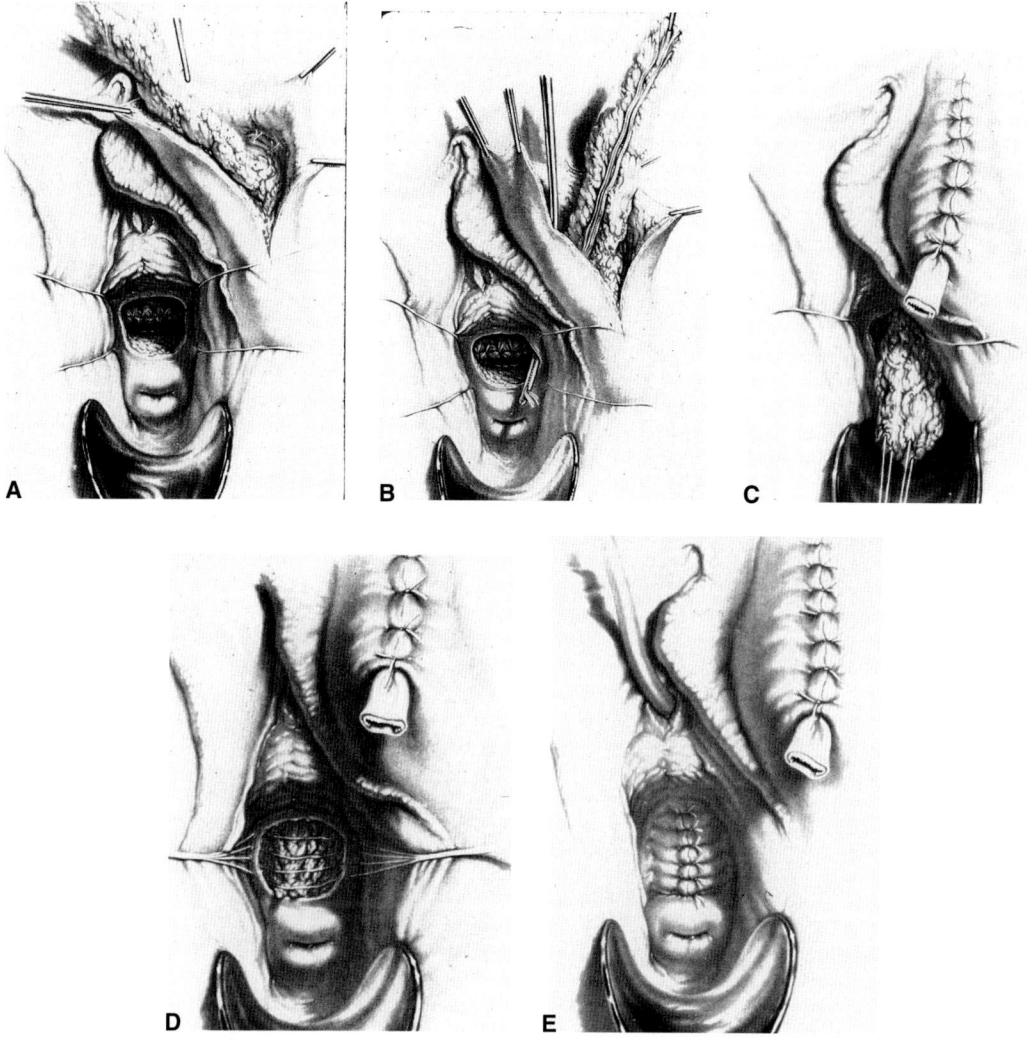

FIGURE 17.2 ● Martius graft. **(A)** The fat pad over the bulbocavernosus muscle is mobilized, maintaining its vascular pedicle from posterior and freed from its superior vascular pedicle. **(B)** A tunnel under the vulvovaginal epithelium is made into the vaginal defect over the fistula and the flap is pulled through with a clamp. **(C)** The vulvar incision is closed; a drain is placed if there is difficulty with hemostasis, and the flap is pulled into the vaginal epithelial defect over the closed fistula. **(D)** The flap is sutured to hold it in place over the defect. **(E)** The vaginal epithelial defect is closed.

Ureteral catheters are placed if needed. The fistula is excised and the bladder muscle is dissected off the anterior vaginal wall, separating both structures. The bladder and vaginal defects are closed in nonopposing fashion using 3-0 or 4-0 polyglactin sutures. This approach may be hampered by limited surgical access to the fistula site.

A posterior bladder wall incision offers greater field of view through an incision over the bladder dome extended down to the fistula site. The fistula is excised, followed by dissection of the bladder off the vagina, and the defects in the vaginal wall and bladder wall are closed separately.

An omental flap may be placed between the bladder and vagina. The use of peritoneal flaps has been described with good results. Omentum is particularly suitable because it has excellent lymphatic drainage and blood supply.

Other Techniques

Various surgeons have reported differing success rates using solutions such as the injection of fibrin sealant into the fistula track (14,15). Fulguration of

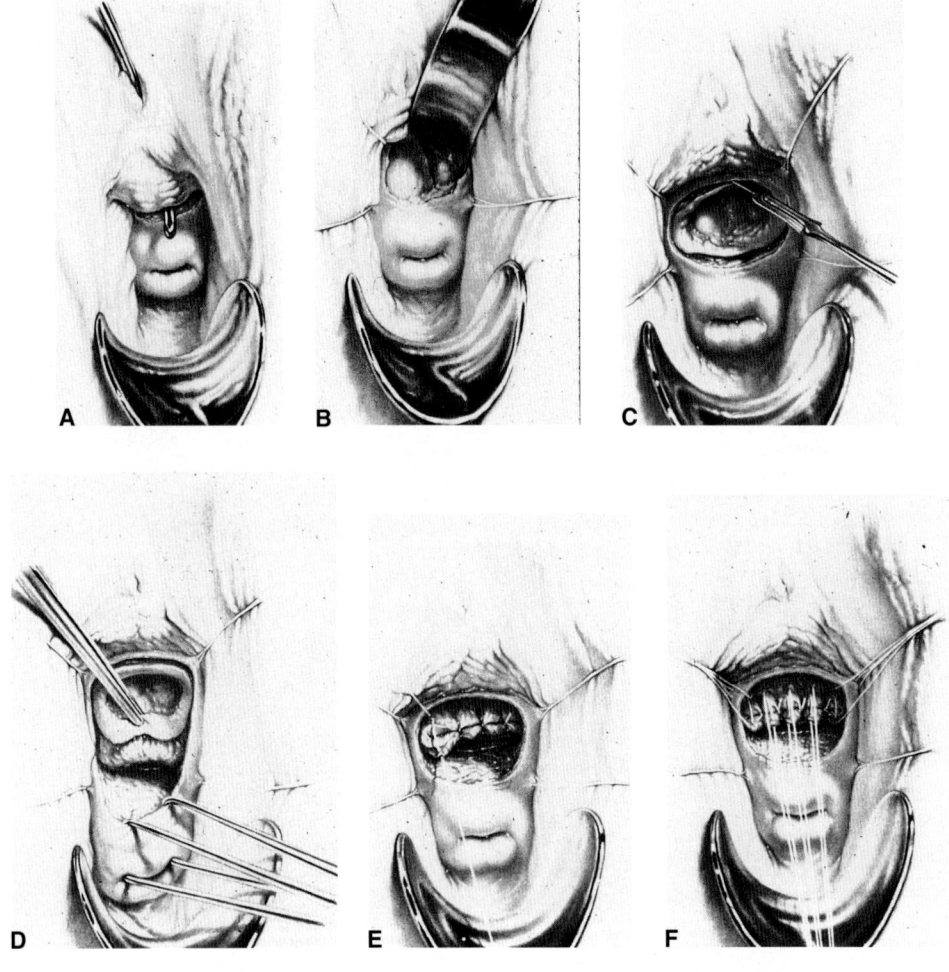

FIGURE 17.3 ● Excision of fistula tract. **(A)** A probe is placed through the urethra into the fistula tract. **(B)** A retractor is placed through the tract to inspect for the location of the ureteral orifices. Stay sutures have been placed; even better is the use of the Lone Star retractor. **(C)** The fistula tract is excised sharply with a knife or Potts scissors. **(D)** The fistula tract is almost excised. **(E)** The first-layer closure with fine interrupted delayed absorbable sutures. **(F)** The second layer is completed and is checked for watertight integrity prior to closure. A Martius flap might also be utilized at this time, also prior to closing the epithelium with interrupted sutures.

the track has also been described (16), but deep fulguration will more likely devitalize tissue and complicate future closure. It may be reasonable to attempt these techniques in very small fistulas.

Postoperative Care

The duration of catheter drainage has not been studied to know the optimal interval. Usually drainage is for 10 to 14 days. Vaginal cases are usually discharged the following day. Antibiotic prophylaxis is given during surgery and is optional thereafter. Patients are to refrain from intercourse or use of tampons for 6 weeks until the vaginal incision is completely healed. Fluids are pushed to keep the urine dilute. If the bladder has been entered (abdominal repair or excision of fistula tract) care must be taken to prevent blood clot formation, and some surgeons will use a large-bore catheter or even combine suprapubic and Foley drainage. Activity is minimized to prevent catheter irritation of the bladder and repair site. Patients should not be working or doing household activities during catheter drainage. Some surgeons will perform a cystogram through the catheter prior to catheter removal to ensure there is no remaining fistula tract, although this

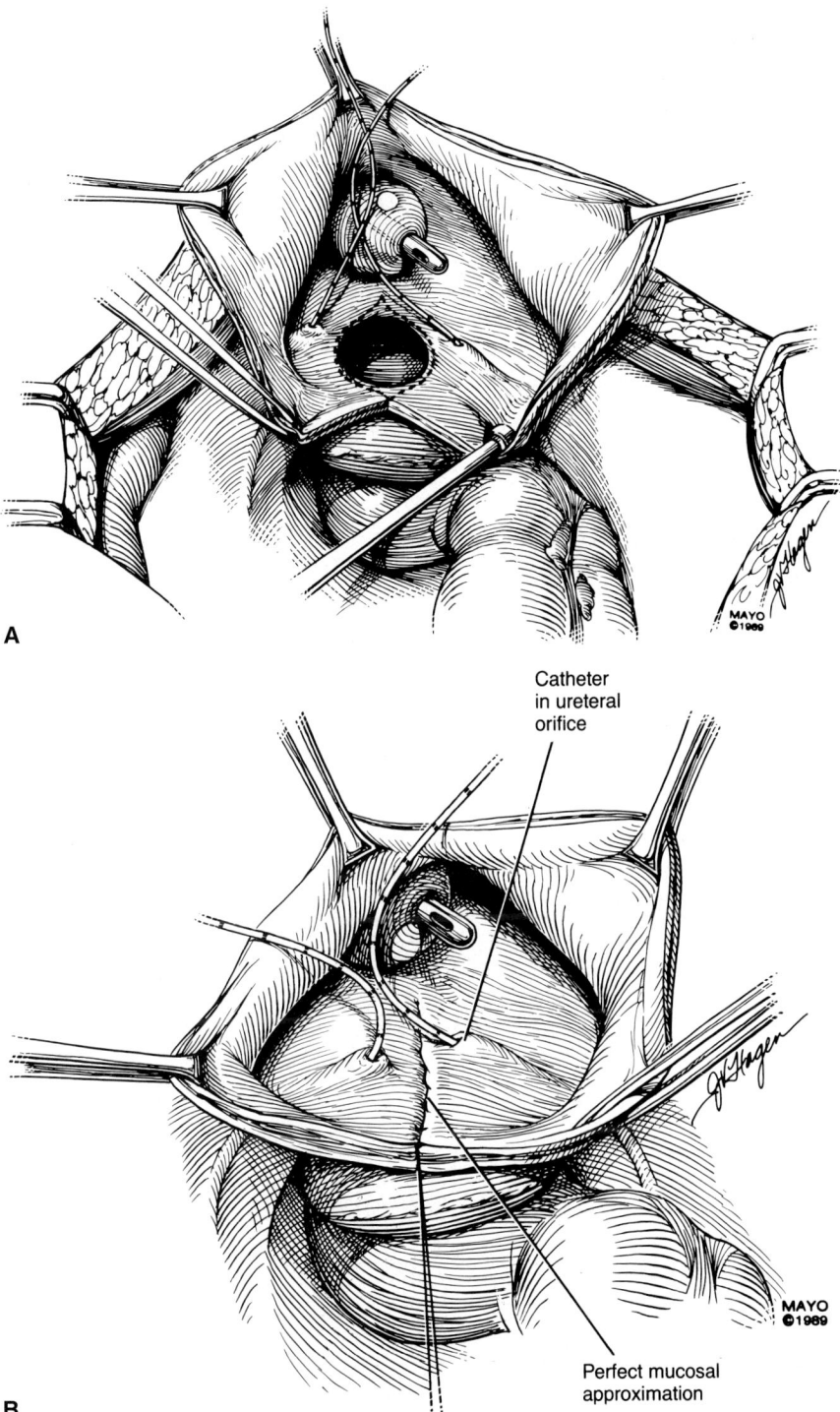

A

B

Catheter
in ureteral
orifice

Perfect mucosal
approximation

FIGURE 17.4 ● Abdominal repair of vesicovaginal fistula. **(A)** Bladder
opened, with outline of area to be resected before placement of initial suture
line. **(B)** Extramucosal approximation by sutures, resulting in approximation of
bladder mucosa. (From Lee RA. *Atlas of gynecologic surgery.* Philadelphia: WB
Saunders, 1992. By permission of Mayo Foundation.)

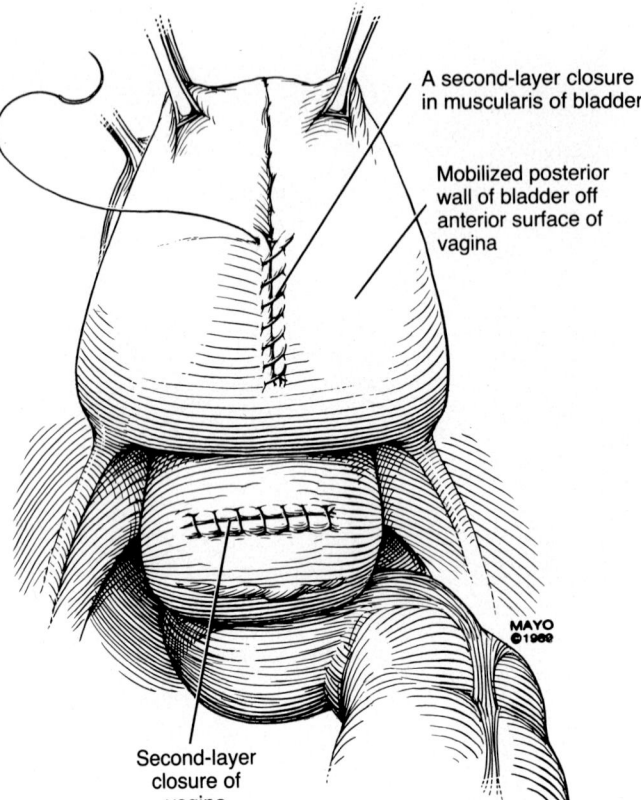

A second-layer closure in muscularis of bladder

Mobilized posterior wall of bladder off anterior surface of vagina

Second-layer closure of vagina

MAYO ©1989

FIGURE 17.5 ● Abdominal repair of vesicovaginal fistula (continued). Previously closed vagina suture line separated from second layer of inverting suture within wall of bladder. (From Lee RA. *Atlas of gynecologic surgery.* Philadelphia: WB Saunders, 1992. By permission of Mayo Foundation.)

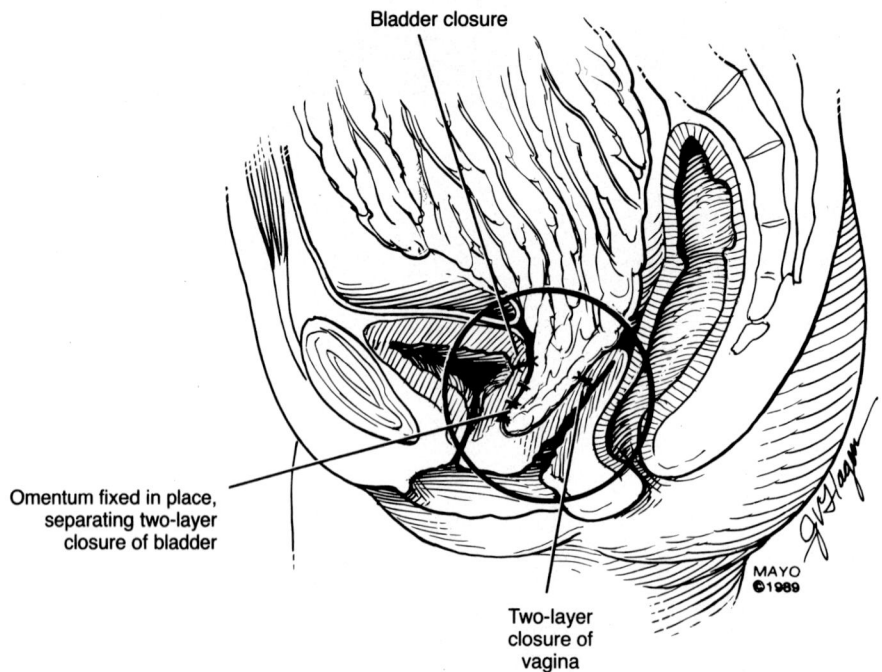

Bladder closure

Omentum fixed in place, separating two-layer closure of bladder

Two-layer closure of vagina

MAYO ©1989

FIGURE 17.6 ● Abdominal repair of vesicovaginal fistula (continued). Mobilized omentum sutured in place between closed bladder and vagina. (From Lee RA. *Atlas of gynecologic surgery.* Philadelphia: WB Saunders, 1992. By permission of Mayo Foundation.)

is not required in most cases. It is important to ensure the patient voids easily on catheter removal and does not develop an overdistended bladder at any point in the postoperative period.

Complications

Success rates as high as 98% have been reported following surgery for simple vesicovaginal fistula repair (6). Complications include recurrence of the fistula, infection, stress urinary incontinence, de novo urge incontinence, and dyspareunia. Radiation-induced fistulas and cancer-related fistulas pose a special problem. These can be difficult to repair and are associated with a higher recurrence and complication rate.

OBSTETRIC FISTULA

Obstetric fistulas are an ancient problem of childbirth. Figure 17.7 is helpful in understanding the etiology of obstetric fistulas in the developing world in the context of the socioeconomic conditions of these countries. Women of many developing countries, especially sub-Saharan Africa, have a very low socioeconomic status. They have few choices in life. Most have little education and are forced to stop school when they are given in marriage at a young age. Childbearing occurs before pelvic growth is completed, and there are almost no medical facilities available. Labor is frequently in the hut of the parents of the father for supposed good luck, and it is only after 1 or 2 days of second-stage labor that an effort may be made to transport the laboring patient to the nearest facility, usually a day away on a wagon or by walking. Help from lay midwives include *gishiri*, the cutting of the vagina in hope of making more space, many times causing the fistula. The stillbirth rate exceeds 75% in these obstructed labors and the maternal mortality approaches 1%. The fistula rate is estimated to be 1%. The injury to the pelvic floor depends on where the head impacts in its descent. Bladder base, trigone, urethra, and rectovaginal tissues are susceptible to breakdown from ischemia. Poor nutrition, chronic anemia, and infections, added to poor hygiene due to a lack of clean water and supplies, accelerates the deterioration of the lesion. The vulva and perineum become constantly exposed to the stream of urine, with subsequent excoriation and maceration of the tissues. Additionally, many have a footdrop that has an unclear etiology. Finally, the worst injury is the social isolation of these patients. Most are divorced and even rejected by their family (7,17,18). They have no resources, with resultant malnutrition, illness, and premature death.

Epidemiology

The socioeconomic conditions of these countries are the main etiology of these fistulas (19). Most patients with fistula are less than 150 cm tall and weigh less than 44 kg. Most have been in labor for at least 2 days prior to being transported for care.

Classification of Fistulas

There is no universally accepted classification system for obstetric vesicovaginal fistula. Using size or location has limitations regarding the outcomes. Old classification systems such as the Hamlin's, which refer to an "easy" fistula or a "difficult" fistula, are not helpful to surgeons who have not done thousands of fistulas (20). Elkins described a classification according to location, but again this is not helpful in prediction of the outcome of repair, though it is helpful in the understanding of vesicovaginal fistula (21) (Fig. 17.8).

Waaldijk based his classification system on the involvement of the closure mechanism and was able to relate advancing stage to poorer results (Table 17.2) (22). Figure 17.9 shows a Waaldjik stage IIB fistula with circumferential defect.

Roenneburg and Wheeless (Table 17.3) presented a classification including size, relation to bladder trigone, and involvement of the closing mechanism that had some correlation to success (International Fistula Conference, July 2005, Johns Hopkins). They looked at the statistics of the International Organization for Women and Development, Inc., mission trips to Niamey, Niger, from 2003 to 2005 (Table 17.4).

Arrowsmith presented a scoring system on 229 patients in Jos, Nigeria, that predicted success of repair (International Fistula Conference, July 2005, Johns Hopkins). After analysis of all factors he found that the amount of scarring and the degree of involvement of the urethral closure mechanism were predictive of success of being dry after surgical repair (Table 17.5). A score of 3 or less had an 85% dry rate. A score of 4 or more had a 41% dry rate.

Previous classification systems were not effective in predicting "success." Fistula closure is not a "success" if the patient has intrinsic sphincter deficiency or intractable urge incontinence from a small contracted bladder. There may be just a pinpoint opening in the vaginal epithelium, but once in surgery there may be no viable tissue for repair until the dissection defines the true size of the fistula. There is a need for an internationally agreed upon classification system. This will allow surgeons to compare their data and help to determine the best approach to the repair.

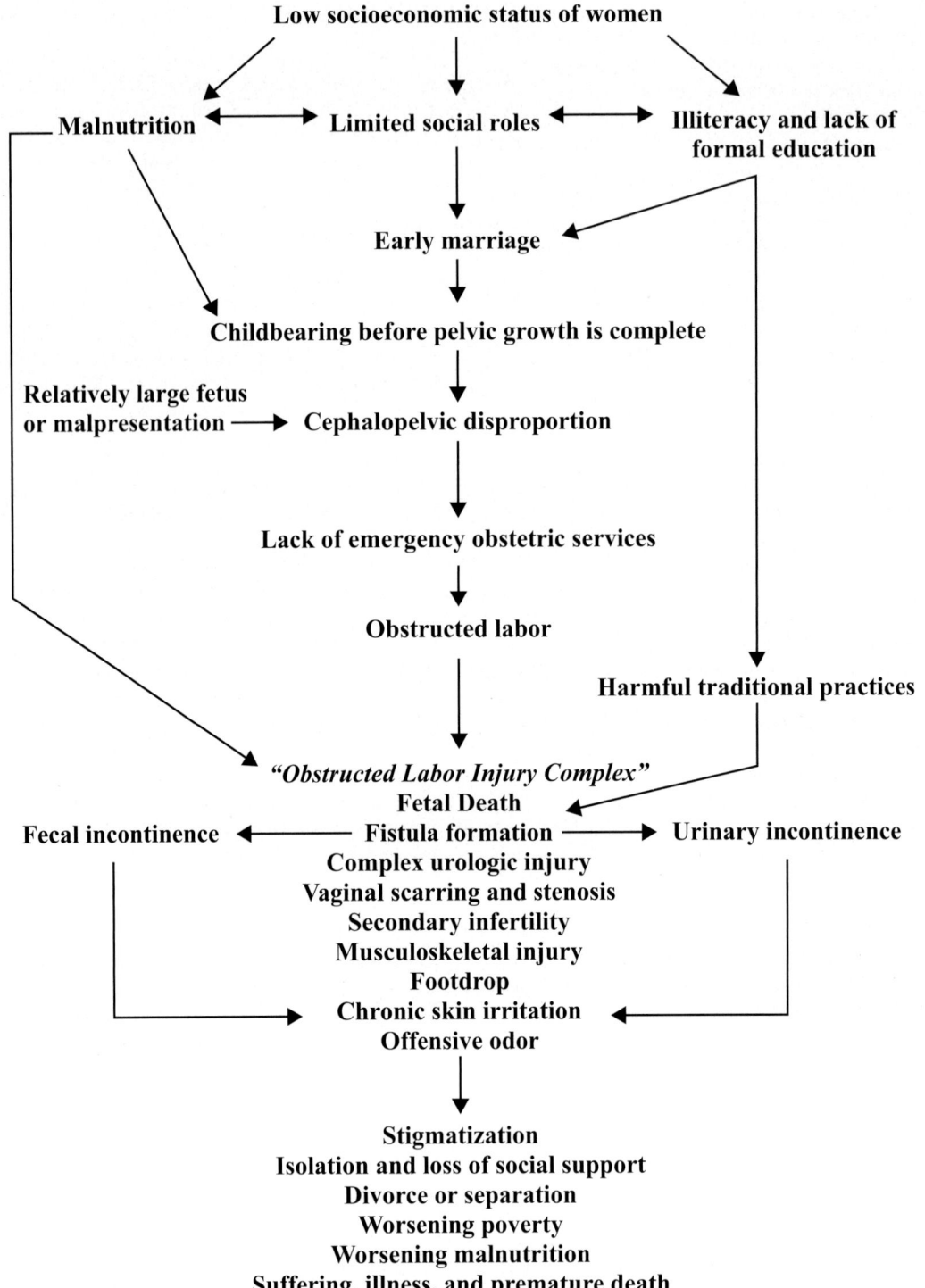

FIGURE 17.7 ● Obstetric fistula pathway: origins and consequences. (From Wall LL, Arrowsmith SD, Briggs ND, et al. The obstetric vesicovaginal fistula in the developing world. *Obstet Gynecol Survey* 2005;60(supp 1):S1–51, by permission.)

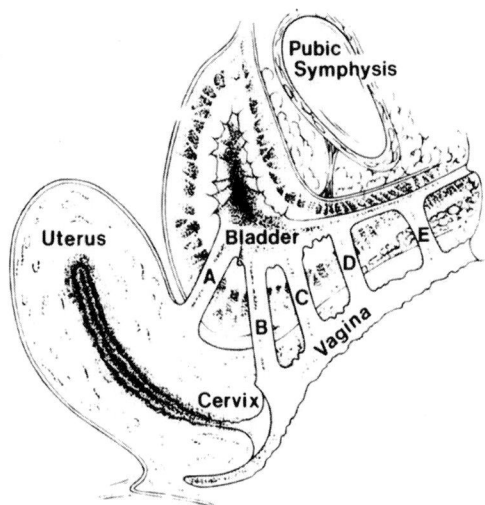

FIGURE 17.8 ● Obstetrical fistula by classification. (From Elkins TE. Surgery for the obstetric vesicovaginal fistula: a review of 100 operations in 82 patients. *Am J Obstet Gynecol* 1994;170(4): 1108–1120, with permission.) **(A)** Vesicocervical fistula. **(B)** Juxtacervical fistula. **(C)** Midvaginal vesicovaginal fistula. **(D)** Suburethral vesicovaginal fistula. **(E)** Urethrovaginal fistula.

TABLE 17.2

Classification of Obstetric Vesicovaginal Fistula According to Waaldijk

Type I: Not involving urethral closure mechanism

Type II: Involving the urethral closure mechanism

A: Without (sub)total urethral involvement

1: Without circumferential defect

2: With circumferential defect

B: With (sub)total urethral involvement

1: Without circumferential defect

2: With circumferential defect

Type III: Miscellaneous ureter/other fistulas

Perioperative Considerations

Evaluation for Other Lesions

The presence and anatomic extent of multiple fistulas must be investigated.

Nutritional Status

Many patients in sub-Saharan Africa with vesicovaginal fistula will have chronic nutritional deprivation. Many will decrease their fluid intake to mini-

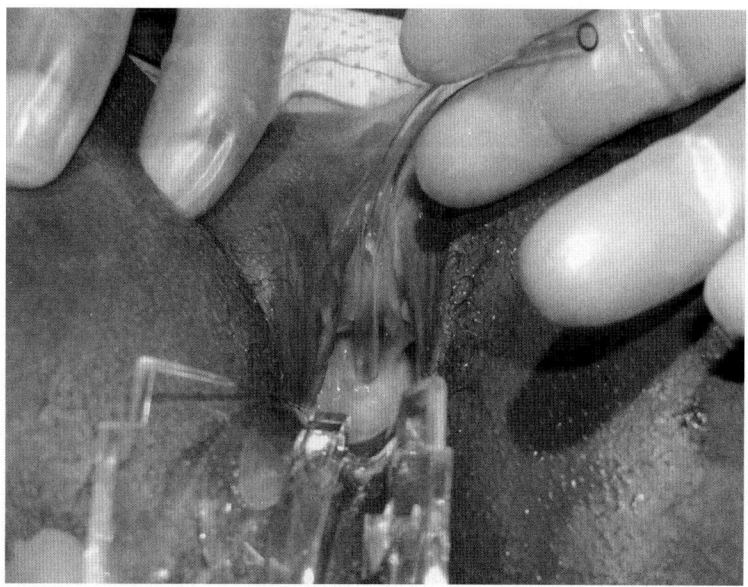

FIGURE 17.9 ● Patient with total circumferential loss of entire urethra. Note the catheter inserted into the bladder at the bladder neck, but no remaining urethra remains except fragments.

TABLE 17.3

Wheeless Classification of Obstetric Vesicovaginal Fistula

Stage I: <2-cm fistula, above the trigone; not involving urethra, trigone, ureteric ridge

Stage II: 2- to 4-cm fistula, above the trigone

Stage III: 4- to 6-cm fistula, above the trigone

OR

Any size fistula involving the continence mechanism of the proximal urethra, urethrovesical junction, trigone, or ureteric ridge

Stage IV: 6-cm fistula or greater

TABLE 17.5

Arrowsmith Fistula Scoring System

Scarring
  None 0
  Mild 1
  Moderate 2
  Severe 3
Status of urethra
  Intact 0
  Partial damage 2
  Complete destruction 3

mize urine leakage. Nutritional build-up prior to surgery should commence in the weeks before surgery, with nutritional supplements (rich in protein, vitamins, and iron) and in some cases blood transfusion. They must also increase their hydration, as this will be important in their surgical care (23).

HIV

The incidence of HIV infection is highest in sub-Saharan Africa compared to the rest of the world and may affect the success because of chronic immunosuppression.

TABLE 17.4

Success Rates of Fistula Closure and Continence (Roenneburg)

Stage I (13 patients)
  57% dry
  33% incontinence
  10% with persistent fistula
Stage II (13 patients)
  54% dry
  23% incontinence
  23% with persistent fistula
Stage III (32 patients)
  75% dry
  10% incontinence
  15% persistent fistula
Stage IV (14 patients)
  50% dry
  29% incontinence
  21% persistent fistula

Timing of Surgery

Controversy exists regarding the optimum time to operate on patients with vesicovaginal fistula. There should be no active infection or necrotic tissue present. A trial of conservative management with bladder drainage for small lesions may be tried. Recent studies have suggested that early repair has an equal success rate (4,23,24).

Surgical Route

Most obstetric fistulas may be closed by the transvaginal approach. The need to reimplant a ureter or bowel diversion for a large rectovaginal fistula may require a dual approach. Severe retropubic scarring may also require an abdominal approach for surgical access.

Tissue Flap Interposition

A Martius flap (see Fig. 17.2) is frequently used in the repair of vesicovaginal fistula. An alternative flap is a gracilis muscle flap, separating the gracilis muscle from the femoral attachment and then rotating it towards the repair site. Limb function is usually not significantly affected. On abdominal cases an omental graft may be utilized.

Ureteral Stent Placement

Ureteral stents are helpful when the trigone is involved in the fistula. The ureter is easy to recognize when the patient is well hydrated or if indigo carmine is available. The catheters are brought out per urethra as cystoscopy equipment is frequently not available to remove the stent at a later time.

Stress Urinary Incontinence

Stress incontinence frequently complicates vesicovaginal fistula repair in these complicated obstetric fistulas, especially when the urethral closure mechanism is compromised. It is unclear whether to place a sling at the time of a urethral reconstruction or to wait until further healing. Use of synthetic midurethral slings in Niamey, Niger, was complicated by frequent mesh erosion, and fascia lata or rectus fascia proved to be better for slings.

Urodynamic equipment is lacking in most of the developing world. Many of these patients have an urge component. Long-term availability of medications for detrusor overactivity is limited.

Antibiotics

The use of antibiotics in vesicovaginal patients varies among surgeons. While prophylactic antibiotics are common in the developed world, they may not be available in the developing world and may be replaced by aggressive hydration (23). Prolonged courses of antibiotics should be reserved for complicated cases, especially when bowel surgery has also been performed.

Anesthesia

Spinal anesthesia is commonly used in environments where limited facilities exist. Equipment for general anesthesia is often very old, with poor reliability. Intubation is frequently blind without proper lighting and should be avoided when possible. Epidural anesthesia would be an improvement, but epidural catheters are generally not available. Repair of complex fistulas involving both rectovaginal and vesicovaginal fistulas may need to be staged because of the limited duration of spinal anesthesia.

Treatment

Nonsurgical

Foley catheter drainage may be successful in obstetric fistula (4,24) in up to 15% of patients in one study and should be tried initially.

Surgical

Most vesicovaginal fistulas are repaired by the transvaginal approach with the excision of the fistula tract as described earlier. The first repair offers the best chance for cure. The Latzko repair is associated with a higher failure rate and should be avoided in the repair of obstetric fistula (24). Surgical techniques include the following:

1. Optimization of the patient's medical and psychological condition prior to surgery
2. Good exposure of the surgical site

3. Meticulous tissue dissection along any natural tissue planes, taking care to avoid the ureters
4. Excision of scarred, fibrotic, or nonviable tissue, as well as complete excision of the fistula track
5. Tension-free reapproximation of the vaginal and bladder defects
6. The use of tissue flaps to improve blood supply when necessary
7. Careful surgical closure of the bladder defect in order to obtain a watertight closure with bladder drainage postoperatively
8. Consideration of staged approach in complex cases

Surgical Techniques
Simple Closure of Obstetric Vesicovaginal Fistula

Excisional transvaginal repair of vesicovaginal fistula as described earlier is used for most obstetric fistulas. Once the patient has been properly positioned and the operative site prepped, the bladder may be catheterized with a urethral catheter if sufficient urethra is present. Ureteral stents are placed if the ureteric ridge is involved. The authors prefer to use a Lone Star retractor with self-retaining hooks for tissue retraction and exposure (Fig. 17.10). The hooks can bring the fistula to the introital opening as shown by attaching to the cervix, improving exposure. The vaginal epithelium is dissected from the underlying fibromuscularis and the fistula tract is excised until there is fibromuscularis and bladder muscularis tissue that is not scarred. The dissection of the epithelium may extend into the retropubic space in order to allow for a tension-free closure of the bladder. Vaginal epithelium may require supplementation from vulvar tissue to allow closure. The bladder defect is closed with 3-0 or 4-0 polyglactin suture with either a small RB or SH needle. Access may also dictate the use of a strongly curved needle like an UR needle. It is important to have a tension-free closure. Instilling dilute methylene blue dye through the urethral catheter into the bladder tests the integrity of the bladder closure. If possible an additional layer may be used. If the repair has poor vascularity, a Martius flap should be performed as described earlier to improve the chance of healing.

Complex Repairs

Urethral involvement will necessitate the reconstruction of the urethra or creation of a neourethra. A flap of anterior or posterior bladder wall may be used as well as vaginal/vulvar tissue to reconstruct the urethra. Many of the reconstructed urethras will require an additional sling after the initial surgery is healed to treat stress incontinence from intrinsic sphincter deficiency. If the repair has poor vascu-

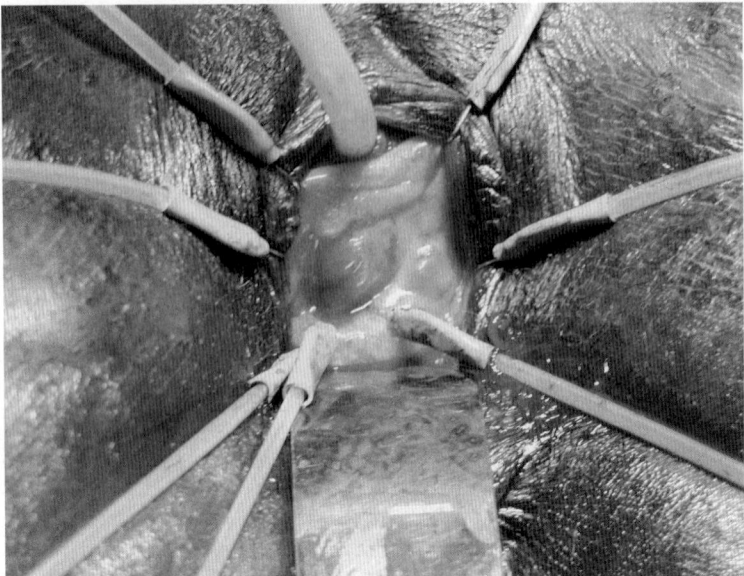

FIGURE 17.10 ● Lone Star retractor on a juxtacervical fistula with the hooks on the cervix, bringing the fistula to the introitus for better exposure.

larity, a Martius flap should be performed. Reconstruction of the urethra may require longer drainage than the standard 10 to 14 days. Neourethras tend to scar, with resultant stenosis, and this may doom the repair to failure if the urethra is not held open with prolonged drainage. Retropubic scarring that extends into the retropubic space might be helped by a dual abdominal and vaginal approach. A second team operating from above may be necessary to maximize anesthesia time.

Postoperative Care

The postoperative care of the obstetric vesicovaginal fistula patient is just as important as the surgical repair. The main principles of postoperative care include:

1. Bladder drainage postoperatively for at least 14 days; however, a longer period of drainage may be required depending on the complexity of the repair. Ureteric stents may be removed the following day if a reimplantation is not involved.

2. Adequate hydration is necessary to maintain a good urine output and keep the urinary catheters patent. Oral fluids can suffice. This may eliminate the need for antibiotics (4).

3. Perineal hygiene is vital. Sitz baths help to provide cleansing and ease discomfort, but facilities are frequently inadequate.

4. The avoidance of sexual activity or other vaginal manipulation should be strictly observed until satisfactory healing has taken place.

5. Repeat vaginal examinations are performed periodically for at least the first 3 months in order to detect and manage any tissue breakdown, infection, or recurrent vaginal stenosis. Gentle dilation may help maintain vaginal caliber. Some patients may require reconstruction of their vagina.

6. Recurrent fistulas should be given time to heal spontaneously with continuous bladder drainage if they are small. If drainage does not work, consider reoperation when inflammation has resolved.

7. Urge incontinence should be treated with anticholinergics if available. If the bladder capacity is inadequate because of scarring, an augmentation cystoplasty may be required.

8. Nutritional status postoperatively should continue to be optimized and anemia should be addressed with oral supplements or in severe cases blood transfusion.

9. Lower limb neuropathy (footdrop) can be managed with physical therapy if available. Most neuropathies associated with vesicovaginal fistula resolve spontaneously with time (25).

10. Education, training, and counseling is necessary to help introduce these patients back into society, since most are divorced and unskilled.

The Incurable Patient and Urinary Diversion

There are a number of patients who may be candidates for urinary diversion because of multiple failures of repair or scarring of the vagina with inadequate tissue for reconstruction. Ureterosigmoidostomy with extramural serous-lined ureterointestinal anastomosis (Mainz type II) has been used (26). Other techniques and tissues have been used. Surgical complications are common even in developed countries (27). Diversions are associated with metabolic disturbances, and medical follow-up may not be available. Malabsorption may lead to electrolyte and vitamin deficiencies (28). Pyelonephritis without medical care may be fatal. The place of continent diversions is still controversial in the developing world. Diversion to the abdominal wall is unsatisfactory because of the lack of access to disposable stoma appliances.

OTHER FISTULAS

Other types of fistula may mimic vesicovaginal fistulas or may coexist with vesicovaginal fistulas. The evaluation of a vesicovaginal fistula includes evaluation for coexisting ureterovaginal, vesicocervical, or vesicouterine fistula. Rectovaginal and colovaginal fistulas may also be present, as well as enterovesical and colovesical fistulas.

Ureterovaginal Fistulas

Ureterovaginal fistulas occur almost exclusively following injury to the ureters during gynecologic surgery. The incidence is believed to be 0.5% to 2.0% following a simple hysterectomy (29). Radical hysterectomy is associated with a higher rate (30), but there is no recent literature to document lower rates.

Recognizing and repairing ureteral injury at the time of the initial injury is the best form of management of injury, but the authors believe that prospective cystoscopy is necessary because of a 1.7% rate of unrecognized injury at the time of hysterectomy (10). Stenting the ureter at the time of injury may prevent the need to reimplant the ureter at a later time. Patients typically present in the postoperative period with leakage of urine from the vagina. They are the fortunate patients, as many ureteral injuries are not discovered until much later with the incidental finding of a nonfunctioning kidney. Immediate postoperative symptoms of injury include flank discomfort and fever and chills. Urosepsis occurs less frequently. There is usually a small increase of about 0.3 in the serum creatinine associated with a blocked ureter, though there has seldom been a reason to measure this at the time of the problem.

The initial investigation is intravenous pyelography. An immediate attempt should be made to pass a stent, either retrograde through cystoscopy or antegrade through a percutaneous nephrostomy. If stenting is accomplished, the fistula may close without further surgery (31). If unable to stent the ureter, a nephrostomy will preserve kidney function until surgical repair. Timing of repair is controversial, with suggestions of repair within 4 weeks (31) to 6 months (30). Delay in surgical repair may increase the probability of a legal suit, but attempts prior to resolution of inflammation from the initial surgery may compromise the repair.

The preferred repair is an ureteroneocystostomy (Fig. 17.11), which may include a psoas hitch, attaching the bladder to the psoas muscle to ensure a tension-free reimplantation of the ureter. Alternatively a Boari (32) flap of bladder muscularis may be used to ensure tension-free reimplantation. If the injury is above the pelvic brim it may be necessary to perform an end-to-end anastomosis of the ureter. The use of an end-to-end anastomosis as well as stenting the injury must be re-evaluated later for ureteral stricture. Transureteroureterostomy is a last-resort procedure, as it may damage the other ureter.

Vesicouterine and Vesicocervical Fistula

First described by Youssef in 1957 (32), vesicouterine and vesicocervical fistulas are becoming more common with the increasing cesarean delivery rate (33). They typically occur as a complication of cesarean section, following the inadvertent placement of sutures in a scarred, poorly developed bladder flap or from postcesarean infection. The patient may have symptoms of menouria or urine leakage from the vagina. Because of differential leakage of urine intra-abdominally through the fallopian tubes, methylene blue may not be appreciated on vaginal examination. Diagnosis may be confirmed by hysterogram or retrograde injection of the cervix at the time of cystoscopy (34). If childbearing is complete, hysterectomy will facilitate the repair. If preservation of the uterus is desired, it might be easier to perform surgery from a transabdominal approach.

Urethrovaginal Fistulas

Urethrovaginal fistulas are relatively uncommon in modern gynecologic practice (35). They occur following surgical procedures such as diverticulectomy, urethropexy, and suburethral sling procedures, as well as procedures involving extensive anterior vaginal wall dissection. Obstetric urethrovaginal fistulas are discussed above in the sec-

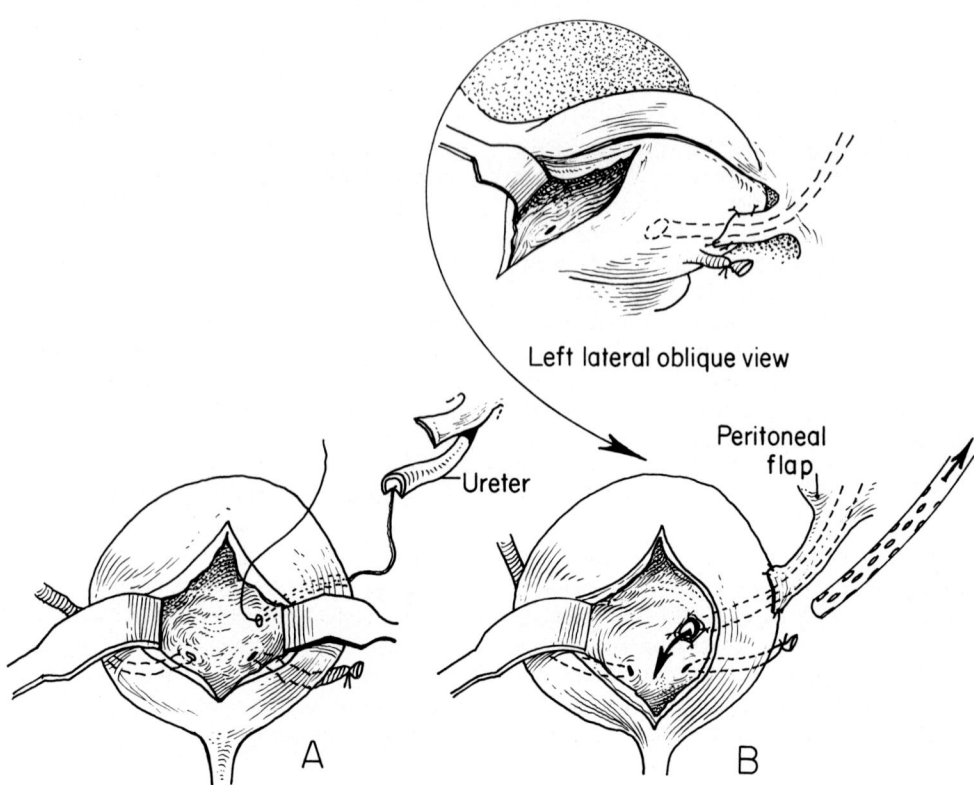

Left lateral oblique view

Ureter

Peritoneal flap

A

B

FIGURE 17.11 ● Abdominal ureteroneocystostomy. **(A)** Abdominal cystotomy in extraperitoneal dome of bladder with traction suture drawing ureter through wall of bladder; ligation of distal ureteral segment. **(B)** Ureter sutured to bladder mucosa; peritoneal flap and adventitial sheath of ureter sutured to bladder muscularis at its site of entry into bladder. (From Symmonds RE. Ureteral injuries associated with gynecologic surgery: prevention and management. *Clin Obstet Gynecol* 1976;19:623–44, with permission.)

tion on obstetric fistula. Distal lesions may have minimal symptoms because the defect is below the urinary sphincter. There may be vaginal retention of urine that dribbles out on standing. Proximal lesions have more symptoms, especially if there is funneling of the bladder neck. A zero-degree urethroscope is valuable in diagnosis, as is the use of a small probe passed per urethra. Wide dissection and a layered tension-free closure are the standard therapy. A Martius flap should be considered for large fistulas and those with poor vascularity. Small asymptomatic lesions may be ignored. Stenting with a urethral catheter for 1 to 2 weeks is the usual postoperative care. Complications include recurrence, stricture formation, and incontinence.

Rectovaginal Fistulas with Vesicovaginal Fistula

Rectovaginal fistulas may also complicate vesicovaginal fistulas, especially in obstetric fistulas and

radiation-associated fistulas. Distal rectovaginal fistula associated with obstetric episiotomy and fourth-degree extensions in the developed world may be closed primarily. Large proximal fistulas and those associated with radiation or Crohn's disease may require fecal diversion to achieve closure (36). In complex cases with rectovaginal and vesicovaginal fistulas, closure of the rectovaginal fistula should be done prior to closure of the vesicovaginal fistula.

Enterovesical and Colovesical Fistulas

Fistulous connections between the small bowel or colon and the urinary bladder are rare; however, they should be suspected in patients who have Crohn's disease or diverticulitis and who complain of dysuria, urinary frequency or urgency, and pneumaturia (37–39). It is generally more prevalent in males since the uterus provides a natural tissue interposition between the bowel and bladder. In a review, diverticulitis was the most common cause (41%) followed by Crohn's disease (17%) and colorectal cancer (16%) (40). Positive urine cultures were obtained in 88% of the patients, with *Escherichia coli* as the most prevalent organism. Cystoscopy is the most effective diagnostic tool but was confirmatory only 67% of the time in the series by Moss (38). Barium study was also useful, being generally abnormal 80% of the time; however, it identified the fistula in only 17% of cases in which it was used. Flexible sigmoidoscopy and computed tomography scan may also be used. The sigmoid colon was the most frequently (53%) involved segment of the bowel in the series by Moss (38).

As in colovaginal fistulas, a one-stage procedure in patients without invasive malignancy is the current approach. A multistage procedure may be needed in the face of severe intra-abdominal disease. Surgery with resection of the affected bowel segment is probably the standard therapy.

Conclusion

Genitourinary fistulas are recognized complications of gynecologic surgery and neglected obstetrics. Prevention of these complications is the goal but will probably not happen in the near future, especially in the developing world. The care of this problem will continue to be a challenge to our specialty. The basic principles of diagnosis and surgical repair have not changed since the first successful case series on vesicovaginal fistula repair over a century and a half ago.

URETHRAL DIVERTICULUM

Introduction

Urethral diverticulum is an uncommon condition first described by William Hey in 1803 (40). Urethral diverticula exist in about 1% to 6% of the population (41–43), though this may be a conservative estimate given that many cases go undiagnosed, untreated, and unreported. The surgical literature contains several references to this condition, highlighting the increase in diagnosed cases when a heightened index of suspicion prompts appropriate workup (44). It is commonly seen in the third to fifth decade of life and does not appear to have any specific ethnic or socioeconomic etiology.

Pathophysiology

Huffman's detailed anatomic study of the urethra and the surrounding paraurethral ducts and glands was the modern review of these structures at the time it was published (45). The urethra can be described as a short tube lined by epithelium and surrounded by numerous tiny glands, some of which are in communication with the urethral lumen via small ostia that range in size from less than 1 mm to several millimeters in diameter. The vast majority of these glands are located in the posterior hemisphere of the distal urethra, typically between the 3 and 9 o'clock positions. Of note is the fact that the embryologic urethra develops in close relation to the vagina, and in the adult female the external meatus and distal urethra may be colonized by vaginal flora. There are several theories on the mechanism of formation of urethral diverticulum. Routh (46) proposed that diverticula were caused by the obstruction of the ostia with secretions, with subsequent dilation of the paraurethral glands. Secondary infection would then cause a rupture of the gland into the urethra, forming a diverticulum. Alternatively, inflammation with or without infection in a paraurethral gland can lead to obstruction of the neck of the gland, with subsequent distention. Diverticula have been shown to be more common after a gonococcal infection (47). Such inflammation may resolve and recur and eventually result in a residual distention of the gland. The diverticulum thus formed may remain asymptomatic, depending on its size, location, and the presence of recurring infection. Urine can accumulate in the more wide-necked glands and stasis can occur, leading to infection. Rarely, stone formation or malignant transformation can occur. Most of the diverticula encountered in urogynecologic practice are acquired and seen in adult females. Urethral diverticula have also been described in neonates, lending support to a congenital etiology (48). Trauma and instrumentation to the urethra, obstetric injury, and infection may be factors predisposing to the development of urethral diverticulum.

Presentation

Patients may harbor a diverticulum for several years before the diagnosis is made. This has resulted from a low index of suspicion by evaluating physicians. The older gynecologic and urologic literature refers to the classic triad of symptoms of dysuria, dyspareunia, and postvoid dribbling in patients presenting with urethral diverticulum. However, recent case series have disputed this and have shown that this classic presentation is rather uncommon. The typical patient with a urethral diverticulum tends to present with a myriad of lower urinary tract symptoms. In Ganabathi's series of 63 patients, 57% presented with stress urinary incontinence, 38% with recurrent urinary tract infections, 21% with dysuria, 18% with urgency, and 16% with urinary frequency. Postvoid dribbling was present in only 5% and dyspareunia in 6% of those patients (49). Other series have had up to a 20% asymptomatic rate, being noticed only at the time of a pelvic examination (50). Purulent discharge from the urethra was noted in only 3% of those patients. Lee reviewed 107 cases of symptomatic urethral diverticula and found that most of the patients were between the ages of 30 and 50 years and presented most commonly with urinary urgency, dysuria, and dyspareunia, with a common history of recurrent urinary tract infections (51). Similarly, Jacoby reviewed 32 cases and the most common presentation was found to be recurrent urinary tract infections, dysuria, urgency/frequency, and stress incontinence (52). However, in Romanzi's report of 46 cases, the most common presenting symptom was pain, which occurred in almost half of the patients, followed by incontinence in 35% (53). Postvoid dribbling was noted in only 8% of the patients and dysuria in 5%. The above series show that the presenting symptoms in patients with urethral diverticulum can be variable and nonspecific. Other complaints include a vaginal lump, which may or may not be painful, hematuria, pelvic pain, and urinary voiding difficulty. The diagnosis of urethral diverticulum should be considered in patients who present with a history of persistent or recurrent nonspecific lower urinary tract symptoms that have failed previous treatment.

Differential Diagnosis

Differential diagnosis includes anterior vaginal wall cysts, which may be embryologic remnants (Gartner's) or large inclusion cysts. Leiomyoma of the anterior vaginal wall has been mistaken for a urethral diverticulum. Leiomyomata tend to be solid masses, but the author had a degenerating leiomyoma of the smooth muscle of the urethra that presented as a soft mass consistent with a diverticulum that did not have an open ostia. Other differential diagnoses include endometriosis as well as malignant lesions such as carcinoma of the urethra.

Diagnosis

In the presence of an obvious anterior vaginal wall swelling, the diagnosis of a diverticulum may be straightforward, and the expression of milky or purulent material from the urethral orifice on compression of the mass is virtually confirmatory. In less obvious cases the surgeon may have to resort to one or more radiologic tests to aid in the diagnosis. Controversy exists as to what test is most appropriate for the initial workup of patients with suspected urethral diverticulum.

Davis in 1958 described the use of a double-balloon catheter for positive-pressure urethrography (PPUG) as a means of diagnosing urethral diverticula (54) (Figs. 17.12 and 17.13). PPUG is probably the best method for diagnosing a urethral diverticulum, although it will miss a noncommunicating diverticulum. A voiding cystourethrogram (VCUG) is used in several centers for the initial investigation of urethral diverticulum. Ultrasound has also been used to confirm the diagnosis, especially with the use of higher-resolution 7- to 10-MHz probes.

Wang and Wang compared PPUG to VCUG in 132 patients and concluded that PPUG is a more

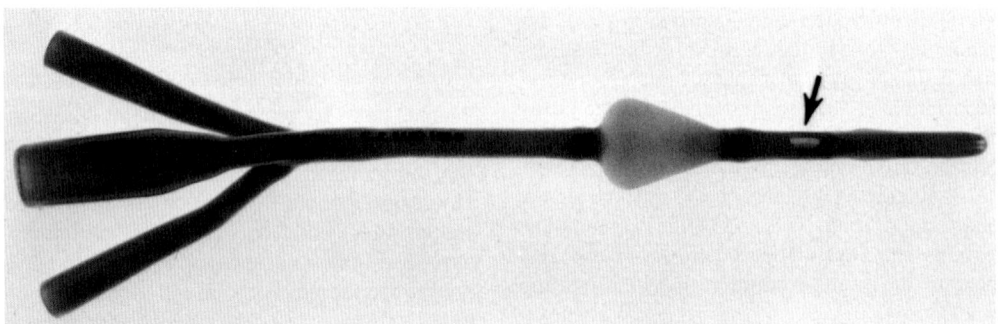

FIGURE 17.12 ● The Trattner catheter. The triple-lumen catheter has a proximal balloon that is filled with water or air once the catheter is placed to keep the catheter in the urethra. The wedge-shaped distal balloon is then filled to trap the urethra between the balloons. The third lumen is then injected with contrast material, which egresses through an opening *(arrow)* between the two balloons, distending the urethra and urethral diverticulum with contrast medium to be seen on fluoroscopy.

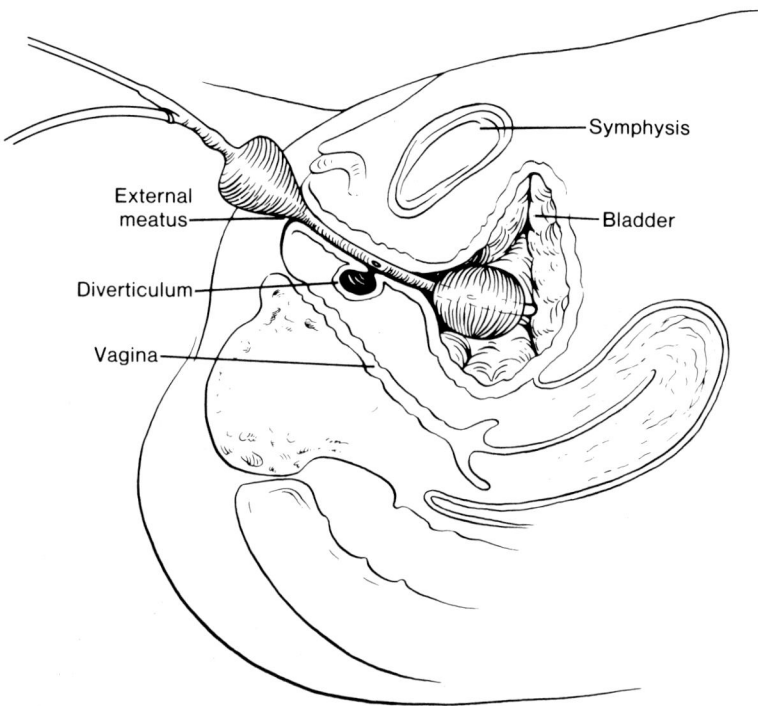

FIGURE 17.13 ● The Trattner catheter in place in the urethra.

sensitive study (55). PPUG diagnosed the urethral diverticulum in 33 out of 120 patients compared with 20 out of 120 patients on VCUG. They also showed that PPUG was more effective in diagnosing smaller diverticula with ostia as small as 1.7 mm in diameter, while VCUG was only effective in outlining diverticula with a minimum ostial diameter of 3 mm. PPUG provides information on the number of diverticula and their relation to the bladder neck. It can also reveal the presence of stones within a diverticulum. However, it may be falsely negative if the ostium is tiny or occluded. Other drawbacks include patient discomfort and exposure to radiation and contrast material. The VCUG has become increasingly popular, as it is easier to perform with less discomfort.

Jacoby directly compared PPUG to VCUG in 32 patients and the results showed that PPUG was more sensitive and proved more valuable in patients with nonpalpable urethral diverticula (13). This is presumably because the positive pressure employed during PPUG aids in distending the diverticulum, rendering it more visible with contrast. Of note, both tests had similar costs.

More recently, the use of endoluminal magnetic resonance imaging (MRI) has been reported to provide even more accurate results. Blander compared endoluminal MRI with VCUG in 27 patients with urethral diverticula (56). MRI accurately showed the diverticulum in all the patients, while VCUG was able to diagnose the lesion in 23 of the 27 patients. Again, MRI provided significantly more accurate detail of the lesions, with better size correlation of the diverticulum when compared to the intraoperative findings. MRI proved vastly superior in providing information on the location and size of the neck of the diverticulum (11 out of 27, compared with none in VCUG). MRI also showed the presence of loculations within the diverticulum in addition to providing accurate anatomic detail of surrounding structures. Another advantage of MRI is that urethral diverticula that do not communicate with the urethral lumen can be seen. It also will show anterior diverticula or horseshoe-shaped diverticula that may be missed on other radiologic tests. This is now considered the gold standard for diagnosis and evaluation of urethral diverticula.

The urethral pressure profile (UPP) has been described in the evaluation of patients with urethral diverticulum (57,58). It typically shows a biphasic profile (Fig. 17.14). The authors do not find UPP to be of value in the overall management of urethral diverticulum, since it is prone to artifact and is operator-dependent. Nevertheless, it does show the relationship of the urethral diverticulum to the area of maximal closure pressure in the ure-

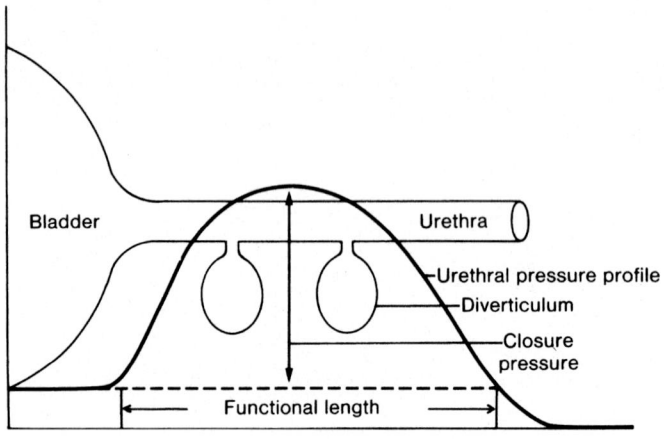

FIGURE 17.14 ● Urethral closure pressure profile with superimposed diverticulum orifices proximal and distal to peak urethral closure pressure.

thra. This provides information on whether the urethral diverticulum exists proximal or distal to the urethral sphincter mechanism. This allows the choice of a marsupialization procedure for a diverticulum distal to the maximum urethral closure pressure, whereas proximal lesions would result in incontinence if marsupialized.

Transvaginal, transrectal, transperineal, and translabial ultrasound studies (59–61) are increasingly employed in the workup of patients with urethral diverticulum. The accuracy of such techniques depends on the experience of the operator and the quality of the equipment. Ultrasound has the advantage of being inexpensive and avoids exposure to radiation. It is readily available and can provide information on the contents of a diverticulum. However, it may not distinguish between urethral diverticulum and other cystic structures.

Cystourethroscopy is a useful adjunct in the workup of patients with urethral diverticulum, providing direct visualization of the bladder and urethral lumen. The ostium of the diverticulum may be visualized on cystoscopy, especially if using a zero-degree scope. Elevation of the anterior vaginal wall during the procedure can help to compress the diverticulum and make the ostium more visible.

The advantages and disadvantages of the various imaging techniques (Table 17.6) and the sensitivity of the various diagnostic modalities (23) are presented for comparison purposes (Table 17.7).

Other Tests

Urinalysis and culture is necessary since up to half of these patients may harbor a urinary tract infection. Cultures may grow mixed anaerobic organisms. In cases of recurrent cystitis, an intravenous pyelogram may be required to exclude upper urinary tract abnormalities or urinary tract stones.

Management of Urethral Diverticulum

A small, asymptomatic urethral diverticulum may be observed. An exception would be a lesion that appeared or felt suspicious for a neoplasm. Patients with mild symptoms can be managed by observation, and antibiotics should be used to treat urinary tract infection. Antibiotics for recurrent infection in a diverticulum are also an option, especially for a patient who is not a surgical candidate. Persistent and troublesome symptoms are best addressed surgically.

Marsupialization

Spence first described a marsupialization technique for the treatment of urethral diverticulum (62) (Fig. 17.15). This involved incising the diverticulum and suturing the wall of the cavity to the surrounding vaginal tissue in an interrupted fashion. It has the advantage of being a simple procedure but may be associated with stress incontinence (63). It should be a distal diverticulum beyond the point of maximal urethral closure pressure. A Skene's duct cyst or abscess is also treated in this manner and is actually another name for a distal diverticulum.

Diverticulectomy

Total excision of a proximal diverticulum is the procedure of choice and offers the best chance of cure. More extensive dissection is required and urethroplasty is usually involved since complete removal of a communicating diverticulum may inevitably leave a defect in the urethra. A urethral or suprapubic catheter may be used to drain the bladder following the procedure.

Traditionally a vertical incision was made in the vaginal epithelium to dissect out the diverticulum (12,64). This incision affords somewhat less

TABLE 17.6

Advantages and Disadvantages of Various Imaging Techniques

Test	Advantages	Disadvantages
Positive-pressure urethrography	• Sensitive • Relatively inexpensive	• Availability of special catheter • Discomfort • Exposure to radiation • Can miss small, noncommunicating diverticula
Voiding cystourethrography	• Relatively inexpensive	• Voiding required and patient may be not be relaxed • Exposure to radiation • May miss small lesions
MRI	• Accurate anatomic detail • Nonionizing radiation • Can diagnose small, noncommunicating diverticula • Endoluminal coil enhances accuracy	• Expensive • Expertise required in interpretation of results
Ultrasound	• Inexpensive • Available • No exposure to radiation • Differentiates cystic from solid contents	• May misdiagnose other cystic lesions
Cystourethroscopy	• Direct visualization of ostia • Diagnose other intraluminal lesions • Evaluation of bladder neck and anterior urethra	• Fail to diagnose anterior urethral diverticula

MRI, magnetic resonance imaging.

TABLE 17.7

Accuracy and Sensitivity of the Various Diagnostic Modalities (70)

Diagnostic Modalities	%
History and physical examination	33%
Voiding cystourethrography	60%
Positive-pressure urethrography	80%
Urethroscopy	60%
Endovaginal sonography	40%
Transrectal sonography	30%
Postvoiding x-ray	22%
Magnetic resonance imaging	70%

exposure over the diverticulum. An inverted-U incision (Fig. 17.16) is made on the anterior vaginal wall over the diverticulum (65). The vaginal epithelium is meticulously dissected away from the underlying pubocervical fibromuscularis and periurethral tissues. The most important step is to dissect these fibromuscular tissues away from the diverticulum, trying not to enter the diverticulum. These tissues will be used to close over the urethral defect created when removing the diverticulum cyst wall. Careful dissection at this stage will provide adequate tissue to close. A Martius bulbocavernosus graft may be necessary to provide adequate tissue closure. Dissection and extirpation of the diverticulum cyst has to include the neck of the diverticulum and the urethral ostium. This creates a urethral defect, which should be repaired over a small urethral catheter using 3-0 or 4-0 delayed absorbable polyglactin suture. The periurethral tissue

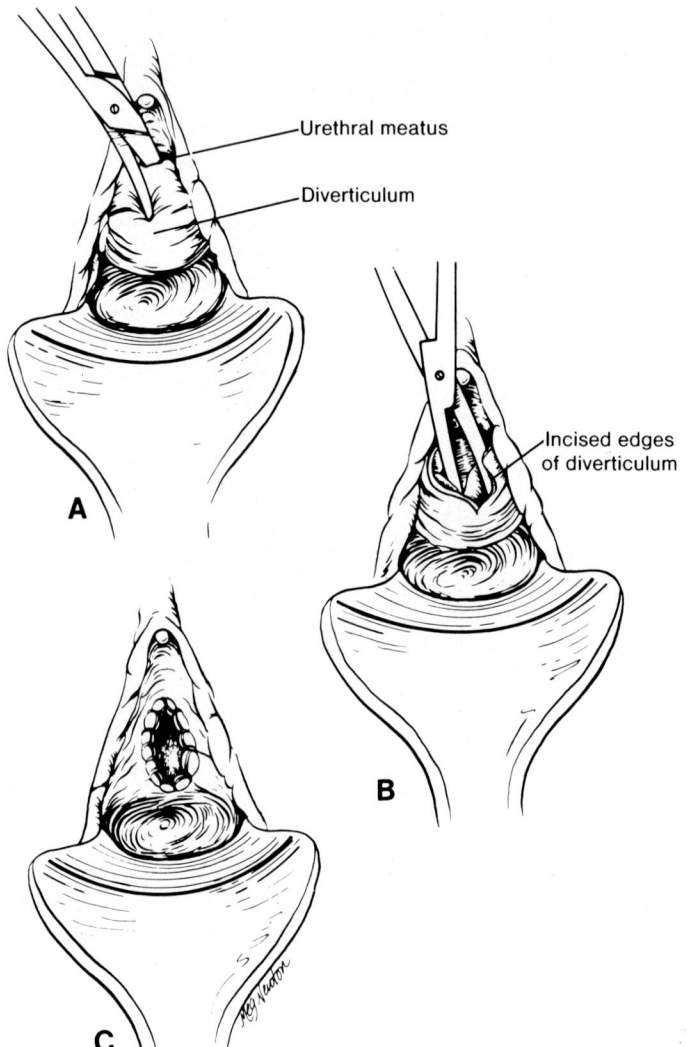

Urethral meatus

Diverticulum

Incised edges
of diverticulum

A

B

C

FIGURE 17.15 ● Spence procedure. The scissors are placed into the diverticulum **(A)** and incise full thickness through to vagina **(B)**. **(C)** A running locked suture secures the edges to prevent bleeding.

developed on the initial dissection is then reapproximated over the urethral repair, overlapping the tissue if adequate, taking care to ensure that the suture lines are not under tension. The vaginal inverted-U–shaped epithelium is closed using the same suture material.

Perioperative Considerations

Stress Urinary Incontinence and Concomitant Urethropexy

Many patients with urethral diverticulum may present with stress urinary incontinence. It is important to evaluate preoperatively for stress incontinence, and urodynamic studies are advisable. The use of concomitant urethropexy at the time of diverticulectomy is controversial. McGuire used a pubovaginal sling at the time of diverticulectomy in patients with concomitant stress urinary incontinence without increased complications (66). There is concern that synthetic materials increase the risk of erosions or fistula. Excessive tension on a sling is also of concern. Finally, the diverticulum may be the etiology of the stress incontinence, and repair of the urethra may cure the incontinence. Slings have their own set of complications that would be avoided. It is probably advisable to allow healing before using one of the many new midurethral mesh slings for incontinence.

Tissue Interposition

Tissue flaps to provide additional blood supply should certainly be employed in patients with a high risk of breakdown from poor healing. These include smokers, patients with chronic medical

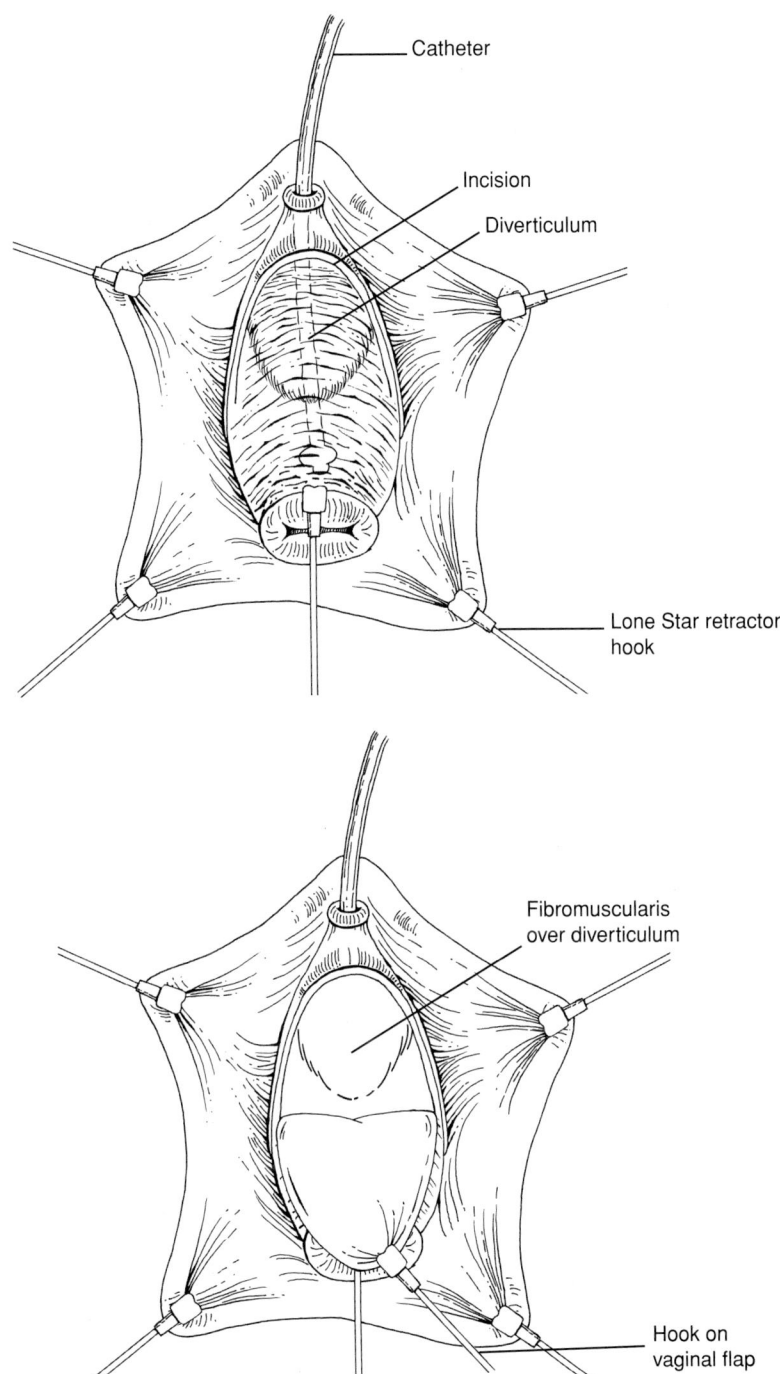

FIGURE 17.16 ● Excision of urethral diverticulum. **(A)** The Lone Star hooks are placed for exposure and on the cervix to bring the fistula closer to the introitus for exposure. An inverted-U incision is made. **(B)** The vaginal epithelium is dissected from over the diverticulum and pubocervical fibromuscularis. *(continued)*

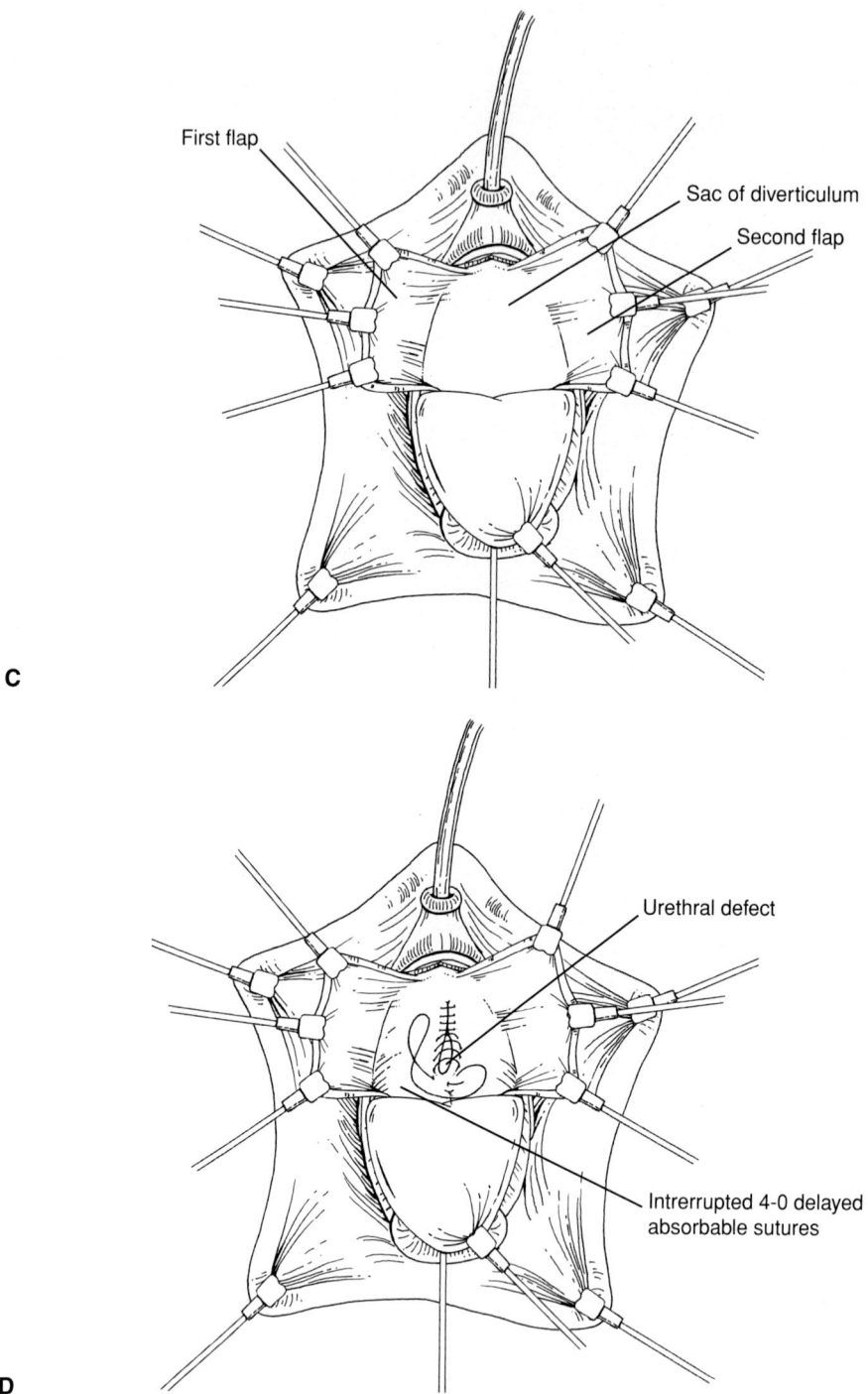

FIGURE 17.16 ● *(continued)* **(C)** Additional incisions are made in the fibromuscularis to mobilize tissue for closing the defect, taking care to try to stay out of the diverticulum if possible. **(D)** The exposed sac is excised and the defect in the urethra is repaired with 4-0 or 5-0 delayed absorbable suture on a small (RB) needle. *(continued)*

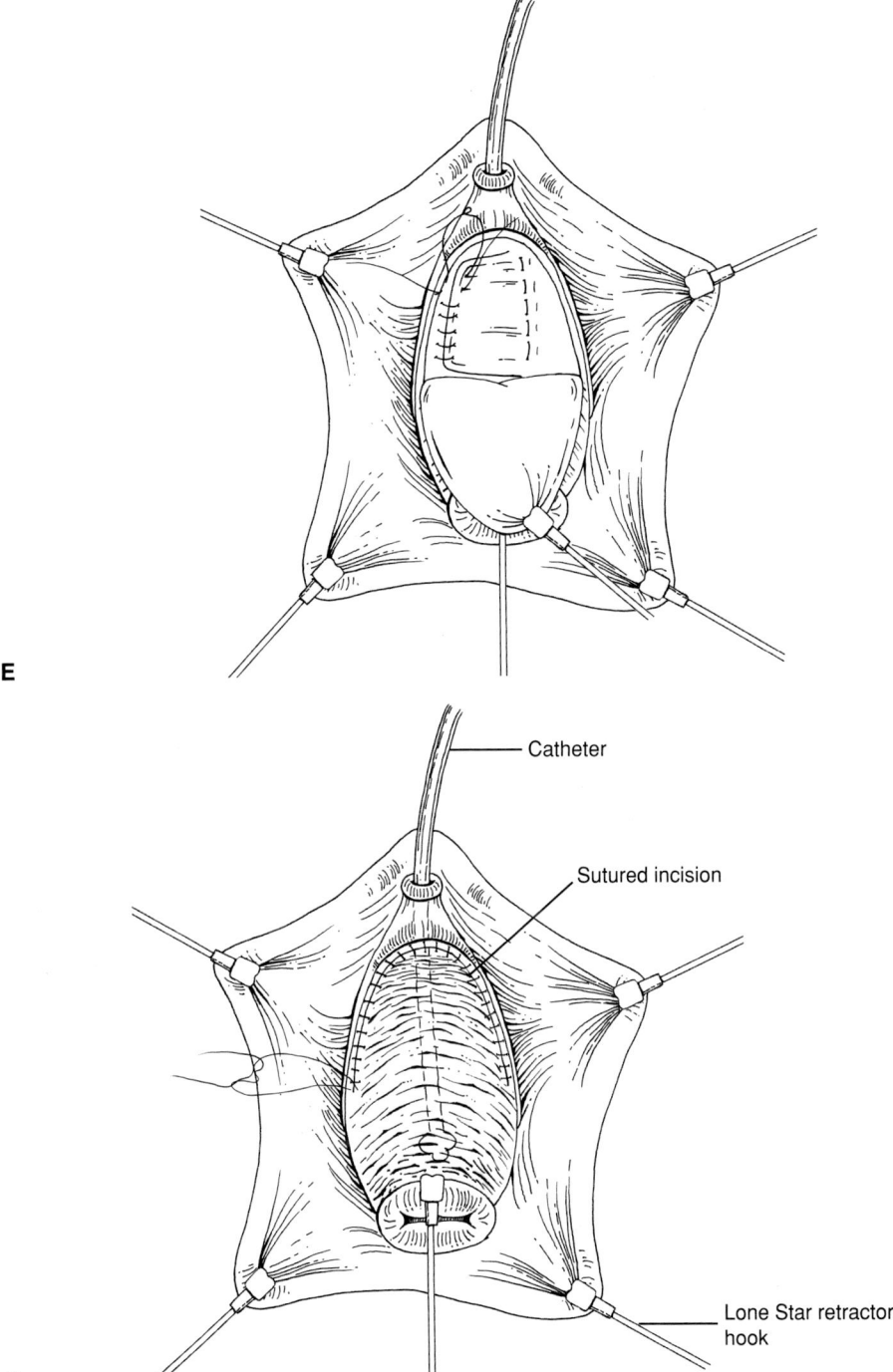

E

F

Catheter

Sutured incision

Lone Star retractor
hook

FIGURE 17.16 ● *(continued)* **(E)** The previous flaps of fibromuscularis are closed over the defect, over-lapping if possible. **(F)** The inverted-U incision is closed, being careful to close the dead space before a running unlocked closure of the vaginal epithelium.

conditions, and when extensive, potentially devascularizing dissection has been performed.

Anterior Diverticula

These occur infrequently and can be tricky to excise because of difficult access. There is no standard excision method, and various techniques have been described in the literature. Exposure of the lesion is key. Vakili described a lateral approach, dissecting along the paraurethral plane into the space of Retzius to expose and resect the diverticulum (67). Spencer described endoscopic drainage of an anterior diverticulum using a pediatric resectoscope (68). However, this procedure mainly involved making an incision to widen the neck of the diverticulum in order to improve its drainage and prevent reaccumulation of the contents. Rovner et al reviewed 41 cases of urethral diverticulum and reported on 9 patients with anterior and circumferential lesions confirmed on MRI (69). They described the technique of end-to-end urethroplasty and the use of the anterior bladder wall as a reconstruction flap.

Postoperative Care

Bladder drainage postoperatively is the normal practice. A suprapubic catheter avoids friction over the site of the urethroplasty. The authors prefer to leave a 12 French urethral Foley catheter in place for 1 to 2 weeks, followed by a voiding trial. The patient should be evaluated after a few weeks to ensure that healing is satisfactory. Cystourethroscopy or a voiding cystourethrogram is appropriate.

Complications

Successful treatment of urethral diverticula is highly dependent on meticulous surgical technique. Complications relate to multiple factors, including infection, smoking, and chronic medical conditions. Difficult dissection and tension on suture lines are additional factors. Recurrent diverticula, stress urinary incontinence, and urethrovaginal fistula are the common complications of diverticulectomy. Voiding dysfunction from strictures may also occur.

The recurrence rate is 3% to 4%, mostly as a result of incomplete excision of the diverticulum, failure to excise multiple lesions, and diverticulum formation from the remaining periurethral glands (26). Reoperation should be undertaken in such situations.

Stress urinary incontinence is estimated to complicate 5% of repairs (26). The exact incidence is unclear, as most series have variable follow-up. Extensive surgical dissection around the bladder neck can interfere with the continence mechanism

and produce stress incontinence. As discussed previously, this problem can be addressed with a urethral sling operation postoperatively once satisfactory healing has occurred. The sling material should most likely be an autologous graft.

Urethrovaginal fistulas may form in patients who experience breakdown of the urethral repair. The incidence is up to 5% (26). Very small fistulas can close spontaneously with continuous bladder drainage, while persistent or large lesions will need to be repaired surgically. A Martius bulbocavernosus graft is recommended.

Urethral stricture may develop postoperatively and cause symptoms such as poor urinary stream, voiding dysfunction, urinary tract infection, or worsening urinary retention. In such cases, careful urethral dilation should be performed.

Sexual dysfunction secondary to dyspareunia may be related to pain at the operative site or recurrence of the diverticulum and infection. The treatment of any underlying problems should be pursued diligently.

Conclusion

Surgeons involved in the treatment of female lower urinary tract complaints must have a high index of suspicion in order to promptly and accurately diagnose urethral diverticulum. The use of PPUG and MRI will increase the diagnostic accuracy. Excision is the standard treatment for proximal diverticula. Distal diverticula may be treated by marsupialization. Management should be individualized, especially in difficult or atypical cases. Proper preoperative evaluation and surgery should minimize complications.

REFERENCES

1. Elkins TE, Thompson JR. Lower urinary tract fistulas. In Walters MD, Karram MM, eds. *Urogynecology and reconstructive pelvic surgery*, 2nd ed. St. Louis: Mosby, 1999:355–366.
2. Mettauer JP. Vesicovaginal fistula. *Boston Med J* 1840;22:154–155.
3. Sims JM. On the treatment of vesicovaginal fistula. *Am J Med Sci* 1852;23:59–82.
4. Waaldijk K. The immediate surgical management of fresh obstetric fistulas with catheter and/or early closure. *Int J Gynecol Obstet* 1994;45:11–16.
5. Harrison KA. Child-bearing, health, and social priorities: A survey of 22,774 consecutive hospital births in Aaria, northern Nigeria. *Br J Obstet Gynaecol* 1985;92:Suppl 5:1–119.
6. Lee RA, Symmonds RE, Williams TJ. Current status of genitourinary fistula. *Obstet Gynecol* 1988;72:313–319.
7. Wall LL, Arrowsmith SD, Briggs ND, et al. The obstetrics vesicovaginal fistula in the developing world. *Obstet Gynecol Survey* 2005;60(7):S3–51.

8. Flores-Carreras O, Cabrera JR, Galeano PA, et al. Fistulas of the urinary tract in gynecologic and obstetric surgery. *Int Urogynecol J* 2001;12:203–214.

9. Meeks GR, Sams JO, Field W, et al. Formation of vesicovaginal fistula: the role of suture placement into the bladder during closure of the vaginal cuff after transabdominal hysterectomy. *Am J Obstet Gynecol* 1997;177(6):1298–1304.

10. Vakili B, Chesson RR, Kyle BL, et al. The incidence of urinary tract injury during hysterectomy: a prospective analysis based on universal cystoscopy. *Am J Obstet Gynecol* 2005;192(5):1599–1604.

11. Angioli R, Penalver M, Muzii L, et al. Guidelines of how to manage vesicovaginal fistula. *Crit Rev Oncol/Hematol* 2003;48:295–304.

12. Blaivas JG, Heritz DM, Romanzi LJ. Early versus late repair of vesicovaginal fistulas: vaginal and abdominal approaches. *J Urol* 1995;153:1110–1113.

13. Latzko W. Postoperative vesicovaginal fistulas: genesis and therapy. *Am J Surg* 1942;58:211–228.

14. Kanaoka Y, Hirai K, Ishiko O, et al. Vesicovaginal fistula treated with fibrin glue. *Int J Gynecol Obstet* 2001;173:147–149.

15. Sharma SK, Perry KT, Turk TMT. Endoscopic injection of fibrin glue for the treatment of urinary tract pathology. *J Endourol* 2005;19(3):419–423.

16. Stovsky MD, Ignatoff JM, Blum MD, et al. Use of electrocoagulation in the management of vesicovaginal fistulas. *J Urol* 1994;152:1443–1444.

17. Onolemhemhen DO, Ekwempu CC. An investigation of sociomedical risk factors associated with vaginal fistula in northern Nigeria. *Women & Health* 1999;28(3):103–116.

18. Muleta M. Sociodemographic profile and obstetric experience of fistula patients managed at the Addis Ababa Fistula Hospital. *Ethiop Med J* 2004;42:9–16.

19. Sanda G (Niamey, Niger). Personal communication.

20. Hamlin RHJ, Nicholson EC. Reconstruction of urethra totally destroyed in labor. *Br Med J* 1969;1:147–150.

21. Elkins TE. Surgery for the obstetric vesicovaginal fistula: a review of 100 operations in 82 patients. *Am J Obstet Gynecol* 1994;170(4):1108–1120.

22. Waaldijk K. Surgical classification of obstetric fistulas. *Int J Gynaecol Obstet* 1995;49(2):161–163.

23. Waaldijk K. The immediate management of fresh obstetric fistulas. *Am J Obstet Gynecol* 2004;191(3):795–799.

24. Elkins TE, Drescher C, Martey JO, et al. Vesicovaginal fistula revisited. *Obstet Gynecol* 1988;72(3 Pt 1):307–312.

25. Waaldijk K, Elkins TE. The obstetric fistula and peroneal nerve injury: an analysis of 947 consecutive patients. *Int Urogynecol J* 1994;a5:12–14.

26. El-Lamie IK. Preliminary experience with Mainz type II pouch in gynecologic oncology patients. *Eur J Gynaecol Oncol* 2001;22(1):77–80.

27. Farnham SB, Cookson MS. Surgical complications of urinary diversion. *World J Urol* 2004;22:157–167.

28. Mills RD, Styderm UE. Metabolic consequences of continent urinary diversion. *J Urol* 1999;161:1057–1066.

29. Everett HS, Mattingly RF. Urinary tract injuries resulting from pelvic surgery. *Am J Obstet Gynecol* 1978;71:502–505.

30. Macasaet MA, Lu R, Nwlaon JH. Ureterovaginal fistula as a complication of radical pelvic surgery. *Am J Obstet Gynecol* 1976;124:757–760.

31. Elabd S, Ghoniem G, Elsharaby M, et al. Use of endoscopy in the management of postoperative ureterovaginal fistulas *Int Urgynecol J* 1997;8:185–190.

32. Youssef AF. Menouria following lower segment caesarean section. *Am J Obstet Gynecol* 1957;73:759–767.

33. Tancer ML. Vesicouterine fistula: a review. *Obstet Gynecol Survey* 1986;41(12):743–753.

34. Shobeiri SA, Chesson RR, Echols KT. Cystoscopic fistulography: a review. *Urol Rev J* 2003;1:20–21.

35. Webster GD, Sihelnik SA, Stone AR. Urethrovaginal fistula: a review of the surgical management. *J Urol* 1984;132:460–462.

36. Saclarides TJ. Rectovaginal fistula. *Surg Clin North Am* 2002;82:1261–1272.

37. Pollard SG, Macfarlane R, Greatorex R, et al. Colovesical fistula. *Ann Roy Coll Surg Engl* 1987;69:163–165.

38. Moss RL, Ryan JA. Management of enterovesical fistulas. *Am J Surg* 1990;159:514–517.

39. Pontari MA, McMillen MA, Garvey RH, et al. Diagnosis and treatment of enterovesical fistulae. *Am Surgeon* 1992;58:258–263.

40. Hey W. *Practical observations in surgery.* Philadelphia: James Humphreys Publishers, 1805:303.

41. Leach GE, Schmidbauer CP, Hadley HR, et al. Surgical treatment of female urethral diverticulum. *Sem Urol* 1986;4:33–38.

42. Davis BL, Robinson DG. Diverticula of female urethra: assay of 120 cases. *Sem Urol* 1970;104:850.

43. Dmochowski R. Surgery for vesicovaginal fistula, urethrovaginal fistula, and urethral diverticulum. In Walsh PC, Retik AB, Vaughan ED, et al, eds. *Campbell's urology,* 8th ed. Philadelphia: WB Sanders, 2002:1195–1217.

44. Davis HJ, Telinde RW. Urethral diverticula: an assay of 121 cases. *J Urol* 1958;80:34–39.

45. Huffman JW. The detailed anatomy of the paraurethral ducts in the adult human female. *Am J Obstet Gynecol* 1948;55:86–101.

46. Routh A. Obstetrical Society of London. Report of Annual Meeting. *Br Med J* 1890;1:361.

47. Peters WA, Vaughan ED. Urethral diverticulum in the female: etiologic factors and postoperative results. *Obstet Gynecol* 1976;47:549–552.

48. Glassman TA, Weinerth JL, Glen JF. Neonatal female urethral diverticulum. *Urology* 1975;5:249.

49. Ganabathi K, Leach GE, Zimmern PE, et al. Experience with the management of urethral diverticulum in 63 women. *J Urol* 1994;152:1445.

50. Palagiri A. Urethral diverticulum with endometriosis. *Urology* 1978;11(3):271–274.

51. Lee RA. Diverticulum of the female urethra: postoperative complications and results. *Obstet Gynecol* 1983;61(1):52–58.

52. Jacoby K, Rowbotham RK. Double-balloon positive pressure urethrography is a more sensitive test than voiding cystourethrography for diagnosing urethral diverticulum in women. *J Urol* 1999;162:2066–2069.

53. Romanzi LJ, Groutz A, Blaivas JG. Urethral diverticulum in women: diverse presentations resulting in diagnostic delay and mismanagement. *J Urol* 2000;164:428–433.

54. Davis HJ, Cian LG. Positive pressure urethrography: a new diagnostic method. *J Urol* 1956;75:753–757.

55. Wang AC, Wang CR. Radiologic diagnosis and surgical treatment of urethral diverticulum in women. A reappraisal of voiding cystourethrography and positive

pressure urethrography. *J Reprod Med* 2000;45:
377–382.

56. Blander DS, Rovner ES, Schnall MD, et al.
    Endoluminal magnetic resonance imaging in the evaluation of urethral diverticula in women. *Urology*
    2001;57(4):660–665.

57. Bhatia NN, McCarthy TA, Ostergard DR. Urethral
    pressure profiles of women with urethral diverticula.
    Obstet Gynecol 1981;58(3):375–378.

58. Summitt RL, Stovall TG. Urethral diverticula: evaluation by urethral pressure profilometry, cystourethroscopy, and the voiding cystourethrogram.
    Obstet Gynecol 1992;80(4):695–699.

59. Fontana D, Porpiglia F, Morra I, et al. Transvaginal
    ultrasonography in the assessment of organic diseases
    of female urethra. *J Ultrasound Med* 1999;18:
    237–241.

60. Vargas-Serranok B, Cortina-Moreno B, Rodriquez-
    Romero R, et al. Transrectal ultrasonography in the diagnosis of urethral diverticula in women. *J Clin
    Ultrasound* 1997;25:21–28.

61. Lee TG, Keller FS. Urethral diverticulum: diagnosis by
    ultrasound. *AJR Am J Roentgenol* 1977;128:690–691.

62. Spence HM, Duckett JW. Diverticulum of the female
    urethra: clinical aspects and presentation of a simple

operative technique for cure. *J Urol* 1970;104:
432–437.

63. Roehrborn CG. Long-term follow-up study of the marsupialization technique for urethral diverticula in
    women. *Surg Gynecol Obstet* 1988;167:191–196.

64. Bennett SJ. Review: urethral diverticula. *Eur J Obstet
    Gynaecol Reprod Biol* 2000;89:135–139.

65. Busch FM, Carter FH. Vaginal flap incision for urethral
    diverticulectomy. *J Urol* 1974;111:773–774.

66. Swierzewski SJ, McGuire EJ. Pubovaginal sling for
    treatment of female stress urinary incontinence complicated by urethral diverticulum. *J Urol* 1993;149:
    1012–1014.

67. Vakili B, Wai C, Nihira M. Anterior urethral diverticulum in the female: diagnosis and surgical approach.
    Obstet Gynecol 2003;102:1179–1183.

68. Spencer WF, Streem SB. Diverticulum of the female
    urethral roof managed endoscopically. *J Urol*
    1987;138:147–148.

69. Rovner ES, Wein AJ. Diagnosis and reconstruction of
    the dorsal or circumferential urethral diverticulum. *J
    Urol* 2003;170:82–86.

70. Fortunato P, Schettini M, Gallucci M. Diagnosis and
    therapy of the female urethral diverticula. *Int
    Urogynecol J* 2001;12:51–57.

CHAPTER 18

Voiding Dysfunction

Jennifer Miles-Thomas and E. James Wright

Normal voiding function relies on complex interactions between the autonomic and somatic nervous systems. Precise coordination allows the lower urinary tract to accomplish the principal tasks of storage and emptying under both volitional and unconscious control. The continuum from normal to abnormal voiding function follows a paradigm that is generally simple to reconcile if reduced to disorders of function (storage and emptying) and disorders of anatomy (the bladder, the bladder outlet/urethra). This chapter will discuss normal voiding and voiding dysfunction, paying attention to relevant aspects of neurophysiology. It will also provide a practical approach to clinical diagnosis and therapy considerations for lower urinary tract disorders.

NORMAL URINARY ANATOMY (1)

Bladder

The urinary bladder is a multifunctional organ. Principal functions include stretch in response to filling without increasing intravesical pressure, urine storage at low pressure, protection of the underlying smooth muscle and nerves from urine, and coordinated expulsion of urine.

The smooth muscle of the urinary bladder allows tension to be developed over a large range of muscle lengths (2). The contractile response is slower and longer than that of cardiac or skeletal muscle, and detrusor muscle uses less energy to maintain tension over longer periods of time. Poor electrical coupling of the bladder smooth muscle is thought to help prevent synchronous activity of the smooth muscle as a whole during the filling phase (3). Bladder contraction during voiding is mediated by parasympathetic stimulation (4).

Collagen types I, III, and IV are most commonly found in the urinary bladder. Collagen, elastin, and proteoglycans located in the stroma account for the mechanical properties of the vesicoelastic bladder wall (5). The urothelium of the bladder is made up of multiple layers. Umbrella cells form the epithelial lining and are covered by a glycosaminoglycans layer. The glycosaminoglycans may inhibit bacterial adherence and prevent large molecule damage to the underlying urothelial layers (6). An intermediate layer and a basal cell layer complete the urothelium (7). Urothelial cells express nicotinic, muscarinic, tachykinin, adrenergic, and capsaicin receptors. They also can release ATP and nitric oxide and have mechanosensitivity and sensitivity to transmitters released from local afferent and efferent nerves. These properties allow the urothelium to respond to the changing environment and communicate with other cells and nerves in the bladder (8–11).

Urethra and Internal Sphincter

The urethra is composed of both striated and smooth muscle. Striated muscle bundles in the walls of the urethra form the rhabdosphincter separate from the pelvic floor musculature. Smooth muscle bundles of the urethra form the thick inner longitudinal and outer circular layer of the urethra, helping to stabilize and occlude the lumen. In females, this extends to the proximal portion. The stroma of the urethra is composed of collagen and elastin. The mucosal lining also provides coaptation to assist in urinary storage (12). The bladder neck (internal urinary sphincter) is a smooth muscle sphincter with α-adrenergic and a few β-adrenergic receptor sites. The bladder neck is thought to be partially controlled by the sympathetic stimulation of the α-receptors.

External Sphincter

In females, the urethra is reinforced by the pelvic floor musculature and connective tissue. Continence is maintained by active contraction and the anatomic compression of the urethra against the posterior pelvic floor. The external sphincter is composed of both slow and fast twitch fibers. In the female urethra, 87% are slow twitch fibers while 13% are fast twitch (6).

NEUROPHYSIOLOGY

Normal voiding is a complex, tightly orchestrated neuromuscular cascade of events coordinating low-pressure storage of urine in the bladder and efficient emptying of stored urine. Understanding the relationship between the central and peripheral nervous systems and the bladder, urethra, and pelvic floor is important for describing both normal and abnormal function of the lower urinary tract.

Central Nervous System Effects

Micturition is the result of supraspinal neurologic pathways that either inhibit or facilitate segmental reflex arcs (13–15). Each anatomic component of the central nervous system plays a role in voiding function. During sustained voluntary pelvic floor straining, the anterior frontal gyrus has been shown on positron emission tomography (PET) studies to be activated (16), supporting the postulate that the frontal lobe is involved in both voluntary micturition and inhibition of the micturition reflex. The pontine mesencephalic reticular formation, also known as Barrington's center, is located in the anterior pons. Two separate areas in the pons play a role in coordinating urine storage and emptying. The M region in the pontine micturition center is also known as Barrington's nucleus. Located in the dorsal pontine tegmentum, it projects to the bladder motor neurons in the sacral parasympathetic nucleus and sphincteric interneurons. Stimulation causes bladder contraction and external sphincter relaxation. Damage to this area leads to urinary retention. The L region is known as the

pontine storage center. It projects to Onuf's nucleus, where motor neurons control the external sphincter. Stimulation of this area causes contraction of the urinary rhabdosphincter and increases urethral resistance (17).

The cerebellum coordinates the force of detrusor contraction and pelvic floor activity. In addition, cerebellar impulses interact with the brain stem reflex centers, including Barrington's nucleus, to coordinate voiding (14,18). The cerebellum plays an inhibitory role during bladder filling and with Barrington's nucleus is involved in rapidly increasing and maintaining bladder pressure during voiding (19,20).

In concert with these central components, sensory afferents travel from the bladder to the brain stem through the spinothalamic tract, providing feedback on bladder filling and voiding cues. In this way, information from the frontal lobes to the pons coordinated in the basal ganglia and cerebellum directs the volitional control of micturition, while pathways from the brain stem to the sacral micturition center coordinate detrusor and sphincter reflexes to allow for bladder evacuation (19,21). While this complex interplay within the central nervous system provides an efficient storage and emptying cycle, it poses multiple sites for injury and subsequent dysfunction.

Autonomic Nervous System Effects

The lower urinary tract has parasympathetic, sympathetic, and somatic innervation. The pelvic nerve supplies the bladder and urethra with efferent parasympathetic input while the hypogastric nerves supply sympathetic components. Both the pelvic and hypogastric nerves return sensory afferent information to the spinal cord. The primary influence of the sympathetic innervation is control of the storage phase of the micturition, while the parasympathetic innervation controls the voiding phase (22–24).

Parasympathetics

Parasympathetic efferents originate in the gray matter of S2–S4 in the lateral aspect of the sacral intermediate matter and exist with preganglionic fibers as the pelvic nerve (6). The pelvic nerve joins the ipsilateral hypogastric nerve to form the pelvic plexus innervating the bladder and urethra. Afferent autonomic nerves travel to the dorsal column of the spinal cord through the pelvic nerve (22–24). The preganglionic neurotransmitter is acetylcholine, which affects nicotinic cholinergic receptors. The primary postganglionic neurotransmitter is also acetylcholine, activating muscarinic receptors. These M2 and M3 receptors are distributed throughout the body, with increased expression in the bladder. They are rare in the bladder neck and urethra. M3 receptors primarily mediate bladder contraction.

Sympathetics

The sympathetic nervous system, is important in bladder filling and storage. Sympathetic nerves (T11–L2) travel in the intermediolateral nuclei of the thoracolumbar spinal cord and in the hypogastric nerve (25–29). Stimulation of B2 receptors in the bladder body promotes relaxation, while stimulation of α-1 receptors in the bladder neck and urethra increases bladder outlet resistance and has inhibitory effects on parasympathetic transmission. Alpha-1 receptors are postsynaptic receptors that stimulate vasoconstriction and smooth muscle contraction. Alpha-2 receptors are presynaptic receptors that inhibit the release of norepinephrine through negative feedback. Beta-adrenergic receptors found in the body of the bladder modulate smooth muscle relaxation. Despite this interaction, β-agonist agents have not been found useful for modulating detrusor overactivity (30).

Afferent Pathways to the Bladder

Afferents from the pelvic nerve consist of (A-delta) myelinated axons and (C-fiber) unmyelinated axons. These fibers monitor the amplitude of bladder contraction and bladder volume. C-fibers are located in the mucosa and mucosa muscularis and are nocioreceptive, responding to stretch and overdistention. Recruitment of C-fibers during inflammation or during neuropathic changes may cause bladder pain or urge incontinence (6). A-delta fibers located in the smooth muscle sense bladder fullness and wall tension.

Neurotransmitters

There are multiple nonadrenergic, noncholinergic neurotransmitters (NANC) present in the central and peripheral nervous systems that affect bladder function. These transmitters, along with various receptor families, offer unique targets for understanding and manipulating lower urinary tract function. Opioids, serotonin, GABA, and dopamine represent a few of these transmitters. Serotonin inhibits the voiding reflex and has some role in increasing urethral tone. ATP acts on purine receptors P2X and P2Y to influence mechanosensory signaling (6,17).

Adenosine (the breakdown product of ATP) has receptors that can modulate afferent and efferent responses. Capsaicin is a vanilloid that stimulates and desensitizes unmyelinated C-fibers to produce pain and additional neuropeptides. Tachykinins (i.e., substance P, neurokinin A, neurokinin B) are released in response to capsaicin and mediate increased excitability of the bladder and bladder contractions and induce vasodilatation. Nitric oxide is a major inhibitory transmitter causing relaxation of urethral smooth muscle during voiding. In addition, it is also released from urothelium during bladder filling and may suppress afferent nerve activity (6,17). Research is ongoing to determine which of these transmitters and receptors can be used to influence lower urinary tract function and dysfunction.

VOIDING DYSFUNCTION

Many classifications exist for defining and stratifying voiding dysfunction. Some address specific neurologic insults while others focus on urodynamic features. Each of these has strengths and limitations. A clinically useful paradigm focuses primarily on defining abnormalities with reference to urine storage and emptying (31). From a functional and anatomic standpoint, the bladder and bladder outlet (bladder neck and urethra) are the key components to normal voiding, and clinical diagnosis and treatment planning can be aided by identifying dysfunction in these elements. A two-by-two matrix can be useful for orienting clinical, urodynamic, and neurologic information, as shown in Tables 18.1 and 18.2.

The following discussion touches on specific causes of voiding dysfunction, many of which are specifically addressed elsewhere in this textbook. The list is not meant to be exhaustive, but serves instead to guide further thought and inquiry into the diagnosis and treatment of voiding dysfunction.

DISORDERS OF URINE STORAGE

Stress Incontinence

Stress urinary incontinence is defined by the International Continence Society as the involuntary leakage of urine with effort or exertion or on sneezing or coughing (32). During urodynamic evaluation, leakage is seen with abdominal contraction in the absence of detrusor contraction. Stress incontinence accounts for approximately 50% of cases of incontinence and is due to urethral dysfunction characterized by urethrovesical hypermobility or intrinsic sphincter deficiency (ISD).

TABLE 18.1

Disorders of Storage

	Bladder Abnormal	Bladder Normal
Outlet abnormal	Radical pelvic surgery Multiple sclerosis Parkinson's disease Shy-Drager	Stress incontinence Intrinsic sphincter deficiency Urethral hypermobility Urethral diverticulum
Outlet normal	Detrusor hyperactivity —Supraspinal neurologic disease —Idiopathic —Decreased compliance —Sensory urgency —Inflammation —Infection —Fistula —Psychological	Ectopic ureter

Urethral hypermobility is due to loss of periurethral support to the pelvic floor musculature. Loss of the native tissue structure allows for mobility, with increases in abdominal pressure preventing adequate anatomic coaptation (33–35). With increasing abdominal pressure, the bladder neck and proximal urethra can be pulled open, allowing for incontinence. ISD is present in the setting of stress incontinence where urethral support is adequate. Poor coaptation of an intrinsic mucosal and muscular seal is thought to allow leakage of urine during increased intra-abdominal pressure.

Both hypermobility and ISD can coexist, and many support that ISD must be present with any degree of stress incontinence. This follows the observation that many women with varying degrees of urethral hypermobility have normal urinary control.

TABLE 18.2

Disorders of Emptying

	Bladder Abnormal	Bladder Normal
Outlet abnormal		Anatomic obstruction Stricture Neoplasm Functional obstruction Hinman's syndrome Fowler's syndrome
Outlet normal	Spinal cord injury Multiple sclerosis Parkinson's disease Myogenic Psychogenic Infectious Idiopathic	

Urodynamic testing with assessment of Valsalva leak point pressure as well as urethral pressure profilometry can provide information on outlet competence. These studies, however, have not been definitively shown to stratify diagnosis or treatment selection in the setting of stress incontinence.

Overactive Bladder/Urge Incontinence

Overactive bladder is defined by the International Continence Society as "the complaint of a sudden compelling desire to pass urine that is difficult to defer" (32). This sensation of urgency is distinguishable from the normal perception of bladder filling. The symptom of urgency is thought to be controlled by the central nervous system as brain activity in the pons and frontal lobes (36). In addition, detrusor overactivity with severe contractions has been found to correlate with the level of urgency (37). Overactive bladder syndrome with incontinence is currently categorized as idiopathic but may have both myogenic and neurogenic causes. Denervation of the detrusor can promote infiltration of connective tissue, stiffening the bladder wall, which in turn leads to muscle hypertrophy and incomplete emptying (38). In addition, ischemia can lead to neuronal injury, changing nerve stimulus response thresholds in the detrusor and causing overactivity (39). This may be a consequence of pregnancy, labor, and other types of pelvic floor injury.

Management of the overactive bladder is multimodal, including among other therapies dietary modification, pelvic floor exercises, and pharmacological treatment with anticholinergic agents (40). These strategies are discussed in detail elsewhere in the text.

Cerebrovascular Accident

After a cerebrovascular accident or other brain injury, voiding dysfunction frequently occurs. Urinary incontinence can be seen in nearly half of patients in the acute phase after a cerebrovascular accident. Urinary retention affects as many as 47% (41). The most common long-term consequence is detrusor hyperreflexia (6). Due to damage to the cerebral cortex and the internal capsule, patients may lose volitional control but maintain sphincteric control. This is primarily a problem of storage, as the voiding mechanism is otherwise normal. True detrusor-sphincter dyssynergia does not occur, as these lesions are above the pons. "Pseudodyssynergia" may be seen as patients try to contract the external sphincter in response to involuntary detrusor contractions (17).

Fistula

Vesicovaginal fistulas most commonly present with continuous urinary drainage from the vagina. In developing countries, they are typically a consequence of complicated vaginal delivery. Where access to adequate obstetrical care is routine, vesicovaginal fistulas are seen after hysterectomy with an incidence of 0.1% to 0.2%. Other sources include pelvic radiation for malignancy. In evaluating vesicovaginal fistulas, it is important to exclude possible ureteral injury with an appropriate imaging study (retrograde pyelogram, computed tomography scan, intravenous pyelography) and cystoscopy.

Urethral Diverticulum

Urethral diverticula are most commonly seen in patients with dysuria, postvoid dribbling, and dyspareunia. It is found in 1% to 5% of the general population and up to a third of patients have a history of recurrent urinary tract infections (42). Patients may have a tender anterior vaginal wall mass on examination. Cystoscopy, urethrography, and pelvic magnetic resonance imaging are helpful for diagnosis and treatment planning. Transvaginal repair includes excision of the diverticulum and tension-free reconstruction of the floor of the urethra. Postoperative stress incontinence can occur, and simultaneous or subsequent pubovaginal sling may be required.

MIXED DISORDERS

Mixed disorders are conditions that may manifest both emptying and storage abnormalities. These most commonly involve neuropathic conditions of traumatic, infectious, inflammatory, or degenerative origin. Two manifestations of this class of disorders require specific explanation. These are detrusor sphincter dyssynergia and autonomic dysreflexia.

Detrusor sphincter dyssynergia is a neuropathic discoordination between normal bladder contraction and urethral sphincter relaxation. This causes functional obstruction, significant elevation of intravesical pressure, and poor emptying. The most significant effect of this condition is possible upper tract injury when intravesical pressures exceed 40 cm H_2O (43). Progression can worsen detrusor hyperreflexia and impair adequate storage. Detrusor sphincter dyssynergia can affect both the internal smooth muscle bladder neck closure mechanism as well as the external striated sphincter. Urodynamic testing with video and electromyography (EMG) monitoring can aid in defining these lesions.

Autonomic dysreflexia is an exaggerated sympathetic response to afferent stimuli at or below a T6 spinal cord lesion. It occurs as a result of sympathetic dysregulation of the viable distal spinal cord. Spinal cord lesions above T6 may trigger sympathetic autonomic outflow from either autonomic or somatic stimulation. Patients typically have bradycardia, headache as a consequence of severe hypertension, and sweating. These symptoms can be triggered by lower urinary tract manipulation such as catheter insertion, overdistention of the bladder, or lower extremity muscle spasm. Treatment begins with immediate removal of the offending factor and pharmacologic control of acute hypertension.

Multiple Sclerosis

Multiple sclerosis is an autoimmune, focal axon-sparing demyelinating disease frequently diagnosed between ages 20 and 50, with a female-to-male predominance of 3:2. Nearly 80% of patients diagnosed with multiple sclerosis have lower urinary tract dysfunction, and 2% to 15% of patients report voiding symptoms at the time of presentation (44). The spectrum of voiding dysfunction includes disorders of both storage and emptying, and both the bladder and outlet can be involved. Consequently, diagnosis of multiple sclerosis–related voiding dysfunction can be challenging. Detrusor hyperreflexia is the predominant voiding pattern, manifesting a spectrum of frequency, urgency, and urge incontinence. Areflexia or hypocontractility can also develop. Detrusor sphincter dyssynergia is seen in up to 60% of multiple sclerosis patients. Magnetic resonance findings do not always correlate with voiding patterns (44–46). Urodynamic testing should be included in the workup and treatment planning of these disorders, and bladder management may be coordinated with other care providers, including urology, neurology, physiatry, and physical therapy. Satisfactory therapy may incorporate behavioral modification, pharmacologic agents, neural stimulation techniques, reconstructive pelvic surgery, and clean intermittent catheterization when necessary.

Spina Bifida Occulta

Spina bifida occulta is a spinal dysraphism with lack of the spinal vertebral arch covering the cord in the lumbosacral region (47). The diagnosis is suggested by physical examination (i.e., sacral hair pattern, sacral dimple, or dermal sinus). Adults may have detrusor hyperreflexia, detrusor areflexia, or a normal examination.

Spinal Cord Injury (17)

Spinal cord injury can be seen as a consequence of trauma and occasionally infection and inflammation (i.e., transverse myelitis, meningitis). The level of the lesion typically gives insight into the type of voiding dysfunction encountered, but wide variability is seen according to injury severity and completeness. As a result, neither the pattern nor the natural history of voiding dysfunction following spinal cord injury can be reliably predicted. Following an acute spinal injury there is an initial period of spinal shock. During this phase of injury and recovery, suppression of autonomic and somatic activity below the level of the lesion leads to urinary retention. This typically continues for up to 6 to 12 weeks after injury.

In presacral spinal cord injuries, patients commonly develop bladder instability (48). After spinal shock resolves, bladder afferents can develop hypersensitivity as the spinal cord attempts repair, leading to bladder instability (49). In suprasacral injury above T7, patients most often experience detrusor hyperreflexia, striated external sphincter dyssynergia, and smooth (internal) sphincter dyssynergia. Detrusor sphincter dyssynergia is most commonly seen in lesions between the pons and the sacral cord. Patients typically lack bladder sensation and are at risk for autonomic dysreflexia. In suprasacral injury below T7, patients experience detrusor overactivity, smooth sphincter synergy, striated sphincter dyssynergia, and absent bladder sensation. In sacral cord injury, the detrusor is areflexic, with normal or high compliance. There is fixed sphincter tone, and urinary incontinence, when seen, is secondary to overflow.

Parkinson's Disease

Parkinson's disease is a neurodegenerative disorder that affects the dopaminergic neurons in the substantia nigra, affecting movement. Symptoms typically include a resting tremor, rigidity, and bradykinesia (50). Urinary symptoms include detrusor overactivity manifesting as urgency, frequency, and nocturia. Patients also may have sphincter bradykinesia with detrusor overactivity, giving a picture of pseudodyssynergia. The smooth internal sphincter is synergic (17). The severity of Parkinson's disease may not correlate with urodynamic findings.

Shy-Drager Syndrome

Also known as multiple system atrophy, this syndrome is characterized by neuronal cell loss and atrophy in the brain, spinal cord, and autonomic ganglia. Patients may present with orthostatic hypotension, anhidrosis, and variable degrees of cerebellar and parkinsonian symptoms (17). The most common urodynamic finding is urinary urgency and frequency. Videourodynamics will reveal the classic finding of an open bladder neck seen with striated sphincter denervation.

Pelvic Surgery (Radical Hysterectomy, Abdominoperineal Resection)

Injury to the hypogastric nerves can occur during dissection of the presacral and periaortic lymph nodes or resection of the rectouterine, uterosacral, cardinal, and vesicovaginal ligaments. The extent of vaginal resection has a direct bearing on bladder dysfunction postoperatively (51–54). A degree of spontaneous recovery is usually seen postoperatively within the first 6 months, while long-term dysfunction is seen in up to 30% (55). Initially, the bladder may be hypertonic with decreased functional capacity postoperatively and over time it may become hypotonic, with poor contractility (56). Sensory function may also be affected due to parasympathetic disruption (57). During resection of the upper portion of the vagina, the structural support of the bladder and bladder neck may be compromised, leading to stress incontinence (58–60).

Colon Resection

Up to 70% of patients after abdominoperineal resection suffer voiding dysfunction. The primary cause is damage to pelvic autonomic nerves (61). The degree of pelvic dissection is once again directly related to the extent of postoperative bladder dysfunction (62). Disruption of the pelvic nerves leads to detrusor areflexia and urinary retention (61). Additional damage to the pudendal nerve can cause urinary incontinence due to sphincteric weakness (63–66). Injury to sympathetic input leads to poor accommodation and decreased bladder compliance. This collection of injuries can create a bladder with poor storage, a weak outlet, and absent contractility. In about 15% to 20% of patients, the resulting dysfunction is permanent (17).

DISORDERS OF EMPTYING

Postoperative Urinary Retention

The underlying cause of postoperative urinary retention is decreased detrusor contractility and increased bladder outlet resistance (67,68). General anesthetics can have a depressant effect on the bladder, while spinal anesthesia rapidly blocks the voiding reflex. Sympathetic stimulation associated with postoperative pain, anxiety, or overdistention of the bladder may stimulate α-1 receptors and increase outlet resistance (68).

Emotional factors may also contribute to retention. As mentioned earlier, neurons in the pontine storage center can be activated by external stimuli. These neurons project to the motor neurons in Onuf's nucleus and require inhibition in order to void (16,69,70).

Pseudomyotonia (Fowler's Syndrome)

Fowler's syndrome is caused by incomplete relaxation of the external urethral sphincter during voiding. EMG studies reveal complex repetitive discharges, which are thought to be direct muscle-to-muscle transmission of excitatory impulses rather than from neuronal pathways (71). Seen more commonly in young women, there is also an association with polycystic ovary syndrome.

THERAPY FOR SELECT CAUSES OF VOIDING DYSFUNCTION

Therapy for voiding dysfunction is based on the premise that the dysfunction symptoms are due to either a failure to store urine or a failure to empty. When considering treatment options for patients, the goal should be to improve storage or facilitate emptying. Therapy to increase storage is directed toward inhibiting bladder contractility, decreasing sensory input from the bladder to the spinal cord, mechanically increasing bladder capacity, or increasing bladder outlet resistance. Therapy to increase emptying should be directed toward increasing intravesical pressure, decreasing outlet resistance, or facilitating the micturition reflex. Tables 18.3 and 18.4 outline some of the options to restore a balanced voiding pattern based on abnormalities of bladder and outlet function.

SUMMARY

Normal voiding requires a series of well-orchestrated neuromuscular events. There must be intact neural circuitry from the brain to the bladder and a constantly changing balance between neuromuscular inhibition and facilitation. Dysfunction in this system can occur at all levels, including cellular epithelial changes in the bladder, anatomic loss of support, and neural miscommunication from the cerebral cortex to the cauda equina.

TABLE 18.3

Therapies to Increase Bladder Storage of Urine (6)

Bladder	Behavioral therapies
	Timed voiding
	Pelvic floor muscle strengthening
	Pharmacology
	Antimuscarinic agents
	Tricyclics
	Neuromodulation
	Sacral nerve stimulation
	Botulinum toxin
	Neurectomy
	Bladder augmentation
Outlet	Behavior therapies
	Pharmacology
	Sympathomimetics
	Vaginal or perineal support devices
	Surgical repair of sphincter
	Urethral bulking
	Suburethral slings
	Colposuspension
	Artificial urinary sphincter

TABLE 18.4

Therapies to Increase Bladder Emptying

Bladder	Bladder pharmacology
	Reduction cystoplasty
	Neuromodulation
	Valsalva and Credé maneuvers
	Intermittent catheterization
Outlet	Pharmacology
	Alpha blockers
	Behavioral therapies
	Intermittent catheterization

When problems arise, correlation between clinical symptoms and a practical understanding of the structure and function of urine storage and emptying can guide diagnosis and therapy.

REFERENCES

1. Awad SA, Downie JW, Lywood DW, et al. Sympathetic activity in the proximal urethra in patients with urinary obstruction. *J Urol* 1976;115:545–547.
2. Uvelius B, Gabella G. Relation between cell length and force production in urinary bladder smooth muscle. *Acta Physiol Scand* 1980;110:357–365.
3. Brading AF, Mostwin JL. Electrical and mechanical responses of guinea-pig bladder muscle to nerve stimulation. *Br J Pharmacol* 1989;98:1083–1090.
4. Andersson K. Pharmacology of lower urinary tract smooth muscles and penile erectile tissues. *Pharmacol Rev* 1993;45.
5. Cortivo R, Pagano F, Passerini G, et al. Elastin and collagen in the normal and obstructed urinary bladder. *Br J Urol* 1981;53:134–137.
6. Chancellor M. In: Walsh PC, Campbell MF, Retik AB, et al. *Campbell's urology*, 8th ed. Philadelphia: WB Saunders, 2002.
7. Kanai A, DeGroat W, Birder L, et al. Symposium report on urothelial dysfunction: pathophysiology and novel therapies. *J Urol* 2006;175:1624–1629.
8. Birder LA, Apodaca G, DeGroat WC, et al. Adrenergic- and capsaicin-evoked nitric oxide release from urothelium and afferent nerves in urinary bladder. *Am J Physiol* 1998;275:F226–229.
9. Birder LA, Kanai AJ, DeGroat WC, et al. Vanilloid receptor expression suggests a sensory role for urinary bladder epithelial cells. *Proc Natl Acad Sci USA* 2001;98:13396–13401.
10. Birder LA, Nealen ML, Kiss S, et al. B-adrenoceptor agonists stimulate endothelial nitric oxide synthase in rat urinary bladder urothelial cells. *J Neurosci* 2002;22:8063–8070.
11. Chopra B, Barrick SR, Meyers S, et al. Expression and function of bradykinin B1 and B2 receptors in normal and inflamed rat urinary bladder urothelium. *J Physiol* 2005;562:859–871.
12. Zinner NR, Sterling AM, Ritter RC. Role of inner urethral softness in urinary continence. *Urology* 1980;16:115–117.
13. De Groat W, Steers WD. Autonomic regulation of the urinary bladder and sexual organs. In: Lowey SK, ed. *Central regulation of the autonomic functions*, 1st ed. Oxford: Oxford University Press, 1990.
14. De Groat W. Nervous control of the urinary bladder in the cat. *Brain Res* 1975;87:201–211.
15. Bradley WE, Rockswold GL, Timm GW, et al. Neurology of micturition. *J Urol* 1976;115:481–486.
16. Blok BF, Willemsen AT, Holstege G. A PET study on brain control of micturition in humans. *Brain* 1997;120(Pt 1):111–121.
17. Boone T. *Physiology of micturition and pathophysiology of voiding dysfunction*. Presented at the AUA Annual Review Course, Dallas, TX, 2005.
18. Bradley W, Scott FB. Physiology of the urinary bladder. In: Harrison GR, Pearlmutter AD, eds. *Campbell's urology*, 4th ed. Philadelphia: WB Saunders, 1978:87–124.
19. Bradley WE, Timm GW, Scott FB. Cystometry. V. Bladder sensation. *Urology* 1975;6:654–658.
20. Sasaki M. Role of Barrington's nucleus in micturition. *J Comp Neurol* 2005;493:21–26.
21. Bradley WE, Timm GW, Scott FB. Innervation of the detrusor muscle and urethra. *Urol Clin North Am* 1974;1:3–27.
22. Keith L. Anatomy of the pelvis and perineum. In: *Clinically oriented anatomy*, 2nd ed. Baltimore: Williams & Wilkins, 1985:359–403.
23. Romanes G. Muscles and fascia. In: *Cunningham's textbook of anatomy*. Oxford: Oxford University Press, 1972:360–364.
24. Clemente C. *Gray's anatomy of the human body*, 30th American ed. Lea & Febiger, 1985.
25. Elbadawi A. Neuromorphological basis of vesicourethral function. Histochemistry, ultrastructure, and function of intrinsic nerves of the bladder and urethra. *Neurourol Urodyn* 1982;1.
26. Elbadawi A. Autonomic muscular innervation of the vesical outlet and its role in micturition. In: Hinman F, ed. *Benign prostatic hypertrophy*. Berlin: Springer-Verlag, 1983:330–348.
27. Elbadawi A. Ultrastructure of vesicourethral innervation. II. Postganglionic axoaxonal synapses in intrinsic innervation of the vesicourethral lissosphincter: a new structural and functional concept in micturition. *J Urol* 1984;131:781–790.
28. Elbadawi A. Ultrastructure of vesicourethral innervation. IV. Evidence for somatomotor plus autonomic innervation of the male feline rhabdosphincter. *Neurourol Urodyn* 1985;4:23–36.
29. Elbadawi A. Ultrastructure of vesicourethral innervation. III. Axoaxonal synapses between postganglionic cholinergic axons and probably SIF-cell derived processes in the feline lissosphincter. *J Urol* 1985;133:524–528.
30. Castleden CM, Morgan B. The effect of beta-adrenoceptor agonists on urinary incontinence in the elderly. *Br J Clin Pharmacol* 1980;10:619–20.
31. Wein A, Barrett DM. *Voiding function and dysfunction: a logical and practical approach*. Chicago: Year Book Medical, 1988.
32. Abrams P, Cardozo L, Fall M, et al. The standardization of terminology in lower urinary tract function: report from the Standardization Subcommittee of the International Continence Society. *Urology* 2003;61:37–49.
33. Constantinou CE, Govan DE. Spatial distribution and timing of transmitted and reflexly generated urethral pressures in healthy women. *J Urol* 1982;127:964–969.
34. DeLancey JO. Structural aspects of the extrinsic continence mechanism. *Obstet Gynecol* 1988;72:296–301.
35. Tanagho E. The ureterovesical junction: anatomy and physiology. In: Chrishold GD, Williams DI, eds. *Scientific foundation of urology*. Chicago: Year Book Medical, 1982:295–404.
36. Athwal BS, Berkley KJ, Hussain I, et al. Brain responses to changes in bladder volume and urge to void in healthy men. *Brain* 2001;124:369–377.
37. Cucchi A, Siracusano S, Guarnaschelli C, et al. Voiding urgency and detrusor contractility in women with overactive bladders. *Neurourol Urodyn* 2003;22:223–226.
38. Abrams P, Blaivas JG, Stanton SL, et al. The standardization of terminology of lower urinary tract function. The International Continence Society Committee on Standardization of Terminology. *Scand J Urol Nephrol Suppl* 1988;114:5–19.

39. Larsson G, Hallen B, Nilvebrant L. Tolterodine in the treatment of overactive bladder: analysis of the pooled phase II efficacy and safety data. *Urology* 1999;53: 990–998.

40. Chu FM, Dmochowski R. Pathophysiology of overactive bladder. *Am J Med* 2006;119:3–8.

41. Ersoz M, Tunc H, Akyuz M, et al. Bladder storage and emptying disorder frequencies in hemorrhagic and ischemic stroke patients with bladder dysfunction. *Cerebrovasc Dis* 2005;20:395–399.

42. Aldridge CW, Jr, Beaton JH, Nanzig RP. A review of office urethroscopy and cystometry. *Am J Obstet Gynecol* 1978;131:432–437.

43. Sullivan M, Yalla SV. Spinal cord injuries and other forms of myeloneuropathies. *Probl Urol* 1992;6:643.

44. Goldstein I, Siroky MB, Sax DS, et al. Neurourologic abnormalities in multiple sclerosis. *J Urol* 1982;128: 541–545.

45. Blaivas JG, Bhimani G, Labib KB. Vesicourethral dysfunction in multiple sclerosis. *J Urol* 1979;122:342.

46. Kim YH, Goodman C, Omessi E, et al. The correlation of urodynamic findings with cranial magnetic resonance imaging findings in multiple sclerosis. *J Urol* 1998;159:972–976.

47. Selzman AA, Elder JS, Mapstone TB. Urologic consequences of myelodysplasia and other congenital abnormalities of the spinal cord. *Urol Clin North Am* 1993;20:485–504.

48. Kaplan SA, Chancellor MB, Blaivas JG. Bladder and sphincter behavior in patients with spinal cord lesions. *J Urol* 1991;146:113–117.

49. de Groat WC, Araki I, Vizzard MA, et al. Developmental and injury–induced plasticity in the micturition reflex pathway. *Behav Brain Res* 1998;92: 127–140.

50. Wein A. Neuromuscular dysfunction of the lower urinary tract and its management. In: Walsh PC, Campbell MF, Retik AB, eds. *Campbell's urology*, 8th ed. Philadelphia: WB Saunders, 2002.

51. Jackson KS, Naik R. Pelvic floor dysfunction and radical hysterectomy. *Int J Gynecol Cancer* 2006;16:354–363.

52. Hockel M. Basic neuroanatomy and neurophysiology of the urethrovesical function with special reference to extended hysterectomy. *J Gynaecol Oncol* 2002;7:32.

53. Ralph G, Tamussino K, Lichtenegger W. Urological complications after radical abdominal hysterectomy for cervical cancer. *Baillieres Clin Obstet Gynaecol* 1988;2:943–952.

54. Zullo MA, Manci N, Angioli R, et al. Vesical dysfunctions after radical hysterectomy for cervical cancer: a critical review. *Crit Rev Oncol Hematol* 2003;48:287–293.

55. Naik R, Nwabinelli J, Mayne C, et al. Prevalence and management of (non-fistulous) urinary incontinence in women following radical hysterectomy for early stage cervical cancer. *Eur J Gynaecol Oncol* 2001;22:26–30.

56. Youseff A, ed. *Gynaecological urology*. Springfield, IL: Thomas, 1960:20–28.

57. Brading AF, Turner WH. The unstable bladder: towards a common mechanism. *Br J Urol* 1994;73:3–8.

58. Lin HH, Sheu BC, Lo MC, et al. Abnormal urodynamic findings after radical hysterectomy or pelvic irradiation for cervical cancer. *Int J Gynaecol Obstet* 1998;63:169–174.

59. Vervest HA, Kiewiet de Jonge M, Vervest TM, et al. Micturition symptoms and urinary incontinence after nonradical hysterectomy. *Acta Obstet Gynecol Scand* 1988;67:141–146.

60. Thomas TM, Plymat KR, Blannin J, et al. Prevalence of urinary incontinence. *Br Med J* 1980;281:1243–1245.

61. Hollabaugh RS Jr, Steiner MS, Sellers KD, et al. Neuroanatomy of the pelvis: implications for colonic and rectal resection. *Dis Colon Rectum* 2000;43:1390–1397.

62. Hojo K, Vernava AM 3rd, Sugihara K, et al. Preservation of urine voiding and sexual function after rectal cancer surgery. *Dis Colon Rectum* 1991;34:532–539.

63. Havenga K, Enker WE, McDermott K, et al. Male and female sexual and urinary function after total mesorectal excision with autonomic nerve preservation for carcinoma of the rectum. *J Am Coll Surg* 1996;182:495–502.

64. Bors E. Effect of electric stimulation of the pudendal nerves on the vesical neck; its significance for the function of cord bladders: a preliminary report. *J Urol* 1952;67:925–935.

65. Power R. An antomical contribution to the problem of continence and incontinence in the female. *Am J Obstet Gynecol* 1950;67:302–314.

66. Hutch JA, Rambo ON Jr. A new theory of the anatomy of the internal urinary sphincter and the physiology of micturition. 3. Anatomy of the urethra. *J Urol* 1967;97:696–704.

67. Tammela T. Postoperative urinary retention—why the patient cannot void. *Scand J Urol Nephrol Suppl* 1995;175:75–77.

68. Wall L, Norton PA, Delancey JL. Bladder emptying problems. In: Wall L, ed. *Practical urogynecology*. Baltimore: Williams & Wilkins, 1993:274–292.

69. Blok BF, Holstege G. The neuronal control of micturition and its relation to the emotional motor system. *Prog Brain Res* 1996;107:113–126.

70. Blok BF, Sturms LM, Holstege G. Brain activation during micturition in women. *Brain* 1998;121(Pt 11): 2033–2042.

71. Fowler CJ, Kirby RS. Electromyography of urethral sphincter in women with urinary retention. *Lancet* 1986;1:1455–1457.

CHAPTER 19

Preoperative and Postoperative Complications and Management

Matthew Fagan

GENERAL CONSIDERATIONS

All surgical procedures involve some risk of intra-operative or postoperative complications, anesthetic risk, and the possibility of long-term morbidity, loss of function, or death. Much of the risk to an individual patient is based on the pathology necessitating surgery and her medical comorbidities. Pelvic organ prolapse and urinary and fecal incontinence are disabling conditions with significant burdens of disease and loss of function. They are not, however, fatal diseases. Every consideration must be made to weigh the risks of surgery against the natural history of the disease being treated. Many interventions are available to both assess and reduce an individual patient's risk of complications during and immediately following surgery. Many of these interventions are backed by sufficient medical evidence that they have been recommended to all surgeons and hospitals. Indeed, agencies such as the Institute for Healthcare Improvement (IHI), Agency for Healthcare Research and Quality (AHRQ), Center for Medicare Services (CMS) and the Joint Commission on the Accreditation of Healthcare Organizations (JCAHO) have identified certain perioperative practices for universal implementation. Table 19.1 lists eleven practices identified by AHRQ with the best evidence to improve patient safety. Four of these relate directly to perioperative care, and three will be discussed below (1). Additionally, there are some time-honored practices and routines that may actually increase the risk of certain complications. It is every surgeon's responsibility to remain current on a set of best practices for perioperative care and to advocate for their implementation in an organized fashion by hospital operating rooms and practices.

The goals of perioperative care are to minimize the risk to individual patients and to maximize the likelihood of a successful surgical outcome and return to normal function. Within this framework are the preoperative medical evaluation, immediate preoperative care, and postoperative care. The goals of the preoperative medical evaluation are to maximize the functional status of individual patients with known disease, and to screen based on history and risk factors for subclinical conditions that may affect their response to surgery. A detailed discussion of the preoperative medical evaluation is beyond the scope of this chapter, but all pelvic surgeons should be familiar with this subject. Surgical clearance by an outside provider does not abdicate the surgeon of his or her primary responsibility for the overall care of the patient. Patients undergoing reconstructive pelvic surgery are often older and have a greater number of comorbidities or risk factors that must be addressed prior to surgery.

Surgery for the correction of pelvic floor dysfunction is common. The lifetime risk of surgery for pelvic organ prolapse or urinary incontinence is estimated to be 11%, with 30% of patients seeking reoperation for recurrent symptoms (2). Rates of operative complications and perioperative morbidity are low in benign gynecologic surgery. The VALUE study estimated the overall risk of major complications in hysterectomies for benign indications to be 3% (3). However, pelvic reconstructive surgery involves a substantially higher risk of in-

TABLE 19.1

Interventions Identified by AHRQ with Best Evidence to Improve Patient Safety, 2001

- Appropriate use of prophylaxis to prevent venous thromboembolism in patients at risk
- Use of perioperative beta blockers in appropriate patients to prevent perioperative morbidity and mortality
- Use of maximum sterile barriers while placing central intravenous catheters to prevent infections
- Appropriate use of antibiotic prophylaxis in surgical patients to prevent postoperative infections
- Asking that patients recall and restate what they have been told during the informed consent process
- Continuous aspiration of subglottic secretions (CASS) to prevent ventilator-associated pneumonia
- Use of pressure-relieving bedding materials to prevent pressure ulcers
- Use of real-time ultrasound guidance during central line insertion to prevent complications
- Patient self-management for warfarin (Coumadin) to achieve appropriate outpatient anticoagulation and prevent complications
- Appropriate provision of nutrition, with a particular emphasis on early enteral nutrition in critically ill and surgical patients
- Use of antibiotic-impregnated central venous catheters to prevent catheter-related infections

AHRQ, Agency for Healthcare Research and Quality.

traoperative and perioperative complications than surgery for other benign gynecologic conditions. The reported rates are similar to those observed in gynecologic oncology procedures. Lambrou et al published a retrospective case series of 100 reconstructive pelvic surgery cases. They reported an overall prevalence of complications of 46% (4,5). Patients undergoing reconstructive pelvic surgery are often older, undergo lengthy surgeries, and have histories of prior pelvic surgery (5–9). All of these are known to increase surgical morbidity and mortality. In addition, patients undergoing reconstructive pelvic surgery often have severely distorted anatomy that also increases the risk of surgical injury.

This chapter will briefly review some topics in perioperative care, including the use of prophylactic antibiotics, perioperative beta blockers, deep vein thrombosis (DVT) prophylaxis, and urinary catheter use. In addition, specific intraoperative complications and management will be discussed. These include lower urinary tract injury, pelvic hemorrhage and hematoma formation, foreign body/mesh-related complications, and postoperative voiding dysfunction.

PERIOPERATIVE CARE

Prophylactic Antibiotics

The use of antibiotics to prevent surgical site infections such as cuff cellulitis and pelvic abscess in hysterectomy patients is well established (10). Moreover, antibiotic prophylaxis is also recommended to prevent surgical site infections in abdominal wounds. Surgical site infections are the second most common source of nosocomial infection in the United States. (11). Their prevention and the appropriate use of prophylactic antibiotics have received much attention in recent years. The Institute for Patient Safety, JCAHO, Centers for Disease Control and Prevention, and CMS have all contributed to new guidelines and performance standards aimed at reducing the incidence of surgical site infections (12). Recent studies indicate significant variation from recommended practices and the need for ongoing efforts to improve compliance. In a review of 34,133 Medicare patients at 2,965 hospitals in the United States, only 55.7% of patients received a dose of antibiotics within 1 hour before incision, and prophylaxis was discontinued within 24 hours of surgery end time for only 40.7% of patients. This study included patients undergoing vaginal and abdominal hysterectomy as well as other general and thoracic surgical procedures (13).

Current guidelines recommend that prophylactic antibiotics be administered within 60 minutes of incision time and be discontinued within 24 hours of surgery. The antimicrobial agent chosen should be active against the likely infectious organisms to be encountered in the surgery performed and should have an appropriate safety profile for the patient (11). For gynecologic surgery, cefazolin and cefotetan are endorsed as appropriate choices for nonallergic patients. For patients unable to tolerate cephalosporins, clindamycin with or without gentamicin or aminoglycosides are recommended regimens. These recommendations are for patients undergoing hysterectomy. Recommendations by the American College of Obstetricians and Gynecologists do not endorse prophylaxis for laparoscopy, urodynamics, and exploratory laparotomy not involving hysterectomy or bowel surgery (10). There is also evidence that antibiotic prophylaxis is not required for office cystoscopy and for urodynamics (14). A study by Cundiff et al demonstrated no difference in the rate of postprocedure urinary tract infection (UTI) between nitrofurantoin and placebo in patients undergoing combined cystourethroscopy and urodynamics.

Several issues related specifically to reconstructive pelvic surgery are not addressed in the literature. Clearly, any patient having reconstructive surgery involving a hysterectomy should receive antibiotic prophylaxis. However, current guidelines do not address abdominal reconstructive operations not involving hysterectomy or vaginal procedures involving neither hysterectomy nor colpotomy. Several examples include abdominal sacral colpopexy, vaginal cystocele and rectocele repairs, midurethral sling operations for urinary incontinence, and the newer minimally invasive total mesh repairs for uterine and vaginal prolapse. In addition, little information in the literature exists regarding the appropriateness and duration of antimicrobial prophylaxis for surgery involving synthetic and biomaterial implants. Most surgeons would favor the use of antibiotic prophylaxis in these cases; however, the question has yet to be studied in a rigorous manner. It has been our practice to use prophylactic antibiotics in all reconstructive procedures, albeit with little evidence to guide our practice. The history of surgical innovation has many stories of time-honored practices failing to show benefit after undergoing scientific study. Given the risks of unnecessary antimicrobial usage, perhaps these issues will receive scrutiny as the discipline of female pelvic medicine and reconstructive surgery continues to mature and develop its scientific base.

Beta Blockers

Beta blockers have been demonstrated to reduce cardiac morbidity and mortality in patients undergoing major noncardiac surgery (15–17). Perioperative cardiac events occur in 1% to 5% of all patients undergoing noncardiac surgery (15). The exact risk in women undergoing reconstructive pelvic surgery is unknown. Lambrou et al reported a 2% rate of cardiac complications in a series of 100 reconstructive pelvic surgery cases, and Waetjen reported a 1.1% rate based on analysis of data from the National Hospital Discharge Summary (4,18). Toglia reported three cases of myocardial infarction in 54 women aged 70 to 85 (5). Although this topic may seem remote from the purview of the gynecologic surgeon, it is important to remember that the operating surgeon is the lead person in the team responsible for patient safety throughout the perioperative period. Furthermore, several patient safety organizations, including AHRQ, have identified perioperative beta blockade as an intervention with sufficiently strong scientific evidence to support implementation (1).

There are several compelling reasons why patients undergoing reconstructive pelvic surgery may be likely to benefit from perioperative beta-blocker therapy. Reconstructive surgery is often performed in older patients who, based on age and other comorbidities, are at increased risk for cardiovascular events perioperatively. Secondly, patients seeking surgery for pelvic floor disorders may have better functional status than age-matched patients undergoing nonelective surgery by other specialties and therefore may not undergo the same in-depth preoperative evaluation as acutely ill patients. Patients with known cardiac disease are usually triaged and treated in a manner to minimize their potential for complications. Undiagnosed, and thus untreated, cardiac disease may represent a large risk in our patient population. Furthermore, cardiac symptoms do not receive the same evaluation in women as they do in men. Cardiac disease is underdiagnosed and undertreated in the female population. Cardiac disease presents with atypical symptoms in women (19). All of these factors may leave our patients especially vulnerable to morbidity or mortality from undiagnosed cardiac disease that comes to light only during the physiologic stress of surgery.

Risk-based algorithms have been devised to identify patients likely to benefit the most from perioperative beta-blocker use. The two algorithms quoted commonly in the literature are in Table 19.2. Based on 1997 data, 42% of patients undergoing surgery for prolapse are over age 60 and 22% are over age 70 (18). Based on age alone, patients undergoing abdominal repairs of pelvic organ prolapse represent a population likely to benefit from intervention.

Metoprolol and atenolol are the two most studied beta blockers used in the perioperative period. Some studies suggest the greatest benefit if started prior to surgery, while others looked at the effects of starting beta blockers at the time of induction of anesthesia. All interventions looked at variable time periods of postoperative treatment (days to 1 month). There are several randomized trials in the literature with some heterogeneity regarding patient populations, medication, intervention, and follow-up periods. However, some conclusions can be

TABLE 19.2

Indications for Beta-Blocker Use

Beta blockers for any TWO of the following:
Age >65
Hypertension
Current smoker
Serum cholesterol >240
Non-insulin-dependent diabetes
Revised Cardiac Risk Index (RCRI)
One point for each of the following:
Intraperitoneal procedure
History of ischemic heart disease
History of cerebrovascular disease
Insulin-dependent diabetes
Serum creatinine >2.0

made. Perioperative beta blockers benefit high-risk patients (Revised Cardiac Risk Index above 2) and are likely to benefit to moderate-risk patients (Revised Cardiac Risk Index above 1) with a low chance for harm. A recent meta-analysis found a benefit for perioperative cardiac mortality (number needed to treat [NNT] = 20), long-term overall mortality (NNT = 11), long-term cardiac mortality (NNT = 10), myocardial infarction (NNT = 14), and myocardial ischemia (NNT = 6). Results of a recent cohort study showed similar results for overall in-hospital mortality. Interestingly, this study also showed that women were less likely than men to receive beta blockers perioperatively (15). A large, well-designed randomized controlled trial with strict inclusion criteria and patients representing the spectrum of noncardiac surgery is needed. Until then, prophylaxis against cardiac events, cardiac mortality, and overall mortality with perioperative beta blockers is recommended for moderate-to high-risk groups, and the criteria in Table 19.2 are reasonable. Patients undergoing reconstructive pelvic surgery are a potentially high-risk group.

DVT Prophylaxis

The risk of DVT following major gynecologic surgery in patients not receiving prophylaxis is estimated to be between 15% and 40%. Risk factors include increasing age, previous venous thromboembolism, and surgery for gynecologic malignancy (20,21). In addition, major reconstructive pelvic surgery should be considered a risk factor. In 2001, Geerts presented a risk stratification

model and recommendations that are endorsed by the American College of Chest Physicians and adopted by the Center for Medicare Services as part of the Surgical Care Improvement Project. These were revised again in 2004. Based on this model, patients between age 40 and 60 undergoing major surgery are at moderate risk and patients over age 60 undergoing major surgery (or age 40 with additional risk factors) are at high risk. Without prophylaxis, moderate-risk patients have a 10% to 20% risk for calf DVT, a 1% to 2% risk of pulmonary embolism (PE), and a 0.5% risk for fatal PE; high-risk patients have a 20% to 40% risk for calf DVT, a 2% to 4% risk for PE, and a 1.0% risk of fatal PE (21). A group-specific model of prophylaxis has been recommended. Individual patients are assigned a group (moderate or high risk) based on age, procedure, and risk factors and appropriate prophylaxis is instituted based on recommendations for that risk group.

Based on 1997 data from the National Hospital Discharge Summary, 42% of patients having surgery for pelvic organ prolapse were over age 60, and an additional 18% were between 50 and 60 years old. The mean age was 55 years (18). Therefore, based on age criteria alone, at least 40% of patients undergoing reconstructive pelvic surgery are in the high-risk category for venous thromboembolism. The above estimates of risk are based on routine benign gynecologic surgical procedures. There is evidence that reconstructive pelvic surgery has a higher inherent risk of complications than routine gynecologic surgery. Lambrou et al showed that reconstructive surgeries have complication rates similar to gynecologic oncology surgeries. Specific to venous thromboembolism risk, they showed a 3% PE rate in their series of patients receiving venous thromboembolism prophylaxis in a university hospital setting. This is 10 times the risk observed in the CREST study of patients undergoing gynecologic surgery for benign disease (4). Based on these considerations, it should be clear that patients undergoing surgery for pelvic floor disorders are at high risk for venous thromboembolism and that the risk estimates for major gynecologic surgery likely represent the lower end of the true risk estimate range.

The American College of Chest Physicians recommends the use of anticoagulant-based prophylaxis, with mechanical prophylaxis being used only in patients considered to be at high risk of bleeding. Anticoagulant prophylaxis for moderate-risk patients includes unfractionated heparin 5,000 U twice per day or low-molecular-weight heparin daily. For higher-risk patients, including reconstructive surgery patients, heparin 5,000 U three times per day or low-molecular-weight heparin with or without sequential compression devices are acceptable choices (21). Continued venous thromboembolism prophylaxis following hospital discharge is largely untested in gynecologic surgery patients and should be considered only in patients who are undergoing cancer surgery and who are over 60 years of age or have previously experienced a venous thromboembolism. Prophylaxis should continue for 2 to 4 weeks after hospital discharge in these highest-risk groups (22).

Catheter Use

UTIs account for about 40% of hospital-acquired (nosocomial) infections, and about 80% of these are associated with urinary catheters (23). Nearly all patients having reconstructive pelvic surgery will have a urinary catheter inserted sometime during their hospital stay. There are no absolute guidelines for catheter care, and often care must be individualized based on specific patient factors and functional status. However, some general principles apply, including aseptic insertion techniques, maintenance of a closed drainage system, and minimizing the duration of catheter usage postoperatively.

With a properly maintained closed drainage system, the risk of infection is between 5% and 10% per day, and up to 50% of patients will remain free of infection after 7 days (24). Management is often complicated in patients undergoing surgery for advanced pelvic organ prolapse or urinary incontinence because of the risk of postoperative urinary retention and the need for voiding trials following surgery. However, early voiding trials are now the norm following reconstructive pelvic surgery, with most patients beginning voiding trials by the second postoperative day. In modern practice, it seems that the majority of patients will be catheterized for less than 2 days. Patients requiring long-term catheterization are best managed with clean intermittent self-catheterization, although suprapubic catheterization remains an option in selected cases.

Investigators have examined several issues related to catheter usage in adults and their potential to reduce the incidence of UTI, including the type of catheter material, the method of catheterization (indwelling transurethral and suprapubic, or intermittent), the duration of catheterization, and the use of prophylactic antibiotics. This topic has also been the subject of several recent Cochrane group reviews (23,25).

With regards to catheterization method (suprapubic versus indwelling urethral versus intermit-

tent urethral), the Cochrane group concluded that there was evidence that suprapubic catheters have advantages over indwelling urethral catheters in terms of bacteriuria, recatheterization, and discomfort (23). However, the clinical significance of bacteriuria in these cases is not clear. Furthermore, there was no information about possible complications or adverse effects during catheter insertion. Severe complications from suprapubic catheter insertion have been reported and include major vascular and bowel injuries. There is limited evidence that the use of intermittent catheterization carries a lower risk of bacteriuria than indwelling urethral catheterization. No clear consensus exists in the literature, especially as it applies to reconstructive pelvic surgery (25). It seems that any benefits in terms of reduced infection rates from the routine use of suprapubic catheters are outweighed by possible complications related to insertion and maintenance. Intermittent clean catheterization is the preferred method of bladder drainage from an infectious standpoint; however, its use is limited in the immediate postoperative period because of cost and patient discomfort. In patients requiring long-term bladder drainage, an attempt should be made to teach intermittent self-catheterization. The balance between risks and benefits favors continuous transurethral bladder drainage for short-term use in the postoperative period in routine cases, with suprapubic catheters reserved for specific situations in individual patients.

There is no evidence to support the use of antibiotics to reduce the incidence of UTIs in postoperative patients requiring transurethral catheterization. The use of prophylactic antibiotics in patients requiring bladder drainage beyond 24 hours does reduce the rate of microbiologic isolates recovered in the urine; however, there is no evidence that this results in fewer clinical UTIs when compared to patients not receiving antibiotics (23,25). Patients managed with clean intermittent catheterization do not require antibiotics. There is evidence that patients managed with suprapubic catheterization may benefit from prophylactic nitrofurantoin, with reduced rates of UTI at catheter removal. In patients managed by suprapubic catheterization, antibiotic prophylaxis may be warranted (26).

The choice of catheter material has also been studied as an intervention to reduce UTI rates in hospitalized patients. Silver alloy–impregnated catheters have been shown to have several benefits, including reducing the incidence of bacteriuria and symptomatic UTI in adults requiring short- and long-term catheterization. Some analyses have also demonstrated a cost savings with the use of such catheters. These catheters are not yet in routine use in most institutions (23).

There is much work remaining to be done to address optimal methods for postoperative urinary catheterization in reconstructive pelvic surgery. The basic principles of a closed drainage system inserted under sterile conditions that remains in place for the shortest duration possible seems the basis standard for appropriate care. Questions regarding optimal method of voiding trial and the timing for the initiation of voiding trials have yet to be answered by high-quality research studies (25).

INTRAOPERATIVE COMPLICATIONS

Lower Urinary Tract Injury

Injury to the bladder or ureter can occur during any pelvic operation. Anti-incontinence procedures and reconstructive surgeries for advanced prolapse increase the risk of such injuries. Unrecognized lower urinary tract injury in gynecologic surgery represents a source of permanent disability to patients and significant litigation risk for hospitals and surgeons (27). The overall incidence rates for urinary tract injury in reconstructive pelvic surgery are difficult to estimate, and only a few studies have looked at such procedures separate from other gynecologic surgery and hysterectomy. A recent review article cited a range of 2% to 12% in surgeries for advanced pelvic organ prolapse (28). The rates of injury for individual procedures vary widely but have been reported as follows: tension-free vaginal tape (TVT) 4% (bladder) (29,30), Burch urethropexy 3% to 6% (bladder, urethra) (31,32), traditional bladder neck slings 3% to 7% (bladder) (33), abdominal sacral colpopexy 3% to 4% (bladder or urethra) (34), sacrospinous suspension 3% to 4% (bladder), and high uterosacral suspension 11% (ureter) (35). Bladder injuries are more common than ureteral injuries. All surgeons performing these procedures must be well trained in techniques necessary for the prevention, detection, and repair of lower urinary tract injuries.

Injury to the bladder can occur at any point during surgery, such as during peritoneal access, during dissection of the vesicovaginal space during abdominal or vaginal surgery, during open retropubic dissection, or during the passage of trocars when performing minimally invasive mid-urethral slings. In a recent study of the long-term follow-up of bladder perforation by Armenakas et al, two thirds of bladder injuries were localized to the anterior wall or dome of the bladder and one third to the base. Risk factors for bladder perforation include prior cesarean section, large fibroid uterus, and laparoscopic hysterectomy (36). The risk of bladder injury can be minimized by careful attention to hemostasis, sharp dissection, and high entry into the peritoneal cavity during laparotomy. In some cases, intentional high, extraperitoneal cystotomy can be used to facilitate further dissection of the bladder and avoid an unintentional or difficult-to-repair injury to the bladder (37). In the past, some authors have advocated the universal use of such a technique in all open retropubic operations. Distention of the bladder can also facilitate identification of the correct tissue planes during difficult dissection. This is easily accomplished by retrograde filling of the bladder transurethrally through either a three-way or conventional Foley catheter. The distention medium is either sterile water or preferably dyed irrigation fluid or sterile infant formula. The use of opaque media also allows for identification of possible small perforations in addition to identification of the correct dissection plane.

Intraoperative detection and immediate repair of bladder injuries is the single most important step in avoiding the risk for long-term sequelae such as fistula formation (38). Direct visual inspection and a high index of suspicion may aid in the recognition of bladder injuries; however, cystoscopic inspection of the bladder mucosa is the preferred method following reconstructive surgical procedures (39). A comprehensive review of the use of cystoscopy in gynecologic surgery was published in 1999 and showed a detection rate for bladder injuries of 10 per 1,000 cases with cystoscopy and only 2.6 per 1,000 cases without intraoperative cystoscopy. With intraoperative cystoscopy, up to 85% of unsuspected bladder injuries were successfully identified and treated intraoperatively (40).

The repair of bladder injuries should include a multilayer closure with delayed absorbable suture material. The closure should be water-tight, tension-free, and hemostatic. The mucosal layer should be included in the initial suture line, followed by one or more additional layers to achieve a water-tight closure. Small perforations such as those following trocar injuries in minimally invasive midurethral sling operations may require no repair (39). Prolonged bladder drainage may be required following cystotomy in dependent areas of the bladder, and ureteral catheterization may be required for injuries involving the trigone. Extraperitoneal cystotomy may be managed with short-term (24 to 48 hours) drainage (41). Suprapubic catheterization and routine cystography prior to catheter removal are not likely to be of benefit in most cases (39). The long-term successful outcome for primary repair of bladder injuries is greater than 98% (36).

Ureteral injury in pelvic surgery most commonly involves laceration and crush injuries from misplaced clamps, and ligation or kinking from sutures. Failure to identify or appreciate the position of the ureter during the operation is frequently involved as a proximal cause (42–44). Knowledge of the anatomy of the ureter from both abdominal and vaginal perspectives is of the utmost importance in avoiding injuries (45). Cadaveric and computed tomography studies have localized the ureter between 1.5 and 3.1 cm lateral to the cervix and approximately 5 cm from the ischial spine (46,47). The surgeon must have familiarity with normal anatomic relationships and be able to appreciate situations where the normal anatomy is distorted. In reconstructive surgery, the most common of these is severe urogenital prolapse. Ureterolysis is an important technique to help identify the course of the ureter during complex abdominal cases. The ability to mobilize the ureter without jeopardizing the blood supply is the key to safely performing ureterolysis. The pelvic ureter receives its blood supply laterally off branches from the hypogastric artery and should always be mobilized in this direction. In addition, blood vessels run parallel to the ureter in the adventitial layer, and this layer should be preserved during dissection to avoid devascularization. The ureter should be identified in all abdominal pelvic operations that involve hysterectomy, adnexal surgery, culdoplasty, or colpopexy. In abdominal surgery, we perform ureterolysis whenever the location of the ureter is in question or normal anatomic relationships are distorted. Anatomic knowledge, sharp dissection, and meticulous hemostasis are critical factors in avoiding injury to the ureter. Preoperative ureteral stent placement does not help prevent ureteral injury but may facilitate location of the ureter in selected cases (48).

In vaginal cases, cystoscopy should be performed at the conclusion of the cases to ensure the integrity of the lower urinary tract. A review of the literature through 1999 showed an intraoperative detection and treatment rate of 90% for ureteral injuries with cystoscopy, compared to 11% in cases without cystoscopy (40).

Ureteral patency should be confirmed postoperatively all cases in which the ureter cannot be directly visualized, such as vaginal reconstructive procedures. In cases of severe uterovaginal prolapse, preoperative assessment of lower urinary tract function with office cystoscopy may aid in the intraoperative and postoperative assessment of ureteral function and is recommended (49–51).

Ureteral patency is easily confirmed postoperatively by the intravenous administration of indigo carmine dye several minutes prior to diagnostic cystoscopy. The direct observation of excretion of blue dye from each ureteral orifice during cystoscopy implies ureteral patency and normal lower urinary tract function. Based on a study of over 700 cases from the Cleveland Clinic, this technique has a reported false-positive rate of 0.4%, with a sensitivity of 94.4% and specificity of 99.5% (52). Rare false-positives have been reported with the use of diuretics to hasten the excretion of the dye (53).

In cases where excretion is not observed or is delayed, or questions arise, ureteral catheterization should be performed. This technique can aid in the intraoperative diagnosis of partial or complete ureteral obstruction during vaginal prolapse repairs. Reconstructive surgeons should be familiar with a technique for ureteral access in order to minimize the risk of undetected ureteral injury. One technique is briefly described below.

Ureteral catheterization can be performed by transurethral cystoscopy or directly via a cystotomy. The former approach is preferred unless a cystotomy has already occurred or is a planned part of the procedure, or when transurethral access is not possible. Indications for ureteral catheterization in reconstructive pelvic surgery may include prophylaxis to aid in the location of the ureter, evaluation of ureteral patency if attempts with intravenous dye have failed, prevention of ureteral stricture or stenosis following extensive ureterolysis or ureteral repair, and protection of the ureteral orifice during repair of bladder injuries or fistulas that are close to the trigone. For evaluation of ureteral patency or short-term catheterization, an open-ended or whistle-tip ureteral catheter is sufficient, and such catheters can be secured to a transurethral catheter or to a separate drainage bag. If the ureteral catheter is to remain for a prolonged period of time postoperatively, a double-J (pigtail) catheter may be required, and its position should be confirmed radiographically following placement. Typical useful catheter sizes are 4 to 7 French and typical lengths are 22 to 24 cm. Placement requires a 30- or 70-degree telescope, a working bridge (22 French), and/or possibly an Albarran (deflecting) bridge. Careful, gentle technique is essential in order to prevent damage to the ureter. In general, with proper technique, complication rates are low.

Intraoperative repair of ureteral injuries involves recognition of the likely mechanism of injury and its location. For complete or partial laceration, extensive devascularization, or segmental resection, ureteroureteral anastomosis or uretero-neocystotomy is indicated. The choice between anastomosis and reimplantation is made based on the level of the injury. The details of these techniques are well described in various references and are beyond the scope of this discussion (44). In vaginal reconstructive surgery cases, ligation of the ureter and kinking of the ureter with a ligature placed in the pelvic sidewall are more common injuries than laceration or devascularization (35). These injuries can often be successfully managed by removal of the offending suture and replacement. A period of ureteral catheterization may be required postoperatively, and this decision should be individualized based on the circumstances surrounding the injury.

If recognized intraoperatively, the majority of ureteral injuries can be successfully managed with little or no long-term loss of function (54). The keys to a successful outcome are early recognition and diagnosis. Based on the likelihood of a successful outcome following immediate diagnosis and repair of lower urinary tract injuries, and the proven efficacy of intraoperative cystoscopy to make the diagnosis, routine intraoperative cystoscopy with assessment of ureteral patency should be a component of any reconstructive pelvic surgery case (50,52,55). The increased litigation rates and permanent disability seen with unrecognized lower urinary tract injury in gynecologic surgery in a recent Canadian study were from cases that did not involve the use of cystoscopy (27). The fellowship training programs in Female Pelvic Medicine and Reconstructive Surgery require training in cystoscopy. Hospital privileges to perform certain reconstructive surgical procedures should also require demonstrated competency in cystoscopy and ureteral catheterization. This would improve patient safety and reduce medicolegal risk.

Pelvic Hemorrhage and Hematoma Formation

Bleeding complications in reconstructive pelvic surgery are rare but do occur with almost any procedure. The rate of hemorrhage, hematoma, or transfusion seems to be similar to that for other benign gynecologic surgery. The risk of hematoma or hemorrhage in vaginal hysterectomy based on a recent European study was 1.2% (3). Other studies found rates of 1% to 4% for vaginal hysterectomy (56). Vascular injury rates or transfusion rates for common reconstructive surgery procedures are reported as follows: traditional pubovaginal slings

2%, TVT 1% to 3%, and sacral colpopexy 4.4% (29,30,34,53,57,58).

Hemorrhage during benign gynecologic surgery is most commonly due to vascular injury. Bleeding can be arterial or venous. Arterial bleeding is usually easy to identify and localize. It will respond invariably to identification and ligation of the offending (or offended) vessel. Major vascular injury is rare in reconstructive pelvic surgery, but damage to the external iliac artery, obturator vessels, and hypogastric artery can occur even with minimally invasive procedures such as the TVT (38).

Venous bleeding presents special challenges because most cases of profuse venous bleeding will not be controlled by identification and ligation of a damaged vein. There are several areas at increased risk for significant venous bleeding during reconstructive pelvic surgery. Two common areas are the retropubic and presacral spaces. Each contains a rich venous plexus that is at risk during procedures such as abdominal sacral colpopexy, open retropubic colposuspension, and pubovaginal slings.

The presacral venous plexus is derived from the medial and lateral sacral veins and from basivertebral veins. These vessels are in close association with the sacral periostium and sacral foramina (59). During injury to these vessels, they can retract into the foramina, and control of bleeding cannot be achieved with conventional means such as ligation, packing, and cautery (59,60). The key to managing hemorrhage in this area is prevention. Detailed anatomic knowledge is important; however, the vascular anatomy of the presacral space is highly variable (61). Therefore, adequate exposure and lighting and meticulous technique are essential. Anatomic keys to avoiding bleeding are to avoid lateral dissection and to avoid extension of the dissection too inferiorly (below S3). When significant bleeding is encountered in the presacral space, a bleeding vessel amenable to cautery, hemoclips, or ligation may be identified, but this is uncommon in cases of massive bleeding. Initial management in these cases should include packing, pressure, and a call for help. Massive blood loss can occur rapidly (60).

If this fails to control bleeding, alternatives such as a sterile thumbtack may be useful. Placement of a sterile thumbtack into a site of bleeding against the sacrum can control difficult bleeding and be a life-saving maneuver. This technique has been well described in the literature and specially designed applicators are available (62–64). In centers performing sacral colpopexy, access to such instruments may be life-saving.

Retropubic space hematoma and hemorrhage is another potential complication from reconstructive surgical procedures and incontinence surgery. The anatomy of the retropubic space makes management of hemorrhage in this area challenging. Important structures within the retropubic space or accessed through the retropubic space include the bladder, anterior vaginal wall, arcus tendineus fascia pelvis, urethra, obturator neurovascular bundle, and venous plexus of Santorini. This potential space extends from the pelvic floor to the umbilicus. The anterior border is the posterior aspect of the rectus sheath, and the pubic bones. The posterior border is the prevesical fascia and the bladder pillars as well as the vesicoumbilical fascia and peritoneum. The inferior border is the anterior vaginal wall. The lateral border is the fascia of the anterior abdominal wall (65). Large amounts of blood can accumulate within this space and track anywhere along these borders. There is a variable amount of loose areolar tissue within the space. In addition, there is a rich venous plexus (Santorini's) below this fatty layer overlying the bladder and anterior vaginal wall. This venous plexus is at risk during open retropubic dissections for colposuspension, pubovaginal sling, or paravaginal repair; and during closed procedures involving the blind passage of trocars, such as minimally invasive mid-urethral slings. Recent studies on female cadavers demonstrate that accessory obturator vessels are present in at least 33% of the population and are found crossing Cooper's ligament, often hidden within a layer of fatty issue (66). This finding is much higher than the 10% to 20% classically taught in anatomy lessons. Accessory obturator veins represent a difficult challenge because they may retract into the obturator canal if injured. An awareness of these potential structures and meticulous dissection are important in avoiding injury to these structures.

Prevention of a retropubic hematoma can be facilitated by adequate exposure, appropriate placement of retractors, and careful blunt and sharp dissection. The use of open gauze sponges can help with blunt dissection. Dissection should be carried out from lateral to medial within the retropubic space, beginning lateral to the pubic symphysis and medial to the obturator notch. A lateral-to-medial approach as the dissection extends in a cephalad direction toward the ischial spine will help avoid disruption of blood vessels (67). Liberal use of electrocautery and hemostatic clips will also help avoid hematoma formation. Sutures placed in the paraurethral tissue during colposuspension should be made in a figure-of-eight fashion and can be tied down in order to control hemorrhage.

The prophylactic use of hemostatic agents such as Gelfoam can also help prevent bleeding.

Immediate management of bleeding in the retropubic space should be directed toward exposure and ligation of the bleeding vessels. Compression sutures placed in the pubocervical fascia lateral to the urethra and bladder can help control bleeding. Packing and manual compression are also effective.

If a hematoma does develop, conservative management is appropriate initially in most instances. Retropubic bleeding can be a self-limited process, as the enlarging hematoma compresses bleeding veins and provides tamponade. However, close observation with serial blood counts and possibly imaging studies may be required. Transfusion may be required and patients should be monitored for the development of disseminated intravascular coagulation. Compression symptoms can develop and include pelvic and vaginal pain or pressure, urinary retention, or neuropathy in the distribution of the obturator nerve.

If a hematoma continues to enlarge, the patient is hemodynamically unstable, severe compression symptoms develop, or there is evidence for infection, the hematoma may require evacuation. Evacuation of a hematoma can be accomplished through the open abdominal route, percutaneously, or transvaginally depending on the presentation and clinical circumstances. In the immediate postoperative period, most surgeons would favor an open approach. For a stable, symptomatic or infected hematoma, successful transvaginal or percutaneous drainage can also been successful. In some instances, a stable hematoma may become infected and a retropubic abscess may develop. The signs of an abscess include fever, elevated white blood cell count, and pain. Examination will reveal an exquisitely tender retropubic mass. Retropubic abscess requires surgical exploration and drainage and may require antibiotics to prevent or treat cellulitis. These cases can be complicated by the presence of foreign material in the case of colposuspension done with permanent suture and pubovaginal slings performed with permanent mesh. The decision to remove a foreign body in the presence of a retropubic abscess is complicated and no clear guidelines exist. Decisions in such cases must be individualized. Fortunately, these occurrences are rare following reconstructive pelvic surgery. Consideration must always be made toward prevention of such complications and should include attention to anatomy, surgical technique, perioperative care, and patient preparation for surgery. In addition, the prudent use of permanent foreign material in light of potential complications should be considered in every case.

POSTOPERATIVE COMPLICATIONS

Foreign Body Complications/Mesh Erosions

The use of synthetic mesh in reconstructive pelvic surgery has become commonplace. Minimally invasive midurethral slings have become first-line operations for urinary incontinence and abdominal sacral colpopexy has gained popularity as a first-line operation for vaginal and uterine prolapse. Total mesh repairs have also become popular in the vaginal approach to prolapse repair. Much controversy exists over the role of mesh in prolapse repairs. For many procedures, questions regarding efficacy and safety have not been rigorously evaluated. Furthermore, the use of biomaterial mesh products also complicates the topic of the proper role of mesh materials in reconstructive pelvic surgery (68–70).

One clear fact that has emerged from this picture is that all mesh materials can erode and cause complications, including autologous tissue grafts. Erosions can occur into the vagina, urethra, or bladder. They can be asymptomatic or be characterized by pelvic pain, dysuria, urinary incontinence, chronic UTI, irritative voiding symptoms, vaginal bleeding, vaginal discharge, or dyspareunia (71–76). These can be minor events, noticeable only to the clinician, or major, life-threatening complications with severe morbidity and permanent loss of function (77,78). Synthetic or biomaterial mesh has proven efficacy in the treatment of urinary incontinence and pelvic organ prolapse; it use is therefore justified based on superior surgical outcomes (29,34). However, the decision to use synthetic or biomaterial mesh must always be weighed against the risk of mesh-related complications such as erosion and chronic sinus tract formation.

Rates of mesh erosion vary according to the type of mesh used, the location of the mesh, and the surgical approach. Overall erosion rates for abdominal sacral colpopexy, the most studied mesh-augmented prolapse repair, are 3% to 4%, but are generally higher in cases where a hysterectomy is also performed (34). Newer transvaginal total mesh repairs have reported erosion rates as high as 13%, and polypropylene used to augment cystocele repairs has a reported erosion rate as high as 20% (79,80). The rate of mesh-related complications in minimally invasive midurethral slings performed with polypropylene is reported to be 1% (29). Permanent suture material used for suspension of the vaginal apex in sacrospinous ligament suspensions and other repairs can also erode into the vagina.

The symptoms of a mesh or suture erosion are variable. Some cases may be asymptomatic and others may present with vaginal discharge, bleeding, pain, or signs and symptoms of infection. Rare events such as an abscess formation may present emergently, with the patient critically ill (77). Attempts to identify risk factors for mesh erosion have not revealed any consistent findings. Mesh erosions are a function of the material, the location of the graft, the route of entry (vaginal or abdominal), and patient comorbidities and concomitant surgeries. The presentation may be in the immediate postoperative period or may be delayed. Erosions have presented years after the initial surgery (81).

There has been much written about the management of mesh-related complications, but there have been no trials comparing alternative treatment strategies. Initial management may be conservative, especially in the case of biomaterial meshes. Vaginal estrogen therapy and antibiotics have been advocated in such cases presenting in the immediate postoperative period. There are reports of spontaneous resolution of erosions with synthetic materials following conservative management alone. However, with synthetic materials, many surgeons would favor local excision and reclosure of the affected vaginal epithelium. There are descriptions of such "mesh trimming" procedures being done in the office setting. Cases that do not respond to conservative management require surgical treatment (81–83).

Some general principles can be applied in these cases, although no single technique has been rigorously studied. Infection should be treated with antibiotics where appropriate, and infected or inflamed tissue should be excised. As much of the foreign material as possible should be excised at the time of reoperation. This may require extensive dissection and risks disruption of the original repair and may cause a return of the patient's original symptoms. In cases involving suburethral slings, however, most patients remain continent following treatment for exposed vaginal mesh, with reported continence rates ranging from 50% to 75% (81,84). Following removal of all infected or chronically inflamed tissue and wide excision of any exposed graft material, the wound should be copiously irrigated. Closure of the wound may involve the creation of advancement flaps or mobilization of adjacent tissue. The final closure should be tension-free and hemostatic. Delayed absorbable monofilament suture is preferred. The use of postoperative antibiotics has not been studied, although there would seem to be no indication for continued antibiotic therapy following surgical repair. In many cases, especially those involving the vaginal apex, exposure and lighting can be difficult. Several authors have described the use of cystoscopic video equipment to aid in difficult cases. We have found this technique to be very helpful in selected cases (85,86). A single surgical repair as described above is sufficient in the majority of cases; however, some patients may require multiple procedures and ultimately removal of the entire graft. Such cases can be associated with significant morbidity and permanent loss of function.

The use of graft materials in reconstructive pelvic surgery has revolutionized the treatment of female pelvic floor disorders and is an area of active investigation. However, as the preceding discussion highlights, the use of any mesh material exposes women to increased risk and potentially devastating complications with short- and long-term morbidity. In many cases, such as midurethral slings, the risk/benefit ratio is in favor of the use of synthetic grafts. However, in other applications, a scientific consensus on the benefits of synthetic or biomaterial mesh augmentation has yet to be reached. All reconstructive pelvic surgeons should be cautious regarding the implementation of new and unproven methods into their practice.

Postoperative Voiding Dysfunction

One of the most troublesome postoperative complications following surgery for the correction of stress urinary incontinence is the development of obstructive voiding symptoms and urge incontinence. Urgency, frequency, and urge incontinence are debilitating and demoralizing symptoms in women whose goal was relief of urine loss with coughing. Any anti-incontinence procedure can result in this complication, and some degree of transient voiding dysfunction is a probably normal during acute convalescence. Published rates for various procedures are listed in Table 19.3. When symptoms persist or are exaggerated, a diagnostic evaluation is warranted. This should include urodynamic evaluation of storage and voiding phases and endoscopy to exclude iatrogenic lower urinary tract lesions.

The causes are not always clear but can include incorrect suture placement in colposuspension, overcorrection of urethrovesical angle, incorrect placement of sling material in pubovaginal sling operations, or excessive tension on a sling. Patients with Valsalva voiding, low flow rates, and hypocontractile bladders preoperatively may be at increased risk for obstructed voiding complications. In some patients, uninhibited detrusor contractility unrelated to outlet obstruction or irritative lesions (infection or injury) may be the cause. These cases may represent misdiagnosis of the original problem and thus failure to recognize preoperative detrusor overactivity. Up to one third of women with stress incontinence symptoms have mixed incontinence (87,88). Women with mixed urinary incontinence have a 45% risk of persistent detrusor overactivity incontinence postoperatively (89). All of these considerations highlight the need for a thorough preoperative evaluation of lower urinary tract function prior to surgery. The evaluation should focus on both the storage and voiding phases in incontinent women. These issues become even more complex in the presence of significant pelvic organ prolapse or prior incontinence surgery. We recommend a thorough urodynamic and endoscopic evaluation of all patients prior to surgery. This will not only confirm the diagnosis

TABLE 19.3

Rate of Postoperative Voiding Dysfunction and Urinary Retention Following Common Anti-Incontinence Procedures

Procedure	Rate	Reference
Traditional pubovaginal sling	2% to 10%	(33)
Burch colposuspension	9% to 12%	(31,32)
Tension-free vaginal tape	6%	(21)
Periurethral collagen injections	Less than 1%	(33)

of stress urinary incontinence but will also evaluate the patient for occult voiding dysfunction and exclude detrusor overactivity as a cause of her symptoms.

The diagnosis of obstructed voiding is complicated in women following surgery for stress incontinence, and the information gained is most useful if comparison can be made to preoperative values. The diagnosis is clinical and cannot be based solely on objective findings. Normal urodynamic parameters in women are not as well defined as they are in men. Most expects agree, however, that a maximum flow rate (Q_{max}) on free uroflow evaluation of less than 12 mL/s or 15 mL/s indicates obstruction. Evaluation of detrusor pressure during the voiding phase in women is also controversial. Detrusor pressure can be only minimally elevated in women during micturition, and different authors have defined abnormally high detrusor pressure using different cutoff values. Values greater than 20 cm H_2O or 50 cm H_2O at maximum flow (P_{det} Q_{max}) have been described. Elevated postvoid ·residual urine may be a late finding and is not necessary for the diagnosis but may be helpful if identified (90,91). Clinical correlation of any urodynamic abnormalities is of the utmost importance. A woman suffering from obstructed voiding seeks a return of normal function, which does not always correlate with normalization of urodynamic parameters. In cases of de novo postoperative detrusor overactivity, overcorrection of the urethrovesical junction may be the cause. The urodynamic correlate of this can be elevated pressure transmission ratios. Women with persistent detrusor overactivity after continence surgery have pressure transmission ratios significantly above 100% (92). As fewer surgeons perform urethropexy in favor of midurethral sling operations, and those who do are less aggressive about elevation of the urethrovesical junction, this diagnosis may become less relevant in clinical practice.

The treatment of obstructed voiding symptoms including urgency, frequency, and urge incontinence in the postoperative period should include surveillance and treatment for UTI, anticholinergic therapy, and clean intermittent self-catheterization. Anticholinergic medications with local anesthetic properties such as oxybutynin are good choices in the immediate postoperative period (88). A period of 6 to 8 weeks of conservative management following traditional operations such as bladder neck slings and colposuspension will likely result in normalization of function in the majority of cases. In a large summary report on bladder neck slings, Leach reported 7 cases of urinary retention lasting greater than 4 weeks in 578 cases (33). Published rates for TVT procedures range from 0.5% to 2.0% (29,93).

Minimally invasive midurethral sling operations such as TVT are an exception to the above-mentioned period of expectant management. Postoperative voiding dysfunction following procedures such as TVT is sufficiently uncommon that immediate reoperation (within 2 to 3 days) has resulted in normalization of function in a majority of cases. Different approaches have been described, but essentially the vaginal incision is reopened and the sling material placed on downward traction in order to loosen the tape without disrupting the sling. Different authors have reported good success with this approach (88,89).

In cases where conservative management has failed, urethrolysis can be performed. Urethrolysis is performed vaginally or abdominally, and the approach may be determined by the initial procedure that was performed. In any case, the goal is mobilization of the bladder neck and urethra and transection or excision of the sling or permanent sutures used in the original operation. Published success rates are between 60% and 90%, with continence rates between 85% and 97% (84,91,94,95). A recent review by Ellerkmann and McBride provides a good summary of the published studies on urethrolysis as well as accurate descriptions of the procedures (91). A recent review of TVT release procedures done in Finland contradicts these results (96). They analyzed 48 cases of postoperative retention from over 9,000 TVT procedures. All patients underwent TVT release, up to 197 days postoperatively. Eighty-eight percent of patients were cured of their retention, but only 49% remained continent. It should be noted that these patients had a longer interval from the index procedure to the release of the sling. This underscores the benefit of early intervention for retention and obstructive voiding after midurethral slings. However, this discrepancy should caution surgeons about being overly optimistic concerning continence rates following urethrolysis, and patients should be counseled about the possibility of recurrent stress urinary incontinence and the need for subsequent treatment. The favorable continence rates from most studies would suggest that a concomitant anti-incontinence procedure is not indicated when performing urethrolysis.

CONCLUSIONS

Surgery for female pelvic floor disorders is common and will likely increase in the years to come. Along with traditional repairs, multiple minimally invasive approaches are currently employed, and the techniques are rapidly evolving. Current approaches are effective and safe. However, adherence to "first do no harm" and expert technique are required to minimize the surgical complications and patient morbidity.

Perioperative care must be evidence-based and comprehensive in scope, especially in geriatric populations. Healthcare quality agencies have made definitive recommendations regarding antibiotic usage, DVT prophylaxis, and beta-blocker use. All surgeons should be familiar with them.

Intraoperative complications occur more commonly in reconstructive surgery cases than in other benign gynecology surgeries. Patients have often had multiple prior surgeries and have complex anatomy. The risk of lower urinary tract injury is high, and thorough intraoperative evaluation is a critical skill that reconstructive pelvic surgeons must master. Intraoperative cystoscopy with assessment of ureteral patency should be performed following all reconstructive surgery, including minimally invasive procedures. In addition, as technology in the field advances, newer procedures will become used in a greater number of patients. New procedures will result in new complications. Reconstructive surgeons must be prepared for this and remain ready to handle unforeseen situations. New technology is not a substitute for rigorous surgical training, fundamental principles, and anatomic knowledge. Prevention may indeed be the best medicine, and our patients will also be best served by a rational, evidence-based approach to the adoption of new procedures and technologies.

There is great demand for reconstructive pelvic surgery, and successful outcomes can transform patient's lives. Good surgical outcomes require good preoperative patient preparation, meticulous attention to surgical details to avoid intraoperative complications, and prompt diagnosis and management of complications when they do occur. This chapter highlights important areas for attention, with specific focus on details relevant to patients and procedures in reconstructive pelvic surgery.

REFERENCES

1. Shojania KG, Duncan BW, McDonald KM, et al, eds. *Making health care safer: a critical analysis of patient safety practices.* Evidence Report/Technology Assessment No. 43 (Prepared by the University of California at San Francisco–Stanford Evidence-based Practice Center under Contract No. 290-97-0013), AHRQ Publication No. 01-E058, Rockville, MD: Agency for Healthcare Research and Quality, July 2001.

2. Olsen A, Smith V, Bergstrom J, et al. Epidemiology of surgically managed pelvic organ prolapse and urinary incontinence. *Obstet Gynecol* 1997;89:501–506.

3. McPherson K, Metcalfe MA, Herbert A, et al. Severe complications of hysterectomy: the VALUE study. *Br J Obstet Gynaecol* 2004;111(3):688–694.

4. Lambrou NC, Buller JL, Thompson JR, et al. Prevalence of perioperative complications among women undergoing reconstructive pelvic surgery. *Am J Obstet Gynecol* 2000;183(6):1355–1358.

5. Toglia M, Nolan T. Morbidity and mortality rates of elective gynecologic surgery in the elderly woman. *Am J Obstet Gynecol* 2003;189:1584–1589.

6. Sultana CJ, Campbell JW, Pisanelli WS, et al. Morbidity and mortality of incontinence surgery in elderly women: an analysis of Medicare data. *Am J Obstet Gynecol* 1997;176(2):344–348.

7. Pollack J, Davila GW, Kopka S. Urogynecological and reconstructive pelvic surgery in women aged 80 and older. *J Am Geriatrics Soc* 2004;52(5):851–852.

8. Moalli P, Jones Ivy S, Meyn L, et al. Risk factors associated with pelvic floor disorders in women undergoing surgical repair. *Obstet Gynecol* 2003;101(5, part 1):869–874.

9. Gordon D, Gold R, Pauzner D, et al. Tension-free vaginal tape in the elderly: is it a safe procedure? *Urology* 2005;65:479–482.

10. American College of Obstetricians and Gynecologists. *Antibiotics prophylaxis for gynecologic procedures.* ACOG practice bulletin No. 23. ACOG, Washington DC, 2001.

11. Bratzler DW, Houck PM, for the Surgical Infection Prevention Guidelines Writers Workgroup. Antimicrobial prophylaxis for surgery: an advisory statement from the National Surgical Infection Prevention Project. *Clin Infect Dis* 2004;38:1706–1715.

12. Centers for Medicare & Medicaid Services. *Surgical infection prevention project description.* Available at: http://www.medqic.org/sip. Accessed 1 March 2006.

13. Bratzler DW, Houck PM, Richards C, et al. Use of antimicrobial prophylaxis for major surgery: baseline results from the National Surgical Infection Prevention Project. *Arch Surg* 2005;140(2):174–182.

14. Cundiff GW, McLennan MT, Bent AE. Randomized trial of antibiotic prophylaxis for combined urodynamics and cystourethroscopy. *Obstet Gynecol* 1999;93: 749–752.

15. Lindenaur P, Pekow P, Wang K, et al. Perioperative beta-blocker therapy and mortality after major noncardiac surgery. *N Engl J Med* 2005;353(4):349–361.

16. Auerbach A, Goldman L. Beta blockers and the reduction in cardiac events in non-cardiac surgery. *JAMA* 2002;287(11):1435–1444.

17. Zaugg M, Tagliente T, Lucchinetti E, et al. Beneficial effects from beta-adrenergic blockade in elderly patients undergoing noncardiac surgery. *Anesthesiology* 1999;91:1674–1686.

18. Waetjen LE, Subak LL, Shen H, et al. Stress urinary incontinence surgery in the United States. *Obstet Gynecol* 2003;101(4):671–676.

19. Wenger NK. Coronary heart disease in women: highlights of the past two years: stepping stones, milestones, and obstructing boulders. *Nat Clin Pract Cardiovasc Med* 2006;3(4):194–202.

20. Gutt C, Oniu T, Wolkener F, et al. Prophylaxis and therapy of deep venous thrombosis in general surgery. *Am J Surg* 2005;189:14–22.

21. Geerts W, Pineo G, Heit J, et al. Prevention of venous thromboembolism: 7th annual ACCP conference on antithrombotic and thrombolytic therapy. *Chest* 2004;126:338–400.

22. Kearon C. Duration of venous thromboembolism prophylaxis after surgery. *Chest* 2003;124:386–392.

23. Neil-Weise BS, van der Broek PJ. Urinary catheter policies for short-term urinary catheterization in adults. *Cochrane Database of Systematic Reviews* 2006(1).

24. Warren JW. Catheter-associated urinary tract infections. *Infect Dis Clin North Am* 1987;1:159–196.

25. Phipps S, Lim YN, McClinton S, et al. Short-term urinary catheter policies following urogenital surgery in adults. *Cochrane Database of Systematic Reviews* 2006(3).

26. Rogers R, Kammerer-Doak D, Olsen A, et al. A randomized, double-blind, placebo-controlled comparison of the effect of nitrofurantoin monohydrate macrocrystals on the development of urinary tract infections after surgery for pelvic organ prolapse and/or stress urinary incontinence with suprapubic catheterization. *Am J Obstet Gynecol* 2004;91:182–187.

27. Gilmour DT, Baskett TF. Disability and litigation from urinary tract injuries at benign gynecologic surgery in Canada. *Obstet Gynecol* 2005;105:109–114.

28. Kim J, Moore C, Jones J, et al. Management of ureteral injuries associated with vaginal surgery for pelvic organ prolapse. *Int Urogyn J* 2006;17(5):531–535.

29. Cody J, Wyness L, Wallace S, et al. Systematic review of the clinical effectiveness and cost-effectiveness of tension-free vaginal tape for treatment of urinary stress incontinence. *Health Technol Assess* 2003;7(21).

30. Karram MM, Segal JL, Vassallo BJ, et al. Complications and untoward effects of the tension-free vaginal tape procedure. *Obstet Gynecol* 2003;101(5 Pt 1):929–932.

31. Lapitan MC, Cody DJ, Grant AM. Open retropubic colposuspension for urinary incontinence in women. *Cochrane Database of Systematic Reviews* 2003(1).

32. Dainer M, Hall CD, Choe J, et al. The Burch procedure: a comprehensive review. *Obstet Gynecol Survey* 1998;54(1):49–60.

33. Leach GE, Dmochowski RR, Appell RA, et al. Female Stress Urinary Incontinence Clinical Guidelines Panel summary report on surgical management of female stress urinary incontinence. *J Urol* 1997;158(3 Pt 1):875–880.

34. Nygaard IE, McCreery R, Brubaker L, et al. Abdominal sacrocolpopexy: a comprehensive review. *Obstet Gynecol* 2004;104(4):805–823.

35. Barber MD, Visco A, Weidner A, et al. Bilateral uterosacral ligament vaginal vault suspension with site-specific endopelvic fascia defect repair for treatment of pelvic organ prolapse. *Am J Obstet Gynecol* 2000;183(6):1402–1411.

36. Armenakas NA, Pareek G, Fracchia JA. Iatrogenic bladder perforations: long-term follow-up of 65 patients. *J Am Coll Surg* 2004;198(1):78–82.

37. Aronson MP, Bose TM. Urinary tract injury in pelvic surgery. *Clin Obstet Gynecol* 2002;45:428–438.

38. Meeks GR, Roth T. In: Rock J, Jones H, eds. *TeLinde's operative gynecology*, 9th ed. Philadelphia: Lippincott Williams & Wilkins, 2003.

39. Alli MO, Singh B, Moodley J, et al. Prospective evaluation of combined suprapubic and urethral catheterization to urethral drainage alone for intraperitoneal bladder injuries. *J Trauma* 2003;55:1152–1154.

40. Gilmour DT, Dwyer PL, Carey MP. Lower urinary tract injury during gynecologic surgery and its detection by intraoperative cystoscopy. *Obstet Gynecol* 1999;94(5 p2):883–889.

41. Karram MM, Partoll L, Miklos J, et al. Suprapubic bladder drainage after extraperitoneal cystotomy. *Obstet Gynecol* 2000;96:234–236.

42. Goodno JA, Powers TW, Harris VD. Ureteral injury in gynecologic surgery: a ten-year review in a community hospital. *Am J Obstet Gynecol* 1995;172:1817–1822.

43. Sakellariou P, Protopapas AG, Voulgaris Z, et al. Management of ureteric injuries during gynecological operations: 10 years experience. *Eur J Obstet Gynecol Reprod Biol* 2002;101:179–184.

44. Montz, FJ, Bristow R, Del Carmen. Operative injuries to the ureter: prevention, recognition, and management. In: Rock J, Jones H, eds. *TeLinde's operative gynecology*, 9th ed. Philadelphia: Lippincott Williams & Wilkins, 2003.

45. Hofmeister FJ. Pelvic anatomy of the ureter in relation to surgery performed through the vagina. *Clin Obstet Gynecol* 1982;25:821–830.

46. Buller J, Thompson JR, Cundiff GW, et al. Uterosacral ligament: description of anatomic relationships to optimize surgical safety. *Obstet Gynecol* 2001;97(6):873–879.

47. Hurd WW, Chee SS, Gallagher KL, et al. Location of the ureters in relation to the uterine cervix by computed tomography. *Am J Obstet Gynecol* 2001;185(4):1009–1010.

48. Kuno K, Menzin A, Kander HH, et al. Prophylactic ureteral catheterization in gynecologic surgery. *Urology* 1998;52:1004–1008.

49. Handa VL, Maddox MD. Diagnosis of ureteral obstruction during complex urogynecologic surgery. *Int Urogynecol J* 2001;12:345–348.

50. Taber K, Visco A, Weidner A, et al. Cost effectiveness analysis of universal cystoscopy at the time of hysterectomy. *Int Urogynecol J* 1999;10:s22.

51. Ferro A, Byck D, Gallup D. Intraoperative and postoperative morbidity associated with cystoscopy performed in patients undergoing gynecologic surgery. *Am J Obstet Gynecol* 2003;189:354–357.

52. Gustilo-Ashby A, Jelovsek J, Barber M, et al. The incidence of ureteral obstruction and the value of intraoperative cystoscopy during vaginal surgery for pelvic organ prolapse. *Am J Obstet Gynecol* 2006;194:1478–1485.

53. Novi JM. Report of case: Partial ureteral obstruction masked by diuretics during intraoperative cystoscopy. *J Am Osteopath Assoc* 2005;105(11):521–522.

54. Ku J, Kim ME, Jeon YS, et al. Minimally invasive management of ureteral injuries recognized late after obstetric and gynaecologic surgery. *Int J Care Injured* 2003;34:480–483.

55. Jabs C, Drutz HP. The role of intraoperative cystoscopy in prolapse and incontinence surgery. *Am J Obstet Gynecol* 2001;185:1368–1373.

56. Makinen J, Johansson J, Tomas C, et al. Morbidity of 10,110 hysterectomies by type of approach. *Hum Reprod* 2001;16(7):1473–1478.

57. Kölle D. Bleeding complications with the tension-free vaginal tape operation *Am J Obstet Gynecol* 2005;193(6):2045–2049.

58. Meschia M, Pifarotti P, Bernasconi F, et al. Tension-free vaginal tape: analysis of outcomes and complications in 404 stress incontinent women. *Int Urogynecol J* 2001;12:(Suppl 2):S24–S27.

59. Qinyao W, Weijin S, Youren Z, et al. New concepts in severe presacral hemorrhage during protectomy. *Arch Surg* 1985;120:1013–1020.

60. Tomacruz R, Bristow R, Montz FJ. Management of pelvic hemorrhage. *Surg Clin North Am* 2001;81(4): 925–948.

61. Flynn MK. Vascular anatomy of the presacral space: a fresh tissue cadaver dissection. *Am J Obstet Gynecol* 2005;192(5):1501–1505.

62. Nivatvongs S, Fang DT. The use of thumbtacks to stop massive presacral hemorrhage. *Dis Colon Rectum* 1986;29(9):589–590.

63. Arnaud JP, Tuech JJ, Pessaux P. Management of presacral venous bleeding with the use of thumbtacks. *Digest Surg* 2000;17:651–652.

64. Timmons MC, Kohler MF, Addison WA. Thumbtack use for control of presacral bleeding, with description of an instrument for thumbtack application. *Obstet Gynecol* 1991;78(2):313–315.

65. Silva W, Karram MM. Anatomy and physiology of the pelvic floor. *Minerva Gynecol* 2004;56(4):283–302.

66. Drewes P, Marinis S, Shaffer J, et al. Vascular anatomy over the superior pubic rami in female cadavers. *Am J Obstet Gynecol* 2005;193:2165–2168.

67. Fitzpatrick C, Elkins T, DeLancey J. The surgical anatomy of needle bladder neck suspensions. *Obstet Gynecol* 1996;87:44–49.

68. Birch C. The use of prosthetics in pelvic reconstructive surgery. *Best Practice & Research Clin Obstet Gynaecol* 2005;19(6):979–991.

69. Vakili B, Huynh T, Loesch H, et al. Outcomes of vaginal reconstructive surgery with and without graft material. *Am J Obstet Gynecol* 2005;193:2126–2132.

70. Silva W, Karram M. Scientific basis for use of grafts during vaginal reconstructive procedures. *Cur Opin Obstet Gynecol* 2005;17:519–529.

71. Visco AG, Weidner AC, Barber MD, et al. Vaginal mesh erosion after abdominal sacral colpopexy. *Am J Obstet Gynecol* 2001;184:297–302.

72. Achtari C, Hiscock R, O'Reilly B, et al. Risk factors for mesh erosion after transvaginal surgery using polypropylene (Atrium) or composite polypropylene/ polyglactin 910 (Vypro II) mesh. *Int Urogynecol J* 2005;16:389–394.

73. Kwong-Pang T, Soo-Cheen N, Yi-Torng T, et al. Complications of synthetic graft materials used in suburethral sling procedures. *Int Urogynecol J* 2005;16(2):165–167.

74. Wai C, Atnip S, Williams K, et al. Urethral erosion of tension-free vaginal tape presenting as recurrent stress urinary incontinence. *Int Urogynecol J* 2004;15(5):353–355.

75. Cosson D, Vinatier R, Rajabally, et al. Rejection of stapled prosthetic mesh after laparoscopic sacropexy. *Int Urogynecol J* 1999;10(5):349–350.

76. Domingo S, Alama P, Ruiz N, et al. Diagnosis, management, and prognosis of vaginal erosion after transobturator suburethral tape procedure using a nonwoven thermally bonded polypropylene mesh. *J Urol* 2005;173: 1627–1630.

77. Goldberg J, Weinstein M, Fagan MJ, et al. Gluteal necrotizing myofasciitis: an unusual delayed complication of abdominal sacral colpopexy. *Am J Obstet Gynecol* 2001;185:1273–1274.

78. Salman MM, Hancock AL, Hussein AA, et al. Lumbosacral spondylodiscitis: an unreported complication of sacrocolpopexy using mesh. *Br J Obstet Gynaecol* 2003;110:537–538.

79. Collinet P, Belot F, Debodinance P, et al. Transvaginal mesh technique for pelvic organ prolapse repair: mesh exposure management and risk factors. *Int Urogynecol J* 2006;17(4):315–320.

80. Deffieux X, de Tayrac R, Huel C, et al. Vaginal mesh erosion after transvaginal repair of cystocele using Gynemesh or Gynemesh-Soft in 138 women: a comparative study. *Int Urogynecol J* 2006;17(5):483–488.

81. Clemmens JQ, DeLancey JOL, Faerber GJ, et al. Urinary tract erosions after synthetic pubovaginal slings: diagnosis and management strategy. *Urology* 2000;56:589–594.

82. Mattox TF, Stanford EJ, Varner E. Infected abdominal sacrocolpopexies: diagnosis and treatment. *Int Urogynecol J* 2004;15:319–323.

83. Huang K, Kung F, Liang H, et al. Management of polypropylene mesh erosion after intravaginal midurethral sling operation for female stress urinary incontinence. *Int Urogynecol J* 2005;16(6):437–440.

84. Bent AE, Ostergard DR, Zwick-Zaffulo M. Tissue reaction to expanded polytetrafluoroethylene suburethral sling for urinary incontinence: clinical and histological study. *Am J Obstet Gynecol* 1993;169: 1198–1204.

85. Fagan MJ, Johnson H. Transvaginal endoscopy in the surgical treatment of vaginal mesh erosion. *J Pelvic Med Surg* 2005;11(suppl1):S25.

86. Chai TC, Sklar GN. The use of the flexible cystoscope as a vaginoscope to aid in the diagnosis of artificial sling erosion. *Urology* 1999;53:617–618.

87. Hampel C, Wienhold N, Benken C, et al. Definition of overactive bladder and epidemiology of urinary incontinence. *Urology* 1997;50 (Suppl. 6A):4–17.

88. Stewart W, Herzog R, Wein A, et al. The prevalence and impact of overactive bladder in the US: results from the NOBLE program. *Neurourol Urodynam* 2001;406–408.

89. Sand PK, Bowen LW, Ostergard DR, et al. The effect of retropubic urethropexy on detrusor stability. *Obstet Gynecol* 1988;71:818–822.

90. Nitti VW, Tu LM, Gitlin J. Diagnosing bladder outlet obstruction in women. *J Urol* 1999;161:1535–1540.

91. Ellerkmann RM, McBride A. Management of obstructive voiding dysfunction. *Drugs of Today* 2003;39(7): 513–540.

92. Bump RC, Fantl JA, Hurt GW. Dynamic urethral pressure profilometry pressure transmission ratio determinations after continence surgery: understanding the mechanism of success, failure, and complications. *Obstet Gynecol* 1988;72:870–877.

93. Klutke C, Siegel S, Carlin B, et al. Urinary retention after tension-free vaginal tape procedure: incidence and treatment. *Urology* 2001;58:697–701.

94. Nitti VW, Raz S. Obstruction following anti-incontinence procedures: Diagnoses and treatment with transvaginal urethrolysis. *J Urol* 1994;152:93–98.

95. Goldman HB, Rackley RR, Appell RA. The efficacy of urethrolysis without resuspension for iatrogenic urethral obstruction. *J Urol* 1999;161:1268–1271.

96. Laurikairen E, Kiilholma. Nationwide analysis of TVT release for urinary retention after tension free vaginal tape procedure. *Int Urogynecol J* 2006;17:111–119.

Disorders of Anus and Rectum

CHAPTER 20

Physiology, Pathophysiology

Robert E. Gutman

INTRODUCTION

Disorders of the anus and rectum are numerous and transcend any individual specialty. Anorectal dysfunction is a nonspecific term referring to any condition that disrupts normal anorectal function. Anorectal dysfunction can be subdivided into conditions that cause defecatory dysfunction and fecal incontinence. This chapter will discuss the physiology of anorectal function, followed by the epidemiology and pathophysiology of defecatory dysfunction and fecal incontinence. Subsequent chapters will focus on the evaluation and management of specific conditions relevant to providers caring for women with pelvic floor dysfunction.

OVERVIEW OF NORMAL COLO-RECTAL-ANAL FUNCTION

The normal physiologic processes of anal continence and defecation are complex, requiring intact and coordinated neurological and anatomical function. The key components for normal function include colonic absorption and motility, rectal compliance, anorectal sensation, and the multifaceted continence mechanism. Providers must have a sound understanding of normal physiology and pathophysiology to properly treat women with anorectal dysfunction.

Stool Formation and Colonic Transit

The colon transfers fecal material to the rectum via peristaltic contractions mediated by the parasympathetic system. The rate of transfer depends on colonic absorption and regulation of water and electrolytes. Under normal conditions, average flow through the colon is approximately 1.5 to 2 liters per day, with only a fraction of that (100 to 150 mL) excreted. However, the colon is capable of absorbing up to 5 liters of water and electrolytes in 1 day. Stool transit is further delayed at the rectosigmoid, allowing for maximal absorption of water and sodium.

Storage

The accumulation of stool in the rectosigmoid triggers a key reflex known as the **rectoanal inhibitory reflex**. Rectal distention results in a transient decrease in internal anal sphincter tone, followed by an increase in external anal sphincter tone. Relaxation of the internal anal sphincter exposes the sensory receptors of the proximal anal canal near the dentate line with a small sample of fecal matter for the purpose of **sampling**. The sensory nerves assess stool consistency in order to differentiate between solid, liquid, or gas. The rectum is normally compliant and relaxes in response to the increased volume, which is known as **accommodation**. Increased rectal distention stimulates an urge to defecate, which can be voluntarily suppressed through cortical control, resulting in further accommodation and activation of the continence mechanism.

Continence Mechanism

Muscles

The anal canal is roughly 4 cm in length, extending from the anorectal angle to the anal verge. Anal canal pressure must exceed rectal pressure for continence to occur. The three muscles responsible for maintaining adequate anal canal pressure are the puborectalis, internal anal sphincter, and external anal sphincter. The puborectalis forms a U-shaped sling around the genital hiatus. Contraction of the puborectalis muscle pulls the anorectal junction toward its origin at the pubic rami (at the arcus tendineus levator ani), narrowing the genital hiatus and developing the anorectal angle. The angle between the lower rectum and upper anal canal should normally be near 90 degrees and is felt to be the critical component for continence of solid stool. This is substantiated by numerous women that are continent of solid stool despite complete disruption of the internal and external anal sphincter. Several theories have been proposed, but the exact mechanism of continence remains uncertain. Kinking of the rectal lumen is implicated in most theories.

Normal external anal sphincter function is critical for abrupt situations that stress the continence mechanism. In the upper anal canal, the puborectalis muscle fibers blend together with the external anal sphincter, which encircles the anal canal and internal anal sphincter. The external anal sphincter inserts posteriorly to the anococcygeal ligament and anteriorly to the perineal body. The puborectalis and external anal sphincter are striated muscles with predominantly type I (slow twitch) muscle fibers that provide constant tone. Rapid contraction of the type II (fast twitch) muscle fibers respond to sudden increases in intra-abdominal pressure. Consequently, the external anal sphincter is ultimately responsible for preventing incontinence associated with fecal urgency and stress incontinence. The puborectalis and external anal sphincter muscles optimize function through a combination of cognitive control and involuntary spinal reflexes.

The internal anal sphincter contributes the majority of resting tone to the continence mechanism. The inner circular layer of the rectum condenses to form the internal anal sphincter, which is made up of smooth muscle. The internal and external anal sphincters are essential for continence of flatus and liquid stool. However, the internal sphincter maintains the majority of resting tone for the sphincter complex through autonomic reflex arcs and is essential for passive continence. The anal cushions (hemorrhoids) serve as the final anatomic barrier by filling with blood to occlude the anal canal.

Nerves

A basic understanding of the neurophysiology is helpful for recognizing and treating anorectal dysfunction associated with denervation. The internal anal sphincter receives its sympathetic supply from L5, which passes through the pelvic plexus via the hypogastric plexus. The parasympathetic supply from S2–4 synapses at the pelvic plexus, where it joins the sympathetic nerves. The internal

anal sphincter is under autonomic control and acts through reflex arcs at the spinal cord. The puborectalis (levator ani) is innervated by branches of the S2–4 sacral roots and does not receive direct innervation from the pudendal nerve (1). The external anal sphincter is innervated bilaterally by the pudendal nerve (S2–4) via Alcock's canal. The pudendal nerve fibers cross over at the level of the spinal cord, allowing for preservation of external anal sphincter function in the event of unilateral damage. The rich sensory supply from the anal canal travels along the inferior rectal branch of the pudendal nerve.

Coordinated muscular control through afferent and efferent nerve supply of the anal canal and receptors in the levator ani muscles is critical to maintain continence. Proper function of these nerves ensures appropriate involuntary responses such as the rectoanal inhibitory reflex, sampling, and accommodation. Sensory nerves of the anal canal distinguish stool consistency and with the help of levator ani sensory nerves establish the degree of rectal distention. Equally important are the voluntary responses to conditions of fecal urgency and increased intra-abdominal pressure.

Evacuation

Initiation of defecation is normally under cognitive control. As previously discussed, delivery of stool to the rectum activates the rectoanal inhibitory reflex, permitting sampling followed by accommodation. Further rectal distention results in an urge to defecate. Voluntary relaxation of the pelvic floor muscles (puborectalis muscle and external anal sphincter) in conjunction with increased intra-abdominal and intrarectal pressure from Valsalva widens the anorectal angle and shortens the anal canal. These actions, along with the coordinated peristaltic activity of the rectosigmoid, facilitate evacuation. After emptying is completed, the closing reflex is initiated through contraction of the pelvic floor muscles and activation of the continence mechanism.

EPIDEMIOLOGY OF ANORECTAL DYSFUNCTION

The epidemiology of anorectal dysfunction is difficult to define as a single entity and is better analyzed in terms of fecal incontinence and defecatory dysfunction. The incidence and prevalence of fecal incontinence has been estimated, but few have done this for defecatory dysfunction. The following sections describe the epidemiology for both fecal incontinence and defecatory dysfunction.

Subsequent sections will consider the vast array of conditions associated with these symptoms.

Defecatory Dysfunction

The term "defecatory dysfunction" is often used synonymously with the symptom of constipation. When patients complain of constipation, they may be referring to a variety of symptoms, including infrequent stools, dyschezia, straining, variation in stool consistency and caliber, incomplete emptying, bloating, and abdominal pain. Therefore, constipation is an imprecise term, with straining and hard stools being the most common associated complaints (2,3). Many physicians focus on stool frequency and define constipation as infrequent stools, less than three bowel movements per week. This definition originates from stool frequency studies in which 95% of women have greater than three bowel movements per week. Based on this definition, the prevalence of constipation should be 5% (4). However, the prevalence of constipation has been estimated to range from 2% to 28%, depending on the definition applied (5–7).

With such a broad range of estimated prevalence, it is not surprising that constipation disproportionately affects certain members of society. Epidemiological studies indicate that constipation is more prevalent among women and elderly individuals (5–7) nonwhites, and people with low income and low education (5).

Constipation negatively impacts quality of life, and caring for this condition contributes to the tremendous economic burden of the health care industry. Based on an estimated 2.5 million U.S. physician visits per year for constipation (8), with an average cost for evaluation of $2,752 per patient (9), the annual cost for evaluation would be approximately $6.9 billion. This estimate is conservative, and the current cost is probably much greater when we consider inflation and the growing elderly population. Additionally, Sonnenberg and Koch estimated that physicians prescribe medications to treat constipation at 85% of these visits, substantially increasing the overall economic impact (8).

For individuals with constipation, studies have confirmed a detrimental effect on health-related quality of life (3,10). Irvine et al discovered decreased mental and physical subscores on the SF-36 for quality of life in a Canadian population-based survey (10).

Fecal Incontinence

Fecal incontinence is a common condition that is underreported because of social stigmata and a lack of public awareness. Over the past decade, individuals and society as a whole have become more comfortable discussing issues related to urinary incontinence. Patients are more likely to seek treatment for urinary incontinence and physicians are more likely to refer them for evaluation and consultation. Commercials about medical treatments and sanitary products frequent televisions across the country. However, this same trend has not occurred for fecal incontinence. Physicians are unlikely to inquire about fecal incontinence and patients are unlikely to volunteer this information. One population-based study showed that women with severe symptoms were more likely to consult a physician than those with mild or moderate symptoms, yet less than half of those with severe symptoms sought assistance (11). The reported prevalence of fecal incontinence varies between 2% and 3% for community-dwelling persons, 3% and 17% with increased age, and 46% and 54% for nursing home residents (12). Boreham et al recently reported a prevalence of 28% among patients seeking benign gynecologic care (13).

Epidemiological studies of fecal incontinence are compromised by the tremendous social stigmata noted above as well as the lack of a uniform definition. There is debate about whether incontinence of flatus constitutes fecal incontinence. Therefore, definitions vary with respect to the type of material passed (solid, liquid, or gas). There is also a lack of consensus regarding the required frequency and duration of incontinent episodes to qualify as having the condition. Is it sufficient to have one or two lifetime episodes in the remote past, or should there be two a week over the past 3 months? Each study sets a different cutoff for the minimum number of incontinent episodes and the duration of events in order to establish the prevalence of fecal incontinence. Also, some consider a negative impact on quality of life essential to the definition of fecal incontinence. Interestingly, in 2002 the International Continence Society removed impact on quality of life from the definition of urinary incontinence (14).

A large U.S. health survey found age, female sex, physical limitations, and poor general health to be independent risk factors associated with fecal incontinence (15). Another study of identical twin sisters indicated that the major risk factors for female anal incontinence are age, menopause, obesity, parity, and stress urinary incontinence (16). The authors discovered a cumulative and persistent detrimental effect on sphincter function with increasing parity. Women tend to develop this condition at a younger age than men because of birth-related trauma. The difference in prevalence between men and women narrows with increasing age. Although the mechanism by which fecal incontinence rates become similar among elderly men and women is uncertain, decreased nerve function has been implicated. This will be discussed further in the pathophysiology section on fecal incontinence.

Similar to defecatory dysfunction, fecal incontinence carries major psychosocial and economic implications for individuals and society as a whole. The loss of such a basic function can be emotionally devastating, leading to poor self-esteem, depression, social isolation, and decreased quality of life (13,17). Fecal incontinence is the second leading reason for nursing home placement in the United States, even though less than one third of individuals with this condition seek medical attention (13,17). The overall annual cost to treat fecal incontinence is difficult to pinpoint, but it accounts for over $400 million per year in adult diapers alone (17). This estimate does not account for physician visits and evaluation, including diagnostic testing, surgical and nonsurgical treatments, management of complications (e.g., skin breakdown, bacteriuria, vaginitis), loss of productivity from missed work or disability, and time costs of health care providers. Thus, annual costs are likely to be grossly underestimated, considering the multitude of indirect and direct costs.

PATHOPHYSIOLOGY/SYMPTOM-BASED APPROACH TO COLORECTAL DISORDERS

There are numerous medical conditions that cause defecatory dysfunction, fecal incontinence, or combined symptoms. This section discusses the breadth of differential diagnosis and proposes a classification system based on systemic factors, anatomical and structural abnormalities, and functional disorders.

Breadth of Differential Diagnosis

Disordered Defecation

The etiology of defecatory dysfunction has traditionally been divided into systemic disorders and idiopathic constipation by the gastrointestinal community. The term "idiopathic constipation" is a nonspecific term used to describe all nonsystemic causes. In this chapter, idiopathic constipation has been divided into anatomical and structural abnormalities plus functional disorders (Table 20.1).

Systemic disorders are subclassified into metabolic/endocrine, neurological, collagen vascular/

muscular disorders, and medications. Of the most common endocrine factors, diabetes, hypothyroidism, and pregnancy all cause some degree of decreased gastrointestinal motility and intestinal transit. Feldman and Schiller discovered gastrointestinal symptoms in 76% of diabetic patients, including constipation in 60% (18). These symptoms are believed to be the result of decreased bowel motility and a delayed or absent gastrocolic reflex from diabetic intestinal autonomic neuropathy. This enteric neuropathy has also been known to cause gastroparesis and diarrhea. Consequently, diabetes should be considered as both an endocrine and neurological cause of constipation. Pregnancy is grouped with these disorders but should not be considered a disease state. Nevertheless, there is an 11% to 38% prevalence of constipation during pregnancy that is primarily attributed to smooth muscle relaxation from elevated progesterone levels (19).

Neurological systemic factors can be divided into central and peripheral processes. Central processes such as spinal cord lesions, multiple sclerosis, and Parkinson's disease affect the autonomic nervous system. Sacral nerve lesions from meningomyelocele, damage to the lumbosacral spine, and pelvic floor trauma often lead to severe constipation secondary to decreased left-sided colonic motility, decreased rectal tone and sensation, and increased distention (20,21). Higher spinal cord lesions result in delayed sigmoid transit and decreased rectal compliance. Colonic reflexes remain intact in upper motor neuron lesions, and defecation can be initiated by digital stimulation of the anal canal (22,23). The lesions associated with multiple sclerosis can cause absence of the gastrocolic reflex, decreased colonic motility, decreased rectal compliance, and even rectosphincteric dyssynergia (24,25). Constipation in those suffering from multiple sclerosis worsens with the duration of illness and may be compounded by the side effects of medical therapy. Similar findings of rectosphincteric dyssynergia and medication side effects are present in Parkinson's disease.

Defecatory dysfunction from peripheral neurogenic disorders originates at the level of the enteric nerves. Congenital aganglionosis (Hirschsprung's disease) is the classic example because it involves absence of intramural ganglion cells in the submucosal and myenteric plexuses of the rectum. This results in loss of the rectosphincteric inhibitory reflex. Individuals with this illness usually present with functional obstruction and proximal colonic dilation. The majority are diagnosed prior to 6 months of age, although milder cases can be seen later in life.

TABLE 20.1

Causes of Defecatory Dysfunction and Fecal Incontinence

Fecal Incontinence		Defecatory Dysfunction
	SYSTEMIC FACTORS	
	Metabolic/Endocrine	
•	Diabetes mellitus	•
•	Thyroid disease	•
	Hypercalcemia	•
	Hypokalemia	•
	Neurological	
•	*Central Nervous System*	•
	Multiple sclerosis, Parkinson's disease, stroke, tumor, dementia	
•	*Peripheral Nervous System*	•
	Hirschprung's disease, spina bifida, autonomic neuropathy, pudendal neuropathy	
	Infectious	
•	Bacterial, viral, parasitic diarrhea	
	Collagen Vascular/Muscle Disorder	
	Systemic sclerosis, amyloidosis, myotonic dystrophy, dermatomyositis	•
	Idiopathic/Autoimmune	
•	Inflammatory bowel disease	
•	Food allergy	
	Medications	
•	Prescription, over-the-counter	•
	ANATOMICAL/STRUCTURAL ABNORMALITIES	
	Pelvic Outlet Obstruction	
•	Pelvic organ prolapse	•
•	Descending perineum syndrome	•
	Anismus/rectosphincteric dyssynergia	•
•	Intussusception, rectal prolapse	•
	Volvulus	•
•	Neoplasia	•
•	Benign strictures	•
•	Hemorrhoids	•
	Anal Sphincter Disruption/Fistula	
•	Obstetrical trauma	
•	Surgical trauma	
•	Anal intercourse	
•	Injury (trauma, radiation proctitis)	

(continued)

TABLE 20.1 (Continued)

Causes of Defecatory Dysfunction and Fecal Incontinence

Fecal Incontinence		Defecatory Dysfunction
	FUNCTIONAL	
	Motility Disorders	
	Global motility disorder	●
	Colonic inertia/slow transit constipation	●
●	Irritable bowel syndrome	●
	Functional constipation	●
●	Functional diarrhea	
	Functional Limitations	
●	Decreased mobility	●
●	Decreased cognition	●

From Gutman RE, Cundiff GW. Anorectal dysfunction. In: Berek J, ed. *Novak's gynecology,* 14th ed. Chapter 25, table 1. Philadelphia: Lippincott Williams & Wilkins, 2006, with permission.

Other systemic factors to consider are collagen vascular/muscular disorders such as systemic sclerosis, amyloidosis, myotonic dystrophy, and dermatomyositis. Pharmacologic agents are commonly overlooked among the systemic factors. In fact, some of the most commonly used prescription and over-the-counter medications result in defecatory dysfunction, including aluminum antacids, beta blockers, calcium channel blockers, anticholinergics, antidepressants, and opiates (Table 20.2). Lifestyle issues related to inadequate fiber intake and insufficient fluid intake can have similar effects independently or in conjunction with other disorders.

The nonsystemic factors, considered by many to be idiopathic causes, are subdivided into anatomical and structural abnormalities and functional disorders. Anatomical and structural abnormalities refer to the obstructive disorders such as pelvic organ prolapse, perineal descent, intussusception, rectal prolapse, anismus, and tumors. Functional disorders, by default, do not have an identifiable anatomical/structural or systemic etiology. The majority of the functional disorders are motility disorders, including slow transit constipation/colonic inertia, irritable bowel syndrome (IBS; constipation-predominant), and functional constipation. Patients also may have functional limitations of decreased mobility and cognition resulting in constipation. Several of the obstructive

TABLE 20.2

Drugs Associated with Constipation

Over-the-counter medications

Antidiarrheals (loperamide, Kaopectate)

Antacids (with aluminum or calcium)

Iron supplements

Prescription medications

Anticholinergics	**Others**
Antidepressants	Iron
Antipsychotics	Barium sulfate
Antispasmodics	Metallic intoxication
Antiparkinsonian drugs	(arsenic, lead, mercury)
	Opiates
	Nonsteroidal anti-inflammatory agents
Antihypertensives	Anticonvulsants
Calcium channel blockers	Vinca alkaloids
Beta blockers	$5\text{-}HT_3$ antagonists
Diuretics	(ondansetron,
Ganglionic blockers	granisetron)

From Gutman RE, Cundiff GW. Anorectal dysfunction. In: Berek J, ed. *Novak's gynecology,* 14th ed. Chapter 25, table 2. Philadelphia: Lippincott Williams & Wilkins, 2006, with permission.

and motility disorders will be reviewed later in this chapter.

It is important to understand the somewhat arbitrary nature of this classification system. Strict lines of demarcation should be avoided as several of these conditions are interrelated and defecatory dysfunction is often multifactorial.

Fecal Incontinence

Anal continence depends on the complex interaction between cognitive, anatomical, neurological, and physiologic processes. The continence mechanism is capable of compensating for a deficiency in one of these processes. However, even a normal continence mechanism can be overwhelmed if the deficiency is of sufficient severity. Similarly, a stable deficiency may result in fecal incontinence if the basic function of the continence mechanism gradually declines over time. Causes of fecal incontinence will be divided into similar categories of systemic factors, anatomical and structural abnormalities, and functional disorders.

Systemic etiologies of fecal incontinence are subclassified into metabolic/endocrine, neurological, infectious, idiopathic/autoimmune, and medications. Disease states that cause diarrhea represent the majority of systemic factors. The rapid transport of large volumes of liquid stool to the rectum can produce urgency and incontinence even in healthy individuals (26). Diabetes mellitus and hyperthyroidism are endocrine factors that can lead to fecal incontinence. In diabetics, diarrhea can develop from autonomic dysfunction, bacterial overgrowth, pancreatic insufficiency, and sugar substitutes causing osmotic diarrhea. Infectious diarrhea caused by bacteria (e.g., *Clostridium, Escherichia coli, Salmonella, Shigella, Yersinia, Campylobacter*), viruses (e.g., Rotavirus, Norwalk, HIV), and parasites (e.g., Entamoeba, Giardia, Cryptosporidium, Ascaris) frequently results in fecal incontinence. Inflammatory bowel disease and food allergies are considered idiopathic/autoimmune factors. Ulcerative colitis and Crohn's disease cause fecal incontinence during exacerbations with bouts of bloody diarrhea. Inflammatory bowel disease is also associated with structural abnormalities like anal fissures, fistulas, abscesses, and operative complications that lead to fecal incontinence. Numerous drugs and dietary items such as laxatives, magnesium antacids, diuretics, prostaglandins, and sugar and fat substitutes cause diarrhea and fecal incontinence (Table 20.3).

As with defecatory dysfunction, neurological etiologies of fecal incontinence are divided into central and peripheral disorders. Among the cen-

TABLE 20.3

Drugs and Dietary Items Associated with Diarrhea

Over-the-counter medications

Laxatives

Antacids (with magnesium)

Prescription medications

Laxatives	Chemotherapy
Diuretics	Colchicine
Thyroid preparations	Cholestyramine
Cholinergics	Neomycin
Prostaglandins	Para-aminosalicylic acid

Dietary items

Dietetic foods, candy or chewing gum, and elixirs with sorbitol, mannitol, or xylitol

Olestra

Caffeine

Ethanol

Monosodium glutamate

From Gutman RE, Cundiff GW. Anorectal dysfunction. In: Berek J, ed. *Novak's gynecology*, 14th ed. Chapter 25, table 3. Philadelphia: Lippincott Williams & Wilkins, 2006, with permission.

tral nervous system disorders, upper motor neuron lesions above the level of the defecation center (located in the sacral cord) cause spastic bowel dysfunction. Impaired cognitive control and sensory deficits occur with disrupted cortical communication. The anal sphincter spastically contracts, but digital stimulation initiates reflex evacuation. Head trauma, neoplasms, and cerebrovascular accidents that damage portions of the frontal lobe result in loss of control of both micturition and defecation. Greater loss of inhibition is observed with lesions in the anterior frontal lobe. Spinal cord trauma and lower motor neuron lesions above the defecation center sever cortical control more permanently. "Spinal shock" occurs for 2 to 4 weeks following spinal cord injury, during which there is a temporary loss of reflexes below the level of the lesion, flaccid bowel function, constipation, and fecal impaction. After the early "shock" phase, spastic paralysis ensues, with hyperactive bowel function. Digital stimulation in conjunction with the gastrocolic reflex initiates reflex evacuation in the absence of cortical inhibition. Fortunately, internal anal sphincter tone is maintained despite the loss of external anal sphincter control for stress and urge situations. Individuals with spinal cord disruption often present with both constipation and fecal incontinence symptoms.

The demyelination of multiple sclerosis is randomly distributed, with lesions occurring at any level of the central nervous system. Somatic disruption transpires similar to spinal cord injury. However, there is additional autonomic dysfunction with multiple sclerosis, leading to decreased colonic motility, absence of the gastrocolic reflex, and even rectosphincteric dyssynergia. In disorders of cognitive impairment (dementia), fecal incontinence frequently results from overflow incontinence. Many nursing home residents have intact sensory nerve function but lack the cognitive ability required to initiate defecation in response to rectal distention or to defer defecation until a socially acceptable time. This results in constipation, fecal impaction, and overflow incontinence.

Lower motor neuron lesions occurring at or below the level of the defecation center in the sacral cord produce flaccid bowel dysfunction. Tumor or trauma to the cauda equina, tabes dorsalis, spina bifida, and peripheral neuropathy all cause lesions at this level, disrupting cortical communication and resulting in impaired cognitive control and sensory deficit. Bowel reflexes that require intact sacral nerve pathways are interrupted, as evidenced by absent bulbocavernosus and anal reflexes on examination. Consequently, digital stimulation does not help to initiate defecation. The anal sphincter is flaccid and fecal retention with overflow incontinence usually occurs. Digital disimpaction and Valsalva are often required for evacuation, and medications tend to work poorly.

As previously discussed, the classic example of peripheral neuropathy is congenital aganglionosis (Hirschsprung's disease), and the most common peripheral neuropathy occurs with diabetes. Approximately 20% of diabetics will have fecal incontinence (27). The cause tends to be multifactorial, with the exact mechanism uncertain. Fecal incontinence can occur with diabetic diarrhea or years later from progressive disease. Diabetics frequently experience intestinal autonomic neuropathy, an abnormal gastrocolic reflex, and chronic constipation. The subsequent pelvic floor denervation causes fecal incontinence by sensory neuropathy, failure of the rectoanal inhibitory reflex, and sphincter dysfunction (28). Therefore, individuals with any type of peripheral neuropathy may develop fecal incontinence because of defective sampling, disrupted rectoanal inhibitory reflex, and/or pudendal neuropathy with sphincter dysfunction. Presenting symptoms may include stress, urge, and overflow incontinence.

Obstetrical and surgical trauma accounts for the majority of anatomical and structural causes of fecal incontinence. The severity of symptoms depends on damage to or dysfunction of the internal anal sphincter, external anal sphincter, and puborectalis muscles. Impaired resting tone from a defective internal anal sphincter results in passive incontinence (incontinence at rest), which is worse during sleep because of decreased external anal sphincter activity (29). External anal sphincter dysfunction limits the ability to respond to sudden increases in rectal pressure and to suppress defecation, resulting in symptoms of urge and stress incontinence. Incontinence of liquid stool is often seen with external and internal sphincter dysfunction, whereas incontinence of solid stool is usually seen with widening of the anorectal angle from damage to the puborectalis muscle. Damage to the anal cushions usually causes only minor soiling or staining. Other anatomical and structural abnormalities associated with fecal incontinence include obstructive disorders such as pelvic organ prolapse, descending perineum syndrome, anismus, and intussusception; fistulas from diverticulitis, inflammatory bowel disease, cancer, or surgical trauma; and decreased rectal compliance from inflammatory bowel disease, cancer, and radiation. Decreased compliance results in higher intraluminal rectal pressures with smaller volumes of stool, poor storage capacity, urgency, and incontinence (30).

Functional disorders associated with fecal incontinence include IBS (diarrhea variant), functional diarrhea, decreased mobility, and decreased cognition.

Combined Disorders of Defecation and Fecal Incontinence

Several of these conditions have the potential to cause both defecatory dysfunction and fecal incontinence (see Table 20.1). This was apparent during the previous discussion reviewing systemic factors (metabolic/endocrine and neurological), anatomical/structural abnormalities (pelvic outlet obstruction), and functional disorders (motility disorders and functional limitations). The majority of these disorders cause combined symptoms through the development of fecal impaction followed by overflow incontinence. The etiology of these symptoms is often multifactorial in nature.

STRUCTURAL VERSUS FUNCTIONAL DISORDERS

The following sections emphasize important anatomical/structural abnormalities and functional motility disorders associated with defecatory dysfunction and fecal incontinence. An understanding of these conditions is highly relevant to those caring for pelvic floor dysfunction. Appropriate evaluation and treatment of several of these conditions will be covered in subsequent chapters.

Disordered Defecation

Outlet Obstruction

Anismus/Rectosphincteric Dyssynergia

Anismus is an obstructive disorder where the puborectalis and external anal sphincter paradoxically contract during defecation, narrowing the anorectal angle. This condition is also commonly referred to as rectosphincteric dyssynergia, pelvic floor dyssynergia, spastic floor syndrome, and paradoxical puborectalis syndrome. Frequent complaints include dyschezia, straining, hard stools, incomplete emptying, and tenesmus (31). A prospective study evaluating 120 consecutive patients with dyssynergic defecation found that approximately half needed digital assistance (digital disimpaction or splinting) to evacuate the rectum (32). The population contained 77% women, supporting the results of other studies that have found a higher prevalence of anismus in women (33). Psychosocial factors such as a history of sexual abuse, depression, eating disorder, obsessive–compulsive disorder, and stress have been implicated in the pathogenesis of this disease. The authors reported a history of sexual abuse in 22% and a history of physical abuse in 31%. Other precipitating factors observed included illness in 15%, surgery in 9%, and pregnancy or childbirth in 5% of the women. Other studies have suggested an even higher prevalence following gynecologic surgery (33). One third believed the problem began during childhood, and anismus should be considered when young children present with symptoms of constipation and dyschezia. The response to biofeedback and pelvic floor physical therapy as well as the above patient characteristics indicate a learned response mechanism.

Pelvic Organ Prolapse

Pelvic organ prolapse is a common condition that will be covered in depth in Section IV, Disorders of Pelvic Support. The following provides a brief assessment of the relationship between prolapse and anorectal dysfunction. Prolapse is inconsistently associated with defecatory dysfunction and many women with prolapse are asymptomatic. Those with symptomatic prolapse may complain of incomplete evacuation, straining, digital disimpaction, and splinting (the need to apply digital pressure to the posterior vaginal wall or perineum to aid in evacuation of stool). Prolapse may also be the result of chronic constipation, straining, and increased intra-abdominal pressure. Therefore, it is important to consider other systemic, anatomical, and functional motility disorders in order to optimize treatment outcomes. Defecatory dysfunction that is associated with pelvic organ prolapse can occur because of rectocele, enterocele, or perineal descent either individually or in combination.

The term *rectocele* refers to posterior vaginal wall prolapse with herniation of the rectal mucosa through a defect in the rectovaginal septum. These site-specific defects can be transverse or longitudinal through the inferior, middle, or superior regions of the rectovaginal septum (34). *Enterocele* is a herniation of a peritoneal sac and bowel through the pelvic floor, typically between the uterus/vaginal cuff and rectum. There are two theories surrounding enterocele formation. The first implicates a defect in the fibromuscular endopelvic fascia of the vagina allowing peritoneum and bowel to herniate, while the second attributes its formation to a support defect permitting full-thickness protrusion of peritoneum, bowel, and endopelvic fascia (35). Ultimately, the mechanism might be a combination of these theories, because some support defects are secondary to superior breaks in the rectovaginal and pubocervical fascia. Enteroceles are more common following hysterectomy and retropubic urethropexy. Women with rectoceles and enteroceles report similar symptoms, including pelvic pain, pressure, vaginal protrusion, obstipation, fecal incontinence, and sexual dysfunction. Although associations have been made between defecatory dysfunction and advanced stages of pelvic organ prolapse, a causal relationship remains to be established. Controversy remains as to whether anatomic herniation is the cause of these symptoms or the effect of underlying colonic dysfunction, chronic constipation, and straining.

Descending perineum syndrome is defined as descent of the perineum (at the level of the anal verge) beyond the ischial tuberosities during Valsalva. Excessive perineal descent was first described in the colorectal literature by Parks and Hardcastle in 1966 (36,37). It occurs due to inferior detachment of the rectovaginal septum from the perineal body. With disease progression, the pudendal nerve stretches and pudendal neuropathy can develop. Perineal descent has been associated with a variety of bowel symptoms, and findings including constipation, fecal incontinence, rectal pain, solitary rectal ulcer, rectocele, and enterocele (38).

Rectal Intussusception

Rectal intussusception or intrarectal prolapse is the circumferential prolapse of the upper rectal wall into the rectal ampulla but not through the anal verge. It is more common in women and typically presents in the fourth and fifth decade. The most common symptoms include incomplete emptying, digital disimpaction, splinting, dyschezia, and rectal bleeding. Bleeding often originates from a solitary rectal ulcer or localized proctitis of the involved bowel segment (39). A recent study of 896 patients referred to a tertiary care center for the assessment of anorectal dysfunction suggests that the only two symptoms, anorectal pain and prolapse (protrusion downward into the rectum or anal canal), were highly predictive of isolated intussusception on evacuation proctography compared to those with combined intussusception and rectocele as well as those with rectocele alone (40). The anatomical disruption of normal physiologic function may result in fecal incontinence, decreased urge to defecate, inability to perform sampling, and pruritus ani from mucous discharge. Intussusception is present in up to one third of women with clinical rectoceles and defecatory dysfunction symptoms of constipation, incomplete emptying with or without fecal incontinence, straining, and splinting (41). However, a small study involving 21 asymptomatic patients found six (29%) cases of intussusception (42). The high prevalence among asymptomatic patients has been confirmed by others (43). Furthermore, the risk of disease progression into total rectal prolapse is minimal, approximately 2% to 3% (44). These findings raise important questions about the association between intussusception and defecatory dysfunction as well as the factors that guide surgical intervention for this condition.

Functional Motility Disorders

Colonic Inertia/Slow Transit Constipation

Severe constipation with less than three stools per week that is refractory to therapy is relatively rare, and health care providers should have a high suspicion for motility disorders such as *global motility disorder* and *colonic inertia* in these individuals. Colonic inertia or slow transit constipation is defined as the delayed passage of radiopaque markers through the proximal colon without retropulsion of markers from the left colon, and absence of systemic or obstructive disorders. Defecatory symptoms are indistinguishable from other obstructive and functional motility disorders. Therefore, imaging studies are required to make the diagnosis. The etiology remains unclear, and women are more commonly affected than men.

Studies have revealed impaired phasic colonic motor activity and diminished gastrocolic reflexes in patients with this disorder (45,46). Laxatives, absorption irregularities, hormones, psychological abnormalities, and endogenous opioids have been implicated in the pathogenesis but the data is inconclusive. Current literature supports a possible neurological and/or smooth muscle disorder as the underlying pathophysiologic mechanism of disease (46,47).

Functional Bowel Disorders

Functional bowel disorders, as defined by the Rome II criteria (48), consist of IBS, functional abdominal bloating, functional constipation, functional diarrhea, and unspecified functional bowel disorders. The primary focus will be on IBS because it is the most prevalent of these disorders.

The prevalence of *IBS* appears to be around 10%; however, estimates range between 3% and 25% (49). IBS sufferers frequently seek health care, and this condition accounts for 25% to 50% of all referrals to gastrointestinal clinics (48). IBS seems to be more common among women and younger individuals. Distinct diagnostic criteria have been developed that require the exclusion of structural or metabolic abnormalities. The Rome II criteria allow for classification of IBS into diarrhea-, constipation- and pain-predominant categories (Table 20.4). The constipation variant is most commonly associated with defecatory dysfunction, whereas the diarrhea variant causes fecal incontinence. The pain or spastic variant causes predominantly abdominal discomfort but can also be associated with both defecatory dysfunction and fecal incontinence. After excluding organic disease, the criteria listed in Table 20.4 have a sensitivity of 65%, specificity of 100%, positive predictive value of 100%, and negative predictive value of 76% (50).

Individuals with IBS often have comorbidity with other gastrointestinal, genitourinary, and psychological illnesses such as gastroesophageal reflux disease, fibromyalgia, chronic fatigue syndrome, headache, backache, chronic pelvic pain, sexual dysfunction, lower urinary tract dysfunction, depression, and anxiety (48,51). Stressful life events seem to correlate with the onset and exacerbation of symptoms. A detailed history frequently reveals past physical or sexual abuse (48). Abdominal pain is the most common complaint, and patients with IBS are at increased risk for potentially unnecessary surgery. A recent analysis of questionnaires from a large health care provider including over 89,000 patients reported significantly higher rates of cholecystectomy (12% vs. 4%), appendectomy (21% vs. 12%), hysterectomy

TABLE 20.4

Diagnostic Criteria of Irritable Bowel Syndrome

At least 12 weeks, which need not be consecutive, in the preceding 12 months of abdominal discomfort or pain that has two out of three features:
(1) Relieved with defecation; and/or
(2) Onset associated with a change in frequency of stool; and/or
(3) Onset associated with a change in form (appearance) of stool.

In the absence of structural or metabolic abnormalities to explain the symptoms.

Supportive Symptoms of IBS
(1) Fewer than three bowel movements a week
(2) More than three bowel movements a day
(3) Hard or lumpy stools
(4) Loose (mushy) or watery stools
(5) Straining during a bowel movement
(6) Urgency (having to rush to have a bowel movement)
(7) Feeling of incomplete bowel movement
(8) Passing mucus (white material) during a bowel movement
(9) Abdominal fullness, bloating, or swelling.

Diarrhea-predominant: 1 or more of 2, 4, or 6 and none of 1, 3, or 5; or: 2 or more of 2, 4, or 6 and one of 1 or 5. (3. Hard or lumpy stools do not qualify.)

Constipation-predominant: 1 or more of 1, 3, 5 and none of 2, 4, or 6; or: 2 or more of 1, 3, or 5 and one of 2, 4, or 6.

From Thompson WG, Longstreth GF, Drossman DA, et al. Functional bowel disorders and functional abdominal pain. In: McLean, ed. *Rome II: the functional gastrointestinal disorders,* 2nd ed. VA: Degnon Associates, 2000:351–432.

(33% vs. 17%), and back surgery (4% vs. 3%) in patients with IBS compared to controls (52). Despite abundant research evaluating cognitive, behavioral, psychological, genetic, dietary, and infectious mechanisms of disease, a single factor has not been identified, and multiple factors probably contribute to this condition. Many believe this to be disordered motility and sensory dysfunction from enteric neuropathy, but data has not substantiated these claims.

Functional constipation is a term created by the Rome II criteria as a unifying definition of constipation (Table 20.5). The rationale for the criteria listed in Table 20.5 stems from the variability in patient definitions of constipation (48).

Fecal Incontinence

Sphincter Disruption

Obstetrical injury is responsible for the majority of fecal incontinence in young females. Birth trauma associated with fecal incontinence results from anatomical disruption of the anal sphincter complex, pelvic floor denervation, or a combination of the two. The risk factors for anal sphincter laceration are primiparity (53,54), birth weight (53–55), forceps delivery (53–56), and episiotomy (54–56). Although there are limited long-term prospective studies demonstrating the progression of anal sphincter injury and pelvic floor neuropathy to the development of fecal incontinence, current literature supports the relationship of early-onset symptoms to sphincter damage and delayed-onset symptoms to neuropathy (57). This accounts for the large discrepancy in the prevalence of fecal incontinence between younger men and women from the effects of obstetrical sphincter trauma. The gender gap narrows with aging secondary to neuropathy, which may stem from a variety of causes (58).

TABLE 20.5

Diagnostic Criteria of Functional Constipation

At least 12 weeks, which need not be consecutive, in the preceding 12 months of two or more of:
(1) Straining >1/4 of defecations;
(2) Lumpy or hard stools >1/4 of defecations;
(3) Sensation of incomplete evacuation >1/4 of defecations;
(4) Sensation of anorectal obstruction/blockage >1/4 of defecations;
(5) Manual maneuvers to facilitate >1/4 of defecations (e.g., digital evacuation, support of the pelvic floor); and/or
(6) <3 defecations per week.

Loose stools are not present, and there are insufficient criteria for IBS.

From Thompson WG, Longstreth GF, Drossman DA, et al. Functional bowel disorders and functional abdominal pain. In: McLean, ed. *Rome II: the functional gastrointestinal disorders,* 2nd ed. VA: Degnon Associates, 2000:351–432.

Obstetrical Trauma

Third- and fourth-degree lacerations at delivery are associated with an increased risk of fecal incontinence (odds ratio 3.09) (57). While the incidence of clinically documented third- and fourth-degree anal sphincter tears is between 0.5% and 5.9% (53,56,59), occult third- and fourth-degree defects are present in 28% to 35% of primiparous women and 44% of multiparous women, with approximately one third of these patients having symptoms of anal incontinence. Patients with occult anal sphincter tears were 8.8 times more likely to have fecal incontinence (56,60). Sultan et al (61) also found that half of patients who underwent immediate repair of a third-degree laceration had symptoms of anal incontinence, and 85% had persistent sphincter defects on endoanal ultrasound. A meta-analysis of five studies with 717 deliveries confirmed these findings, with a 26.9% incidence of anal sphincter defect in primiparous women and an 8.5% incidence of new sphincter defect in multiparous women (62). The probability of postpartum fecal incontinence due to a sphincter defect was high, at 77% to 83%.

The magnitude of these findings is alarming and the results cannot be ignored but must be interpreted with caution. Misinterpretation of the normal physiological split of the proximal external anal sphincter merging with the puborectalis muscle as a sphincter tear can result in an increased prevalence of reported defects. Nevertheless, the high prevalence of persistent defects following repair and the increased risk of fecal incontinence symptoms associated with these defects indicates the permanent and detrimental effects of obstetrical sphincter trauma and a need to focus on prevention. A recent prospective study also discovered a higher rate of bowel symptoms with fourth-degree lacerations compared to third-degree lacerations (63). Those with fourth-degree tears were more likely to have persistent combined defects of the internal and external anal sphincter on ultrasound. These findings emphasize the importance of the internal anal sphincter for maintaining continence.

Specific obstetrical factors have been identified that increase the risk of sphincter laceration, including primiparity (53,54), birth weight (53–55), forceps delivery (53–56), and episiotomy (54–56), as noted above. Forceps-assisted vaginal delivery significantly increases the risk of sphincter trauma, but the data on vacuum-assisted delivery is less conclusive (55,64,65). Some have hypothesized that elective cesarean section prevents anal incontinence compared to emergent cesarean section; however, studies argue against any protective effect with cesarean section irrespective of timing (56,64,66,67). Midline episiotomy is strongly linked to sphincter damage (55) and fecal incontinence (55,68). Handa et al reported conflicting results, with an overall protective effect seen with episiotomy (odd ratio 0.89) in their large population study. There was an increased likelihood of fourth-degree laceration (odds ratio 1.12) and a decreased likelihood of third-degree laceration (odds ratio 0.81) (53). A Cochrane review supports restricting the use of both midline and mediolateral episiotomy (69). A recent retrospective study found an approximately 50% reduction in anal sphincter laceration rate with the use of restrictive episiotomy (54).

Surgical Trauma

Iatrogenic injury is the second most common cause of direct sphincter damage, behind obstetrical trauma. Surgical procedures associated with fecal incontinence include anal fistula repair, anal sphincterotomy, hemorrhoidectomy, and anal dilation. Of these procedures, fistulotomy is the most common cause of sphincter damage and fecal incontinence. Rectovaginal or anovaginal fistulas can develop from obstetrical injury, operative complications during pelvic surgery, inflammatory bowel disease exacerbations, rectal cancers, and spontaneously without an identifiable etiology. Fistulas cause fecal incontinence as stool escapes through the path of least resistance. The degree of postoperative dysfunction following repair depends on preoperative sphincter function and pudendal nerve function as well as the location of the fistula and the amount of sphincter that is disrupted during the surgical repair. Anal sphincterotomy to treat painful anal fissures can lead to incontinence by disruption of rectal sensory innervation, anal cushions, and transection of the anal sphincter (70,71). Hemorrhoidectomy often results in minor soiling due to resection of the anal cushions, which act as the final mucosal barrier. Similar to sphincterotomy, rectal sensory innervation can be disrupted, and there can also be injury to the internal sphincter during sharp dissection (71,72).

Sphincter Denervation

Idiopathic (primary neurogenic) fecal incontinence results from denervation of both the anal sphincter and pelvic floor muscles. Denervation injury related to obstetrical trauma accounts for approximately three out of every four cases of idiopathic fecal incontinence and is the most common overall cause of fecal incontinence (73,74).

Obstetrical Trauma

The two proposed mechanisms of pudendal neuropathy are stretch injury during the second stage of labor and compression of the nerve as it exits Alcock's canal (73,75). Established risk factors for pelvic floor neuropathy include multiparity (76), birth weight, forceps delivery, prolonged active second stage, and third-degree laceration (77). Several studies have shown increased pudendal nerve terminal motor latencies following vaginal delivery, especially after sphincter laceration (56,74,78). The majority of women will recover function within a few months postpartum, while others will have evidence of injury several years out, the effects of which may be cumulative with subsequent deliveries (74,79). However, only a fraction of these patients with neuropathy will develop fecal incontinence (77). The reason for the low predictive value of neuropathy toward the development of fecal incontinence is uncertain, but one theory suggests that intact anatomical and physiologic function compensates for the neurological deficit. Those who develop fecal incontinence may have additional dysfunction that overwhelms the continence mechanism.

Descending Perineum Syndrome

As noted earlier, prolonged straining for any reason can cause descending perineum syndrome. This syndrome is defined as descent of the perineum beyond the ischial tuberosities during Valsalva (36,37). Pudendal neuropathy results from stretching and entrapment of the pudendal nerve. This is supported by findings of elongation of the pudendal nerve, prolonged pudendal nerve motor terminal latency, and decreased anal sensation in women with perineal descent (80–82). The progression of the pudendal neuropathy ultimately leads to fecal incontinence (38,83).

Functional Bowel Disorders

IBS epidemiology and pathophysiology have been previously discussed with respect to disordered defecation. The diarrhea variant of IBS is often associated with fecal incontinence. Increased bowel motility, decreased transit time, and resultant fecal urgency can overwhelm a normal continence mechanism. The criteria for diagnosis are in Table 20.4.

Functional diarrhea is defined by the Rome II criteria in order to create a unifying definition of diarrhea (Table 20.6). The rationale for the criteria listed in Table 20.6 stems from the variability in patient definition of diarrhea (48).

SUMMARY

In conclusion, the physiology of anorectal function, including anal continence and defecation, is complex, requiring intact neurological and anatomical function. The pathophysiology of

TABLE 20.6

Diagnostic Criteria of Functional Diarrhea

At least 12 weeks, which need not be consecutive, in the preceding 12 months of:

(1) Loose (mushy) or watery stools;

(2) Present >3/4 of the time; and

(3) No abdominal pain.

From Thompson WG, Longstreth GF, Drossman DA, et al. Functional bowel disorders and functional abdominal pain. In: McLean, ed. *Rome II: the functional gastrointestinal disorders,* 2nd ed. VA: Degnon Associates, 2000:351–432.

anorectal dysfunction consists of many disorders that may lead to defecatory dysfunction, fecal incontinence, or a combination of the two. Specialists in the field of pelvic floor dysfunction must strive to gain a better understanding of the various etiologies underlying these disorders. We must have a systematic and logical approach to evaluating patients with these complaints and remain current in our diagnostic criteria and modalities. We should approach patients with anorectal dysfunction by considering general categories such as systemic factors, anatomical and structural abnormalities, and functional (motility) disorders.

Important pitfalls for reconstructive pelvic surgeons to consider involve malignancy and pelvic organ prolapse. Care must be taken not to overlook or misinterpret signs and symptoms of anorectal dysfunction, and any acute change in bowel habits must be thoroughly evaluated. Malignancy must be ruled out even in the presence of chronic disease. Persistent symptoms after an empiric trial of medical therapy should prompt further evaluation such as a colonoscopy or flexible sigmoidoscopy. Care should also be taken when attempting to determine if prolapse is the cause or the result of defecatory dysfunction. This can be extremely challenging but is important because surgical correction of defecatory dysfunction mistakenly attributed to prolapse will have little lasting benefit if the underlying bowel disorder remains untreated.

Equally important is the need for further research into both defecatory dysfunction and fecal incontinence. For example, advances in genetics may someday explain the wide overlap of symptoms in functional gastrointestinal disorders. Further advances in gastrointestinal evaluation and pelvic floor imaging may improve our understanding of pelvic floor anatomy and sensorimotor dysfunction. This chapter provides a foundation for understanding the complex nature of anorectal physiology and pathophysiology. The symptoms of constipation and fecal incontinence are nonspecific and underlying etiologies are often multifactorial. The specialist dealing with pelvic floor dysfunction should be able to formulate a differential diagnosis that can be further evaluated and treated according to the principles discussed in the following chapters.

REFERENCES

1. Barber MD, Bremer RE, Thor KB, et al. Innervation of the female levator ani muscles. *Am J Obstet Gynecol* 2002;187:64–71.
2. Harari D, Gurwitz JH, Avorn J, et al. How do older persons define constipation? Implications for therapeutic management. *J Gen Intern Med* 1997;12:63–66.
3. Glia A, Lindberg G. Quality of life in patients with different types of functional constipation. *Scand J Gastroenterol* 1997;32:1083–1089.
4. Cundiff GW, Nygaard I, Bland DR, et al. Proceedings of the American Urogynecologic Society Multidiscipinary Symposium on Defecatory Disorders. *Am J Obstet Gynecol* 2000;182:S1–10.
5. Higgins PD, Johanson JF. Epidemiology of constipation in North America: a systematic review. *Am J Gastroenterol* 2004;99:750–759.
6. Sonnenberg A, Koch TR. Epidemiology of constipation in the United States. *Dis Colon Rectum* 1989;32:1–8.
7. Drossman DA, Li Z, Andruzzi E, et al. U.S. household survey of functional gastrointestinal disorders: prevalence, sociodemography, and health impact. *Dig Dis Sci* 1993;38:1569–1580.
8. Sonnenberg A, Koch TR. Physician visits in the United States for constipation: 1958 to 1986. *Dig Dis Sci* 1989;34:606–611.
9. Rantis PC Jr, Vernava AM 3rd, Daniel GL, et al. Chronic constipation: is the work-up worth the cost? *Dis Colon Rectum* 1997;40:280–286.
10. Irvine EJ, Ferrazzi S, Pare P, et al. Health-related quality of life in functional GI disorders: focus on constipation and resource utilization. *Am J Gastroenterol* 2002;97:1986–1993.
11. Bharucha AE, Zinsmeister AR, Locke GR, et al. Prevalence and burden of fecal incontinence: a population-based study in women. *Gastroenterology* 2005;129:42–49.
12. Nelson RL. Epidemiology of fecal incontinence. *Gastroenterology* 2004;126:S3–S7.
13. Boreham MK, Richter HE, Kenton KS, et al. Anal incontinence in women presenting for gynecologic care: Prevalence, risk factors, and impact upon quality of life. Am J Obstet Gynecol 2005;192:1637–1642.
14. Abrams P, Cardozo L, Fall M, et al. The standardization of terminology of lower urinary tract function: report from the Standardization Subcommittee of the International Continence Society. *Am J Obstet Gynecol* 2002;187:116–126.
15. Nelson R, Norton N, Cautley E, et al. Community-based prevalence of anal incontinence. *JAMA* 1995; 274:559–561.
16. Abramov Y, Sand PK, Botros SM, et al. Risk factors for female anal incontinence: new insight through the Evanston-Northwestern Twin Sisters Study. *Obstet Gynecol* 2005;106:726–732.
17. Johanson JF, Lafferty J. Epidemiology of fecal incontinence: the silent affliction. *Am J Gastroenterol* 1996;91:33–36.
18. Feldman M, Schiller LR. Disorders of gastrointestinal motility associated with diabetes mellitus. *Ann Intern Med* 1983;98:378–384.
19. Jewell DJ, Younge G. Interventions for treating constipation in pregnancy. *Cochrane Database Syst Rev* 2001;(2):CD001142.
20. Devroede G, Lamarche J. Functional importance of extrinsic parasympathetic innervation to the distal colon and rectum in man. *Gastroenterology* 1974;66:273–280.
21. Devroede G, Arhan P, Duguay C et al. Traumatic constipation. *Gastroenterology* 1979;77:1258–1267.
22. Read NW, Timms JM. Defecation and the pathophysiology of constipation. *Clin Gastroenterol* 1986;15:937–965.
23. Glick ME, Meshkinpour H, Haldeman S, et al. Colonic dysfunction in patients with thoracic spinal cord injury. *Gastroenterology* 1984;86:287–294.
24. Weber J, Grise P, Roquebert M, et al. Radiopaque markers transit and anorectal manometry in 16 patients with multiple sclerosis and urinary bladder dysfunction. *Dis Colon Rectum* 1987;30:95–100.
25. Glick ME, Meshkinpour H, Haldeman S, et al. Colonic dysfunction in multiple sclerosis. *Gastroenterology* 1982;83:1002–1007.
26. Barnett JL. Anorectal diseases. In: Yamada T, ed. *Textbook of Gastroenterology*, 3rd ed. Philadelphia: Lippincott Williams & Wilkins, 1999.
27. Wald A, Tunuguntla AK. Anorectal sensorimotor dysfunction in fecal incontinence and diabetes mellitus: Modification with biofeedback therapy. *N Engl J Med* 1984;310:1282–1287.
28. Schiller LR, Santa Ana CA, Schumulen AC, et al. Pathogenesis of fecal incontinence in diabetes mellitus: Evidence for internal-anal-sphincter dysfunction. *N Engl J Med* 1982;307:1666–1671.
29. Harris RL, Cundiff GW. Anal incontinence. *Postgrad Obstet Gynecol* 1997;17:1–6.
30. Ihre T. Studies on anal function in continent and incontinent patients. *Scand J Gastroenterol* 1974;9:1–80.
31. Rao SS. Dyssynergic defecation. *Gastroenterol Clin North Am* 2001;30:97–114.
32. Rao SS, Tuteja AK, Vellema T, et al. Dyssynergic defecation: demographics, symptoms, stool patterns, and quality of life. *J Clin Gastroenterol* 2004;38:680–685.
33. Talley NJ, Weaver AL, Zinsmeister AR, et al. Functional constipation and outlet delay: A population-based study. *Gastroenterology* 1993;105:781–790.
34. Richardson AC. The rectovaginal septum revisited: its relationship to rectocele and its importance in rectocele repair. *Clin Obstet Gynecol* 1993;36:976–982.
35. Tulikangas PK, Walters MD, Brainard JA, et al. Enterocele: Is there a histologic defect? *Obstet Gynecol* 2001;98:634–637.
36. Parks AG, Porter NH, Hardcastle J. The syndrome of the descending perineum. *Proc R Soc Med* 1966;59:477–482.
37. Henry MM, Parks AG, Swash M. The pelvic floor musculature in the descending perineum syndrome. *Br J Surg* 1982;69:470–472.
38. Cundiff GW, Harris RL, Coates K, et al. Abdominal sacral colpoperineopexy: A new approach for correction of posterior compartment defects and perineal descent

associated with vaginal vault prolapse. *Am J Obstet Gynecol* 1997;177:1345–1355.

39. Ihre T. Intussusception of the rectum and the solitary ulcer syndrome. *Ann Med* 1990;22:419–423.

40. Dvorkin LS, Knowles CH, Scott SM, et al. Rectal intussusception: characterization of symptomatology. *Dis Colon Rectum* 2005;48:824–831.

41. Thompson JR, Chen AH, Pettit PD, et al. Incidence of occult rectal prolapse in patients with clinical rectoceles and defecatory dysfunction. *Am J Obstet Gynecol* 2002;187:1494–1500.

42. Freimanis MG, Wald A, Caruana B, et al. Evacuation proctography in normal volunteers. *Invest Radiol* 1991;26:581–585.

43. Dvorkin LS, Gladman MA, Epstein J, et al. Rectal intussusception in symptomatic patients is different from that in asymptomatic volunteers. *Br J Surg* 2005;92: 866–872.

44. Mellgren A, Schultz I, Johansson C, et al. Internal rectal intussusception seldom develops into total rectal prolapse. *Dis Colon Rectum* 1997;40:817–820.

45. Bassotti G, Imbimbo B, Betti C, et al. Impaired colonic motor response to eating in patients with slow-transit constipation. *Am J Gastroenterol* 1992;87:504–508.

46. Rao SS. Constipation: evaluation and treatment. *Gastroenterol Clin North Am* 2003;32:659–683.

47. Knowles CH, Martin JE. Slow-transit constipation: a model of human gut dysmotility. Review of possible etiologies. *Neurogastroenterol Mot* 2000;12:181–196.

48. Thompson WG, Longstreth GF, Drossman DA, et al. Functional bowel disorders and functional abdominal pain. In: McLean, ed. *Rome II: The Functional Gastrointestinal Disorders,* 2nd ed. VA: Degnon Associates, 2000:351–432.

49. Cremonini F, Talley NJ. Irritable bowel syndrome: epidemiology, natural history, health care seeking, and emerging risk factors. *Gastroenterol Clin North Am* 2005;34:189–204.

50. Vanner SJ, Depew WT, Paterson WG, et al. Predictive value of the Rome criteria for diagnosing the irritable bowel syndrome. *Am J Gastroenterol* 1999;94:2912–2917.

51. Whitehead WE, Palsson O, Jones KR. Systemic review of the comorbidity of irritable bowel syndrome with other disorders: what are the causes and implications? *Gastroenterology* 2002;122:1140–1156.

52. Longstreth GF, Yao JF. Irritable bowel syndrome and surgery: a multivariable analysis. *Gastroenterology* 2004;126:1665–1673.

53. Handa VL, Danielsen BH, Gilbert WM. Obstetric anal sphincter lacerations. *Obstet Gynecol* 2001;98:225–230.

54. Clemons JL, Towers GD, McClure GB, et al. Decreased anal sphincter lacerations associated with restrictive episiotomy use. *Am J Obstet Gynecol* 2005;192: 1620–1625.

55. Fenner DE, Genberg B, Brahma P, et al. Fecal and urinary incontinence after vaginal delivery with anal sphincter disruption in an obstetrics unit in the United States. *Am J Obstet Gynecol* 2003;189:1543–1550.

56. Sultan AH, Kamm MA, Hudson CN, et al. Anal-sphincter disruption during vaginal delivery. *N Engl J Med* 1993; 329:1905–1911.

57. De Leeuw JW, Vierhout ME, Struijk PC, et al. Anal sphincter damage after vaginal delivery: functional outcome and risk factors for fecal incontinence. *Acta Obstet Gynecol Scand* 2001;80:830–834.

58. Nygaard IE, Rao SS, Dawson JD. Anal incontinence after anal sphincter disruption: a 30-year retrospective cohort study. *Obstet Gynecol* 1997;89:896–901.

59. Kamm MA. Fecal incontinence. *Br Med J* 1998; 316:528–532.

60. Faltin DL, Boulvain M, Irion O, et al. Diagnosis of anal sphincter tears by postpartum endosonography to predict fecal incontinence. *Obstet Gynecol* 2000;95: 643–647.

61. Sultan AH, Kamm MA, Hudson CN, et al. Third-degree obstetric anal sphincter tears: risk factors and outcome of primary repair. *Br Med J* 1994;308:887–891.

62. Oberwalder M, Connor J, Wexner SD. Meta-analysis to determine the incidence of obstetric anal sphincter damage. *Br J Surg* 2003;90:1333–1337.

63. Nichols CM, Lamb EH, Ramakrishnan V. Differences in outcomes after third- versus fourth-degree perineal laceration repair: A prospective study. *Am J Obstet Gynecol* 2005;193:530–536.

64. MacArthur C, Glazener CM, Wilson PD, et al. Obstetric practice and fecal incontinence three months after delivery. *Br J Obstet Gynaecol* 2001;108:678–683.

65. Sultan AH, Johanson RB, Carter JE. Occult anal sphincter trauma following randomized forceps and vacuum delivery. *Int J Gynecol Obstet* 1998;61:113–119.

66. Lal M, Mann CH, Callender R, et al. Does cesarean delivery prevent anal incontinence? *Obstet Gynecol* 2003;101:305–312.

67. McKinnie V, Swift SE, Wang W, et al. The effect of pregnancy and mode of delivery on the prevalence of urinary and fecal incontinence. *Am J Obstet Gynecol* 2005;193:512–518.

68. Signorello LB, Harlow BL, Chekos AK, et al. Midline episiotomy and incontinence. *Br Med J* 2000;320: 86–90.

69. Carroli G, Belizan J. Episiotomy for vaginal birth. *Cochrane Database Syst Rev* 2000;(2):CD000081.

70. Walker WA, Rothenberger DA, Goldberg SM. Morbidity of internal sphincterotomy for anal fissure and stenosis. *Dis Colon Rectum* 1985;28:832–835.

71. Zbar AP, Beer-Gabel M, Chiappa AC, et al. Fecal incontinence after minor anorectal surgery. *Dis Colon Rectum* 2001;44:1610–1623.

72. Read MG, Read NW, Haynes WG, et al. A prospective study of the effect of haemorrhoidectomy on sphincter function and fecal incontinence. *Br J Surg* 1982;69: 396–398.

73. Snooks SJ, Henry MM, Swash M. Fecal incontinence due to external anal sphincter division in childbirth is associated with damage to the innervation of the pelvic floor musculature: A double pathology. *Br J Obstet Gynaecol* 1985;92:824–828.

74. Snooks SJ, Setchell M, Swash M, et al. Injury to the innervation of the pelvic floor sphincter musculature in childbirth. *Lancet* 1984;1:546–550.

75. Lien KC, Morgan DM, Delancey JO et al. Pudendal nerve stretch during vaginal birth: a 3D computer stimulation. *Am J Obstet Gynecol* 2005;192:1669–1676.

76. Ryhammer AM, Bek KM, Laurberg S. Multiple vaginal deliveries increase the risk of permanent incontinence of flatus and urine in normal premenopausal women. *Dis Colon Rectum* 1995;38:1206–1209.

77. Handa VL, Harris TA, Ostergard DR. Protecting the pelvic floor: Obstetric management to prevent incontinence and pelvic organ prolapse. *Obstet Gynecol* 1996;88:470–478.

78. Allen RE, Hosker GL, Smith AT, et al. Pelvic floor damage and childbirth: A neurophysiological study. *Br J Obstet Gynaecol* 1990;97:770–779.

79. Smith ARB, Hosker GL, Warrell DW. The role of partial denervation of the pelvic floor in the etiology of

genitourinary prolapse and stress incontinence of urine: a neurophysiologic study. *Br J Obstet Gynaecol* 1989;96:24–28.

80. Henry MM, Parks AG, Swash M. The anal reflex in idiopathic fecal incontinence: an electrophysiological study. *Br J Surg* 1980;67:781–783.

81. Ho YH, Goh HS. The neurophysiological significance of perineal descent. *Int J Colorectal Dis* 1995;10:107–111.

82. Gee AS, Mills A, Durdey P. What is the relationship between perineal descent and anal mucosal electrosensitivity? *Dis Colon Rectum* 1995;38:419–423.

83. Berkelmans I, Heresbach D, Leroi AM, et al. Perineal descent at defecography in women with straining at stool: a lack of specificity or predictive value for future anal incontinence. *Eur J Gastroenterol Hepatol* 1995;7:75–79.

CHAPTER 21

Evaluation of Colorectal Dysfunction

Marc R. Toglia

INTRODUCTION

Colorectal disorders occur commonly among adult women and are associated with diverse symptoms, including abdominal pain and bloating, constipation, incomplete defecation, and fecal incontinence. To adequately care for women with these disorders, clinicians must have an adequate understanding of the physiology and pathophysiology of the colon and anorectum.

OVERVIEW OF NORMAL COLORECTAL FUNCTION

Stool Formation and Colonic Transit

Voluntary storage and evacuation of the stool is a complex neuromuscular mechanism that involves many physiologic processes. Intestinal transit and absorption, colonic transit, rectal compliance, anorectal sensation, and sphincteric mechanism all play an important role in normal colorectal function. An understanding of how each of these variables affects continence is essential in the proper diagnosis and treatment of the women with colorectal disorders.

A major function of the colon is the final regulation of water and electrolyte absorption. The colon is capable of absorbing up to 5 L of water and associated electrolytes in 24 hours. Stool content is propelled along the large intestine via contractile waves know as peristalsis. Colonic motility is complex, with great regional heterogeneity. Functionally, the colon can be divided into three segments: the proximal colon, the segment from the midtransverse colon to the proximal rectosigmoid, and the rectosigmoid. The rectosigmoid is uniquely adapted for sodium and water absorption. The transit of the stool content is significantly delayed in this region to permit complete reabsorp-

tion of fecal water and electrolytes before final elimination.

Anorectal Continence

The voluntary storage and evacuation of solid waste is a complex physiologic process involving learned social behavior, voluntary cortical control, and a series of involuntary reflexes. When stool content first enters into the rectal vault, several physiologic events take place. The arrival of stool in the rectum is associated with a transient decrease in internal anal sphincter tone and an increase in external sphincter activity; this is known as the *rectoanal inhibitory reflex*. This allows the sensory-rich anal canal to come in contact with the rectal contents to determine whether it contains solid, liquid, and/or gas. This physiologic event is known as *sampling*. This is followed by a relaxation of the rectum to store the increased rectal volume in a process known as *accommodation*. The rectum, like the bladder, is a highly compliant reservoir that facilitates storage of waste. As rectal volume increases, an urge to defecate is experienced. If this urge is voluntarily suppressed, the rectum relaxes further to continue the accommodation of stool. Rectal compliance may be decreased in certain disease states such as ulcerative proctitis or radiation proctitis. A loss in compliance may decrease the ability of the rectal wall to stretch, and as a result, rectal pressure remains high. This may compromise this first part of the continence mechanism and place an increased demand on the sphincteric mechanism.

The anal canal is primarily responsible for preventing leakage of stool during this phase of rectal storage. The anal canal remains closed as the result of the interactions between three distinct muscles: the puborectalis portion of the levator ani, the external anal sphincter, and the internal anal sphincter. The puborectalis and external anal sphincter comprise a unique type of striated muscle that is capable of maintaining a constant resting tone that is proportional to the volume of the rectal content and that relaxes at the time of defecation. Both of these muscles contain a majority of type I (slow-twitch) muscle fibers, which are ideally suited to maintaining a constant tone over time. Each muscle group also contains a smaller proportion of type II (fast-twitch) fibers, which allows them to respond quickly during sudden increases in intra-abdominal pressures (1).

Continence of solid stool is maintained primarily by the actions of the puborectalis. This muscle originates from the pubic rami on either side of the midline at the level of the arcus tendineus levator ani. The muscle fibers pass laterally to the vagina and form a U-shaped sling that cradles the rectum. The constant resting tone of the puborectalis pulls the anorectal junction towards the pubic symphysis, creating a 90-degree angle between the anal and rectal canals referred to as the anorectal angle (Fig. 21.1).This angulation is easily palpated on digital rectal examination. It was once proposed that this acute angulation creates a

"flap-valve" effect in which an increase in intra-abdominal pressure compresses the anterior rectal wall against the pelvic floor, and that this action was critical to maintaining continence. However, more recent physiologic studies have failed to demonstrate that such a mechanism exists (2,3), and successful surgical restoration of anal continence does not appear to depend upon the restoration of this angle (4,5). Defecation of solid stool is initiated by the voluntary relaxation of the puborectalis, which together with intestinal peristalsis, a voluntary increase in intra-abdominal pressure, and relaxation of the external and internal anal sphincters, allows for the passage of stool downward through the anal canal. The effectiveness of the puborectalis muscle in maintaining continence without the external or internal anal sphincter is illustrated by the relative continence that women with a chronic fourth-degree laceration have over solid stool.

The internal and external anal sphincters maintain continence below the level of the puborectalis (Fig. 21.2). These two structures are critical in the control of flatus and liquid feces, as the puborectalis mechanism is ineffective in this regard. The shape of the combined internal and external

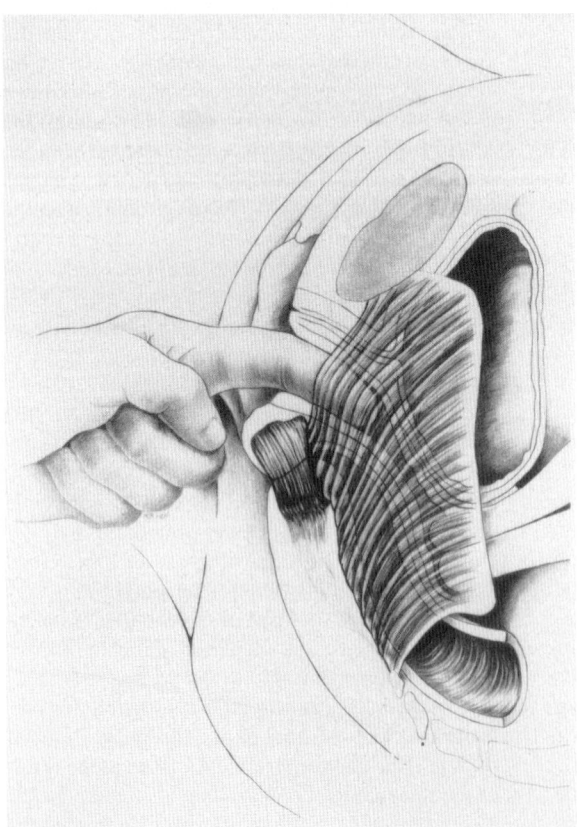

FIGURE 21.1 ● Lateral view of the external anal sphincter and levator ani muscles showing palpation of the medial border of the levator ani muscle (puborectalis–pubococcygeus portion). Note the approximately 90-degree angle between the anal canal and the axis of the rectum. (From Toglia MR, DeLancey JOL. Anal incontinence and the obstetrician gynecologist. *Obstet Gynecol* 1994;84;4(2):731–740, with permission.)

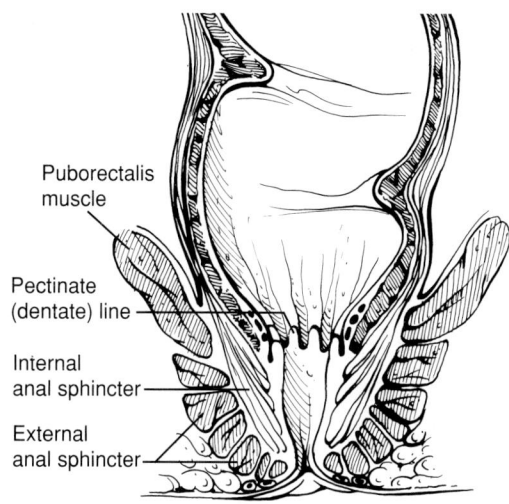

Puborectalis
muscle

Pectinate
(dentate) line

Internal
anal sphincter

External
anal sphincter

FIGURE 21.2 ● Schematic representation of the anal canal illustrating the relationship of the internal and external anal sphincter in coronal section. Note how the internal anal sphincter extends somewhat cephalad to the external anal sphincter. The dentate line separates the anal canal from the rectum. (From Weber AM, Brubaker L, Schaffer J, et al, eds. *Office urogynecology.* New York: McGraw Hill, 2004, with permission.)

sphincter muscles is nearly cylindrical as it encircles the anal canal and, measured in the midline, is approximately 18 mm thick and 28 mm long (6). It is critical that clinicians recognize that 50% of the anterior thickness of the sphincter complex is attributable to the internal anal sphincter. The anatomic and functional importance of the internal anal sphincter is often underappreciated in most textbooks on obstetric and gynecologic surgery, but it is believed to be critical in the proper repair of obstetric sphincter lacerations as well as the surgical correction of anal incontinence.

The internal anal sphincter is a thickened, downward continuation of the circular smooth muscle layer of the colon and is innervated by sympathetic nerves from the presacral complex. Unlike the external anal sphincter and puborectalis muscle, the internal anal sphincter is not under voluntary control, and its function is mediated largely by reflex arcs at the spinal cord level. At rest, the anal canal is kept closed by the constant tonic activity of both the internal and external anal sphincters. Physiologic studies suggest that the internal anal sphincter is responsible for 75% to 85% of the resting tone of the anal canal (7,8). As the intestinal content passes into the rectum, the internal anal sphincter relaxes reflexively to allow the upper anal canal to "sample" the contents and to discriminate between solid, liquid, and gas. Once

the intestinal contents have been determined, the internal anal sphincter contracts again to augment closure of the anal canal. Thus, it is currently believed that continence at rest (particularly for liquid stool and flatus) is largely the responsibility of the internal anal sphincter, whereas continence during sudden distention of the anal canal is principally maintained by the external anal sphincter (9).

Anal sensation is also thought to play a critical role in the normal continence mechanism. Sensory receptors located within the anal canal and within the levator ani muscles detect the presence of stool in the rectum as well as the degree of rectal distention. The upper anal canal is capable of distinguishing between solid, liquid, and gaseous forms of stool, and feedback from these sensory organs is important in coordinating the actions of the sphincteric musculature.

The anal canal cushions (hemorrhoids) are thought to assist in the continence mechanism by facilitating mucosal coaptation. These vascular channels fill with blood and may occlude the lower anal canal. Supporters of this theory suggest that the loss of these structures following hemorrhoidectomy may account for the reported incidence of incontinence following this procedure.

Defecation

Defecation is a highly coordinated physiologic action that involves neuromuscular regulation by the central nervous system. Distention of the rectum by the stool content initiates the rectoanal inhibitory reflex discussed previously and allows the sensory-rich upper anal canal to sample stool content. The act of defecation is initiated by a Valsalva maneuver to raise intra-abdominal and intrarectal pressure. Voluntary inhibition of the external anal sphincter and puborectalis enables the rectum to empty. This is assisted by coordinated peristaltic activity of the rectosigmoid. When evacuation is completed, the external anal sphincter and puborectalis contract (termed the closing reflex) and the continence mechanism is initiated again.

SYMPTOM-BASED APPROACH TO COLORECTAL DISORDERS

Clinicians who care for women with pelvic floor disorders are commonly asked to evaluate patients with two separate syndromes involving colorectal disorders. The first syndrome involves symptoms suggestive of disordered defecation, and the second syndrome involves symptoms of fecal incontinence.

Disordered Defecation

Women with disordered defecation will typically refer to their symptoms as "constipation." Constipation frequently has different meanings to different people. Commonly accepted definitions include infrequent stools (less than three per week), passing stool that is too hard or too small, difficulty or prolongation of the act of defecation ("straining"), or a feeling of rectal fullness or incomplete evacuation. Abdominal pain and bloating are frequently the predominant complaint in constipated patients. Therefore, the first step in managing constipation is to understand what the patient means by using that term. It may be helpful to classify patients with constipation into one of three categories: (a) those with colonic motility disorders, (b) those with pelvic outlet obstructive symptoms, and (c) those with a combination of both (10) (Table 21.1). History, physical examination, and ancillary testing can distinguish them.

Clinicians should question the patient carefully to determine the following historical data: number of bowel movements per week, length of time spent on the commode, pain associated with defecation, sensation of incomplete evacuation or a false sense of the need to evacuate, need to digitally assist defecation by either splinting the perineum or extracting feces from the anus directly, and presence of a bulge, either vaginal or rectal. Physical examination may reveal the presence of pelvic organ prolapse, including a rectocele, ente-rocele, or rectal prolapse; fecal impaction; poor sphincter tone; or spasm of the puborectalis muscle. Proctoscopy is helpful in the detection of anal fissures, edema, internal hemorrhoids, or a solitary rectal ulcer. The presence of rectal bleeding should prompt referral to an appropriate specialist. Ancillary testing will be discussed later.

Systemic Factors

After inadequate dietary fiber, drug therapy is probably the most common cause of constipation. Common prescription and over-the-counter medications that may cause constipation are listed in Table 21.2. Many systemic factors may affect normal colonic factors and cause constipation. The prevalence of constipation during pregnancy is well recognized. Hypothyroidism, diabetes, hyperparathyroidism, and severe electrolyte abnormality can also cause constipation. Uncommon diseases such as scleroderma and amyloidosis can cause structural changes in the intestine that can lead to constipation. Neurologic diseases involving the central nervous system such as multiple sclerosis and Parkinson's disease are frequently associated with constipation.

Colonic Motility Disorders

A deficiency in dietary fiber has long been thought to be an important cause of constipation. Fiber may shorten whole gut transit and increase stool weight. Primary therapy for constipation consists of a diet trial with approximately 30 g of dietary

---

TABLE 21.1

Causes of Constipation

Systemic factors
  Drug therapy
  Metabolic and endocrine disorders
  Neurologic disease
  Pregnancy
Motility disorders
  Inadequate fiber intake
  Colonic inertia
  Global motility disorder
Anorectal outlet obstruction
  Intrarectal prolapse
  Rectocele
  Enterocele
  Paradoxical puborectalis syndrome
  Descending perineum
Irritable bowel syndrome

TABLE 21.2

Drugs Commonly Associated with Constipation

Over-the-counter medication
  Antidiarrheals such as loperamide and Kaopectate
  Antacids (calcium and aluminum products)
  Iron therapy
Prescription medication
  Antidepressants
  Anticholinergics
  Anticonvulsants
  Calcium channel blockers
  Beta-blockers
  Diuretics
  Opiates
  Nonsteroidal anti-inflammatory agents
  Phenothiazines
  Psychotherapeutic agents

fiber per day for 4 to 6 weeks coupled with an adequate intake of fluid.

Colonic inertia, or slow transit constipation, is a condition of chronic idiopathic constipation in which patients are found to have no organic cause for their symptoms and have diffuse, pancolonic marker delay on transit study. Megacolon or megarectum may or may not be present in association with colonic inertia. Colonic inertia is found almost exclusively in women, and some studies suggest an unusually high prevalence of psychiatric disturbances among these patients (11). Some patients with megacolon have a loss of the normal myenteric plexus ganglion cells, which is considered diagnostic of Hirschsprung's disease and usually presents in childhood or early adulthood.

Anorectal Outlet Obstruction Syndromes

Functional outlet obstruction is common cause of constipation in women. These patients typically have no obvious organic cause for their symptoms. Colonic transit studies reveal normal pancolonic transit time but delayed transit through the rectum. Anorectal outlet obstruction may be the manifestation of a variety of pelvic floor disorders listed in Table 21.1.

Intrarectal prolapse, also referred to as rectal intussusception, is characterized by a circumferential intussusception of the upper rectal wall into the rectal ampulla. It occurs most commonly among women with an age of onset between 40 and 50 years. Symptoms include a sensation of obstruction, incontinence, pain on defecation, bleeding, and a mucus discharge (12). Patients with obstructive defecation typically complain of the sensation of incomplete evacuation. Bleeding is usually related to localized proctitis or a solitary rectal ulcer that occurs as the result of the intussusception. Diagnosis is most reliably confirmed by cinedefecography and proctosigmoidoscopy.

A rectocele represents a detachment of the rectovaginal septum and subsequent herniation of the rectum and anal canal anteriorly against the posterior vaginal wall. Breaks in the rectovaginal fascia can occur transversely either at its attachment to the perineal body or at the apex of the vagina. Longitudinal breaks may exist laterally at the point where the lateral vagina attaches to pubococcygeus. Many rectoceles are clinically asymptomatic; however, in some patients they are the cause of obstructed defecation (13). Patients typically complain of incomplete evacuation and "pocketing" of stool into the vagina during attempts at defecation. Patients often report using their fingers to splint the vagina during defecation or applying pressure to the posterior vaginal wall

to complete evacuation. It is important to rule out other causes of constipation prior to contemplating surgical repair because as many as 54% of women continue to have significant constipation postoperatively in several published series (14,15). Most rectoceles can be characterized by vaginal and rectal examination, but cinedefecography is the preferred method of imaging the rectocele radiographically as well as confirming that the rectocele is responsible for trapping the stool. It should be kept in mind that a rectocele by itself is not a common cause of constipation but rather presents as obstructed defecation. Therefore, a proper evaluation for other causes of anorectal outlet obstruction should be considered prior to proceeding with surgical correction.

Enterocele may be best described as a herniation of a peritoneal sac through the fibromuscular layer at the apex of the vagina. It is typically located posterior to the uterus and anterior to the rectum. On examination, the sac is typically filled with small intestine, omentum, and/or sigmoid colon. Enteroceles are thought to be a significant cause of symptoms following hysterectomy and anterior urethropexies. The best way to diagnose an enterocele is with the patient standing and straining. The examiner should place one finger in the vagina and another in the rectum. Although radiologic studies are often unnecessary, they may help to distinguish a true enterocele from a high rectocele or large cystocele. Symptoms include pelvic pressure, low back pain, and a feeling of perineal protrusion. In general, enteroceles are an uncommon cause of constipation.

Descending perineal syndrome is often associated with pronounced difficulty with defecation leading to prolonged straining efforts. First described by Sir Alan Parks, the syndrome is now clinically defined as when the plane of the perineum (at the level of the anal verge) descends beyond the ischial tuberosities during Valsalva maneuvers (16). Excessive descent of the perineum is typically readily apparent on physical examination and can be objectively quantified by defecography. Patients with this syndrome may also complain of deep-seated pain that is precipitated by prolonged standing and relieved by lying down. Neurologic damage to the pudendal nerve is thought to occur as the result of stretching, which may eventually result in denervation of the anal sphincter and may, in time, lead to anal incontinence.

Constipated patients who have no structural abnormalities of the anorectum or dysfunction of colonic motility may experience dysfunction of the pelvic floor musculature. Electromyography (EMG) and anal manometry studies have identified a subgroup of patients who complain of constipation who experience a paradoxical contraction of the anal sphincter and the levator ani at the time of attempted defecation (17,18). This syndrome has been termed anismus, pelvic floor dyssynergia, and paradoxical puborectalis syndrome. The failure of the pelvic floor to relax at the time of straining to defecation results in a physiologic anorectal outlet obstruction. The typical patient is a young woman who suffers from constipation that fails to respond to fiber therapy and laxatives. Symptoms include pain with defecation, excessive straining, and the sensation of incomplete evacuation. Definitive diagnosis can be made by anorectal manometry, EMG, or cinedefecography. Patients with anismus who undergo cinedefecography are unable to evacuate barium and retain a prominent impression of the puborectalis muscle on lateral films during attempts to evacuate the rectum. This suggests that the pelvic floor remains contracted during straining and prevents rectal emptying. Anal manometry studies may include a balloon expulsion test in which the patient attempts to evacuate a 30-mL intrarectal balloon. EMG studies actually measure neuromuscular action potentials, looking for normal silencing before defecation. Anal manometry and EMG are superior to cinedefecography studies because they show evidence of nonrelaxation of the anal sphincters and levator ani at the time of attempted defecation. EMG studies are currently thought to be the most sensitive technique for diagnosing anismus.

Functional Bowel Disorders

Constipation is a frequent symptom in patients with irritable bowel syndrome (IBS). IBS is thought by many to be the most common disorder of the digestive tract. About two thirds of those affected are women, and it occurs most commonly in younger adults. One study has suggested that 5% to 11% of patients with IBS present with constipation (19). Stress has long been felt to contribute to the symptoms of IBS, and patients with IBS frequently have a history of depression.

The Rome criteria for functional bowel disorders have established criteria for the diagnosis of IBS (Table 21.3)(20). IBS is a symptom-based diagnosis, and the physical examination in these patients is primarily directed at ruling out other etiologies of disordered defecation. Key symptoms include abdominal pain usually relieved by a bowel movement as well as a subjective change in bowel frequency or consistency. Complaints of blood in the stool or nocturnal stool are highly unlikely with IBS. Episodes of IBS are often associated with stress, including anxiety or depression. Patients should be referred for a thorough gastrointestinal (GI) workup including rigid or flexible sigmoidoscopy.

A growing body of evidence links constipation with psychological factors in some patients. Personality factors, self-esteem, psychological distress, and anxiety have all been linked to stool frequency and constipation. Studies suggesting that constipation is responsive to psychological intervention further support the theory that not all constipation has an organic cause.

TABLE 21.3

Rome Criteria for Irritable Bowel Syndrome (20)

At least 12 weeks or more, which need not be consecutive, in the preceding 12 months, of abdominal discomfort or pain that has two out of three features:
- Relieved with defecation; and/or
- Onset associated with a change in frequency of stool; and/or
- Onset associated with a change in form of stool

Supportive Symptoms
- Abnormal stool frequency (greater than 3 bowel movements a day or less than 3 bowel movements per week);
- Abnormal stool form (lumpy/hard or loose/watery stool);
- Abnormal stool passage (straining, urgency, or feeling of incomplete evacuation);
- Passage of mucus;
- Bloating or abdominal distention

Fecal Incontinence

Fecal incontinence, the involuntary loss of flatus or feces, is rapidly gaining recognition as a condition that occurs more frequently than previously thought. In most studies, it is reported to occur most frequently in multiparous women and has its highest incidence in adults over 65 years of age, although some recent studies have shown a surprisingly high prevalence in men (21). Unfortunately, the symptoms of anal incontinence are frequently underreported by patients and commonly unrecognized by the clinician. The emotional, psychological, and social problems created by this condition can be both devastating and debilitating.

The most common cause of fecal incontinence in healthy women is related to obstetrical trauma. It is widely recognized that vaginal delivery can damage the anal continence mechanism by direct injury to the anal sphincter muscles or damage to the motor innervation of the sphincters and pelvic floor. Recent studies have reported that injury to the anal continence mechanism is much more common following a vaginal delivery than previously recognized. In a prospective study of 200 pregnant women evaluated both before and after delivery, Sultan et al (22) reported that 13% of women develop incontinence or urgency following their first vaginal delivery and that 30% have unrecognized structural injury to the internal and external anal sphincter detected by anal endosonography. Women who suffered a traumatic rupture of the anal sphincter at the time of vaginal delivery appear to have a greater risk of anal incontinence than previously recognized. Several investigators have reported that 36% to 63% of women develop symptoms of incontinence following primary sphincter repair (23–26).

There is strong evidence to suggest that vaginal delivery results in significant injury to the innervation of the pelvic floor muscles. Snooks et al (27) noted a significant increase in the mean pudendal nerve motor latencies (PNTMLs) 48 hours after delivery in primiparous women who had a forceps delivery compared with controls and with multiparous patients. In a study of 128 women in whom PNTMLs were measured both during pregnancy and after delivery, PNTMLs were significantly prolonged 6 weeks postpartum in 32% of women who delivered vaginally (28). Two thirds of those women with an abnormally prolonged PNTML at 6 weeks postpartum had a PNTML within the normal range when restudied after 6 months, suggesting that nerve damage is permanent in 19% of women following vaginal delivery.

Although obstetrical trauma is a leading cause of fecal incontinence in women, it can also result from a variety of other conditions (Table 21.4). Several operations performed frequently by colorectal surgeons can result in fecal incontinence, including internal sphincterotomy, fistulectomy and fistulotomy. Several disease states have been associated with fecal incontinence. These include diabetes, multiple sclerosis, Parkinson's disease, spinal cord injury, and myotonic dystrophy. Fecal impaction is a leading cause of fecal incontinence among the elderly and institutionalized individuals.

Illnesses causing diarrhea are another important cause of fecal incontinence. IBS is frequently associated with incontinence, as is inflammatory bowel disease. Infectious diarrheal states are also commonly associated with incontinence. Radiation proctitis can lead to fecal incontinence through a variety of mechanisms, including decreases in rectal compliance and neurogenic injury to the sphincter complex.

TABLE 21.4

Causes of Fecal Incontinence

Obstetric
  Rupture of anal sphincter
  Chronic third- and fourth-degree perineal laceration
  Rectovaginal and anovaginal fistulas
Surgical
  Internal sphincterotomy
  Fistulectomy
  Low anterior resection
Traumatic sphincter rupture
Diarrheal states
  Inflammatory bowel disease
  Radiation enteritis
  Infectious enteritis
  Laxative abuse
Neurologic conditions
  Congenital abnormalities
  Parkinson's disease
  Systemic sclerosis
  Spinal cord injury
  Stroke
  Dementia
  Diabetic neuropathy
Congenital anorectal malformation
Pelvic floor denervation
  Rectal prolapse
  Chronic straining
  Descending perineum syndrome

From Toglia MR. Pathophysiology of anorectal dysfunction. *Obstet Clin North Am* 1998;25:771–781, with permission.

ELEMENTS OF THE PHYSICAL EXAMINATION

The basis for evaluating colorectal dysfunction begins with a good history and careful physical examination. The clinician must specifically address colorectal symptoms, as patients seldom offer this information voluntarily. It is important to ask specific questions regarding the onset, duration, and frequency of symptoms and to identify associated exacerbating factors such as diet and activity.

The evaluation of colorectal dysfunction requires a focused examination of the abdomen and pelvis. Routine examination of the abdomen involves inspection, palpation, and auscultation to rule out the presence of masses, organomegaly, and areas of peritoneal irritation. This should be followed by a detailed evaluation of the vagina and anorectum. Visual and digital inspection of the vagina and anus will identify structural abnormalities such as prolapse, fistulas, fissures, hemorrhoids, or prior trauma. A simple neurologic examination should test for the intactness of the motor component of S2 through S4. The anal wink, bulbocavernosus, and cough reflexes all test the integrity of the motor innervation of the external anal sphincter. Sensation over the inner thigh, vulva, and perirectal areas should be tested for symmetry by light touch and pinprick. Pelvic muscle strength can be subjectively graded by digital palpation of the puborectalis sling with voluntary contraction.

The integrity of the external anal sphincter and puborectalis muscle can be evaluated by observation and palpation of these structures during voluntary contraction. When a patient is asked to contract her pelvic floor, two motions should be present. First, the external anal sphincter should contract concentrically and the anal verge should be pulled inward. These actions should also be readily apparent on digital rectal examination. The firm and resilient muscular sling of the puborectalis should be readily palpable posteriorly as it creates a 90-degree angle between the anal and rectal canals. Voluntary contraction of this muscle "lifts" the examining finger anteriorly toward the insertion of this muscle on the pubic rami. An external anal sphincter muscle that is intact but lax at rest as well as a weak voluntary contraction of this muscle often indicates pudendal neuropathy. Neuropathy affecting the puborectalis can likewise be recognized if the anorectal angle is obtuse and if there is a palpable weakness with voluntary contraction. The presence of fecal material in the anal canal may suggest fecal impaction or neuromuscular weakness of the anal continence mechanism.

Finally, defects in the anterior aspects of the external anal sphincter may be detected by digital examination. The patient should then be asked to strain or bear down with a finger still within the anus. Both the puborectalis and external anal sphincter should relax during such activity. Patients suffering from anismus may have a paradoxical contraction of these muscles during straining.

ANCILLARY TESTING

Disordered Defecation

Colorectal screening should be discussed with all women 50 years and older. It is obviously important to reinforce this with any woman in this age range who is currently experiencing colorectal complaints such as bleeding, constipation, changes in bowel habits, or abdominal pain. Alarm symptoms such as bleeding, weight loss, or sudden changes in bowel habits should prompt immediate referral for colonoscopy.

Patients presenting with symptoms suggestive of disordered defecation should undergo a standard gastrointestinal evaluation including colonoscopy to eliminate colorectal malignancy from the differential diagnosis. Anoscopy should be considered as part of the office examination because it may reveal anorectal pathology such as prolapsing hemorrhoids or anal fissures. Rigid proctosigmoidoscopy should also be performed to exclude intrarectal prolapse, ulcerative or radiation proctitis, or a solitary rectal ulcer.

In women who fail a conservative trial of therapy for disordered defecation, referral to an anorectal physiology laboratory may be helpful in order to differentiate between patients with colonic motility disorders and those with predominant pelvic outlet symptoms. Standard evaluation in these laboratories may include colonic transit studies, cinedefecography, anorectal manometry, anorectal ultrasound, and electromyography.

Cinedefecography is a radiologic examination of the anatomy and function of the pelvic floor and anorectum. It is useful in the diagnosis of intrarectal prolapse, rectocele, enterocele, paradoxical puborectalis syndrome (anismus), and perineal descent. A series of lateral still films and, in some laboratories, cinevideography are made with fluoroscopy while the patient sits on a radiolucent commode. The patient is filmed at rest, during defecation, and while squeezing the anal sphincters. Measurements are taken of the size of the rectal ampulla, length of the anal canal, size of the anorectal angle, motion of the puborectalis, and degree of pelvic floor descent. The procedure is more fully described in Chapter 26.

Anal manometry is performed as described earlier to determine maximum resting pressure, maximum squeeze pressure, and rectal sensation. The role of manometry is to evaluate sphincteric function, although it is also helpful in diagnosing Hirschsprung's disease. Surface EMG of the anal sphincter is helpful in excluding anismus as a cause of obstructed defecation. Normally, the anal sphincter relaxes at the time of defecation. Patients with anismus typically show an increase in electrical activity in both the external sphincter and the puborectalis with attempted defecation (29).

Colonic transit studies involve the use of ingested radiopaque markers followed by abdominal radiographs or scintigraphic studies performed serially over a period of several days. Patients are asked to observe a high-fiber diet over the test period. Twenty to 24 markers are ingested initially and abdominal radiographs are taken either daily or on the fourth day, the seventh day, and every 3 days until all the markers are gone. Segmental transit times are then calculated using a mathematical formula. On the basis of colonic transit studies, patients suffering from constipation can be divided into those with delayed colonic transit, those with anorectal outlet obstruction, and those with normal studies.

Fecal Incontinence

Sophisticated diagnostic testing is currently being used in clinical research and in anorectal physiology laboratories to quantify the structure and function of the anorectum.

Transanal ultrasonography is a technique that allows for the accurate imaging of both the internal and external anal sphincters. Transanal ultrasound is currently the single best method of identifying defects in the anal sphincters. In this technique, continuity of the muscle is assessed, as is thickness of the muscle. Transanal ultrasound is commonly performed using a Bruel-Kjaer (Copenhagen, Denmark) ultrasound scanner with a 360-degree rectal endoprobe (type 1850) with 7.0-MHz transducer (focal length 2 to 5 cm) housed within a plastic cone (Fig. 21.3). The normal internal anal sphincter is observed as a continuous hypoechoic band. A thick layer of mixed echogenic-

ity outside of the internal anal sphincter is the striated layer of the normal external anal sphincter (Fig. 21.4). Discontinuity of the muscle bands is considered evidence of a sphincteric defect. Defects can be measured in degrees of circumference as well as distance from the anal verge (Fig. 21.5).

EMG has been used to evaluate the integrity of external anal sphincter innervation following a traumatic injury such as during childbirth, as well as to document the presence of pelvic floor neuropathy (30). EMG is a study of electrical activity arising in muscle fibers during contraction and at rest. Many different electrodes may be used to measure electrical activity in the muscles. Surface electrodes applied near or within the anal canal record electrical activity within the area adjacent to the electrode and can give a general record of anal sphincter activity. Surface electrodes are typically used in conjunction with biofeedback therapy. Concentric needle electrodes are most commonly used in anorectal physiology laboratories. The recording electrode consists of a thin steel wire contained within a thin, needle-like cannula. The area surveyed by the electrode is small and therefore records selectively from individual muscles. Single-fiber EMG electrodes contain extremely small electrodes and record the activity of single muscle fibers. Quantification of single-fiber EMG results allows for calculation of fiber density.

Denervation injury to a muscle is accompanied by subsequent reinnervation of the affected motor unit, which is reflected by an increase in fiber density. Thus, single-fiber EMG studies provide indirect evidence of neurologic injury by measuring the amount of reinnervation. Single-fiber EMG can be utilized to map the external anal sphincter and to identify areas of injury. Unfortunately, this requires multiple needle punctures around the anus and can be uncomfortable for the patient. This technique has largely been replaced by transanal ultrasound in clinical practice for the detection of disruption to the external anal sphincter, based both on increased patient comfort and more reliable results.

Motor nerve conduction studies offer a way of measuring neuropathic injury to the muscles of the pelvic floor. These studies are performed by stimulating the axon of a nerve and measuring the speed that it takes for the action potential to reach

FIGURE 21.3 ● Bruel-Kjaer (Copenhagen, Denmark) ultrasound probe (type 1850), with a 7.0-MHz transducer (focal length 2 to 5 cm) housed within a plastic cone.

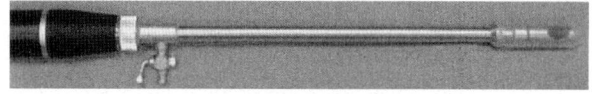

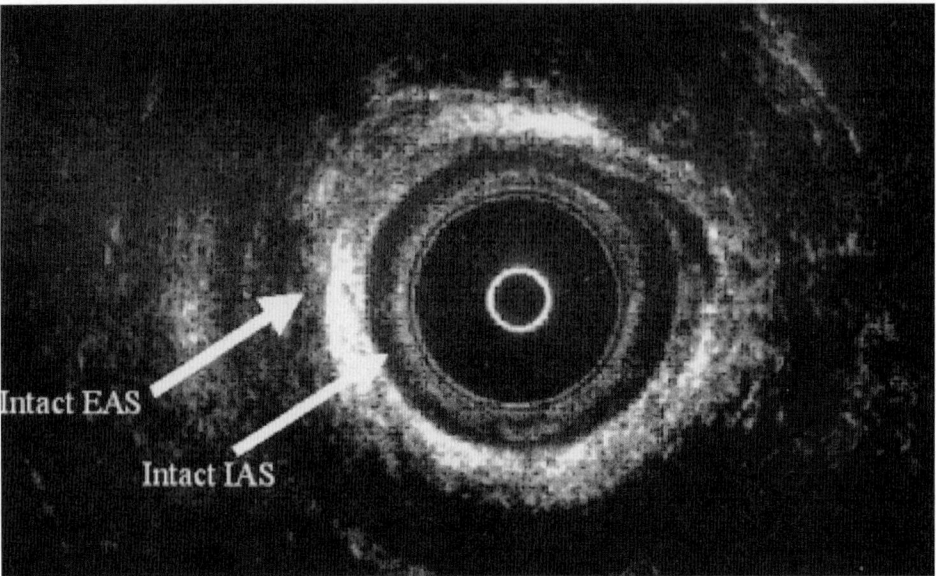

FIGURE 21.4 ● Endoanal ultrasound image from the midsphincter demonstrating the intact hypoechoic internal anal sphincter and hyperechoic external anal sphincter.

the muscle supplied by the nerve. The delay between stimulation and the response is called the nerve latency. Pudendal nerve motor terminal latency (PNTML) can be determined by transrectal stimulation of the pudendal nerve (31). These studies are performed using a nerve stimulator mounted on an examination glove at the fingertip (Fig. 21.6). The nerve stimulator is positioned transrectally over the pudendal nerve at each ischial spine. A transrectal stimulus of 0.1 milliseconds duration and up to 50 mV is given and the latency of the external anal sphincter muscle contraction is measured. A value of 2.2 milliseconds or less is considered normal. Prolongation of the pudendal nerve terminal motor latency is indicative of damage to that nerve. A normal or near-normal PNTML study is a significant predictor for successful surgical repair of traumatic sphincter injuries (32).

Anal manometry can be used to quantify function of the anal sphincter mechanism. Pressures in the anal canal can be measured by a variety of techniques and catheters. Water-perfused manometry catheters and water-filled balloons are the most commonly used methods (Fig. 21.7). Resting anal canal pressure is mostly a reflection of the activity of the internal anal sphincter, and mechanical defects in this structure can be inferred indirectly from the measurement of a low resting anal pressure. Anorectal pressures measured in the lower anal canal during maximal voluntary contraction reflect external anal sphincter function. Vector analysis of the manometric pressures consists of computerized analysis of data and can be used to determine symmetry or asymmetry within the anal sphincter. The pressure measurements obtained by anal manometry provides indirect evidence of sphincter injury: a low resting tone is often an indication of subclinical injury to the internal anal sphincter, whereas a decrease in the maximum squeezing pressure tends to reflect activity of the external anal sphincter. A variety of factors influence anal pressure measurements, including tissue compliance and muscular tone. These measurements do not distinguish between the activities of the individual sphincter muscles and often lack specific anatomic correlation. Interpretation of anal canal pressures is difficult and there is a wide variation of "normal pressures" that varies with age and parity. There is a wide overlap between manometric values obtained from incontinent patients and normal controls. Anal manometry may therefore be of limited value in helping the clinician determine proper therapy.

FUTURE AREAS OF RESEARCH

Traditional concepts of anorectal dysfunction have followed a polarized paradigm in which constipation and fecal incontinence represent opposite extremes of abnormal function. This may be

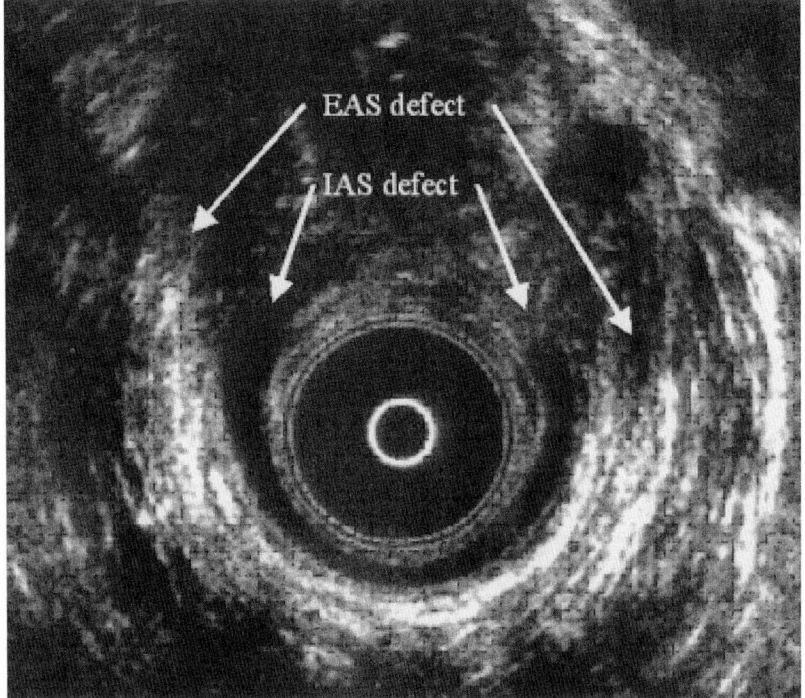

A

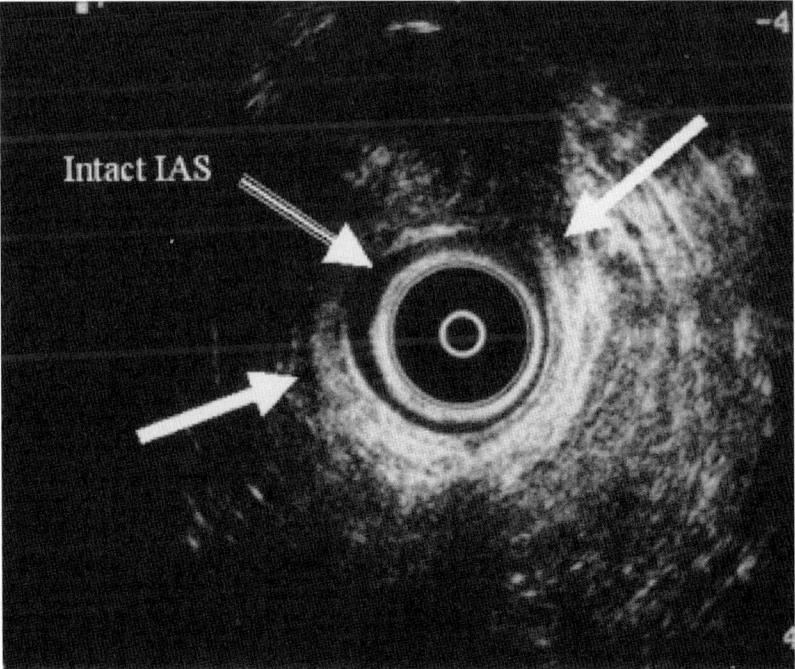

B

FIGURE 21.5 ● **(A)** Endoanal ultrasound image from the midsphincter demonstrating defects in both the internal and external anal sphincters from 10 to 2 o'clock. **(B)** Endoanal ultrasound image from cranial sphincter demonstrating an intact internal anal sphincter (*broken arrow*) and defect in external anal sphincter from 8 to 2 o'clock (*solid arrows*).

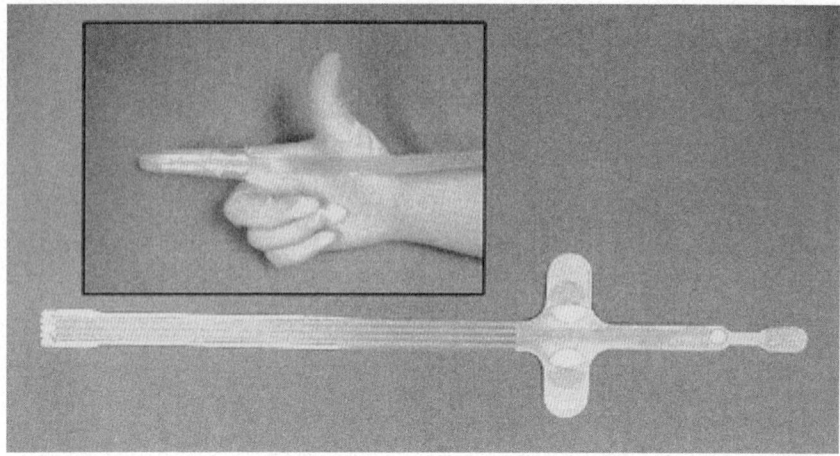

FIGURE 21.6 ● St. Mark's electrode used for measuring pudendal nerve motor terminal latency. The stimulating electrode is on the fingertip and the receiving electrode is on the proximal finger near the knuckle (*inset*).

oversimplistic, as there are data suggesting that certain etiologies of constipation will progress to anal incontinence if untreated. Abnormal perineal descent at evacuation proctography, with or without rectocele or enterocele, has been shown to be related to the later development of fecal incontinence. Clarifying the relationship between fecal incontinence, perineal descent, and constipation is another important area of future research. The relationship between pelvic organ prolapse and fecal incontinence is also poorly understood and thus demands investigation.

Technical developments over the past decade have significantly improved our understanding of the effect of vaginal delivery on the anal continence mechanism. At the same time, the adequacy of our current techniques for primary sphincter repair at the time of delivery has been questioned. In the past, insufficient attention has been paid by obstetricians toward the anatomic repair of third- and fourth-degree obstetrical lacerations, and it is widely recognized that standard repairs for these lacerations are possibly inadequate (33). Additional research is needed to refine surgical techniques and improve adjuvant therapies such as biofeedback to enable clinicians to offer more effective treatments for fecal incontinence.

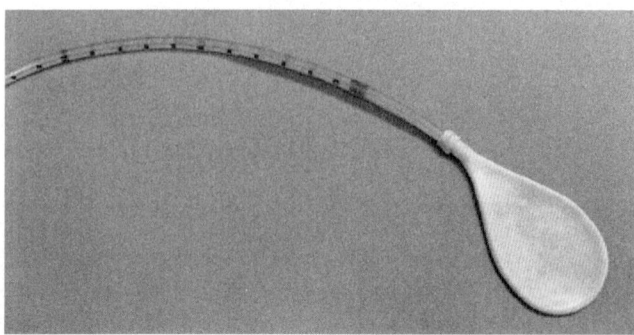

FIGURE 21.7 ● Manometry catheter with balloon.

REFERENCES

1. Gosling JA, Dixson JS, Critchey HOD, et al. A comparative study of the human external sphincter and periurethral levator ani muscles. *Br J Urol* 1983;53:35–41.
2. Bartolo DCC, Roe AM, Locke-Edmunds JC, et al. Flap-valve theory of anorectal continence. *Br J Surg* 1986;73:1012–1014.
3. Bannister JJ, Gibbons C, Read NW. Preservation of fecal continence during rises in intraabdominal pressure: is there a role for the flap valve? *Gut* 1987;28:1241–1245.
4. Miller R, Bartolo DCC, Locke-Edmunds JC, et al. Prospective study of conservative and operative treatment of fecal incontinence. *Br J Surg* 1988;75:101–105.
5. Miller R, Orrom WJ, Cornes H, et al. Anterior sphincter plication and levatorplasty in the treatment of fecal incontinence. *Br J Surg* 1989;75:1058–1060.
6. Aronson MP, Lee RA, Berquist TH. Anatomy of anal sphincters and related structures in continent women studied with magnetic resonance imaging. *Obstet Gynecol* 1990;76:846–851.
7. Sweiger M. Method for determining individual contributions of voluntary and involuntary anal sphincters to resting tone. *Dis Colon Rectum* 1979;22:415–416.
8. Frenckner B, Euler CV. Influence of pudendal block on the function of the anal sphincters. *Gut* 1975;16:482–489.
9. Read NW, Bartolo DCC, Read MG. Differences in anal function in patients with incontinence to solids and in patients with incontinence to liquids. *Br J Surg* 1984;71:39–42.
10. Modesto VL, Gold RP, Gottesman L. Pelvic floor abnormalities. In: Mazler WP, Levien DH, Luchtefeld MA, et al, eds. *Surgery of the colon, rectum, and anus.* Philadelphia: Saunders,1995:1075–1090.
11. Varma JS, Smith AM. Neurophysiological dysfunction in young women with intractable constipation. *Gut* 1988;29:963.
12. Ihre T, Seligson U. Intussusception of the rectum—internal procidentia: treatment and results in 90 patients. *Dis Colon Rectum* 1975;18:391.
13. Weber AM, Walters MD, Ballard LA, et al. Posterior vaginal prolapse and bowel function. *Am J Obstet Gynecol* 1998;179(6 Pt 1):1446–1450.
14. Arnold MW, Stewart WR, Aquilar PS. Rectocele repairs: Four years' experience. *Dis Colon Rectum* 1990;3:684.
15. Kodner IJ, Fry RD, Fleshman JW. Rectal prolapse and other pelvic floor abnormalities. *Surg Annu* 1992;2:157.
16. Henry MM. Descending perineum syndrome. In: Henry MM, Swash M, eds. *Coloproctology and the pelvic floor,* 2nd ed. Oxford: Butterworth-Heinemann, 1992:299–305.
17. Turnbull GK, Lennard-Jones JE, Bartrum CI. Failure of rectal expulsion as a cause of constipation: why fiber and laxatives sometimes fail. *Lancet* 1986;1:767–769.
18. Read NW, Timms JM, Barfield LJ, et al. Impairment of defecation in young women with severe constipation. *Gastroenterology* 1986;90:53–60.
19. Everhart JE, Renault PF. Irritable bowel syndrome in office-based practice in the United States. *Gastroenterology* 1991;100:998–1005.
20. Thompson WG, Longstreth G, Drossman DA, et al. Functional bowel disorders and functional abdominal pain. In: Drossman DA, ed. *Rome II: the functional gastrointestinal disorders,* 2nd ed. McLean, VA: Degnon Associates, 2000:360.
21. Campbell AJ, Reinken J, McCosh L. Incontinence in the elderly: Prevalence and prognosis. *Age Aging* 1985;14:65–70.
22. Sultan AH, Kamm MA, Hudson CN, et al. Anal sphincter disruption during vaginal delivery. *N Engl J Med* 1993;329:1905–1911.
23. Sorenson M, Tetzschner T, Rasmussen OO, et al. Sphincter rupture in childbirth. *Br J Surg* 1993;80:393–394.
24. Bek KM, Laurberg S. Risks of anal incontinence from subsequent vaginal delivery after a complete obstetric anal sphincter tear. *Br J Obstet Gynaecol* 1992;99:724–726.
25. Haadem K, Dahlstrom JA, Ling L, et al. Anal sphincter function after delivery rupture. *Obstet Gynecol* 1987;70:53–56.
26. Haadem K, Ohrlander S, Lingman G. Long-term ailments due to anal sphincter rupture caused by delivery—a hidden problem. *Eur J Obstet Gynecol Reprod Biol* 1988;27:27–32.
27. Snooks SJ, Swash M, Henry MM, et al. Risk factors in childbirth causing damage to the pelvic floor innervation. *Int J Colorect Dis* 1986;1:20–24.
28. Sultan AH, Kamm MA, Hudson CN. Pudendal nerve damage during labor: prospective study before and after childbirth. *Br J Obstet Gynaecol* 1994;101:22–28.
29. Preston DM, Lennard-Jones JE. Is there a pelvic floor disorder in slow-transit constipation? *Gut* 1981;22:A890.
30. Swash M. Eletromyography in pelvic floor disorders. In: Henry MM, Swash M, eds. *Coloproctology and the pelvic floor,* 2nd ed. Oxford: Butterworth-Heinemann, 1992:184–195.
31. Swash M, Snooks SJ. Motor nerve conduction studies of the pelvic floor innervation. In: Henry MM, Swash M, eds. *Coloproctology and the pelvic floor,* 2nd ed. Oxford: Butterworth-Heinemann, 1992:196–206.
32. Laurberg S, Swash M, Henry MM. Delayed external sphincter repair for obstetric tear. *Br J Surg* 1988;75:786–788.
33. DeLancey JOL, Toglia MR, Peruccchini D. Internal and external anal sphincter anatomy as it relates to midline obstetric lacerations. *Obstet Gynecol* 1997;90:924–927.

CHAPTER 22

Anal Incontinence

Mikio A. Nihira and Okechukwu A. Ibeanu

INTRODUCTION

Defecation is normally a private function, which is performed at socially acceptable times chosen by the individual. Bowel control is learned in early childhood, and failure of bowel control may be associated with loss of independence, reduced self-esteem, social isolation, a sense of inadequacy or helplessness, and clinical depression.

EPIDEMIOLOGY AND ETIOLOGICAL FACTORS

The incidence and prevalence of anal incontinence (AI) is difficult to estimate. Surveys report widely differing figures. Sampling biases may result in significant underestimation in some populations and overestimation in others. For example, embarrassment may cause anally incontinent individuals to deny their symptoms in self-reporting surveys. On the other hand, surveys in which people over the age of 65 are represented by nursing home occupants may overestimate the prevalence in geriatric populations (1). Similarly, the reported prevalence of AI in younger, obstetric populations is suspected to be underestimated because a proportion of these patients may have injuries that go unrecognized, or these individuals experience transient fecal incontinence. Lastly, a standardized definition of AI does not exist. Currently, the reported prevalence varies according to the definition used. In several papers, "fecal incontinence" refers to the exclusive loss of feces, while the term "anal incontinence" is used for incontinence inclusive of flatus and stool (1). In addition, the threshold for the frequency of incontinence varies. Some surveys include individuals who admit to any anal incontinence in the past 1 year, while other surveys focus only on individuals who report incontinence of liquid or solid stool in the past month. Data col-

lection methods also affect the quality of information obtained. Although face-to-face interviews offer the greatest potential for accurate data collection, some individuals are uncomfortable disclosing private information to a live examiner. Conversely, paper questionnaires can be difficult to complete for impaired patients.

Macmillan et al (1) performed a systematic literature review on the prevalence of AI (including flatal incontinence) and fecal incontinence in community-dwelling individuals. These investigators retrieved 1,517 articles and identified 16 that fit their inclusion and exclusion criteria. Overall, these studies estimate the prevalence of AI to be 2% to 24% and the prevalence of fecal incontinence to be 0.4% to 18%. Only 3 of the 16 studies employed a design that minimized significant sources of bias; these studies focused on fecal incontinence and had a much smaller prevalence variation than the other 13. The estimated prevalence of fecal incontinence in these particular trials ranged from 11% to 15%.

Fecal incontinence has a multifactorial etiology, and in gynecologic practice, the majority of patients with AI have obstetric trauma as the principal cause of their symptoms. Many of these women have anal sphincter defects (2). However, patients typically present years after the presumed obstetrical insult, which implies that compensatory continence mechanisms degrade with time.

Sultan et al (3) reported that 35% of a group of primiparous women who were demonstrated to have had intact sphincters antepartum had sphincter defects observed on endoanal ultrasound 6 weeks after vaginal delivery. More concerning was their observation that 13% of the primiparous women developed fecal incontinence or fecal urgency after delivery. Pretlove et al (4) followed a cohort of postpartum patients and found that 61% of patients with recognized sphincter defects were symptomatic postpartum. The patients were not stratified according to parity or age. Faltin et al (5) performed immediate postpartum endoanal ultrasound in 150 primiparous women. They identified clinically undetected anal sphincter tears in 42 of 150 women (28%). In a postal questionnaire 3 months postpartum or more, fecal incontinence was reported by 22 women (15%). The odds ratio of those who had clinically undetected sphincter tears was 8.8 for the development of fecal incontinence.

In addition to sphincter defects, vaginal delivery is associated with pudendal neuropathy, particularly during a prolonged or difficult second stage of delivery. A proposed mechanism of injury is that nerve damage results from traction or compression. This damage may develop into impaired rectal evacuation with the need to strain, perineal descent, and subsequent fecal and urinary incontinence. Other common conditions seen by an obstetrician-gynecologist that are associated with fecal incontinence are presented in Table 22.1.

While there is no universally accepted scoring system for AI at present, several scoring systems have been described and used in different trials. These include the Cleveland Clinic Florida Fecal Incontinence Scale (Wexner) (6), Fecal Incontinence Severity Index (FISI) (7), Fecal Incontinence Quality of Life Score (FIQL) (8), Gastrointestinal Quality of Life Index (GIQLI) (9), as well as non–disease-specific instruments such as the Short Form-36 (10).

PATHOPHYSIOLOGY

The detailed pathophysiology and evaluation of AI are covered in Chapters 20 and 21.

The maintenance of fecal incontinence involves complex interaction between higher centers (frontal cortex) and intact neural pathways between the spinal cord and pelvic muscles and sphincters. These, together with several other physiologic mechanisms, work to result in bowel control, allowing defecation to occur voluntarily at socially acceptable times. Degeneration or injury at any of these levels can result in fecal incontinence; hence there are a variety of etiological factors (Tables 22.2 and 22.3).

Specifically, obstetric-related fecal incontinence can result from pudendal nerve damage by compression or stretching, in addition to physical disruption of the anal sphincter mechanism from perineal lacerations. Postmenopausal estrogen deficiency may also affect levator muscle and pelvic floor strength.

CLINICAL EVALUATION

The goal of the evaluation process is to understand the specific pathophysiology in the individual patient in an effort to identify any easily treatable contributing condition and develop an appropriate treatment plan. Thorough assessment begins with a detailed history and physical examination. Prior instrumented deliveries, gastrointestinal disease, and neurological history should be noted. Levator strength should be assessed, as well as the presence of pelvic or rectal prolapse, hemorrhoids, fistulas, and any abnormal or absent reflexes or sensation. A focused neurological examination is essential as well as an appropriate assessment of any suspected diarrheal disease.

TABLE 22.1

General Causes of Anal Incontinence Encountered by the Gynecologist

Obstetric trauma	Injury to the sphincter
	Injury to the levator ani
	Pudendal neuropathy (stretch injury)
Pelvic organ prolapse	Descending perineal syndrome
Anorectal surgical trauma	Sphincter disruption
	Sphincter dilatation
Functional etiologies	Fecal impaction
	Diarrhea

TABLE 22.2

Factors That Contribute to the Continence of Stool and Flatus

Colonic factors	Normal stool consistency and volume Normal colonic accommodation and capacity
Muscular factors	Intact anal sphincters and resting anal tone
Neurologic factors	Normal mentation and social behavior Intact levator muscle innervation Intact external sphincter mechanism Normal anal sensory mechanism (sampling)
Anorectal factors	Normal rectal capacity and compliance Intact anal seal of the vascular cushions

Investigative tools for the evaluation of AI include anorectal manometry, endoanal ultrasound, defecography, endoscopy, and pudendal nerve latency tests; a description of these tests can be found in Chapter 21.

PREVENTION

Because obstetrical trauma is the most common etiology of AI in women, prevention should be focused on the management of labor and delivery. There is an association between sphincter disruption and episiotomy (both midline and mediolateral). When episiotomy must be performed for obstetrical indications, the mediolateral approach should be preferred in an effort to avoid direct injury to the anal sphincters (11). There is also a well-established association between operative delivery using forceps and anal sphincter trauma. Avoidance of episiotomy and use of vacuum-assisted vaginal delivery (as opposed to forceps) when operative delivery is indicated, as well as maintaining a low threshold for cesarean delivery for labor dystocia, may be protective (12).

MANAGEMENT

Before embarking on an extensive work-up and committing to specific treatments for AI, it is prudent to identify and address any gastrointestinal conditions that may contribute to fecal incontinence.

Treatments for AI include medical therapy, behavioral therapy in the form of biofeedback therapy, and surgery. A significant issue in the management of AI is the differing opinion on what constitutes successful treatment. This is due to a lack of consistent outcome measures. The use of post-treatment questionnaires in some studies relies on vague and subjective quantification such as "improved," while in other studies there is variation in the inclusiveness of the definition of incontinence with respect to gas, liquid, or solid stool.

NONSURGICAL THERAPY

Dietary Modification

The initial approach to conservative treatment of AI is to manipulate and improve the consistency and volume of bowel movements by increasing dietary fiber intake to generate well-formed stools. Formed stool is easier to control than liquid stool, which tends to seep out from the incompetent anal sphincter and produces soiling. Fiber supplements are easily available without prescription. Dosage should be titrated to stool consistency by the patient. The use of bulking agents should be monitored in the elderly because excessive use can predispose such patients to fecal impaction, especially if fluid intake is inadequate. A common side effect of high fiber consumption is increased flatus. The avoidance of highly spiced foods and bowel irritants like pepper and caffeine, lactose, beer, and some citrus fruits, all of which may produce diarrhea, can improve continence for many patients.

Pharmacotherapy

In addition to dietary manipulation, constipating agents can be useful in patients with chronic loose stools, which are hard to control.

Loperamide is a popular drug that reduces bowel motility, hence increasing stool transit time.

TABLE 22.3

Differential Diagnosis of Anal Incontinence

Anatomic derangements	**Developmental** (congenital abnormalities)
	Traumatic (obstetric trauma, hemorrhoidectomy, anal sphincterotomy, or dilatation)
	Fistula, rectal prolapse, sequelae of inflammatory bowel disease
Neurologic disorders	**Central nervous system process** Dementia, sedation, mental retardation Stroke, brain tumor, spinal cord lesion, multiple sclerosis Tabes dorsalis
	Peripheral nervous system process Cauda equina lesions Polyneuropathies Diabetes mellitus, toxic neuropathy Shy-Drager syndrome
	Traumatic neuropathy Obstetric trauma Perineal descent
	Altered rectal sensation (unknown lesion) Fecal impaction Delayed sensation syndrome Skeletal myopathies Myasthenia gravis Muscular dystrophies
Smooth muscle dysfunction	**Abnormal rectal compliance** Proctitis due to inflammatory bowel disease, radiation Rectal ischemia
	Internal anal sphincter weakness Radiation proctitis Diabetes mellitus Childhood encopresis

Modified from Johanson JF, Lafferty J. Epidemiology of fecal incontinence: the silent affliction. *Am J Gastroenterol* 1996;91:33–36, with permission.

A 4-mg dose before meals has been demonstrated to improve continence (13). The main side effect is constipation, which is usually better tolerated than AI. A balance between continence and constipation can usually be achieved with careful dose titration and with attention to the precise timing of administration.

Codeine phosphate may also be used to induce constipation in divided daily doses of 30 to 120 mg. It can cause drowsiness. Lomotil (codeine with diphenoxylate and atropine) is a good alternative, but anticholinergic side effects may limit its use (14).

Fecal incontinence secondary to fecal impaction or constipation should be treated with laxatives. Again, caution must be used in elderly patients, because excessive use can cause diarrhea and electrolyte imbalances. The goal of this therapy is to clear hard stool and maintain predictable, regular bowel evacuations, leaving the rectum empty between bowel movements.

Alpha-adrenergic agonists theoretically appeared promising as a means of increasing the resting tone of the internal anal sphincter, but unfortunately a preparation of topical phenylephrine was disappointing in clinical practice (14).

Enemas and Rectal Irrigation

Rectal washout by irrigation and enema treatments using water is used mainly for patients with fecal incontinence resulting from fecal impaction and constipation. Patients can safely perform these treatments at home by themselves after initial instruction. The aim is to evacuate the rectum periodically in order to control fecal soiling. Crawshaw et al reported their findings on 48 patients who were managed with rectal irrigation and followed up for a median period of 11 months. Forty-eight percent of patients with fecal incontinence and 53% with constipation noticed improvement in their symptoms. Interestingly, the use of anal manometry was not helpful in predicting patients who responded to treatment (15).

Biofeedback Therapy

This form of behavioral therapy is frequently added to dietary management and drug treatment when simple measures fail to satisfactorily improve continence. There are two proposed mechanisms through which biofeedback improves anal continence:

- *Efferent training:* Voluntary contraction of the external anal sphincter may be enhanced through training, allowing the patient to recruit more motor units and stimulate muscle hypertrophy.
- *Afferent training:* Impaired sensation in the anorectal canal may be improved through practice that recruits adjacent neurons to decrease the sensory threshold of volume stimulation.

Although there are few long-term data to support the efficacy of biofeedback for the treatment of fecal incontinence, some investigators have observed success rates as high as 70% to 80%. Patients may be taught to contract the sphincters and the levators voluntarily in response to rectal distention. This strategy serves two purposes: one is to improve voluntary contraction of the puborectalis and the anal sphincters (efferent training); the other is to improve sensory discrimination for rectal filling (afferent training) (16).

One of the most important elements of biofeedback is patient education. An explanation of the influence of stool consistency or levator ani tone permits the patient to modify these parameters to improve continence. Similarly, an explanation of the physiology of the rectoanal inhibitory reflex can help patients with fecal urgency (17).

There are several different modalities of biofeedback therapy. These may each be utilized individually or in combination:

- **Intra-anal electromyographic sensor with anal manometric probe**: The patient is taught how to improve continence by squeezing the external anal sphincter muscle. Correct isolation of the muscle is reinforced with the use of pressure measurements as objective evidence of correct technique. Importantly, the goal includes improving duration of squeeze rather than achieving a high pressure peak during squeeze.
- **Three-balloon system for rectal distention**: The patient is taught to identify and respond to rectal distention and filling with squeezing of the external anal sphincter. One of the important goals of this method is to improve the response time to the stimulus, and hence reduce delay in rectal sensation.
- **Rectal sensory threshold training using a rectal balloon**: Rectal distention to different volumes helps the patient to recognize the sensation of rectal filling at even relatively small volumes; the aim is to gradually build tolerance to greater volumes of distention and improve the symptom of fecal urgency.

A recent randomized study by Norton et al (18) involved the stratification of patients into four therapy groups—education only, with sphincter exercises added, with computer-assisted biofeedback, and lastly, with biofeedback and a home electromyographic device. Patient demographics and pretreatment symptomatology were similar across all groups. There was no significant difference among the groups in improvement outcomes such as bowel control as rated by the patients, number of soiling accidents and bowel movements, and objective anorectal physiologic measurements. Overall, 47% of patients reported no accidents for a period of 1 week in diary records. Interestingly, there were no reliable predictors of response to treatment. Anal sonography findings, continence scores, and anal manometric measures of sphincter function were not useful predictors of outcome. Patients, however, did continue to experience improvement at 1-year posttreatment.

The limitations in truly assessing the overall effectiveness of biofeedback therapy in the published literature are a lack of standardized techniques in trials, nonuniform outcome data, and nonhomogenous patient groupings.

SURGICAL THERAPY

Anal Sphincteroplasty

Anal sphincteroplasty is the most commonly performed operation to treat fecal incontinence in the United States (2). Specifically, the overlapping sphincteroplasty technique is generally favored over the end-to-end repair of the disrupted external anal sphincter distant from obstetric injury.

Sphincteroplasty is generally reserved for patients who have significant anterior defects of the external anal sphincter. These may be demonstrable on preoperative physical examination and confirmed with endoanal ultrasound.

The procedure begins with wide mobilization of the ruptured external anal sphincter without excision of the scarred ends. This is accomplished through an inverted semilunar perineal incision or a transverse incision at the posterior vaginal fourchette with inferolateral extension in patients who have damage to the perineal body or rectovaginal septum. The latter incision facilitates repair of the perineal body and rectovaginal fascial attachments. Patients with external anal sphincter defects may have fibrous scar tissue intervening between the viable muscular ends of the sphincter, or they may have complete separation with scar tissue present only on the ruptured ends of the sphincter. In the latter case, the perineal body is usually compromised and a complete reconstruction is indicated. It is recommended that the scar tissue between the separated muscle bundles be transected but not excised from the viable muscle, as scar may hold suture better than muscle. A Pena muscle stimulator is invaluable in identifying the distal ends of the external anal sphincter and differentiating viable muscle from scar tissue before and during the dissection. In dissecting out the external anal sphincter, care should be taken to avoid excessive lateral dissection because the hemorrhoidal branches of the pudendal nerve that supply the external anal sphincter enter at the 3 and 9 o'-clock positions. Because this dissection can be bloody, needle point electrocoagulation can help to achieve hemostasis.

There is controversy about dissecting the external anal sphincter from the internal anal sphincter before repair of the external sphincter. This is done by identifying the intersphincteric groove and dissecting in this plane to avoid damage to either sphincter. If the internal sphincter is also ruptured, its ends are identified and plicated before repair of the external sphincter. This can be difficult because the internal sphincter is intimately associated with the rectal mucosa, but a finger in the anal canal should help. The primary goal is to repair at least 2 to 3 cm of the external sphincter to ensure that the anal canal is enclosed by an adequate bulk of muscular sphincter. Closure of the internal sphincter and reconstruction of the perineal body and rectovaginal septum are also indicated to maximize the continence mechanism.

Copious irrigation is recommended between layer closures. The external sphincter is overlapped with three or four stitches of 2-0 delayed absorbable or permanent suture placed through the distal scar tissue. The muscle ends are overlapped sufficiently to create snugness around a finger placed in the anal canal.

Finally, the perineal skin is closed with interrupted absorbable monofilament suture. This frequently requires modification of the initial incision because of changes in the perineal architecture that result from repair of the sphincter. The most common approach is a Y closure of the skin. Some surgeons recommend the overlapping technique regardless of the timing of the repair. In the case of delayed repairs, it is recommended to wait 3 to 6 months before surgery to allow postpartum inflammation and swelling to resolve.

Postoperative bowel confinement with constipating agents has not been demonstrated to improve functional outcomes and is associated with an increased frequency of bowel complications. Nessim et al (19) randomized 54 patients who underwent reconstructive anorectal surgery to receive either a clear liquid diet with constipating drugs until the third postoperative day or a regular diet commencing the day of surgery. The first postoperative bowel movement was at 3.9 days for the bowel confinement group and 2.8 days for the regular diet group. There were no differences in either morbidity or functional success rates.

Other issues regarding pre- and postoperative management remain unresolved. Some authors recommend only prophylactic antibiotic coverage (20). Others recommend regimens of antibiotic regimens of metronidazole and ciprofloxacin for 1 week after surgery (21). Most experts recommend sitz baths and stool softeners after sphincteroplasty, but there is no consensus as to the duration or frequency of these maneuvers.

No randomized trials have directly compared sphincteroplasty to other treatments like biofeedback or neuromodulation. Again, differences in the assignment of outcome measures and variable durations of follow-up make it difficult to systematically evaluate the effectiveness of sphincteroplasty. Recently published research demonstrates that sphincteroplasty has good short-term benefit, but unfortunately it tends to deteriorate over time. Gutierrez et al (2) reported on the long-term (10 years) evaluation of the results of sphincteroplasty on 191 patients (29% contacted). Overall, 61% had a poor outcome and 57% had incontinence of solid stool, up from 36% at the 3-year follow-up. Despite this, 74% of patients overall remained happy with the results of their surgery. Age and severity of fecal incontinence as assessed by the Fecal Incontinence Quality of Life Score (8) were found to be predictors of poor outcome. Anorectal physiologic measurements were not predictive of outcome.

The role of additional therapies such as biofeedback in improving the results of sphincteroplasty is not known, but they may be helpful. Eight of the 18 patients in Gutierrez's study underwent additional biofeedback therapy and reported some improvement. The same study also affirmed the strong link between obstetric trauma and anal sphincter injury. Not unexpectedly, a recent study evaluating sexual function after sphincter repair found that fecal incontinence does negatively impact sexual intimacy in postpartum patients who had third- or fourth-degree perineal tears. Questionnaire responses demonstrated an improvement in sexual satisfaction after sphincteroplasty (22).

Other Treatment Modalities

Gracioplasty

The transposition of the gracilis muscle for augmentation of the external sphincter was first described in the 1950s by Pickrell et al. Adynamic gracioplasty refers to gracilis transposition without additional electrical stimulation, the so-called passive gracilis wrap. Dynamic gracioplasty (with electrical stimulation) has the advantage of maintaining contraction of the muscle, and tone, over longer periods. The goal of this procedure is to convert the fatigable fast twitch (type II) muscle fibers of the gracilis to fatigue-resistant slow twitch (type I) fibers (23) in an effort to gain an improved functional result.

Gracioplasty carries significant morbidity; the main complication is infection. The Dynamic Gracioplasty Therapy Study Group trial on 123 patients reported an infection rate of 14%; 74% of the patients experienced an adverse event (24). In successful cases, lower limb function does not appear to be adversely affected following transposition of the gracilis muscle. Because there are no approved electrical stimulators in the United States, dynamic gracioplasty is not routinely performed in the United States.

Artificial Anal Sphincter

The artificial sphincter (Acticon Neosphincter®, American Medical Systems, Minneapolis, MN) is a modification of the device developed as an artificial urethral sphincter. It consists of three parts: (a) a Silastic inflatable cuff that encircles the anal canal, (b) a reservoir balloon, and (c) a patient-activated poppet valve that permits deflation of the cuff when the patient desires to defecate. The reservoir is placed in the retropubic space, and the poppet valve is placed in the labia majora. The sphincter cuff is placed through a perineal incision.

Experience with this device remains limited to a few, highly specialized researchers. At present, the literature consists only of pilot studies. Madoff (25) reported on the results of 28 patients who received artificial anal sphincters between 1997 and 1999. Seven artificial sphincters were removed (25%), six for infection. An additional six patients required surgical revision. One year after surgery, 9 of 12 patients were considered to have had a successful procedure as measured by reduced incontinence scores and improved quality-of-life scores.

Lehur et al (26) described their implantation experience in 24 patients. At a median follow-up of 20 months, 20 patients had an activated implanted device. Incontinence scores improved drastically, and 75% of the patients had satisfactory results in terms of incontinence avoidance and ability to defecate. O'Brien et al studied 14 patients and reported significant improvements in fecal incontinence scores in the study group of 7 patients (13). One of the seven patients had the device removed because of infection.

Christiansen et al (27) have the longest documented experience with the artificial anal sphincter. They have a cohort of patients 5 years or more (median 7 years) after implantation. Originally, 17 patients were implanted. During the follow-up period, two died from unrelated conditions, three implants were removed secondary to infectious complications, and an additional four were removed secondary to malfunctions. Eight of the implants remained (47%). Four of these patients were continent of solid and liquid stool. The other four had "occasional" episodes of incontinence of liquid. O'Brien et al randomized 14 patients to placement of an artificial sphincter or a program of supportive care. These investigators observed significant improvements in continence as well as quality of life in the artificial sphincter group 6 months postoperatively (28). One of the seven patients had the device removed because of infection.

Despite the challenges of postoperative infection and erosion that require device removal, the artificial sphincter appears to be relatively safe when under the care of an experienced specialist and offers the potential for good bowel control to a significant number of patients whose alternative may be fecal diversion. The drawbacks of this treatment are the increased chance of fecal impaction and constipation. Also, it requires some dexterity on the part of the patient.

EMERGING TREATMENTS

Novel therapeutic modalities continue to be developed in the effort to expand the treatment options for patients with AI. These are particularly welcomed by patients with intractable AI, in which the only further options hitherto available were to undergo fecal diversion or live with their symptoms indefinitely.

Sacral Neuromodulation

Sacral neuromodulation was first used for the treatment of bladder dysfunction in 1981. Following the observation of simultaneous improvement in bowel symptoms in some patients, it has since been used to treat fecal urgency and incontinence, typically in patients with an intact external sphincter (29).

The procedure of sacral nerve stimulation is described in Chapter 12. The original technique has evolved to a simplified percutaneous procedure of lead insertion into the third sacral foramina with minimal dissection, and it employs tined leads to prevent displacement. Following initial implantation, an external stimulator carried by the patient is used to temporarily test for symptom improvement. If the patient experiences at least a 50% reduction in incontinence episodes, she becomes a candidate for an implantable pulse generator or pacemaker (Interstim™, Medtronic, Minneapolis, MN).

The main complications of this approach are infection, buttock pain, and lead displacement. Patients with infection should have the device removed. A new generator and stimulator leads may be reimplanted after infection and inflammation have been controlled. Lead displacement usually requires repositioning. Patients typically experience a tingling sensation in the buttock, anus, or vagina, and the generator settings are often adjusted according to the intensity of these sensations. Frequency, pulse width, and amplitude are all adjustable according to response. The patient can turn the device on or off using a magnetized switch. Patients must not undergo an MRI with this appliance in situ due to concerns regarding generator heating, lead displacement, and reprogramming of the device.

A review of six series from various centers in Europe involving 266 patients reported on 149 patients who went on to have permanent implantation of a generator (29). Nineteen adverse events occurred: lead displacement, pain over the implantation site, infection, and wound dehiscence. A range of 41% to 75% of patients were reported as having full continence of liquid and solid stool, while 75% to 100% of patients were reported to have experienced at least 50% reduction in the frequency of fecal incontinence. It is difficult to generalize the results of these trials to different populations of patients suffering from AI due to variations in patient populations, together with the differences in etiology of these patients' AI. However, it appears that sacral nerve stimulation did result in improvement in the quality of life and fecal incontinence scores by reducing fecal urgency and incontinence episodes.

The exact mode of action of sacral neuromodulation remains unclear. It is thought that neuromodulation may alter autonomic nerve activity and also stimulate sensory neurons in the pelvis. Observed end-organ effects include increased rectal mucosal blood flow and increased rectal sensitivity to distention, as well as a reduction in anal relaxation waves and fecal urgency. The effect on anal squeeze pressure varies in different trials.

Overall, sacral neuromodulation has the potential to be an effective treatment modality for AI that has not responded to more conventional approaches. It is currently not approved for the indication of AI in the United States (Table 22.4). No randomized trials that have compared neuromodulation to other modalities such as surgery or biofeedback are currently published. In addition, long-term efficacy data are lacking. Nevertheless, it does represent an option for patients with intact external anal sphincters who have failed nonsurgical therapies for fecal incontinence and do not want to undergo fecal diversion.

Radiofrequency

Radiofrequency collagen remodeling has been used effectively in the treatment of gastroesophageal reflux disease and was recently adapted to the treatment of fecal incontinence using the same basic principle.

The controlled delivery of radiofrequency energy to the mucosa causes tissue heating that results in collagen alteration with subsequent tissue remodeling and contraction. In the treatment of fecal incontinence, the energy is delivered through an anoscope with four 7-mm needle electrodes that are deployed from within. The radiofrequency device (SECCA®, Curon Medical, Inc., Freemont, CA) is placed under direct vision. The needles are fed by an energy source (generator) and have temperature sensors to monitor mucosal and deeper tissue temperatures; simultaneous cooling is achieved by means of cold water irrigation delivered to the bases of the needles. The mucosal temperature is regulated at a constant 85°. The energy is delivered in quadrants through the needle points,

TABLE 23.2

Drugs Associated with Constipation

Analgesics
Anticholinergics
  Antispasmodics
  Antidepressants
  Antipsychotics
  Antiparkinsonian drugs
Neurally active agents
  Opiates
  Antihypertensives
  Ganglionic blockers
  Vinca alkaloids
  Anticonvulsants
  Calcium-channel blockers
  Diuretics
Cation-containing agents
  Iron supplements
  Aluminum (antacids, sucralfate)
  Calcium (antacids, supplements)
  Barium sulfate
  Metallic intoxication (arsenic, lead, mercury)
Other
  5-HT$_3$ antagonists
  Granisetron
  Ondansetron

From Wald A. Approach to the patient with constipation. In: Yamada T, Alpers DH, Owyang C, et al, eds. *Textbook of gastroenterology*, 3rd ed. Philadelphia: Lippincott Williams & Wilkins, 1999;911, with permission.

tions of incomplete emptying. In one study, only one third of patients complaining of constipation related this complaint to infrequent defecation. More common complaints included the inability to defecate when desired (34%), the passage of hard stools (44%), and straining associated with defecation (52%) (10). Given the range of symptoms related to constipation as well as the subjectivity of self-reporting, attempts have been made over the years to classify bowel dysfunction in terms of functional gastrointestinal disorders (FGIDs) that are identified only by symptoms. To this end, the recently revised Rome III criteria are proposed to classify the functional bowel disorders, including functional diarrhea. The FGIDs will be discussed in more detail later in this chapter.

Idiopathic Constipation

In approaching the differential diagnosis of constipation, it is necessary to consider and exclude con-

ditions that could contribute to the symptom. When concurrent disease processes, diet, medications, and psychological factors cannot be identified, attempts to classify constipation as idiopathic may be based on age of presentation, colonic transit times, or anorectal sensory and motor dysfunction. Commonly, colonic transit times are used based on the presumption that there is some underlying colonic or anorectal motor dysfunction responsible for the disorder. To characterize constipation on this basis, four subtypes have been classified: (a) normal colonic and rectal transit time; (b) slow colonic transit time only; (c) slow rectal transit time only; (d) slow colonic and rectal transit times (11) (Table 23.3).

Age and Constipation

In children, chronic constipation may involve both physiologic and psychological factors. Children may present with symptoms of abdominal pain and distention when constipation is associated with fecal impaction with or without rectal (megarectum) and sigmoid (megacolon) dilation. Affected children may report the absence of a defecatory urge. Alternatively, they may demonstrate a conscious inhibitory or withholding reflex (learned response) related to previous experiences with dyschezia (possibly related to anal fissures or attempts to evacuate large stools) (7). Although decreased transit times localized to the distal colon and rectum have been demonstrated in many children with chronic constipation (12), manometric thresholds for rectal sensation and resting anal sphincter pressures are often normal (13,14). With the exception of children with Hirschsprung's disease, manometry usually demonstrates normal relaxation of the internal anal sphincter. Conversely, studies suggest that roughly two thirds of constipated children with encopresis suffer from anismus or rectosphincteric dyssynergia (failure to relax the puborectalis and external anal sphincter) (7,15) (Fig. 23.1). The role of dietary fiber appears to be important; several studies have demonstrated that fiber alone is independently negatively correlated with chronic constipation and that an inadequate daily intake of fiber is a risk factor for chronic constipation in children (16,17).

Idiopathic constipation is twice as common in females as males in the young to middle-aged population (10). Of the patients who remain refractory to therapeutic intervention, 30% have normal colonic transit studies (18). Several studies have suggested that this subset of individuals has more psychopathology, including depression, than those individuals with delayed transit times (19,20), but there appears to be little efficacy in using psycho-

TABLE 23.3

Diagnostic Algorithm for Idiopathic Constipation

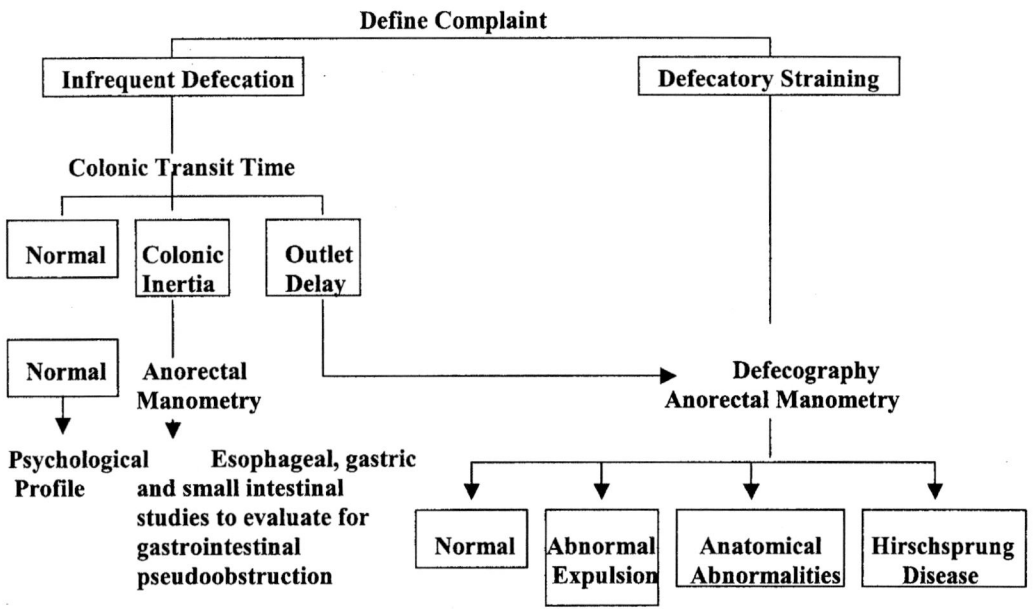

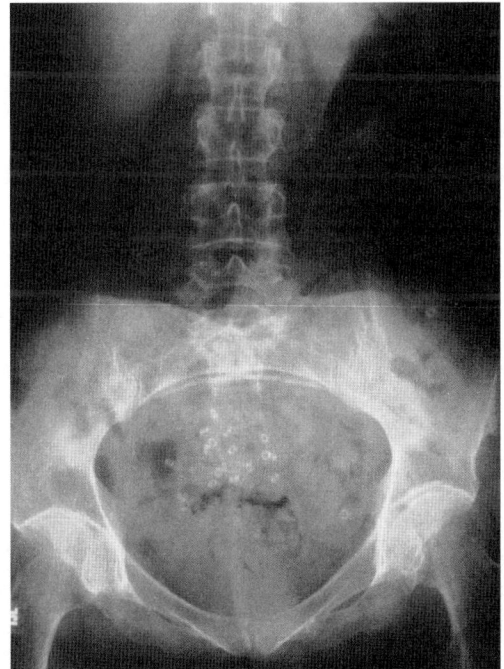

FIGURE 23.1 ● Colonic transit study of a patient with rectosphincteric dyssynergia or colonic stricture on day 5 after ingestion of one Sitzmark capsule. The progression of markers to the rectum was normal.

logical factors to characterize subtypes of idiopathic constipation (21).

There is an exponentially increased prevalence of constipation after the age of 65 years (10). Although it is generally accepted that age does not significantly affect colonic motor function in healthy individuals, this increase in prevalence could result from chronic stress to the enteric nervous system resulting in denervation and neuronal loss. This may be secondary to underlying systemic or colonic disorders or side effects from medications (7). Conditions affecting elderly patients, such as changes in mental status (dementia, Alzheimer's disease, confusion) and factors associated with mobility and bathroom access, may contribute to delayed defecation, which, in turn, may contribute to fecal impaction, a significant problem in elderly patients (22). Longstanding dilation of the rectum and rectosigmoid may contribute to denervation, diminished sensation, and worsening constipation.

Evaluation

The evaluation of the constipated patient begins with a careful history, with special consideration to the age of onset and duration of symptoms. Symptoms present since birth or childhood suggest an underlying congenital etiology. In contrast, constipation occurring later in life tends to be an acquired disorder. A sudden or recent change in bowel habits suggests an underlying organic lesion, whereas chronic symptoms usually represent a functional bowel disorder. A review of symptoms with respect to defecatory dysfunction must include questions regarding frequency and consistency of bowel movements, the presence of melena or hematochezia, the time required for a bowel movement, and the need to strain or digitally facilitate evacuation. Associated symptoms of dyschezia, obstipation, encopresis, incomplete defecation, anismus, fecal incontinence, abdominopelvic pain, or bloating must also be reviewed.

Medications (prescription, nonprescription, and alternative) should be reviewed in detail because many have constipating side effects (see Table 23.2). Chronic laxative use or abuse is a common precipitating factor contributing to chronic constipation. Stimulant laxatives such as the anthraquinones (aloe, senna, cascara), bisacodyl/castor oil, and the polyphenolic derivatives can cause degeneration of Meissner's and Auerbach's plexuses through neurotoxicity (10,23).

Patients should be questioned regarding a family history of both benign and malignant intestinal disorders. Psychosocial issues must also be addressed to detect any concurrent psychological diagnoses, history of emotional disorders, physical or sexual abuse, familial dysfunction, and other life stressors. A careful review of past medical, surgical, gynecologic, and obstetric history is essential.

Physical examination should include a focused abdominal, pelvic, and neurologic evaluation to rule out extraintestinal causes of constipation. Abdominal examination should include an assessment of previous incision sites and a search for ventral and inguinal hernias. Distention, tympany, and the presence of masses or hepatosplenomegaly should be documented. The presence of bowel sounds and any abdominal discomfort should be quantified and the location and quality described.

Rectal and pelvic examinations are essential. Typically performed in the dorsal or semi-Fowler's lithotomy position, a careful systematic evaluation of pelvic organ support is undertaken using the Pelvic Organ Prolapse Quantification (POPQ) method. An overall stage of prolapse and compartment-specific stages are assigned. If present, attempts should be made to qualify and describe site-specific defects, especially with respect to anterior and posterior compartments. An assessment for perineal descent and rectal prolapse

should be done, and when present the type of rectal prolapse should be documented. Perineal examination should also look for any deformity, presence of surgical or traumatic scarring, ongoing sepsis, "dovetail sign" or flattening of the bilateral gluteal creases, or atrophy of the gluteal or perineal muscles. Rectal examination may reveal a stricture from previous anorectal surgery or trauma or may detect a neoplasm. The texture and amount of stool in the rectal vault should be noted. A large, hard mass of feces suggests impaction. Sphincter tone and symmetry should be assessed. With the patient straining, the presence of a paradoxical contraction of the puborectalis may indicate rectosphincteric dyssynergia. Neurologic examination should include an assessment of autonomic function and reflexes, including lower extremity deep tendon reflexes as well as pelvic and perineal sensation and bulbocavernosus and clitoral–anal reflexes.

In the patient with acute complaints of altered bowel habits, with a family history of colorectal cancer, or in the age group appropriate for colorectal cancer screening, colonoscopy, double-contrast barium enema, or computed tomographic colonography should be performed.

If there is no evidence suggesting an underlying systemic or organic etiology, conservative therapy may be pursued. For patients failing to respond to initial therapy, a 1- to 2-week bowel diary and a measurement of colonic transit time with either radiopaque markers or scintigraphic techniques are the most useful diagnostic investigations (24). Further testing and diagnostic studies should be tailored to the specific complaint (see Table 23.3).

Treatment

Most patients presenting with uncomplicated idiopathic constipation may be treated conservatively with modifications in diet and toileting behavior, fiber supplementation, and laxatives. If fecal impaction was diagnosed on initial evaluation, the patient must first be disimpacted. Twice-daily enemas or oral polyethylene glycol may be used to facilitate this. For severe constipation, biofeedback and other pharmacologic agents may be used. If symptoms persist after failure of escalating medical therapy, diagnostic studies evaluating colonic and anorectal function should be undertaken.

Conservative Behavioral Therapy

Conservative therapy begins with patient education. Most patients require reassurance that their condition is not life-threatening and can be successfully managed. Regular toileting strategies to prevent impaction are often used with children as well as with patients suffering from dementia, physical handicaps, and neurogenic constipation. Postprandial colonic motility can be enhanced, with behavior modification aimed at encouraging morning and postprandial defecation. Other initial recommendations include reducing excessive use of laxatives or cathartics, increasing daily fluid and fiber intake, and behavioral modification, including daily exercise. Biofeedback using visible or audible signal recordings from rectal manometric or electromyographic monitoring may be useful in treating chronic constipation related to pelvic floor dyssynergia (25).

Fiber

Fiber is a bulking agent that increases fecal volume and density. Fiber consists of insoluble and soluble components that vary depending on the source. The cell wall in fiber resists digestion and contributes to the physical bulking property. It may also serve as a substrate for bacterial proliferation and gas production, which may stimulate colonic motility. It is hypothesized that the therapeutic effect of fiber on large bowel function is multifactorial. First, through enhancing bacterial metabolism and fermentation, fiber may enhance the absorption of bacterial metabolites, such as secondary bile acids. Second, gas production leads to colonic distention and increases in intraluminal pressures, which triggers peristaltic activity. Third, the presence of fiber promotes intraluminal water absorption, increasing fecal bulk and consistency (26).

Burkitt et al first advocated the efficacy of dietary fiber in the early 1970s (27). Bowel frequency, stool weight, and intestinal transit times were compared between African and British cohorts. The authors concluded that the high prevalence of constipation in Western societies was associated with a diminished intake of dietary fiber. The role of fiber in the pathogenesis and prevention of constipation has been difficult to ascertain. Several studies have failed to detect a difference in dietary fiber intake in constipated patients versus healthy controls (28–30). Most studies demonstrate a beneficial effect of bran in treating constipation in patients with IBS (31–33) and diverticular disease (34–36). A meta-analysis of 27 studies investigating the relationship between dietary fiber and bowel function found that constipated patients continued to have lower stool weights and longer transit times despite being maintained on high-fiber diets (37). In another meta-analysis of 36 separate trials evaluating laxative and fiber therapy for the treatment of chronic constipation, Tramonte et al found improved stool consistency,

decreased abdominal pain, and an increase in weekly bowel movement frequency in patients treated with both daily fiber supplements and laxatives (38). The data could not determine, however, whether fiber was superior to laxatives or whether one type of laxative was better than another.

The accurate assessment of fiber intake is often difficult. Although the recommended daily intake of fiber is 25 to 35 g, or 10 to 13 g per 1,000 kcal (39), the average American typically consumes only 14 to 15 g daily. Fiber therapy may be recommended for patients who have constipation without evidence of impaction, megacolon or megarectum, or obstructing gastrointestinal lesions (Table 23.4). Patients may be started on a high-fiber cereal and should be encouraged to continue daily fiber consumption, increasing the amount to 25 to 35 g/d. Intake of six to eight 8-oz glasses of water per day is recommended with this fiber load. Bloating can be a side effect that typically resolves

TABLE 23.4

Fiber Content

Cereals	Amount of Fiber (g)
All Bran-Extra Fiber (1/2 c)	15
Fiber One (1/2 c)	14
Bran Buds (1/2 c)	10
100% Bran (1/3 c)	9
Raisin Bran (1/2 c)	7
All Bran (1/2 c)	6
Fruit & Fiber (2/3 c)	5
Frosted Mini Wheats (1/2 c)	3
Frosted Flakes (1 oz)	1
Breads	
Whole wheat (1 slice)	2.0
White bread (1 slice)	0.5
Bagel (1)	1.0
Fiber supplements	
Konsyl (1 tsp)	6.0
Perdiem (1 tsp)	4.0
Konsyl D (1 tsp)	3.4
Maalox w/fiber (1 tbs)	3.4
Mylanta w/fiber (1 tsp)	3.4
Metamucil (1 tsp)	3.4
Citrucel (1 tbs)	2.0
Vegetables	
Lettuce (1 c)	1.4
Celery (1)	0.5
Tomato, raw (1)	1.0

over weeks. If bloating persists, a different type of fiber supplement or type of cereal may be substituted.

Laxatives

The use of laxatives is widespread in Western society, especially in the elderly population (40). Laxatives may be classified by their mechanism of action and content (Table 23.5). Bulk-forming laxatives include both natural (psyllium) and synthetic (methylcellulose, polycarbophil) components, which increase the water content and bulk volume of stool. The mechanism of action is similar to that of fiber, and the net effect of bulk-form-

ing laxatives is demonstrated by decreased colonic transit times, increased stool mass and density, and improved stool consistency (11).

Emollient laxatives include docusate salts and mineral oil. The anionic action of docusate salts decreases stool surface tension, thereby enhancing the penetration and absorption of intestinal fluids, which results in softened stools. Docusate salts may also alter intestinal mucosal permeability, promoting absorption of other laxatives. Their overall efficacy in the treatment of chronic idiopathic constipation has been questioned because studies have failed to demonstrate objective improvement in defecatory frequency, colonic transit

TABLE 23.5

Laxatives: Mechanism of Action and Content

Type of Laxative	Adult Dose	Onset of Action	Side Effects
Bulk-forming laxatives			
Natural (psyllium)	7 g PO	12–72 h	Impaction above strictures
Synthetic (methylcellulose)	4–6 g PO	12–72 h	Fluid overload
Emollient laxatives			
Ducusate salts	50–500 mg PO	24–72 h	Skin rashes
Mineral oil	15–45 mL PO	6–8 h	Decreased vitamin absorption
			Lipid pneumonia
Hyperosmolar laxatives			
Polyethylene glycol	3–22 L PO	1 h	Abdominal bloating
Lactulose	15–60 mL PO	24–48 h	Abdominal bloating
Sorbitol	120 mL 25% sol. PO	24–48 h	Abdominal bloating
Glycerine	3 g suppository	15–60 min	Rectal irritation
	5–15 mL enema	15–30 min	Rectal irritation
Saline laxatives			
Magnesium sulfate	15 g PO	0.5–3 h	Magnesium toxicity
Magnesium phosphate	10 g PO	0.5–3 h	Magnesium toxicity
Magnesium citrate	200 mL PO	0.5–3 h	Magnesium toxicity
Stimulant laxatives			
Castor oil	15–60 mL PO	2–6 h	Nutrient malabsorption
Diphenylmethanes			
Phenolphthalein	60–100 mg PO	6–8 h	Skin rashes
Bisacodyl	30 mg PO	6–10 h	Gastric irritation
	10 mg PR	0.25–1 h	Rectal stimulation
Anthraquinones			
Cascara sagrada	1 mL PO	6–12 h	Melanosis coli
Senna	2 mL PO	6–12 h	Degeneration of Meissner
			and Auerbach plexuses
Aloe (casanthrol)	250 mg PO	6–12 h	
Danthron	75–150 mg PO	6–12 h	Hepatotoxicity (w/docusate)

From Wald A. Approach to the patient with constipation. In: Yamada T, Alpers DH, Owyang C, et al, eds. *Textbook of gastroenterology,* 3rd ed. Philadelphia: Lippincott Williams & Wilkins, 1999; 921, with permission.

times, and stool weights (7). Mineral oil, administered orally or rectally as an enema, also works as an emollient to penetrate and soften stool.

Hyperosmolar laxatives include nonabsorbable sugars, such as lactulose and sorbitol, as well as glycerine and polyethylene glycol (GoLYTELY). These agents work by increasing intracolonic osmolarity, which promotes water absorption by stool with subsequent softening. Sorbitol and lactulose are poorly absorbed and are ultimately hydrolyzed by colonic coliform bacteria. Through hydrolysis, lactic, acetic, and formic acids are created and increase intracolonic osmolarity. Side effects include abdominal bloating and flatulence. Polyethylene glycol is not hydrolyzed and is typically associated with fewer symptoms of bloating and flatulence. Polyethylene glycol is usually used for preoperative bowel preparation; however, it may also be used in cases of severe constipation (11).

Saline laxatives include magnesium-containing solutions such as magnesium sulfate, phosphate, and citrate. Saline laxatives increase colonic osmolarity, which, in turn, results in increased water absorption and subsequent stool softening. Administered by enema or suppository, saline laxatives can give rise to mineral and metabolic imbalances and, in patients with renal insufficiency, magnesium toxicity (11).

Stimulant laxatives are typically indicated if bulk or osmotic laxatives are not effective. They include castor oil, the diphenylmethanes (phenolphthaleins, bisacodyl), and the anthraquinones (senna, aloe, cascara sagrada, and danthron). Castor oil, after intestinal conversion to ricinoleic acid, stimulates intestinal secretion and motility. The diphenylmethanes act directly to stimulate colonic motility and small intestine water absorption. The anthraquinones, in contrast, are catalyzed by intestinal microorganisms and promote colonic peristalsis by altering intraluminal fluid and electrolyte composition (7). Stimulant laxatives may be abused, and chronic daily use may lead to diarrhea, electrolyte abnormalities, and dehydration. However, use up to two or three times per week may be undertaken for longer periods.

Prokinetic agents include drugs that directly stimulate gastrointestinal motor activity. The efficacy of metoclopramide, cisapride, cholinergic agonists such as bethanechol, cholinesterase inhibitors such as neostigmine, and serotonin agonists in the treatment of chronic idiopathic constipation is questionable. Metoclopramide, for example, appears to be more effective in treating upper gastrointestinal motor disorders, whereas studies addressing the efficacy of cisapride report conflicting results. Current research is examining the facilitatory role of serotonin agonists on enteric cholinergic transmission and opioid receptor antagonist therapy in the treatment of chronic constipation (7).

MOTILITY DISORDERS

Megacolon and Megarectum

Megacolon and megarectum may occur separately or together and may be divided into either primary or secondary entities (7). Primary megacolon or megarectum is usually present from birth and is associated with an underlying neurologic pathology. Although Hirschsprung's disease is the most classic example, other possibilities include meningomyelocele and other lumbosacral spinal cord lesions. Secondary megacolon or megarectum is an acquired disease state usually found in children and elderly people. It may follow bowel surgery resulting in an anastomotic stricture (see Fig. 23.1) and is usually associated with constipation or defecatory dysfunction. Diagnostic criteria are based on radiographic (Fig. 23.2) and manometric findings, including increased rectal compliance and elasticity, decreased rectal sensation, increased sensory thresholds, and diminished internal anal sphincter relaxation (41).

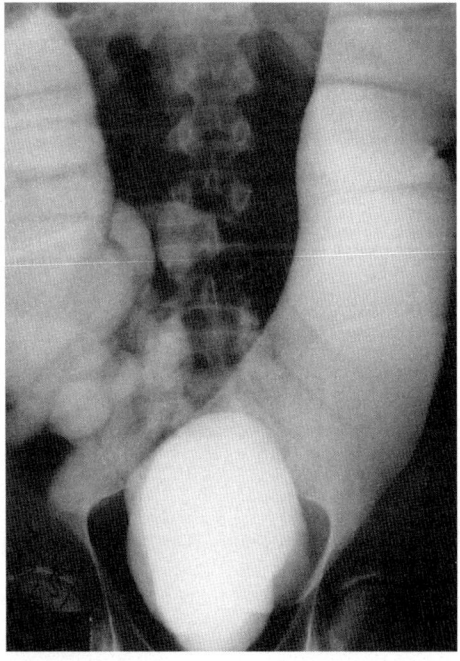

FIGURE 23.2 ● Contrast enema showing megacolon above an anastomotic stricture.

Functional Gastrointestinal Disorders

Attempts to characterize IBS date back to 1820, when Powell first described a triad of pain, bowel dysfunction, and flatulence (42). It was not until 1962 that the syndrome was described in more detail (43), with the first classification of all the FGIDs appearing in 1979 (44). The Manning criteria (45) and the Kruis criteria (46) formed the basis for the first internationally recognized classification system for IBS, the Rome criteria. Since their introduction in 1988, the Rome criteria have become the gold standard for the diagnosis of FGIDs (47). The FGIDs are identified only by symptoms. Rome I criteria recommended that the diagnosis of IBS be based on the presence of abdominal pain or discomfort associated with a chronic change in bowel habit and two or more supporting criteria. Rome II criteria recommend that the diagnosis of IBS be based on the presence of two of the three main diagnostic criteria alone and provide consensus statements for each of the 25 FGIDs located throughout five anatomic regions (48). In 2006, a further revision of the Rome II criteria was published (Rome III) that further refined the diagnostic criteria for the FGIDs and their respective treatment options (49).

The category of functional bowel disorders includes symptoms related to the middle and lower gastrointestinal tract. This group is further subclassified by Rome II and III criteria into the following categories:

1. IBS
2. Functional abdominal bloating
3. Functional constipation
4. Functional diarrhea
5. Unspecified functional bowel disorders

By definition, these diagnoses presume the absence of biochemical or structural etiologies, and symptoms must have occurred for the first time at least 6 months before the patient presents and their presence on at least 3 days per month during the past 3 months would indicate current activity (49).

IBS is a poorly understood, chronic disorder characterized by episodic abdominal pain and changes in bowel habits. In addition to gastrointestinal and defecatory dysfunction, individuals with IBS may also suffer from sleep disturbances, sexual and lower urinary tract dysfunction, and other nongastrointestinal pain syndromes (50). About 60% of patients report abdominal pain or discomfort as their primary complaint. Symptoms characterizing defecatory dysfunction appear to be equally divided between diarrhea-predominant IBS, constipation-predominant IBS, and a variation of the two (51).

Similar to other chronic functional syndromes, a conceptual model involving the interplay of cognitive, behavioral, psychological, genetic, infectious, dietary, and physiologic components has been developed to serve as a framework for understanding the multiple possible factors that may contribute to IBS symptoms. Because there is no single biochemical, physiologic, neurologic, or psychological marker for IBS, researchers have stressed the interrelationship of these multiple components.

Cognitive factors, including abnormal coping mechanisms; misconceptions regarding disease, nutrition, and medications; and illness behavior are common in patients with IBS. Behavioral factors, such as traumatic or stressful events, are often correlated to the first onset of IBS symptoms and have been associated with changes in stool pattern, abdominal pain, and defecation frequency (52,53). IBS is diagnosed more frequently in patients with a history of prior psychological trauma or physical or sexual abuse, especially if incurred during childhood (54,55). Concurrent psychological disorders have been diagnosed in 42% to 61% of patients and include depression, anxiety, panic, and somatization disorders (50,56). Genetic factors may also play a role in the development of IBS because symptoms also appear to be more common in first-degree relatives (57). Infectious disease may in some way be responsible for triggering IBS because several studies have shown an increased risk for IBS symptoms after gastrointestinal infection (58,59). Histologic and biochemical studies have demonstrated evidence of long-term, persistent mucosal inflammation and changes in mucosal permeability in predisposed individuals suffering from IBS symptoms following an initial infectious insult.

There is little evidence to support a causal relationship between specific diet and the development of IBS. Patients intolerant or allergic to specific foods do not necessarily experience improvement of IBS symptoms when these food types are removed from their diets (50,60).

Many symptoms of IBS are consistent with dysfunction of the sensory and motor function of the enteric nervous system. These include dysfunction of neuroenteric regulation resulting in altered intestinal motility, myoelectrical activity, tone and compliance, sensation, and fluid and electrolyte absorption. Unfortunately, correlations between these alterations and IBS symptoms remain weak, raising the question of clinical relevance.

Diagnostic Criteria

Irritable Bowel Syndrome

IBS is characterized by abdominal pain or discomfort associated with defecation or a change in bowel habit. Often having a chronic, relapsing course, symptoms of IBS often overlap with those of other FGIDs, and the diagnostic criteria are listed in Table 23.6 (49). Supporting symptoms may help to classify patients, according to Rome II criteria, further into diarrhea- or constipation-predominant IBS. These include the following (61):

1. Fewer than three bowel movements per week
2. Greater than three bowel movements per day
3. Hard or lumpy stools
4. Loose (mushy) or watery stools
5. Straining during a bowel movement
6. Urgency (having to rush to have a bowel movement)

TABLE 23.6

Functional Gastrointestinal Disorders

Irritable Bowel Syndrome	
Diagnostic Criteria[a]	Recurrent abdominal pain or discomfort at least 3 days per month, which need not be consecutive, in the preceding 3 months, associated with two or more of the following three features:
	Is relieved with defecation
	Has onset associated with a change in frequency of stool
	Has onset associated with a change in form (appearance) of stool
Functional Bloating	
Diagnostic Criteria[a]	Must include **both** of the following:
	Recurrent sensation of bloating or visible distension at least 3 days/month for 3 months
	Insufficient criteria for a diagnosis of IBS, functional dyspepsia or other functional disorders
Functional Constipation	
Diagnostic Criteria[a]	Must include **2 or more** of the following:
	Straining in at least 25% of defecations
	Lumpy or hard stools in at least 25% of defecations
	Sensation of incomplete evacuation in at least 25% of defecations
	Sensation of anorectal obstruction or blockade in at least 25% of defecations
	Manual maneuvers to facilitate at least 25% of defecations (e.g., digital evacuation, support of the pelvic floor)
	Fewer than 3 defecations per week
	Loose stools are rarely present without the use of laxatives.
	There are insufficient criteria for IBS.
Functional Diarrhea	
Diagnostic Criteria[a]	Loose (mushy) or watery stools without pain occurring in at least 75% of stools.
	Diagnostic Criterion for Unspecified Functional Bowel Disorders
Diagnostic Criteria[a]	Bowel symptoms that cannot be attributed to organic pathology and which do not meet criteria for the previously defined FGID categories.
	Diagnostic Criteria for Pelvic Floor Dyssynergia
Diagnostic Criteria[a]	The patient must satisfy all criteria for functional constipation.
	There must be manometric, electromyographic, or radiologic evidence of inappropriate contraction or failure of pelvic floor muscle relaxation during repeated attempts to defecate.
	There must be evidence of adequate propulsive defecatory forces.
	There must be evidence of incomplete evacuation.

[a]Criteria fulfilled for the past 3 months with symptom onset at least 6 months prior to diagnosis.

7. Feeling of incomplete bowel movement
8. Passing mucus (white material) during a bowel movement
9. Abdominal fullness, bloating, or swelling
   Diarrhea-predominant IBS: *1 or more of 2, 4, or 6 and none of 1, 3, or 5*
   Constipation-predominant IBS: *1 or more of 1, 3, or 5 and none of 2, 4, or 6*

Collaborators involved with the Rome III criteria for the FGIDs have recommended subtyping IBS by predominant stool pattern: (a) IBS with constipation (IBS-C); (b) IBS with diarrhea (IBS-D); (c) IBS with both diarrhea and constipation (i.e., mixed stool patterns [IBS-M]); and (d) unsubtyped IBS (Table 23.7).

Functional Bloating

Functional bloating is a recurrent symptom of abdominal distension, which may or may not be objectively measurable. Symptoms are typically less severe in the morning and tend to worsen as the day progresses. Symptoms suggestive of other functional bowel disorders, however, are lacking. Diagnostic criteria for functional bloating are listed in Table 23.6 (49).

Functional Constipation

Functional constipation is characterized by symptoms of abnormal defecation, with respect to either frequency of bowel movements or the act of defecation itself. Symptoms of persistently difficult and infrequent defecation, possibly accompanied by the sensation of incomplete evacuation, that do not meet IBS criteria define functional constipation (49) (see Table 23.6).

Functional Diarrhea

Functional diarrhea is characterized by the recurrent or continuous painless passage of watery or loose stools. The diagnosis depends on the exclusion of other diagnoses, such as pseudodiarrhea

(defecation of solid stools associated with symptoms of urgency and frequency) and underlying organic disease. The diagnostic criteria for functional diarrhea are listed in Table 23.6 (49).

Unspecified Functional Bowel Disorders

Unspecified functional bowel disorders are characterized by functional bowel symptoms that do not meet the criteria for the previously defined categories (49).

In summary, the Rome criteria currently serve as a standardized classification system for FGIDs. The development of the Rome criteria continues to be an ongoing process, with each revision revealing new areas of required research, validation, and debate (see Table 23.6).

Evaluation

Diagnosis is based on identifying symptoms and differentiating IBS from other organic disease (Table 23.8). Once underlying organic diseases are excluded, the Rome criteria demonstrate a sensitivity of 63%, a specificity of 100%, a positive predictive value of 100%, and a negative predictive value of 76% (62). Longitudinal studies examining a diagnosis of IBS based on symptoms and minimal diagnostic testing have shown that over time, fewer than 5% of IBS patients have other diagnoses responsible for their symptoms (63).

A detailed history and physical examination can usually exclude most organic diseases. Warning signs, including fever, weight loss or gain, anorexia, early satiety, anemia, intestinal bleeding, and palpable masses, must be ruled out and a differential diagnosis considered. Attention to stool consistency, defecatory frequency, and relationship of pain and bloating to activity and defecation can help to classify IBS. A symptom diary may be helpful in characterizing symptoms.

TABLE 23.7

IBS Subtyping by Predominant Stool Pattern[a]

1. IBS with constipation (IBS-C)
   Hard or lumpy stools at least 25% and loose (mushy) or watery stools less than 25% of bowel movements.
2. IBS with diarrhea (IBS-D)
   Loose (mushy) or watery stools at least 25% and hard or lumpy stools less than 25% of bowel movements.
3. Mixed IBS (IBS-M)
   Hard or lumpy stools at least 25% and loose (mushy) or watery stools at least 25% of bowel movements.
4. Unsubtyped IBS
   Insufficient abnormality of stool consistency to meet criteria for IBS-C, IBS-D, or IBS-M.

[a]All four subtypes are defined in the absence of use of antidiarrheals or laxatives.
IBS, irritable bowel syndrome; C, constipation; D, diarrhea; M, mixed.
Adapted from Longstreth GW, Thompson WG, Chey WD, et al. Functional bowel disorders. *Gastroenterology* 2006;130:1481.

TABLE 23.8

Differential Diagnosis of Irritable Bowel Syndrome

Chronic intestinal idiopathic pseudo-obstruction
Colorectal carcinoma
Diabetes
Endocrine tumors
Gastrointestinal infections
  Viral enteritis
  Parasitic (*Giardia species, Entamoeba histolytica*)
  Bacterial (*Clostridium, Salmonella, Yersinia, Campylobacter* species)
Inflammatory bowel disease
Lactose intolerance
Malabsorption syndromes/endocrine
  Celiac sprue
  Pancreatic insufficiency
Medications (constipating or diarrhea-provoking)
Microscopic colitis
Psychiatric disorders
Thyroid disease

From Wald A. Approach to the patient with constipation. In: Yamada T, Alpers DH, Owyang C, et al., eds. *Textbook of gastroenterology*, 3rd ed. Philadelphia: Lippincott Williams & Wilkins, 1999; 921, with permission.

Additional consideration should be given to reviewing psychosocial issues, including the patient's concerns and fears, possible stressors, the role of family support or dysfunction, reason for the visit including possible hidden agenda (e.g., disability or narcotic seeking), screening for previous psychological trauma, physical or sexual abuse, and history of concurrent psychological diagnoses.

Laboratory evaluation and diagnostic procedures should be undertaken in the initial evaluation to exclude structural lesions and systemic disease. These include a complete blood count and erythrocyte sedimentation rate, serum chemistries and metabolic profile, urine analysis, thyroid panel, and stool evaluation for occult blood, ova, and parasites. Further diagnostic studies should be tailored to address the patient's predominant symptoms and may be considered for those patients who are older than 50 years of age, have a positive family history of colon cancer, present with sudden onset of symptoms, or have symptoms that appear overly severe or disabling.

Current Rome criteria differentiate subtypes of IBS based on predominant symptoms. Patients who present with complaints of infrequent bowel movements, hard and lumpy stools, sensation of incomplete rectal emptying, or need to strain or splint to facilitate defecation are classified as having constipation-predominant IBS. These patients also tend to have a higher frequency of other specific symptoms, including sexual and sleep dysfunction, anorexia, depression, dyspepsia, and musculoskeletal complaints. Patients presenting with symptoms of increased defecatory frequency and urgency and with loose, watery stools are classified as having diarrhea-predominant IBS. Finally, patients may present with chief complaints of abdominal pain rather than with changes in bowel habits. In this pain-predominant IBS subcategory, pain is commonly accompanied by abdominal bloating, distention, and gas.

After a preliminary diagnosis of IBS is made, basic therapy should be initiated. If no improvement is seen within 2 to 3 weeks, further studies, including colonic transit times (colonic inertia), flexible sigmoidoscopy (functional rectal outlet obstruction, organic lesions), and evaluation of stool weight and composition (malabsorption syndromes, steatorrhea), osmotic gap, and pH (secretory or osmotic diarrhea), can be helpful (63).

Treatment

Therapy for IBS is divided into dietary, pharmacologic, psychological, and behavioral approaches that focus on predominant symptoms and cofactors. Diet should be considered first, although attempts to modify dietary intake may be met with resistance. Avoidance of symptom-provoking agents, such as caffeine, alcohol, sorbitol, and gas-producing foods, including beans, raisins, apricots, carrots, celery, and onions, should be stressed (64). Dietary fiber (20 to 30 g/d) has been widely recommended and may be beneficial in the treatment of constipation-predominant IBS. By promoting free water absorption into the large bowel, fiber acts as a stool-bulking agent that facilitates defecation. Fiber has been shown to decrease intestinal transit time and intracolonic pressure (65). Current literature and meta-analyses evaluating the role of dietary and supplemental fiber in treating IBS reveal significant controversy regarding its long-term efficacy and effectiveness in treating diarrhea-predominant or pain-predominant subtypes (66).

Pharmacologic therapy for IBS is tailored toward alleviating predominant symptoms (Table 23.9). Prokinetic agents, such as cisapride, that stimulate colonic smooth muscle may be helpful as adjuvant therapy in constipation-predominant IBS. Conversely, in patients with diarrhea-predominant IBS, loperamide is the drug of choice. Cholestyramine may also be added because bile acid malabsorption may contribute to the diarrhea. For predominant symptoms of pain and bloating,

antispasmodics, anticholinergics, and antidepressants have commonly been prescribed. Unfortunately, well-designed clinical studies are lacking, and outcome studies evaluating the efficacy of various drugs in these classes have shown conflicting results. In the class of antispasmodics or smooth muscle relaxants, many are anticholinergic. Although Klein's (67) frequently cited 1988 meta-analysis offered no convincing evidence of antispasmodic efficacy, Poynard et al (68) reported on five antispasmodics (mebeverine, trimebutine, cimetropium, pinaverium bromide, octylonium) that were superior to placebo in alleviating IBS symptoms. Dicyclomine and hyoscyamine are commonly prescribed in the United States, and newer agents in this class, including zamifenacin and darifenacin, both M3-receptor antagonists, are showing promise in the treatment of IBS (69). Research evaluating the efficacy of peppermint oil, a natural antispasmodic, remains inconclusive (70).

Historically, antidepressants were used to treat IBS because a large percentage of these patients were thought to be clinically depressed. The neuromodulatory, anticholinergic, and analgesic proper-

TABLE 23.9

Dosage Guidelines for Drugs Commonly Used to Treat the Irritable Bowel Syndrome

Drug	Dose
Anticholinergic agents	
Dicyclomine hydrochloride	20 mg every 6 h; can be increased to 40 mg every 6 h if tolerated
Hyoscyamine sulfate	0.125–0.25 mg sublingually every 4 h (0.375-mg extended-relief tablets: 1 or 2 tablets every 12 h)
Antidiarrheal agents	
Loperamide	4 mg/d initially, with a maintenance dose of 4–8 mg/d, in a single or divided dose
Diphenoxylate (2.5 mg) + atropine sulfate (0.025 mg)	2 tablets 4 times a day
Cholestyramine resin	1 packet (9 g) mixed with fluid and taken once or twice a day
Osmotic laxatives	
Lactulose	10 mg/15 mL of syrup; 15–30 mL/d (usual dose), up to 60 mL/d
Polyethylene glycol solution	17 g dissolved in 240 mL (8 oz) of water, taken daily
Tricyclic compounds	
Amitriptyline	25–75 mg/d
Nortriptyline	25–75 mg/d
Desipramine	25–75 mg/d

From Horwitz BJ, Fisher RS. The irritable bowel syndrome. *N Engl J Med* 2001;344(24):1846–1850, with permission. (Copyright © 2001, Massachusetts Medical Society. All rights reserved.)

ties of selected psychotropics provided some alleviation of IBS symptoms. Tricyclic antidepressants were the first to be used, and numerous studies have since demonstrated their varying degrees of efficacy in treatment of diarrhea- and pain-predominant IBS. Amitriptyline, doxepin, and imipramine are commonly prescribed, albeit usually in doses lower than those typically used for depression (66). More recently, the role of serotonin reuptake inhibitors in the treatment of IBS is being investigated, and preliminary results are promising (71).

Newer agents, including the 5-HT$_3$ antagonists (granisetron, ondansetron, and alosetron) and 5-HT$_4$ agonists (prucalopride and tegaserod), that may have peripheral visceral antinociceptive actions have also shown promise in treating diarrhea- and pain-predominant IBS subtypes. Several studies have shown fewer pain episodes, firmer stools, and fewer episodes of defecatory urgency and frequency in patients treated with these agents (72). Other substances that influence sensation and sensory thresholds to colonic distention include opioid receptor agonists. These include the kappa-opioid receptor agonist fedotozine, and trimebutine, a mu-receptor agonist (73). Pinaverium bromide and octylonium are calcium-channel blockers that have been shown to blunt intestinal motor activity. In contrast, motilin agonists provoke colonic motor activity and thereby reduce gut transit times and promote gastric emptying (66).

Psychological and alternative intervention has also been used to varying degrees of success in treating patients with IBS. Psychotherapy, hypnotherapy, and behavioral and cognitive therapy, as well as therapeutic massage and acupuncture, have undergone study with lack of scientific rigor. Factors that appear to correspond with a favorable response after psychotherapy include diarrhea- and pain-predominant IBS symptoms, especially when associated with and exacerbated by stress. In a recent review (74) evaluating the efficacy of hypnotherapy, relaxation training, and stress management for IBS, the authors found all three modalities effective (reduction in symptom scores; improvement in anxiety, pain, and bowel function; and decrease in gastric acid production and colonic motility). Based on their findings, it would appear that hypnotherapy leads to significant improvement in patients with poorly controlled IBS and that this therapy should be offered to all patients who fail conventional medical therapy.

Colonic Inertia

In the absence of outlet obstruction and following confirmatory transit studies, constipation refractory to fiber and laxative therapy is often referred to as idiopathic slow-transit constipation (STC). The underlying pathophysiology of this condition, representing a disorder of colonic motor function or ineffective colonic propulsion, is poorly understood. Schouten et al (75) documented diminished neurofilament concentration in enteric ganglia, and others have confirmed similar findings with respect to the myenteric plexus in patients with this disorder (76). Other research has focused on neuropeptide composition, transmission, and abnormal hormonal responses to gastrin and motilin secretion. The term "colonic inertia" has been used to describe the failure of a meal or colonic stimulant, such as bisacodyl or neostigmine, to increase colonic activity. The term "cathartic colon" has been used by radiologists to describe abnormal barium enema studies demonstrating significant colonic dilation and redundancy, absence of haustral folds, and incompetent ileocecal valves. It was initially proposed that these findings were secondary to chronic stimulant laxative that had led to myenteric plexus neuropathy (77). The etiology is now less clear, and this term has fallen out of favor.

Women appear to be commonly affected by STC, with symptoms often beginning in childhood (28). Characterized by infrequent bowel movements, STC is also associated with many symptoms that are similar to those of constipation-predominant IBS. These include abdominal bloating and discomfort, flatulence, and defecatory dysfunction characterized by dyschezia, splinting, incomplete emptying, and lumpy, hard stools. Typically, abdominal pain is not a prominent feature in STC. After organic causes and underlying systemic disorders are excluded, the diagnosis of STC can be based on colonic transit measurements by radiopaque markers (Fig. 23.3) or scintigraphic techniques. Both procedures demonstrate good correlation with each other and are sensitive in demonstrating both overall and regional colonic transit delay. Further testing may be required to rule out concurrent outlet obstruction (secondary to dyssynergic defecation or mechanical obstruction) or chronic intestinal pseudo-obstruction, an entity typically characterized by more pronounced abdominal distress, including distention, pain, nausea, and vomiting.

Pharmacologic Treatment

After an empiric trial of fiber supplementation, patients with persistent STC may be treated with laxatives, usually beginning with bulk-forming types such as psyllium and methylcellulose, followed by emollients or stimulant laxatives (see Table 23.5).

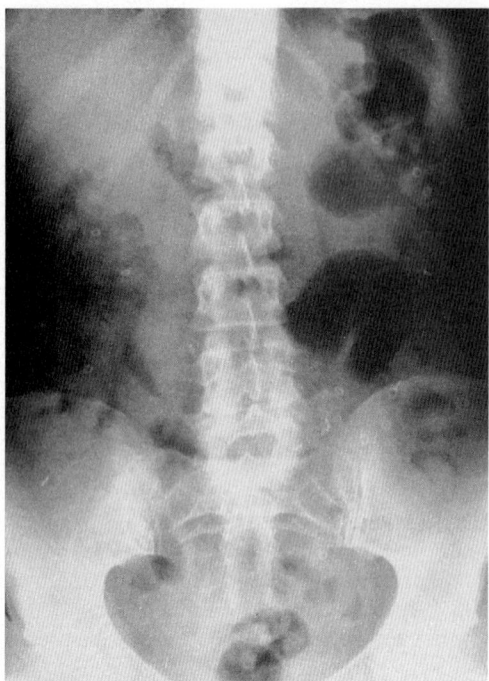

FIGURE 23.3 ● Colonic transit study of a patient with slow-transit constipation on day 5 after ingestion of one Sitzmark capsule.

Caution should be used in prescribing laxatives for long-term use because some literature suggests that chronic stimulant laxative abuse may compromise myenteric plexus innervation, leading to further impairment of colonic motility (77). Enemas may also be used with caution to induce evacuation through colonic distention and mechanical lavage. Prokinetic agents such as the serotonin 5-HT$_4$ agonists, cisapride and metoclopramide, have not been proved effective in treating STC. In contrast, preliminary research involving prucalopride and tegaserod, both newer serotonin 5-HT$_4$ agonists, is encouraging. Both agents promote acceleration of colonic transit times (78). Investigational work involving selective recombinant human neurotrophic agents that enhance sensory neuronal growth and synaptic transmission may also lead to effective therapy for STC (79).

Surgical Treatment

Total abdominal colectomy with ileorectal anastomosis (IRA) may be curative for patients who have exhausted medical therapy. Before considering surgery, mechanical and other functional causes, such as Hirschsprung's disease, volvulus, rectal prolapse, tumors, anastomotic strictures, and pseudo-obstruction, must be excluded. Additionally, concomitant extraintestinal and pelvic floor–related causes must be addressed. Wald proposes that at least four crite-

ria be met before surgery: (a) chronic, disabling symptoms related to constipation refractory to medical therapy; (b) demonstration of slow proximal colonic transit; (c) no evidence or intestinal pseudo-obstruction or mechanical obstruction; (d) normal anorectal function (11).

Lane was the first to publish his results on subtotal colectomy and to advocate this approach for the treatment of refractory constipation (80). Since then, subtotal colectomy with IRA has become the operation of choice for refractory STC, with success rates ranging from about 80% to 94%. Most authors attribute failures to preexisting or postoperative rectal dysfunction or to a more profound generalized intestinal motility disorder (81,82).

The largest series of long-term results of surgery for STC has been published by Nyam et al from the Mayo Clinic (83). In this series, patients underwent extensive evaluation before surgical referral, and of 1,009 patients studied, only 53 with STC underwent colectomy with IRA. An additional 22 patients had STC with coexisting pelvic floor dysfunction and underwent pelvic floor retraining before IRA. At a mean follow-up of 56 months, all patients who underwent IRA were able to defecate spontaneously without the need of enemas, laxatives, or manual assistance. Of these patients, 97% were satisfied with surgery, and 90% reported an improvement in quality of life.

Other authors have reported similarly low operative rates after evaluation of patients for refractory constipation. Wexner et al operated on only 16 of 163 patients initially evaluated for STC, with a reported success rate of 94% (84). The importance of preoperative assessment and diagnosis was also emphasized by Sunderland et al, who operated on only 18 of 228 patients evaluated for STC, with an 88% success rate (85). Redmond et al further categorized patients into those with colonic inertia alone and those with a more generalized intestinal dysmotility problem (82). After subtotal colectomy, the authors found improved success rates in those patients in the STC group (90%) compared with those with generalized intestinal dysmotility (13%).

In addition to abdominal colectomy with IRA, more and less aggressive procedures have been studied. Hosie et al reported results of 13 patients with intractable constipation who underwent restorative proctocolectomy (ileal pouch–anal anastomosis), 8 of whom had previously failed colectomy with IRA (86). Despite a high complication rate, 85% of patients reported symptomatic improvement 20 months after surgery. Anorectal myectomy, an accepted procedure for short-segment Hirschsprung's disease, has also been used in patients with refractory idiopathic constipation. Although initial results were encouraging, long-term results are poor, with one study showing 70% of patients with no functional improvement at 30 months of follow-up (87).

Finally, initially encouraging experience with the Malone antegrade continence enema (ACE) in the pediatric population has prompted some investigators to apply this option to adults with constipation and incontinence. In one study by Krogh et al, time required for defecation was significantly reduced after ACE therapy, and 75% of patients reported overall satisfaction (88). Initially requiring an operative appendicostomy or exteriorization of other tubularized bowel, this procedure can be easily performed under fluoroscopic or colonoscopic guidance. Finally, a trapdoor cecostomy appliance (Fig. 23.4) allows for easy access to the proximal large intestine for antegrade colonic lavage.

OUTLET OBSTRUCTION

First described by Martelli et al in 1978 (89), outlet obstruction has come to represent a subtype of STC in which there is normal passage of colonic transit Sitz markers until the level of the rectum (see Fig. 23.1). A number of functional (rectosphincteric dyssynergia, perineal descent, megarectum, mucosal intussusception, Hirschsprung's disease) or structural (rectocele or enterocele, hemorrhoids, anal fissure, anorectal neoplasia, rectal prolapse, fecal impaction) causes can lead to obstructive defecation. Numerous terms have been used to describe constipation associated with anorectal dysfunction. Anismus, for example, was coined by Preston and Lennard-Jones to describe defecatory dysfunction related to paradoxical anal sphincter contraction (rectosphincteric dyssynergia) (90). Other terms, such as spastic floor syndrome, paradoxical puborectalis contraction syndrome, and pelvic floor dyssynergia, have been used to include the dysfunction of other muscles in the pelvic floor contributing to outlet obstruction. Currently, pelvic floor dyssynergia and resulting dyssynergic defecation are the preferred terms in the gastrointestinal literature (91,92).

Dyssynergic Defecation

In normal defecation, cortical inhibition of the spinal reflex is required to allow relaxation of the external anal sphincter. In patients with rectosphincteric dyssynergia, there is a paradoxic contraction of the puborectalis and external anal sphincter at the time of desired defecation. This is analogous to detrusor–sphincter dyssynergia in pa-

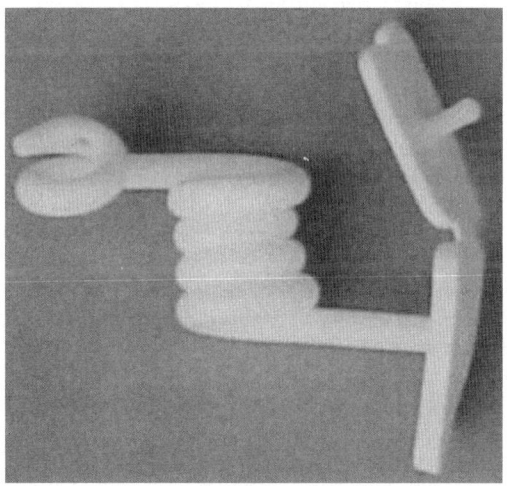

A

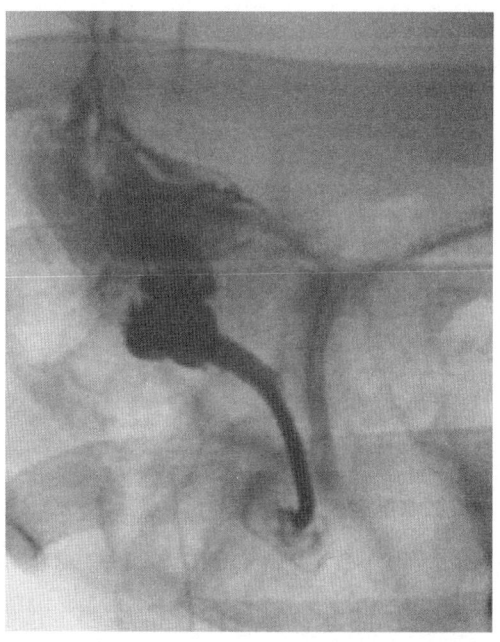

B

FIGURE 23.4 ● **(A)** Cecostomy button with trapdoor. **(B)** Fluoroscopic confirmation of proper cecostomy placement.

tients with voiding dysfunction. The result is a narrowing of the anorectal angle and an increase in anal canal pressures leading to impaired evacuation. Rectosphincteric dyssynergia may be found in patients with both normal and decreased colonic transit times as well as in those with other causes for outlet obstruction (93). Although the etiology of dyssynergic defecation is unknown, psychosocial factors, including a history of sexual abuse, depression, eating disorders, obsessive-compulsive disorders, stress, and childhood constipation and dyschezia, appear to be important. Preliminary data in one survey by Rao et al (94) suggest that dyssynergic defecation begins in childhood about one third of the time and is associated with a precipitating event in about 30% of individuals with this problem. The pathophysiology contributing to rectosphincteric dyssynergia (characterized by either paradoxic anal contractions or involuntary anal spasm during defecation) is likely multifactorial. The premise that this disorder is due only to the spasm of the external anal sphincter has been challenged by studies documenting minimal improvement after botulinum toxin injection or myectomy of the external sphincter (95,96). It seems more likely that multiple areas of rectoanal dysfunction are involved. In a study by Rao et al (97), 35 patients with obstructive defecation were evaluated with anorectal manometry and rectal balloon expulsion. The authors found impaired rectal contraction in 61% and paradoxic anal contractions in 78%, whereas others demonstrated inadequate anal relaxation and impaired rectal sensation. Paradoxic muscle contraction is likely a learned acquired response, because therapies using biofeedback and pelvic floor physical therapy have demonstrated improved defecation patterns (98,99).

The diagnosis is based on history, clinical findings, and diagnostic testing. Patients usually complain of impaired defecation associated with tenesmus and constipation. Other symptoms that may be present with any cause of outlet obstruction include the feeling of incomplete evacuation, anorectal pain or sensation of perianal heaviness, excessive straining with defecation, digital disimpaction, or vaginal splinting. In one survey evaluating symptoms associated with dyssynergic defecation, excessive straining was reported by 85% of patients, the need to facilitate defecation digitally by 66%, and the sensation of incomplete evacuation by 75% (94). Symptomatic criteria (Rome II) for the diagnosis of dyssynergic defecation have recently been published (100).

Symptoms alone, however, are not helpful in differentiating between the different causes of outlet obstruction (101). The diagnosis of a dyssynergic anorectal disorder is one of exclusion. Metabolic, systemic, and structural etiologies must first be ruled out with laboratory testing and sigmoidoscopy. The first clue to dyssynergic defecation may be perceived with a digital rectal examination in which there is a paradoxical contraction of the external sphincter. Rather than experiencing relaxation of the external sphincter, the clinician will appreciate a contraction of the puborectalis and external sphincter when the patient is asked to bear down to imitate a bowel movement. Confirmatory testing with anorectal manometry will demonstrate a heightened rather than diminished external sphincter pressure at the time of defecation that will coincide with increases in electromyographic recording activity from the puborectalis and external sphincter. Balloon expulsion testing and defecography have also been used diagnostically, with manometric correlation approximating 67% of cases (102). In addition to the symptom criteria listed previously, Rao has advocated using additional physiologic criteria based on manometry, balloon expulsion testing, and colon transit times to identify patients with dyssynergic defecation (103).

Treatment

Initial therapy should be aimed at addressing and alleviating constipation, a complaint usually always associated with this disorder. Standard therapies, including adequate fiber and fluid intake, avoidance of constipating medicines, scheduled toileting to maximize postprandial gastrocolonic and early morning waking responses, and laxative and prokinetic agents, should be tried first. In addition to addressing constipation, therapy must also be aimed at improving impaired rectal sensation and dyssynergic function of the abdominal, rectal, and anal sphincters that characterize this disorder. Biofeedback using manometry or electromyographic recording to provide visual or audible displays has been used successfully in the treatment of dyssynergic defecatory dysfunction. Defecatory simulation with balloon expulsion and rectal sensory threshold conditioning are also used.

Using the concept of operant conditioning, biofeedback enables patients to moderate motor and sensory function in response to desired visual displays representing ideal neuromuscular behavior. The efficacy of biofeedback in the treatment of dyssynergic defecation is difficult to access because randomized controlled trials are lacking and methodology, including study design and treatment end points, does not allow for good comparison or firm conclusions. In one meta-analysis by Ernst and Resch (104), the authors were unable to make any conclusions regarding the clinical effectiveness of biofeedback for the treatment of anismus, even though the results of subjective success rates in the 11 studies they reviewed ranged between 18% and 100%. Two other reviews (105,106) have suggested cure rates ranging between 67% and 80%, with another suggesting 89% symptomatic improvement (107). Ho et al reported on the results of biofeedback in patients with dyssynergic defecation, both with and without measurable paradoxic puborectalis contractions. Clinical and anorectal physiologic parameters were evaluated, and subjective improvement was reported in 90% of patients after therapy (108).

For patients who fail to improve with biofeedback, several other options exist. The use of botulinum toxin type A has been used with varying results in the treatment of spastic disorders of smooth muscle in the upper and lower gastrointestinal tract. Injection of botulinum toxin into the external anal sphincter or puborectalis muscle has shown promising short-term results in the treatment of dyssynergic defecation (109). Surgical options as a last resort include sphincteric myectomy, obturator internus muscle auto-transfer (110), sacral nerve modulation (off-label indication), and diverting colostomy.

Anatomic Obstruction

Chronic idiopathic constipation may be secondary to an underlying colonic motility disorder, an outlet obstructive disorder, or a combination of the two. In considering outlet obstruction, it is helpful to think in terms of either a mechanical etiology, such as POP, rectal prolapse, intussusception, or fecal impaction, or a neuromuscular disorder, such as Hirschsprung's disease, dyssynergic defecation, or anismus, as discussed previously. Constipation appears to be an important factor in the pathogenesis of uterovaginal prolapse because a history of chronic straining has been shown to be an independent risk factor for tissue attenuation and abnormal pudendal nerve function (111).

Pelvic Organ Prolapse

The true prevalence of POP has been difficult to quantify, primarily because of difficulties related to data collection and, until recently, a universally accepted grading system. Samuelsson et al (112) recently reported a 31% overall prevalence of prolapse in a Swedish population, with that number increasing to 56% in women aged 50 to 59 years. Swift described the distribution of POP stages in

women seen for routine gynecologic care as representing a bell-shaped curve, with most women having stage 1 (43%) and stage II (48%) prolapse (113). Unfortunately, there is little published literature addressing symptoms related to POP, especially when related to defecatory dysfunction.

It is commonly perceived that defecatory dysfunction related to outlet obstruction is secondary to posterior compartment defects. Rectoceles or herniations of the rectum through attenuated or site-specific breaks in the rectovaginal fascia are common forms of POP. Enteroceles are also common and may play an as-yet-undefined role in outlet obstruction. Because the definition of an enterocele is controversial and its diagnosis clinically challenging, the prevalence is difficult to quantify. It is estimated that enteroceles are found in 0.1% to 16% of women undergoing gynecologic surgery for POP (114).

Associated Symptoms

Rectoceles and enteroceles have commonly been associated with symptoms of bowel and defecatory dysfunction. This belief presumably stems from the direct involvement of the bowel and rectum in these defined areas of pelvic floor herniation. Symptoms usually attributed to rectocele and enterocele include pelvic pain and pressure, vaginal protrusion, constipation and splinting, sensation of incomplete evacuation, obstipation, fecal incontinence, and sexual dysfunction. However, a causal relationship between symptoms and posterior compartment prolapse has yet to be defined. Some researchers postulate that trauma to or intrinsic weakness of the rectovaginal fascia leads to rectocele formation and subsequent defecatory dysfunction. In contrast, others believe that the primary insult is related to chronic colonic dysfunction (i.e., idiopathic constipation, dyssynergic defecation), which then leads to rectocele or enterocele formation.

Although symptoms related to defecatory dysfunction may coexist with POP, they have not been consistently correlated. Weber et al (115) compared symptoms of bowel dysfunction with stage of posterior compartment prolapse and reported no clinically significant association. The authors did, however, find a weakly positive correlation between more advanced posterior vaginal prolapse and bowel dysfunction severity. Ellerkmann et al (116) prospectively evaluated 273 patients and attempted to correlate symptoms with stage and location of POP. Although they found weak correlations between splinting and incomplete evacuation and worsening posterior compartment prolapse, they were not able to determine a specific stage of POP at which these symptoms became more pronounced. The use of proctography has also failed to show a correlation between rectocele size and defecatory symptoms (117,118). In a recent subanalysis of the Colpopexy and Urinary Reduction Efforts (CARE) study by Bradley et al evaluating bowel symptoms in women planning surgery for pelvic organ prolapse, the researchers found no linear association with stage of posterior prolapse and bowel symptoms as evaluated by Colorectal-anal Distress Inventory and Impact Questionnaires (119). This lack of correlation was further demonstrated by Da Silva et al. In their study of 132 patients with posterior vaginal wall prolapse, the researchers found no correlation between anorectal symptoms and stage of rectocele; furthermore, physiologic studies showed no association between rectal capacity, first sensation and urgency, and prolapse stage (120).

Weidner et al (121) also attempted to characterize symptoms of defecatory dysfunction, including constipation and fecal incontinence, in 352 patients with urinary incontinence and POP, and found that symptoms of constipation were more likely reported in patients with advanced stages of POP (stage III or IV). Interestingly, these authors also found a higher prevalence of fecal incontinence in patients with worsening stage of anterior and posterior vaginal wall prolapse. Jackson et al (122) also reported significant correlations between POP and fecal incontinence.

The effect of hormonal status on colorectal function is not clear. The effect of estrogen on the posterior compartment and concurrent fecal incontinence, for example, was examined by Donnelly et al, who found improvement in anorectal physiologic parameters and improvement in quality of life after estrogen replacement therapy (123). In evaluating enteroceles and concurrent defecatory dysfunction, Chou et al (114) found no association between symptoms of bowel function and the presence or absence of enterocele.

Treatment

Pessary

Treatment for POP may be thought of in terms of either surgical or nonsurgical approaches. Dating back to antiquity, pessaries have remained the mainstay of nonsurgical intervention for POP. Unfortunately, there is a paucity of literature regarding pessaries, with much being anecdotal and controversial. It has traditionally been advocated that pessaries should be used as a second-line therapy, reserved for those patients who either decline or have contraindications to surgery (124,125). In a recent survey of the American Urogynecologic Society, Cundiff et al (126) confirmed this sentiment among gynecologic surgeons who had greater than 20 years of experience. In contrast, the same survey found that younger gynecologists reported using pessaries more frequently as a first-line therapy for POP. The reason for this difference in inclination toward pessary use is not known.

The choice of pessary and its relative indications and contraindications are based primarily on subjective opinion rather than level I or II data. With the exception of one prospective study (127), which attempted to establish clinical parameters associated with successful pessary use, the large number of different pessaries and absence of uniform guidelines or recommendation have led to a lack of consensus regarding their use.

With respect to posterior compartment defects, the efficacy of conservative pessary treatment is debated (128,129). Cundiff et al recently presented data evaluating relief of prolapse symptoms in the only randomized crossover trials comparing ring with Gellhorn pessaries. They found that both the Gellhorn and ring with support pessaries showed statistically significant and clinically important improvements in protrusion symptoms and symptoms related to urinary and defecatory obstruction. Additionally, posterior-predominant prolapse was positively associated with improvement in the defecatory symptoms (130).

Posterior Colporrhaphy

The surgical repair of rectocele evolved in the 19th century, with the first procedures attempting to correct perineal tears by way of simple perineal closure. More aggressive approaches were soon undertaken to address prolapse, specifically elytrorrhaphy of the posterior compartment, which denuded the posterior vaginal mucosa, followed by closure and narrowing of the vaginal caliber. The traditional posterior colporrhaphy, advocated by Heidelberg and Simon in 1867, attempted to reduce rectoceles and uterovaginal prolapse by plicating the levator ani muscles and the inferior aspect of the vagina. This served to create a rigid inferior shelf that reduced herniations of the posterior compartment and prevented apical and uterine descensus. In 1870, Hegar introduced the concept of the colpoperineorrhaphy, which, by creating a tight introital band, sought to address all types of POP (131). The traditional posterior colporrhaphy has a reported success rate of 76% to 96% (132,133) for reducing actual rectocele herniation. Unfortunately, this approach appears to be less successful at alleviating defecatory dysfunction and may, in fact, exacerbate symptoms and contribute to de novo sexual dysfunction. Francis and

Jeffcoate were the first to publish a significant correlation between posterior colporrhaphy and sexual dysfunction. In their series of 243 women, they reported postoperative dyspareunia in 50% of their patients (134). In a retrospective study by Kahn and Stanton, dyspareunia and defecatory dysfunction, including fecal incontinence, constipation, and incomplete evacuation, all increased postoperatively after posterior colporrhaphy (133). In one prospective study of posterior colporrhaphy, Mellgran et al found a 48% prevalence of postoperative constipation in 25 patients 1 year after surgery (132). In this study, abnormal preoperative transit studies and dyssynergic defecation were risk factors for persistent postoperative constipation. In contrast, Pariaso et al at the Cleveland Clinic postoperatively followed 124 women at 12 and 24 months following traditional posterior repair with validated questionnaires and analog scales evaluating bowel and sexual function. They found improvement in defecatory dysfunction and related quality of life, specifically noting increases in bowel movement frequency and diminished straining and need for manual evacuation. Unfortunately, they also found significant postoperative dyspareunia rates of 25% (135).

Transanal Repair

Colorectal surgeons traditionally approach rectocele repair through a transanal approach. The technique, popularized by Sullivan et al (136), includes plication of the rectal muscularis and attachment of this plicated tissue to the levator ani fascia bilaterally. Although this approach appears to alleviate constipation in 22% to 85% of patients (137,138), it makes it difficult to address concurrently perineal descent, high rectocele, or enterocele. In one comparative study reviewing transanal and transvaginal approaches, Arnold et al found no difference in surgical outcome with respect to fecal incontinence, constipation, or dyspareunia (139). Similar findings have also been published by Kahn et al, who prospectively evaluated both approaches and found few differences with respect to postoperative defecatory dysfunction (140).

Defect-Directed Repair

In the 1970s, Richardson popularized the concept of discrete fascial breaks rather than tissue attenuation as the primary cause of POP (141). With attention to the posterior compartment, he described five sites at which the rectovaginal fascia could be broken and advocated a site-specific repair for rectocele reduction. This concept allowed for a deviation from the traditional nonanatomic repair while still maintaining the basic principle of hernia repair. The site-specific repair does not attempt to plicate the levator ani fascia and, as such, may be

associated with a lower incidence of postoperative morbidity. Cundiff et al reported on their series of 69 women who underwent defect-directed repair for symptomatic rectocele (142). After this surgical approach, they reported resolution of several symptoms thought to be associated with rectocele, including constipation in 84%, splinting in 55%, and dyspareunia in 66%. The improved symptom outcome in this series was attributed to the defect-directed repair, which reestablished the normal integrity and anatomy of the rectovaginal fascia.

Other authors have supported this premise. Porter et al (143) and Glavind and Madsen (144) noted significant improvement in bowel symptoms after site-specific posterior colporrhaphy, and Kenton et al (145) reported similar findings in patients undergoing rectovaginal fascia reattachment.

Although these reports suggest that the discrete site-specific repair may be preferable to the traditional posterior colporrhaphy in preventing postoperative dyspareunia and alleviating symptoms related to defecatory dysfunction, other studies have challenged this idea. In a retrospective review comparing the anatomic and functional outcomes of these two surgical techniques, Abramov et al evaluated 124 patients who had undergone site-specific repair and 183 patients who had undergone standard posterior colporrhaphy without levator ani plication. Although preoperative baseline characteristics, including prolapse stage, between the two groups were similar, the authors found that recurrence of rectocele, recurrence of symptomatic bulge, and postoperative Bp point (POPQ -2.2 vs. -2.7 cm, $p = 0.001$) were significantly higher after site-specific rectocele repair. Interestingly, rates of postoperative dyspareunia, constipation, and fecal incontinence were not significantly different between the two study groups (146).

Posterior Fascial Replacement

Attempts to augment rectocele repair with synthetic or allogenic material have met with varying results. Most initial reports involving permanent synthetic mesh have focused on anterior compartment support. Julian reported on his experience with Marlex mesh in the repair of recurrent anterior compartment prolapse. Although he reported no recurrence, the follow-up was relatively short, and the mesh erosion rate of 25% proved unacceptable (147).

Numerous authors have confirmed the high erosion and infection rates with permanent types of mesh used in this application. As a result, others have attempted to use absorbable synthetic mesh material to prevent recurrent prolapse. Sand et al recently published their results from a prospective randomized trial using polyglactin 910 (Vicryl) mesh in cystocele and rectocele repair (148). Although they found that the addition of mesh reduced the rate of recurrent central cystocele, there was no significant effect on the incidence of recurrent rectocele. Additionally, they reported no postoperative mesh erosions. Others have attempted to bolster attenuated rectovaginal fascia with biological grafts, including autologous and allograft fascia lata, allogenic dermal grafts, and xenografts. Introduced in 1995, dermal allografts such as Alloderm™ and Repliform™ (Lifecell Corp., Branchburg, NJ), are acellular cadaveric dermal products that are marketed to surgeons on the premise that they allow native tissue ingrowth, revascularization, and tissue remoldeling. One of the first reports was by Oster and Astrup, in which the authors reported on their experience with dermal graft augmentation in rectocele repair in 15 patients (149). With a follow-up period of 1 to 4 years, they reported no recurrent prolapse and alleviation of most symptoms related to defecatory dysfunction, although five patients experienced persistent constipation. Other authors have reported using dermal allografts successfully in augmenting rectovaginal fistula (150).

Alternatives to synthetic materials and allografts for use in augmentation include a plethora of xenografts that are now available. Porcine-derived products enjoy a large market share, including Pelvicol™ (CR Bard, Covington, GA) and InterGraft™ (American Medical Systems, Minnetonka, MN), which are both acellular, porcine dermal matrixes. SurgiSIS (Cook Ob/Gyn, Indianapolis, MN), an extracellular matrix derived from the submucosa of porcine small intestine, has also been a popular product for graft augmentation. Bovine xenografts, such as Veritas™ (Synovis, St. Paul, MN), an acellular matrix matufactured from bovine pericardium, have also been used for rectocele augmentation. Although preliminary results suggest that these biomaterials are safe in vaginal applications, there are no data supporting that they add any additional strength or durability to the repair. Most published reports to date are nonrandomized case series, typically not powered to demonstrate any significance difference with respect to clinical and functional outcomes. It remains unknown whether the use of these materials will independently affect defecatory symptoms.

Although the majority of recent literature suggests that the defect-directed repair has better symptom-based outcomes than the traditional posterior colporrhaphy, controversy remains regarding the actual diagnosis of site-specific defects and the longevity of these repairs. The proponents of posterior fascia replacement augmentation maintain that these materials will add further durability to the repair with no increase in morbidity. The results of the first of several prospective randomized studies comparing these various approaches to posterior compartment prolapse were recently presented, and other studies are underway in an effort to establish which repair provides better symptom relief and durable surgical results.

In 2006, Paraiso et al presented data from the Cleveland Clinic's randomized trial of three surgical techniques for rectocele repair, including one with graft augmentation with a porcine small intestinal submucosa bioengineered collagen matrix (Fortagen™). The authors randomized 106 women with stage II or greater posterior vaginal wall prolapse to one of three treatments: traditional posterior repair, site-specific repair, or site-specific rectocele repair augmented with Fortagen. Subjective and objective outcome measures were evaluated postoperatively, with a mean follow-up of 16 months. The authors concluded that traditional posterior colporrhaphy and site-specific rectocele repair resulted in similar anatomic and functional outcomes; in contrast, the graft augmentation cohort experienced a greater anatomic failure rate. All three methods of rectocele repair, however, did result in significant improvements in prolapse and bowel symptoms, quality of life, and sexual function (151).

Recently, there has been a resurgence in the use of synthetic mesh for vaginal prolapse repair including rectocele. Surgical innovation by gynecologic surgeons in France has led to the development and marketing of polypropylene mesh products such as GyneMesh/Prolift™ (Gynecare, Ethicon, Johnson & Johnson, New Brunswick, NJ), Apogee™ and Perigee™ (American Medical Systems, Minnetonka, MN), and Atrium™ (Atrium, Hudson, NH). These surgical devices employ curvilinear trocars to facilitate transvaginal mesh placement in a minimally invasive manner. The anatomic placement of the nonsutured polypropylene "arms" of the mesh at the level of the ischial spines allow for a high level II support of the vaginal apex.

The initial experience of de Tayrac et al was published in 2006. The authors reported their 2-year experience with transvaginal rectocele repair using polypropylene mesh involving bilateral sacrospinous suspension and attachment of the mesh from the sacrospinous ligaments to the perineal body. In their cohort of 26 women, only one patient experienced a recurrent stage II rectocele, and all but one patient reported improvement in defecatory symptoms and quality of life. Vaginal mesh erosion occurred in 12% and de novo dyspareunia in 7.7% (152).

Milani et al also reported on the functional and anatomical outcomes of anterior and posterior vaginal prolapse repair with polypropylene mesh augmentation. In their series, 63 women were followed for a mean of 17 months, for an anatomic success rate of 94%. Of the 31 patients who underwent rectocele repair, constipation improved in 15% and anal incontinence in 4%. However, dyspareunia also increased in 63% (153). Similar results were also published by Dwyer et al in their retrospective review of women who had underegone vaginal prolapse sugery, including rectocele repair, with Atrium mesh reinforcement. With a mean follow-up of 29 months, mesh erosion rates were noted 9% (154).

The majority of literature regarding polypropylene vaginal mesh placement for the correction of POP suggests a relatively high mesh erosion rate in the range of 3% to 13% as well a high de novo rate of dyspareunia. With modifications of surgical technique and mesh design, there have been improvements in these two complications. For example, avoiding concurrent hysterectomy (OR 5.17, p <0.001) and limiting the extent of colpotomy incisions (OR 6.06, p <0.01) reduce the risk of mesh erosion (155). As there is currently little to no published information regarding polypropylene mesh rectocele repair and its impact on defecatory dysfunction, randomized controlled studies are needed to evaluate the efficacy of these surgical vaginal mesh devices in this and other domains.

Perineal Descent

Sir Allan Parks and colleagues first described the syndrome of the descending perineum in 1966 (156). The anatomic derangements that produce characteristic bulging of the pelvic floor with anterior displacement of the urethral axis and posterior displacement of the anal canal coexist with a variety of physiologic disturbances in the anorectum, vagina, and distal urinary tract. Associated clinical conditions may include symptomatic constipation, obstructed defecation, fecal incontinence, urinary incontinence, and anatomic abnormalities with single or multicompartmental POP (157,158). Because the endopelvic fascial support is often attenuated and significant pudendal neuropathy may coexist with descent, many surgeons consider perineal descent to be a nonoperative condition despite often disabling sequelae. This problem is compounded by the association of this syndrome with poor outcomes following other reconstructive anorectal procedures (159,160).

Biofeedback and behavioral modification with pelvic floor retraining have been the most common forms of nonoperative therapy for perineal descent and should be exhausted before pursuing operative repair. The avoidance of straining is of paramount importance, and early improvement in up to 64% of patients has been reported after intensive pelvic floor retraining (161). Unfortunately, the results are usually not durable, and defecatory disorders recur with behavioral relapse to chronic straining. With recurrence, the progression of symptoms may include obstructed defecation, fecal and urinary incontinence, POP, and rectal prolapse, leading to a very poor quality of life in severely affected women.

Early results presented by several groups may offer surgical alternatives for the management of perineal descent. Cundiff et al modified the abdominal sacral colpopexy (162) (for apical prolapse) by extending the mesh support down to the perineal body in association with rectocele repair in patients with rectocele and perineal descent (163). The intent of this procedure, the abdominal sacral colpoperineopexy, is to restore and replace disrupted central perineal body support from the rectovaginal fascia and uterosacral-cardinal ligaments. The results of 19 patients who underwent abdominal sacral colpoperineopexy with Mersilene mesh have been reported. Postoperative stage of prolapse was significantly reduced, with no patient having greater than stage II prolapse on postoperative POPQ examination. Bowel symptoms improved in 8 of 11 women. Despite these encouraging early results, erosion of Mersilene mesh into the posterior vaginal wall occurred in up to 40% of patients (164). Alternatively, mesh erosion into the vault had only been reported in 3% of patients who underwent more apical mesh placement for abdominal sacral colpopexy (162). In a 2004 literature review by Nygaard et al, the incidence of mesh erosion following abdominal sacral colpopexy ranged from 0% to 5.5%, depending on the type of mesh used to support the vagina. The overall rate of mesh erosion was 3.4%.

Total pelvic mesh repair has been described by Sullivan et al for the treatment of advanced POP (165). A trapezoidal sheet of Marlex mesh is attached to the perineal body through an abdominal approach, brought to the left of the rectum, and secured to the sacral periosteum at S1 to S2 (Fig. 23.5). A 2-cm strut of Marlex is secured from each side of the trapezoid to Cooper's ligament. A fourth strut is placed between the two anterior struts to support the bladder and vagina in patients with anterior prolapse.

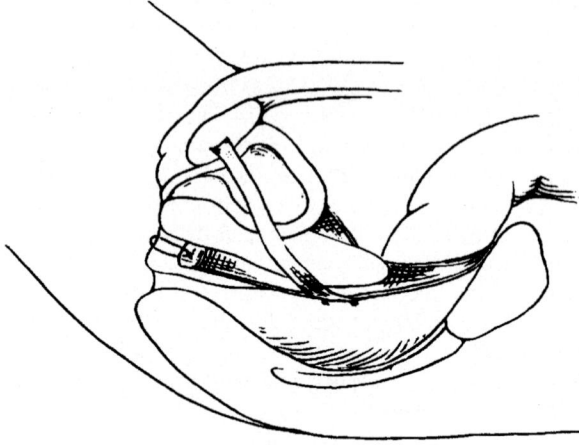

FIGURE 23.5 ● Position of the trapezoidal and anterolateral mesh struts in the total pelvic mesh repair. (From Sullivan ES, Longaker CJ, Lee PY. Total pelvic mesh repair: a 10-year experience. *Dis Colon Rectum* 2001;44:857–863, with permission.)

The long-term follow-up on 236 patients operated on by total pelvic mesh repair from 1990 to 1999 has been reported (165). Indications included patients with previously failed conventional techniques of prolapse surgery and those with combined rectal and genitourinary prolapse. Rectal prolapse was common (74%) and included women with mucosal to full-thickness disease. Perineal descent was present in 64% of patients. There were no cases of recurrent stage IV vaginal vault prolapse or full-thickness rectal prolapse. Data were not reported on recurrence of perineal descent. Marlex erosion into the rectum or vagina occurred in 5% of patients. Additional procedures were subsequently performed for persistent urinary symptoms in 36% and anorectal symptoms in 28% of patients at a median interval of 197 days from the initial repair. Overall satisfaction rate was reported at 74% in patients followed more than 6 years.

The rectovaginopexy with polytetrafluoroethylene (PTFE, Gore-Tex) has been proposed for the treatment of constipation and fecal incontinence with concomitant apical or posterior POP (Fig. 23.6). Although perineal descent was not specifically addressed by the authors, the attachments of the synthetic support may serve a similar purpose. The midpoint of a 20- $\times$ 1-cm strip of PTFE is sutured to the sacral promontory, with the legs of this graft attached to the lateral rectum and uterosacral ligaments. Despite the absence of a separate rectocele or enterocele repair, these defects decreased from 74% and 33% preoperatively to 30% and 0%, respectively. There were no reports of PTFE erosion into pelvic viscera. Improvement in constipation was 76% at 1 year ($p = 0.0015$) and 71% at 4 years ($p = 0.005$). At 1 year, incontinence improved by 87% ($p = 0.0015$), and this figure decreased to 53% at 4 years ($p = 0.09$).

Given the high rate of mesh erosion into the vagina when a transvaginal rectocele repair is performed in association with abdominal sacral colpoperineopexy, autologous fascia and other biomaterials have been used for attachment of the perineal body to the sacrum. Kaufman et al used Alloderm as a graft in 11 women who did not desire autologous fascial harvest (166). Coexisting full-thickness or internal rectal prolapse or poor mesorectal fixation was documented by dynamic magnetic resonance imaging or cystocolpoproctography (167) in these patients with coexisting defecatory dysfunction. Simultaneous rectopexy (with or without sigmoid resection) was performed in association with abdominal sacral coloperineopexy in these patients for severe perineal descent with defecatory dysfunction (Fig. 23.7).

Highlights of this procedure include two teams beginning simultaneously, with the perineal surgeon performing a transvaginal rectocele repair (defect-directed or posterior colporrhaphy) and the abdominopelvic team beginning with sigmoid resection (if indicated) and rectal mobilization. The mesorectal plane is developed down to the pelvic floor posteriorly, with care taken to identify and preserve the hypogastric nerves. Avoiding lateral dissection and lateral ligament division preserves the more distal autonomic pelvic plexus. Sutures are placed from the fascia propria of the rectum to the sacral periosteum at S1 to S3 for the rectopexy. These sutures are not tied until the coloproctostomy is completed if the sigmoid has been resected. A 4- $\times$ 16-cm strip of nonmeshed Alloderm is sutured to the perineal body overlying the rectocele repair and passed into the pelvis through a defect made in the cul-de-sac. The proximal portion of this graft is secured to the sacrum by the right-sided rectopexy sutures, along with a

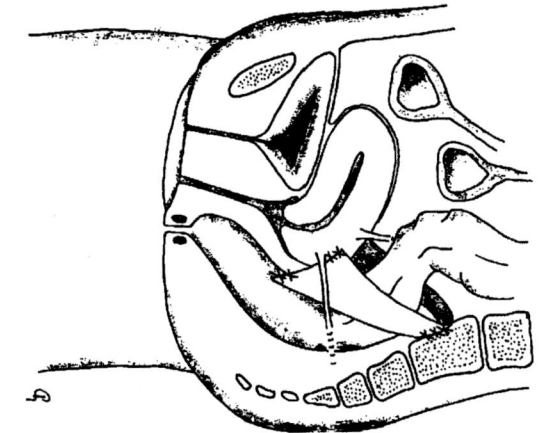

FIGURE 23.6 ● Position of the polytetra-fluoroethylene (PTFE) strip in the recto-vaginopexy. The midpoint of the PTFE strip is sutured to the sacral promontory with the legs attached to the anterolateral aspects of the rectum and uterosacral ligaments. (From Silvis R, Goosen HG, van Essen A, et al. Abdominal rectovaginopexy: modified technique to treat constipation. *Dis Colon Rectum* 1999;42(1):82–88, with permission.)

smaller anterior graft attached distally to the pub-ocervical fascia.

In follow-up (12.5 ± 7.7 months), 9 of 11 patients (82%) remained free of perineal descent, whereas 2 patients had recurrences (166). Significant symptomatic improvement was noted in constipation, incomplete evacuation, and need for assisted evacuation. Overall, 8 of 11 patients reported an improvement in their quality of life, and there were no cases of erosion of Alloderm through the vaginal mucosa or into the rectum or bladder.

This study notwithstanding, there are numerous case reports of abdominal sacral colpopexy and abdominal sacral coloperineopexy utilizing other biomaterials in lieu of synthetic mesh. In the first randomized controlled trial to be published evaluating synthetic versus biological graft for abdominal sacral colpopexy, Culligan et al evaluated 100 patients prospectively with an average of 1-year follow-up. The authors found significant differences between the mesh and fascia groups with respect to postoperative POPQ stage and points Aa and C, with a higher objective anatomic cure rate in the polypropylene mesh group (91% versus 68%, $p < 0.007$) (168).

Rectal Prolapse

Rectal prolapse results when the full thickness of the rectum intussuscepts through the anal canal. In adults, this syndrome most often affects elderly people, with the earliest onset usually occurring

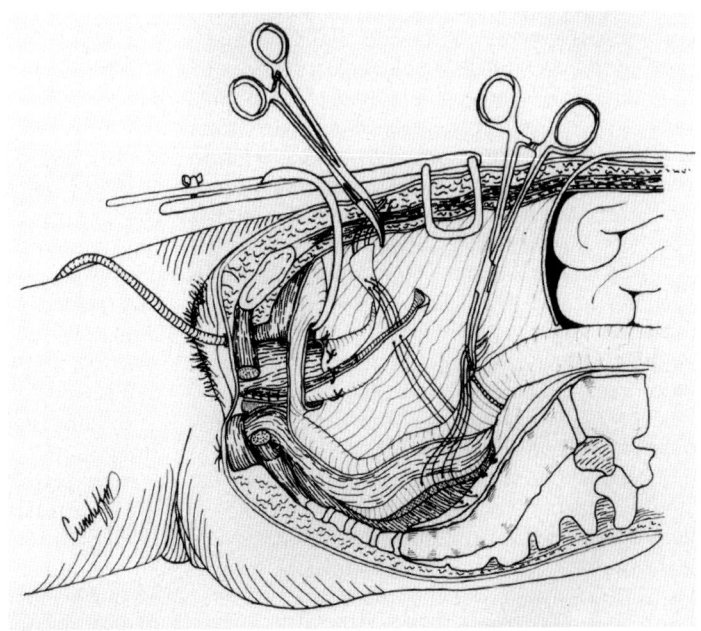

FIGURE 23.7 ● Abdominal sacral coloperineopexy with sigmoid resection and suture rectopexy. This sagittal view shows the posterior Alloderm graft sutured to the rectovaginal fascia and perineal body after defect-directed rectocele repair. The anterior sheet of Alloderm is sutured to the pub-ocervical fascia. Both sheets will be secured to the sacral periosteum to the right of the rectum. Rectopexy sutures (*left*) have not yet been tied and secured. (Courtesy of Geoffrey W. Cundiff, MD.)

during the fifth decade. The female-to-male ratio is 5:1. Numerous congenital and acquired conditions have been implicated in the etiology of rectal prolapse and include chronic constipation, neurologic disease (congenital anomaly, spinal cord trauma, cauda equina lesion, dementia), weak anal sphincter (due to injury, denervation), and previous surgery (fistulotomy, sphincterotomy, hemorrhoidectomy, coloanal anastomosis). Anatomic findings associated with this process include a deep pouch of Douglas, patulous anus, redundant rectosigmoid, levator ani diastasis, and poor mesorectal fixation to the presacral tissues and pelvic sidewalls. A rectosigmoid lesion may also serve as a lead point for intussusception.

Patients usually present with a chief complaint of protrusion of the rectum, most often with attempts at defecation or with the Valsalva maneuver. With progression of disease, prolapse may occur without increases in intra-abdominal pressure. Constipation has been reported in 25% to 50% of patients (169), and up to 75% of patients report fecal incontinence (170). Incontinence usually improves after surgical management of prolapse without any intervention directed at the anal sphincter.

On physical examination, the surgeon must differentiate between full-thickness rectal prolapse, mucosal prolapse, and prolapsing hemorrhoids. Except for the most profound cases, patients often can only demonstrate rectal prolapse by sitting on a commode and straining to stool. A pelvic examination should be performed to rule out other POP.

More than 100 surgical procedures have been described to treat full-thickness rectal prolapse. These procedures may be broadly classified into those performed through the abdominal route and those performed through a perineal approach. Some surgeons prefer a perineal approach for nearly all patients; however, given overall lower recurrence rates after abdominal procedures, perineal procedures have classically been reserved for more debilitated patients.

Ripstein described the modern anterior sling rectopexy in 1965 (171). Although Ripstein anecdotally reported a very low recurrence rate, the details of his personal series of more than 1,500 patients were never published. Unfortunately, a relatively high constipation rate has been found in long-term follow-up of these patients. Erosion of mesh and obstructed defecation secondary to a complete anterior wrap have been the major morbidities associated with this procedure. Subsequent modification to a two-thirds posterolateral wrap has led to improvements in postoperative defecatory dysfunction. Tjandra et al reported the results

of 142 Ripstein procedures performed over a 27-year period (172). The recurrence rate of complete prolapse was 8% and within the range reported from other series (5% to 10%) (171,172). Recurrence rates of 0% to 2% have been reported by others, but with shorter postoperative follow-up (173). Other related suspensions and fixation procedures include the Wells procedure, direct suture rectopexy, posterior Ivalon sponge rectopexy, and resection rectopexy (Frykman-Goldberg procedure) (170,174). Most series of prolapse surgery are retrospective, and there have been no data to suggest that the addition of a foreign sling provides any advantage to simple suture fixation alone. Debate continues about the value and extent of resection when combined with rectopexy (175).

Perineal operations for rectal prolapse have usually been reserved for more infirm and unfit patients who cannot tolerate an abdominal approach. Although easily tolerated, perianal encirclement procedures such as the Thiersch wire have largely been abandoned owing to poor success rates and high rates of recurrence and fecal impaction. Alternatively, the Altemeier procedure (Fig. 23.8), a full-thickness rectosigmoidectomy with or without levatorplasty, can be performed with minimal morbidity in this patient population. Although the incidence of recurrent rectal prolapse varies widely (3% to 60%) (176) after the Altemeier procedure, this operation can be easily repeated if necessary.

The Delorme procedure (Fig. 23.9), first described by a French army surgeon in 1900, entails mucosal stripping of the prolapsed rectum with subsequent rectomucosectomy and plication of the distal rectal wall (177). There was little interest in Delorme's procedure until the 1970s, when several small series were reported. Senapati et al published the results of this procedure in 32 patients (178). There was no mortality. At a mean follow-up of 24 months, 12.5% of patients developed a recurrence. Incontinence improved in 46%, and constipation improved in 50%. Oliver et al reported their experience of 41 patients who underwent Delorme's procedure over a 10-year period (179). Twenty-two percent of patients developed a recurrence. Thirty-two patients (68%) claimed that their continence was enhanced after this procedure.

In conclusion, rectal prolapse is a multifactorial disease affecting mostly elderly people. For younger and fit patients, abdominal approaches offer low recurrence rates. Recently, laparoscopic approaches to suture rectopexy, sling rectopexy, and resection rectopexy have been described with satisfactory results (180). Regardless of the abdominal technique, continence is usually improved

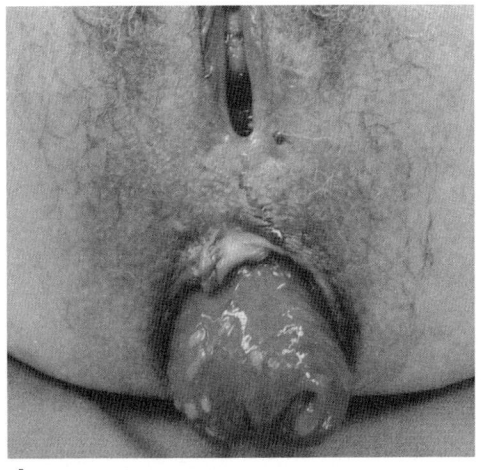

A

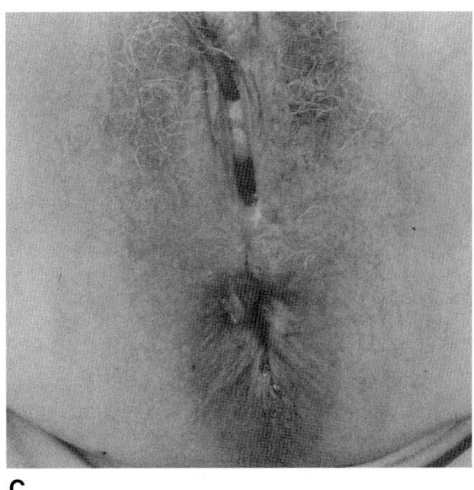

C

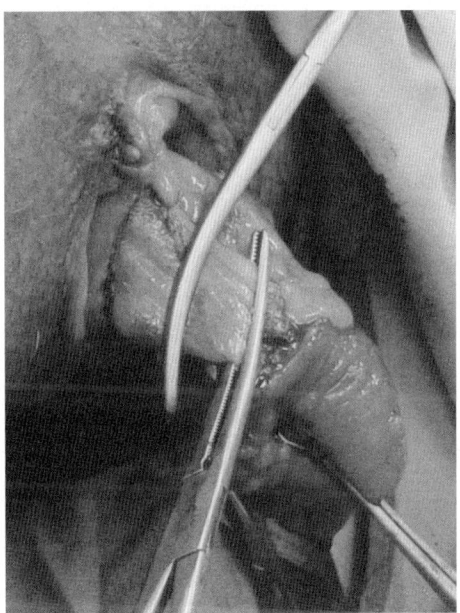

B

FIGURE 23.8 ● Altemeier procedure (perineal rectosigmoidectomy). **(A)** Preoperative appearance revealing full-thickness rectal prolapse. **(B)** Mesorectal division and ligation. **(C)** Postoperative view after end-to-end coloanal anastomosis.

after repair. Elderly and debilitated patients, as well as younger patients with multiple medical problems, are best served by a perineal procedure.

CONCLUSIONS

In summary, defecatory dysfunction encompasses many disorders that are manifested by gastrointestinal symptoms, including but not limited to difficulty with evacuation. Epidemiologic studies attempting to characterize the prevalence of

defecatory dysfunction have been difficult to perform because of the all-encompassing nature of the term and the lack of defining criteria.

In approaching this subject, it is helpful to consider general etiologic factors. As we have seen, these include lifestyle issues such as the effect of diet, exercise, medications, and patient mobility; systemic diseases, including underlying diabetes mellitus, thyroid dysfunction, and neuromuscular disorders such as multiple sclerosis and Hirschsprung's disease; functional disorders, such

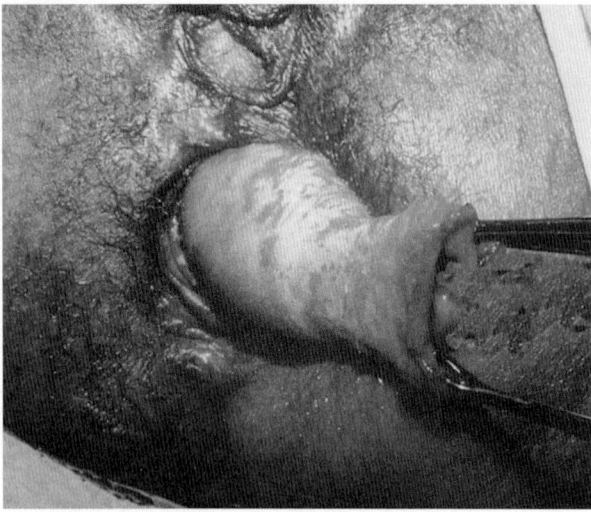

FIGURE 23.9 ● Delorme's procedure. After mucosal stripping to the full extent of the prolapse, the circular smooth muscle of the rectum is plicated. A mucosa-to-mucosa anastomosis is then performed.

as IBS, colonic inertia, and idiopathic constipation; obstructive disorders resulting from either mechanical causes such as malignancy, POP, and impaction or from pelvic floor dyssynergia; and finally, psychiatric causes, such as depression, eating disorders, and dementia. Although considerable overlap exists within the subcategories of defecatory dysfunction, constipation is a common denominator.

Further research is needed to address many aspects of defecatory dysfunction. Most important is the need for a validated, disease-specific quality-of-life instrument to assist in clarifying the potential interrelationships between symptoms and their etiologies and respective therapies. Equally important are the development and standardization of normative data regarding normal physiologic defecation stratified by age, gender, and parity. Once established, these normal ranges will assist in defining diagnostic criteria and etiologies for various aspects of pelvic floor dysfunction, including important subcategories such as pelvic floor dyssynergia. Further advances in gastrointestinal diagnostic testing techniques and pelvic floor imaging will enhance our understanding of underlying pathology as it relates to both sensorimotor and pelvic support dysfunction. Further research is needed, for example, in defining the indications for and the utility of magnetic imaging in the evaluation and management of patients with POP. Advances in surgical innovation and biomaterial availability may ultimately enhance the longevity of surgical procedures addressing POP.

In the field of FGIDs, a better understanding of the enteric nervous system is needed. Factors influencing neural regulation and modulation are currently being defined that will clarify relationships between symptom subgroups. This information will also shed light on the natural history of sensorimotor dysfunction and its respective relationship to the evolution of respective FGID symptoms. It is hoped that this, along with further research in genetics, will explain why there is such a broad range and overlap in FGID symptoms and their severity. Advances in pharmacologic research have led to the development of drugs that modulate visceral sensitivity, an important aspect of IBS therapy. Further research is needed to elucidate visceral afferent pathways, their respective neurotransmitters, and the gut–brain connection. The psychosocial aspects of the FGIDs also warrant further investigation, and validated instruments controlling for gender, sociocultural factors, and clinical settings are needed to assess psychosocial traits and bowel symptoms. Once these are established, the impact of psychological intervention and other similar treatment modalities (such as biofeedback) can be critically analyzed.

REFERENCES

1. Jewell DJ, Younge G. Interventions for treating constipation in pregnancy (Cochrane review). In: *The Cochrane Library*, Issue 2. Oxford: Update Software, 2001.
2. Perry E, Shields R, Turnball AC. The effect of pregnancy on the colonic absorption of sodium, potassium and, water. *J Obstet Gynecol Br Commonw* 1970;77:900.
3. Devroede G, Lamarche J. Functional importance of extrinsic parasympathetic innervation to the distal colon and rectum in man. *Gastroenterology* 1974;66: 273–281.
4. Devroede G, Arhan P, Duguay C, et al. Traumatic constipation. *Gastroenterology* 1979;77:1258.
5. Weber J, Grise P, Roquebert M, et al. Radiopaque markers transit and anorectal manometry in 16 patients with multiple sclerosis and urinary bladder dysfunction. *Dis Colon Rectum* 1987;30:95.

6. Metzger PP, Alvear DT, Arnold GC, et al. Hirschsprung's disease in adults: report of a case and review of the literature. *Dis Colon Rectum* 1978;21:113.

7. Wald A. Approach to the patient with constipation. In: Yamada T, Alpers DH, Owyand C, et al, eds. *Textbook of gastroenterology,* 3rd ed. Philadelphia: Lippincott Williams & Wilkins, 1999.

8. MacIver AG, Whitehead R. Zonal colonic aganglionosis: a variant of Hirschsprung's disease. *Arch Dis Child* 1972;47:233.

9. Wood JD, Alpers DH, Andrews PLR. Fundamentals of neurogastroenterology. *Gut* 1999;45(Suppl II):6–16.

10. Johanson JF, Sonnenberg A, Koch TR. Clinical epidemiology of chronic constipation. *J Clin Gastroenterol* 1989;11:525–536.

11. Wald A. Advances in gastroenterology. *Med Clin North Am* 2000;84(5):1231–1246.

12. Corazzari E, Cucchiara S, Staiano A, et al. Gastrointestinal transit time, frequency of defecation, and anorectal manometry in healthy and constipated children. *J Pediatr* 1985;106:379.

13. Molnar D, Taitz LS, Urwin OM, et al. Anorectal manometry results in defecation disorders. *Arch Dis Child* 1983;58:257.

14. Loening-Baucke VA, Younoszai MK. Effect of treatment on rectal and sigmoid motility in chronically constipated children. *Pediatrics* 1983;71:774.

15. Loening-Baucke VA, Cruikshank B, Savage C. Defecation dynamics and behavior profiles in encopretic children. *Pediatrics* 1987;80:672.

16. Roma E, Adamidis D, Nikolara R, et al. Diet and chronic constipation in children: the role of fiber. *J Pediatr Gastroenterol Nutr* 1999;29(4):487.

17. Moarais MB, Vitolo MR, Aguiire AN, et al. Measurement of low dietary fiber intake as a risk factor for chronic constipation in children. *J Pediatr Gastroenterol Nutr* 1999;29(2):132.

18. Wald A. Colonic transit and anorectal manometry in chronic idiopathic constipation. *Arch Intern Med* 1986; 146:1713.

19. Wald A, Hinds JP, Caruana BJ. Psychological and physiological characteristics of patients with severe idiopathic constipation. *Gastroenterology* 1989;97:932–937.

20. Wald A, Burgio K, Holeva K, et al. Psychological evaluation of patients with severe idiopathic constipation: which instrument to use. *Am J Gastroenterol* 1992; 87:977–980.

21. Grotz RL, Pemberton JH, Talley NJ, et al. Discriminant value of psychological distress, symptom profiles, and segmental colonic dysfunction in outpatients with severe idiopathic constipation. *Gut* 1994;35: 798–802.

22. Wald A. Constipation and fecal incontinence in the elderly. *Gastroenterol Clin North Am* 1990;19:405.

23. Odenthal KP, Ziegler D. In vitro effects of anthraquinones on rat intestine and uterus. *Pharmacology* 1988;36(Suppl 1):57–65.

24. Ashraf W, Park F, Lof J, et al. An examination of the reliability of reported stool frequency in the diagnosis of idiopathic constipation. *Am J Gastroenterol* 1996;1:26.

25. Koutsomanis D, Lennard-Jones JE, Roy AJ, et al. Controlled randomized trial of visual biofeedback versus muscle training without a visual display for intractable constipation. *Gut* 1995;37:95–99.

26. Davies GJ, Crowder M, Reid B, et al. Bowel function measurements of individuals with different eating patterns. *Gut* 1974;27:1068–1074.

27. Burkitt DP, Walker ARP, Painter NS. Effect of dietary fiber on stools and transit times and its role in the causation of disease. *Lancet* 1972;ii:1408–1411.

28. Preston DM, Lennard-Jones JE. Severe chronic constipation of young women: idiopathic slow transit constipation. *Gut* 1986;27:41–48.

29. Watier A, Devroed G, Duranceau A, et al. Constipation with colonic inertia: a manifestation of systemic disease? *Dig Dis Sci* 1983;28:1025.

30. Lee AJ, Evans CJ, Hau CM, et al. Fiber intake, constipation, and risk of varicose veins in the general population: Edinburgh vein study. *J Clin Epidemiol* 2001; 54(4):423–429.

31. Manning AP, Heaton KW, Harvey RF, et al. Wheat fiber and irritable bowel syndrome: a controlled trial. *Lancet* 1977;2:417–418.

32. Arffmann S, Andersen JR, Hegnhay J, et al. The effect of coarse bran in the irritable bowel syndrome: a double-blind cross-over study. *Scand J Gastroenterol* 1985; 20:295.

33. Cann PA, Read NW, Holdsworth CD. What is the benefit of coarse wheat bran in patients with irritable bowel syndrome? *Gut* 1984;25:168.

34. Findlay JM, Smith AN, Michell WD, et al. Effects of unprocessed bran on colon function in normal subjects and in diverticular disease. *Lancet* 1974;1:146–149.

35. Brodribb AJM. Treatment of symptomatic diverticular disease with a high-fiber diet. *Lancet* 1977;2:664–666.

36. Ornstein MH, Littlewood ER, McLean Baird I, et al. Are fiber supplements really necessary in diverticular disease of the colon? A controlled clinical trial. *Br Med J* 1981;282:1353–1356.

37. Müller-Lissner S. Effect of wheat bran on weight of stool and gastrointestinal transit time: a meta-analysis. *Br Med J* 1988;296:615–617.

38. Tramonte SM, Brand MB, Mulrow CD, et al. The treatment of chronic constipation in adults: a systematic review. *J Gen Intern Med* 1997;12(1):15–24.

39. Slavin JL. Implementation of dietary modifications. *Am J Med* 1999;106:46S–49S.

40. Everhart JE, Go VLW, Johannes RS, et al. A longitudinal survey of self-reported bowel habits in the United States. *Dig Dis Sci* 1989;34:1153–1162.

41. Verduron A, Devroede G, Bouchoucha M, et al. Megarectum. *Dig Dis Sci* 1988;33:1164–1174.

42. Powell R. On certain painful affections of the intestinal canal. *Med Trans Coll Physicians* 1820;114:841.

43. Chaudhury NA, Truelove SC. The irritable colon syndrome. *Q J Med* 1962;32:307.

44. Thompson WG. *The irritable gut.* Baltimore: University Park Press, 1979.

45. Manning AP, Thompson WD, Heaton KW, et al. Towards positive diagnosis in the irritable bowel syndrome. *Br Med J* 1978;2:653–654.

46. Kruis W, Thieme CH, Weinzierl M, et al. A diagnostic score for the irritable bowel syndrome: its value in the exclusion of organic disease. *Gastroenterology* 1984;87:1–7.

47. Drossman DA, Richter JE, Talley NJ, et al, eds. *The functional gastrointestinal disorders: diagnosis, pathophysiology, and treatment,* 1st ed. McLean, VA: Degnon Associates, 1994.

48. Drossman D, Corazziari E, Talley NJ, et al., eds. *Rome II: the functional gastrointestinal disorders*, 2nd ed. McLean, VA: Degnon Associates, 2000.

49. Longstreth GW, Thompson WG, Chey WD, et al. Functional bowel disorders. *Gastroenterology* 2006; 130:1480–1491.

50. Mayer EA. Emerging disease model for functional gastrointestinal disorders. *Am J Med* 1999;107(5A): 12S.
51. Talley NJ, Zinsmeister AR, Melton LJ. Irritable bowel syndrome in a community: symptom subgroups, risk factors, and health care utilization. *Am J Epidemiol* 1995;142:76–83.
52. Drossman DA, Sandler RS, McKee DC. Bowel patterns among subjects not seeking health care. *Gastroenterology* 1982;83:529–534.
53. Whitehead WE, Crowell MD, Robinson JC, et al. Effects of stressful life events on bowel symptoms: subjects with irritable bowel syndrome compared with subjects without bowel dysfunction. *Gut* 1992;33:825–830.
54. Talley NJ, Fett SL, Zinsmeister AR, et al. Gastrointestinal tract symptoms and self-reported abuse: a population-based study. *Gastroenterology* 1994;107: 1040–1049.
55. Drossman DA, Leserman J, Nachmann G, et al. Sexual and physical abuse in women with functional or organic gastrointestinal disorders. *Ann Intern Med* 1990; 113:828–833.
56. Walker EA, Katon WJ, Jemelka RP, et al. Comorbidity of gastrointestinal complaints, depression, and anxiety disorders in the epidemiologic catchment (ECA) area study. *Am J Med* 1992;92(1A):26S–30S.
57. Locke GR III, Talley NJ, Zinsmeister AR, et al. The irritable bowel syndrome and functional dyspepsia: familial disorders? [abstract] *Gastroenterology* 1996;110: A26.
58. Rodriguez LAG, Ruigomez A. Increased risk of irritable bowel syndrome after bacterial gastroenteritis: cohort study. *Br Med J* 1999;318:565–566.
59. Gwee KA, Graham JC, McKendrick MW, et al. Psychometric scores and persistence of irritable bowel after infectious diarrhoea. *Lancet* 1996;347:150–153.
60. Zwetchkenbaum J, Burakoff R. The irritable bowel syndrome and food hypersensitivity. *Ann Allergy* 1988;62:47–49.
61. Thompson WG, Longstreth GF, Drossman DA, et al. Functional bowel disorders and functional abdominal pain. *Gut* 1999;45(Suppl 2):43–47.
62. Vanner S, Glenn D, Paterson W. Diagnosing irritable bowel syndrome: predictive values of Rome criteria [abstract]. *Gastroenterology* 1997;112:A47.
63. Schmulson MW, Chang L. Diagnostic approach to the patient with irritable bowel syndrome. *Am J Med* 1999;107(5A):20S–26S.
64. Almoundjed G, Drossman DA. Newer aspects of the irritable bowel syndrome. *Prim Care* 1996;23(3): 477–495.
65. Camilleri M. Clinical evidence to support current therapies of irritable bowel syndrome. *Aliment Pharmacol Ther* 1999;13:48–53.
66. Camilleri M. Therapeutic approach to the patient with irritable bowel syndrome. *Am J Med* 1999;107(5A): 27S–32S.
67. Klein KB. Controlled treatment trials in the irritable bowel syndrome. *Gastroenterology* 1988;95:232–241.
68. Poynard T, Naveau S, Mory B, et al. Meta-analysis of smooth muscle relaxants in the treatment of irritable bowel syndrome. *Aliment Pharmacol Ther* 1994;8: 499–510.
69. Rothstein RD. Irritable bowel syndrome. *Med Clin North Am* 2000;84:1247–1257.
70. Pittler MH, Ernst E. Peppermint oil for irritable bowel syndrome: a critical review and meta-analysis. *Am J Gastroenterol* 1998;93(7):1131–1135.
71. Clouse RE. Antidepressants for functional gastrointestinal syndromes. *Dig Dis Sci* 1994;39:2352–2363.
72. Gunput MD. Review article: clinical pharmacology of alosetron. *Aliment Pharm Ther* 1999;70(Suppl 2):70.
73. Corazziari E. Role of opioid ligands in the irritable bowel syndrome. *Can J Gastroenterol* 1999;13(Suppl A):71A.
74. Vicker AJ. *Hypnotherapy for irritable bowel syndrome: a report commissioned by North East Thames Regional Health Authority.* London: Research Council for Complementary Medicine, 1994.
75. Schouten W, ten Kate F, de Graaf E, et al. Visceral neuropathy in slow-transit constipation: an immunohistochemical investigation with monoclonal antibodies against neurofilament. *Dis Colon Rectum* 1993;36: 1099–1101.
76. Krishnamurthy S, Schuffler M, Rohrmann C, et al. Severe idiopathic constipation is associated with a distinctive abnormality of the colonic myenteric plexus. *Gastroenterology* 1985;88:26–34.
77. Bharucha AE, Phillips SF. Slow transit constipation. *Gastroenterol Clin North Am* 2001;30(1):77–95.
78. Camilleri M, McKinzie S, Burton D, et al. Prucalopride accelerates small bowel and colonic transit in patients with chronic functional constipation or constipation-predominant irritable bowel syndrome. *Gastroenterology* 2000;118:A845.
79. Coulie B, Szarka LA, Camilleri M, et al. Recombinant human neurotrophic factors accelerate colonic transit and relieve constipation in humans. *Gastroenterology* 2000;119(1):41–50.
80. Lane W. Remarks on the results of the operative treatment of chronic constipation. *Br Med J* 1908;1:126–130.
81. Christiansen J, Rasmussen OO. Colectomy for severe slow-transit constipation in strictly selected patients. *Scand J Gastroenterol* 1996;31(8):770–773.
82. Redmond JM, Smith GW, Barofsky I, et al. Physiological tests to predict long-term outcome of total abdominal colectomy for intractable constipation. *Am J Gastroenterol* 1995;90:748–753.
83. Nyam DCNK, Pemberton JH, Ilstrup DM, et al. Long-term results of surgery for chronic constipation. *Dis Colon Rectum* 1997;40:273–279.
84. Wexner SD, Daniel N, Jagelman DG. Colectomy for constipation: physiologic investigation is the key to success. *Dis Colon Rectum* 1991;34:851–856.
85. Sunderland GT, Poor FW, Lauder J, et al. Video-proctography in selecting patients with constipation for colectomy. *Dis Colon Rectum* 1992;35:235–237.
86. Hosie KB, Kmiot WA, Keighley MR. Constipation: another indication for restorative proctocolectomy. *Br J Surg* 1990;77(7):801–802.
87. Pinho M, Yoshioka K, Keighley MRB. Long-term results of anorectal myectomy for chronic constipation. *Br J Surg* 1989;76:1163–1164.
88. Krogh K, Laurberg S. Malone antegrade continence enema for faecal incontinence and constipation in adults. *Br J Surg* 1998;85:974–977.
89. Martelli H, Devroede G, Arhan P, et al. Mechanisms of idiopathic constipation: outlet obstruction. *Gastroenterology* 1978;75:623.
90. Preston DM, Lennard-Jones J. Anismus in chronic constipation. *Dig Dis Sci* 1985;30:413–418.
91. Whitehead WE, Wald A, Diamant N, et al. Functional disorders of the anorectum. In: Drossman DA, ed. *International Working Party consensus: Rome criteria II.* McLean, VA: Degnon, 2000:482–532.

92. Rao SSC. Dyssynergic defecation. *Gastroenterol Clin North Am* 2001;30(1):97.
93. Read NW, Timms JM. Defecation and the pathophysiology of constipation. *Clin Gastroenterol* 1986;15:937.
94. Rao SSC, Vellema T, Kempf J, et al. Symptoms, stool patterns and quality of life in patients with dyssynergic defecation. *Gastroenterology* 2000;118:A782.
95. Joo JS, Agachan F, Wolff B, et al. Initial North American experience with botulinum toxin type A for treatment of anismus. *Dis Colon Rectum* 1991;35: 145–150.
96. Pinho M, Yoshioka K, Keighley MRB. Long-term results of anorectal myectomy for chronic constipation. *Br J Surg* 1989;76:1163–1164.
97. Rao SSC, Welcher K, Leistikow J. Obstructive defecation: a failure of rectoanal coordination. *Am J Gastroenterol* 1998;93:1042–1050.
98. Enck P. Biofeedback training in disordered defecation: a critical review. *Dig Dis Sci* 1993;38:1953.
99. Bleijenberg G, Kuiipers HC. Treatment of the spastic pelvic floor syndrome with biofeedback. *Dis Colon Rectum* 1987;30:108.
100. Whitehead WE, Wald A, Diamant NE, et al. Functional disorders of the anus and rectum. *Gut* 1999;45: 1143–1147.
101. Rao SSC. Dyssynergic defecation. *Gastroenterol Clin North Am* 2001;30(1):101.
102. Wald A, Cauana BJ, Friemanis MG, et al. Contributions of evacuation proctography and anorectal manometry to evaluation of adults with idiopathic constipation. *Dig Dis Sci* 1990;35:481.
103. Rao SSC. Dyssynergic defecation. *Gastroenterol Clin North Am* 2001;30(1):107.
104. Ernst E, Resch KL. A meta-analysis of biofeedback treatment for anismus. *Eur J Phys Med Rehabil* 1995, 5(5):157–159.
105. Enck P. Biofeedback training in disordered defecation: a critical review. *Dig Dis Sci* 1993;38:1953–1960.
106. Rao SSC, Loening-Baucke V, Enck P. Biofeedback therapy for defecation disorders. *Dig Dis Sci* 1997; 15(Suppl 1):78–92.
107. Rao SSC. Dyssynergic defecation. *Gastroenterol Clin North Am* 2001;30(1):109.
108. Ho YH, Tan M, Goh HS. Clinical and physiologic effects of biofeedback in outlet obstruction constipation. *Dis Colon Rectum* 1996;39(5):520–524.
109. Joo JS, Agachan F, Wolff B, et al. Initial North American experience with botulinum toxin type A for treatment of anismus. *Dis Colon Rectum* 1996;39(10): 1107–1111.
110. Farag A. Obturator internus muscle autotransfer: a new concept for the treatment of anismus. Clinical experience. *Eur Surg Res* 1997;29(1):42–51.
111. Spence-Jones C, Kamm MA, Henry MM, et al. Bowel dysfunction: a pathogenic factor in uterovaginal prolapse and urinary stress incontinence. *Br J Obstet Gynecol* 1994;101:147–152.
112. Samuelsson EC, Arne Victor FT, Tibblin G, et al. Signs of genital prolapse in a Swedish population of women 20 to 59 years of age and possible related factors. *Am J Obstet Gynecol* 1999;9:961–964.
113. Swift SE. The distribution of pelvic organ support in a population of female subjects seen for routine gynecologic health care. *Am J Obstet Gynecol* 2000;183: 277–285.
114. Chou Q, Weber AM, Piedmonte MR. Clinical presentation of enterocele. *Obstet Gynecol* 2000;96(4):599–603.
115. Weber AM, Walters MD, Ballard LA, et al. Posterior vaginal prolapse and bowel function. *Am J Obstet Gynecol* 1998;179(6 Pt 1):1446–1449.
116. Ellerkmann RM, Cundiff GW, Bent AE, et al. Correlation of symptoms with location and severity of pelvic organ prolapse. *Am J Obstet Gynecol* 2001; 185(6):1332–1337.
117. Goei R. Anorectal function in patients with defecatory disorders and asymptomatic subjects: evaluation with defecography. *Radiology* 1990;174:121–123.
118. Yoshioka K, Matsui Y, Yamada O, et al. Physiologic and anatomic assessment of patients with rectocele. *Dis Colon Rectum* 1991;34:704–708.
119. Bradley CS, et al. Bowel symptoms in women planning surgery for pelvic organ prolapse. Presented at the 32nd Annual Meeting of the Society of Gynecologic Surgeons, Tucson, AZ, 2006.
120. DaSilva G, Gurland B. Posterior vaginal prolapse does not correlate with fecal symptoms or objective measurements of anorectal function. Presented at the 32nd Annual Meeting of the Society of Gynecologic Surgeons, Tucson, AZ, 2006.
121. Weidner AC, Coates KW, Cundiff GW, et al. Dysfunctional bowel symptoms in women with urinary incontinence and pelvic organ prolapse (Submitted for publication).
122. Jackson SL, Weber AM, Hull TL, et al. Fecal incontinence in women with urinary incontinence and pelvic organ prolapse. *Obstet Gynecol* 1997;89(3):423–427.
123. Donnelly V, O'Connell PR, O'Herlihy C. The influence of estrogen replacement on fecal incontinence in postmenopausal women. *Br J Obstet Gynaecol* 1997;104(3):311–315.
124. Sulak PJ, Kuehl TJ, Shull BL. Vaginal pessaries and their use in pelvic relaxation. *J Reprod Med* 1993;38: 919–923.
125. Zeitlin MP, Lebherz TB. Pessaries in the geriatric patient. *J Am Geriatr Soc* 1992;40:635–639.
126. Cundiff GW, Weidner AC, Visco AG, et al. A survey of pessary use by members of the American urogynecology society. *Obstet Gynecol* 2000;95(6 Pt 1): 931–935.
127. Wu V, Farrell SA, Baskett TF, et al. A simplified protocol for pessary management. *Obstet Gynecol* 1997; 90:990–994.
128. Davila GW. Vaginal prolapse. *Postgrad Med* 1996;99: 171–185.
129. Sulak PJ, Kuehl TJ, Shull BJ. Vaginal pessaries and their use in pelvic relaxation. *J Reprod Med* 1993;38: 919–923.
130. Cundiff GW, Amundsten CL, Bent AE, et al. Randomized crossover trial of ring and Gellhorn pessaries: symptom outcomes. Presented at the 25th Annual Meeting of the American Gynecologic and Obstetrical Society, Williamsburg, VA, 2006.
131. Jeffcoat TNA. Posterior colpoperineorrhaphy. *Am J Obstet Gynecol* 1959;77:490–502.
132. Mellgren A, Anzén B, Nilsson BY, et al. Results of rectocele repair: a prospective study. *Dis Colon Rectum* 1995;38:7–13.
133. Kahn MA, Stanton SL. Posterior colporrhaphy: its effects on bowel and sexual function. *Br J Obstet Gynaecol* 1997;104:882–886.
134. Francis WJA, Jeffcoate TNA. Dyspareunia following vaginal operations. *J Obstet Gynaecol Br Emp* 1961; 68:1–10.
135. Paraiso M, Weber A, Walters M. *J Pelv Med Surg* 2001;7:335–339.

136. Sullivan ES, Leaverton GH, Hardwick CE. Transrectal perineal repair: an adjunct to improved function after anorectal surgery. *Dis Colon Rectum* 1968;11:196–214.

137. Sehapayak S. Transrectal repair of rectocele: an extended armamentarium of colorectal surgeons. A report of 355 cases. *Dis Colon Rectum* 1985;28:422–433.

138. Khubchandani AT, Clancy JP, Rosen L, et al. Endorectal repair of rectocele revisited. *Br J Surg* 1997;84:89–91.

139. Arnold MW, Stewart WRC, Aguilar PS. Rectocele repair: four year's experiences. *Dis Colon Rectum* 1990; 33:684–687.

140. Kahn MA, Stanton SL, Kumar DA. *Randomized prospective trial of posterior colporrhaphy versus transanal repair of rectocele.* Presented at American Urogynecologic Society, September 1997.

141. Richardson AC, Lyon JB, Williams NL. A new look at pelvic relaxation. *Am J Obstet Gynecol* 1976;568: 568–573.

142. Cundiff GW, Weidner AC, Visco AG, et al. An anatomic and functional assessment of the discrete defect rectocele repair. *Am J Obstet Gynecol* 1998;179(6 Pt 1):1451–1456.

143. Porter WE, Steele A, Walsh P, et al. The anatomic and functional outcomes of defect-specific rectocele repairs. *Am J Obstet Gynecol* 1999;181(6):1353–1359.

144. Glavind K, Madsen H. A prospective study of the discrete fascial defect rectocele repair. *Acta Obstet Gynecol Scand* 2000;79(2);145–147.

145. Kenton K, Shott S, Brubaker L. Outcome after rectovaginal fascia reattachment for rectocele repair. *Am J Obstet Gynecol* 1999;181:1360.

146. Abramov Y, Gandhi S, Goldberg RP, et al. Site-specific rectocele repair compared with standard posterior colporrhaphy. *Obstet Gynecol* 2005;105(2):314–318.

147. Julian TM. The efficacy of Marlex mesh in the repair of severe, recurrent vaginal prolapse of the anterior midvaginal wall. *Am J Obstet Gynecol* 1996;175: 1472–1475.

148. Sand PK, Koduri S, Lobel RW, et al. Prospective randomized trial of polyglactin 910 mesh to prevent recurrence of cystoceles and rectoceles. *Am J Obstet Gynecol* 2001;184(7):1357–1362.

149. Oster S, Astrup A. A new vaginal operation for recurrent and large rectoceles using dermis transplants. *Acta Obstet Gynecol Scand* 1981;60(5):493–495.

150. Miklos JR, Kohli N. Rectovaginal fistula repair utilizing a cadaveric dermal allograft. *Int Urogynecol J Pelvic Floor Dysfunct* 1999;10(60):405–406.

151. Paraiso MR, Barber MD, Muir TW, et al. Rectocele repair: a randomized trial of three surgical techniques including graft augmentation. Presented at the 32nd Annual Meeting of the Society of Gynecologic Surgeons, Tucson, AZ, 2006.

152. de Tayrac R, Picone O, Chauveaud-Lambling A, et al. A 2-year anatomical and functional assessment of transvaginal rectocele repair using a polypropylene mesh. *Int Urogynecol J Pelvic Floor Dysfunct* 2006; 17(2):100–106.

153. Milani R, Salvatore S, Soligo M, et al. Functional and anatomical outcome of anterior and posterior vaginal prolapse repair with prolene mesh. *Br J Obstet Gynaecol* 2005;112(8):1164.

154. Dwyer PL, O'Reilly BA. Transvaginal repair of anterior and posterior compartment prolapse with Atrium polypropylene mesh. *Br J Obstet Gynaecol* 2004; 11(8):831–836.

155. Collinet P, Belot F, Debodinance P, et al. Transvaginal mesh technique for pelvic organ prolapse repair: mesh exposure management and risk factors. *Int Urogynecol J Pelvic Floor Dysfunct* 2006;17(4):315.

156. Parks AG, Porter NH, Hardcastle J. The syndrome of the descending perineum. *Proc R Soc Med* 1966;59: 477–482.

157. Bartolo DC, Read NW, Jarett JA, et al. Differences in anal sphincter function and clinical presentation in patients with pelvic floor descent. *Gastroenterology* 1982;85:68–75.

158. Mackle EJ, Parks TG. Clinical features in patients with excessive perineal descent. *J R Coll Surg Edinb* 1989;34:88–90.

159. Yoshioka K, Hyland G, Keighley MR. Anorectal function after abdominal rectopexy: parameters of predictive value in identifying return of continence. *Br J Surg* 1989;76:64–68.

160. Korsgen S, Deen KI, Keighley MR. Long-term results of total pelvic floor repair for postobstetric fecal incontinence. *Dis Colon Rectum* 1997;40:835–839.

161. Harewood GC, Coulie B, Camilleri M, et al. Descending perineum syndrome: audit of clinical and laboratory features and outcome of pelvic floor retraining. *Am J Gastroenterol* 1999;94:126–130.

162. Addison WA, Cundiff GW, Bump RC, et al. Sacral colpopexy is the preferred treatment for vaginal vault prolapse. *J Gynecol Tech* 1996;2:69–74.

163. Cundiff GW, Harris RL, Coates KW, et al. Abdominal sacral colpoperineopexy: a new approach for correction of posterior compartment defects and perineal descent associated with vaginal vault prolapse. *Am J Obstet Gynecol* 1997;177:1345–1355.

164. Visco AG, Wiedner AC, Barber MD, et al. *Vaginal erosion with abdominal sacral colpoperineopexy.* Presented at the 20th Annual Scientific Meeting of the American Urogynecologic Society, San Diego, October 1999.

165. Sullivan ES, Longaker CJ, Lee PY. Total pelvic mesh repair: a ten-year experience. *Dis Colon Rectum* 2001; 44:857–863.

166. Kaufman H, Cundiff G, Thompson J, et al. Suture rectopexy and sacral colpoperineopexy with Alloderm® for perineal descent. *Dis Colon Rectum* 2000;43:A16.

167. Kaufman HS, Buller JL, Thompson JR, et al. Dynamic pelvic magnetic resonance imaging and cystocolpoproctography alter surgical management of pelvic floor disorders. *Dis Colon Rectum* 2001;44: 1575–1584.

168. Culligan PJ, Blackwell L, Goldsmith LJ, et al. A randomized controlled trial comparing fascia lata and synthetic mesh for sacral colpopexy. *Obstet Gynecol* 2005;106(1):29–37.

169. Jurgeleit HC, Corman ML, Coller JA, et al. Procidentia of the rectum: Teflon sling repair of rectal prolapse, Lahey Clinic experience. *Dis Colon Rectum* 1975;18:464.

170. Duthie GS, Bartolo DCC. Abdominal rectopexy for rectal prolapse: a comparison of techniques. *Br J Surg* 1992;79:107–113.

171. Ripstein CB. Surgical care of muscle rectal prolapse. *Dis Colon Rectum* 1965;8:34–38.

172. Tjandra JJ, Fazio VW, Church JM, et al. Ripstein procedure is an effective treatment for rectal prolapse without constipation. *Dis Colon Rectum* 1993;36:501–507.

173. Gordon PH, Hoexter B. Complications of the Ripstein procedure. *Dis Colon Rectum* 1978;21:277–280.

174. Frykman HM, Goldberg SM. The surgical treatment of rectal procidentia. *Surg Gynecol Obstet* 1969;129: 1225–1230.

175. Kuijpers HC. Treatment of complete rectal prolapse: to narrow, to wrap, to suspend, to fix, to encircle, to plicate, or to resect? *World J Surg* 1992;16:826–830.
176. Wassef R, Rothenberger D, Goldberg S. Rectal prolapse. *Curr Probl Surg* 1986;23:402.
177. Delorme R. Sue le traitement des prolapses du rectum totavx pour l'excision de la mucueuse rectele ou recto-colique. *Bull Mem Soc Chir Paris* 1900;26:498.
178. Senapati A, Nicholls RJ, Thomson JPS, et al. Results of Delorme's procedure for rectal prolapse. *Dis Colon Rectum* 1994;37:456–460.

179. Oliver GC, Vachon D, Eisenstat TE, et al. Delorme's procedure for complete rectal prolapse in severely debilitated patients. *Dis Colon Rectum* 1994;37:461–467.
180. Graf W, Stefansson T, Arvidssom D, et al. Laparoscopic suture rectopexy. *Dis Colon Rectum* 1995; 38:211–212.

suggest a definite benefit to elective cesarean, although there may be an association between vaginal delivery and a worsening of postpartum vaginal support (35,36). Clearly this is an area for further study.

In addition to injuries associated with childbirth, injuries might also occur with recreational or occupational exposures to forces (37–39). However, we do not know what activities have a significant impact. Therefore, clinicians cannot currently provide evidence-based recommendations for primary or secondary prevention.

Disruption of pelvic muscle function is viewed as another potential initiating factor for prolapse. After a single vaginal delivery, gaps in the levator ani muscle are seen in 20% of women (1,40). We know that the levator hiatus is transiently widened after childbirth (41) and also widened in women with prolapse (17–20). Peripheral neuropathy has been observed after childbirth and might contribute to muscle dysfunction and atrophy. In one of the first studies of peripheral neuropathy in pelvic floor disorders, Sharf et al (42) found electromyographic evidence of levator ani denervation in 50% of women with prolapse. Subsequent investigators have confirmed an association between denervation and pelvic floor disorders, including prolapse (43,44). The role of pelvic muscle injury or denervation in the genesis of prolapse remains uncertain. Similarly, it is not known whether pelvic floor muscle exercises can reduce the incidence or progression of prolapse in susceptible individuals.

Environmental and lifestyle exposures may also play an important promoting role. For example, obesity has been associated with the development of prolapse as well as with the worsening of prolapse over time (23,45,46). There is some suggestion that body morphology might be a stronger risk factor than obesity (45), raising the possibility of metabolic as well as mechanical effects of obesity. Chronic straining and chronic increased intra-abdominal pressure may also play a role (26), potentially as a result of the impact on connective tissue supports.

In cross-sectional studies, hysterectomy has been associated with prolapse (46,47). Until recently, this was viewed as a likely causal association, attributed to disruption of connective tissue supports at the time of surgery. However, recent data from two large randomized trials of supracervical hysterectomy suggests that preserving the cervix does not reduce the risk of prolapse (48,49). Thus, it is likely that the association between hysterectomy and prolapse is due either to preexisting prolapse among women undergoing hysterectomy or to other confounding factors associated with hysterectomy (e.g., parity). More research is needed to investigate whether other hysterectomy techniques have an impact on prolapse risk.

Urethropexy has also been blamed for subsequent development of prolapse (50,51). Again, it's unclear whether this is due to undiagnosed prolapse at the time of bladder neck suspension, to the impact of confounding factors, or to a true causal association. It has been hypothesized that urethropexy deflects the vagina anteriorly, resulting in an increased mechanical load on the posterior vaginal wall. It is not known whether the long-term risk of prolapse is independently increased by urethropexy and whether this outcome can be minimized with other surgical treatments for stress incontinence, such as midurethral slings.

Finally, we cannot dismiss the important impact of aging. The prevalence of prolapse increases with age. Aging affects connective tissue properties and muscle function (52). The hormonal changes of menopause may play a role, although there is no evidence that hormone treatment halts the progression of pelvic organ prolapse. It is hard to separate the impact of aging from other confounding factors, such as parity, obesity, vascular changes, and lifestyle changes.

CONCLUSIONS

While we are learning more about the mechanisms of normal pelvic organ support and the pathophysiology of prolapse, many questions remain unanswered. Identification of the specific anatomic causes will improve surgical treatments. Additional key questions include whether prolapse can be prevented (or its progression halted) by lifestyle modifications, whether elective cesarean could affect the incidence of prolapse, and whether susceptible individuals can be identified early in life. These questions are essential to understanding the pathophysiology of prolapse and critical to primary and secondary prevention.

REFERENCES

1. Wei JT, De Lancey JO. Functional anatomy of the pelvic floor and lower urinary tract. *Clin Obstet Gynecol* 2004;47(1):3–17.
2. Tulikangas PK. Defect theory of pelvic organ prolapse. *Clin Obstet Gynecol* 2005;48(3):662–667.
3. Weber AM, Walters MD. Anterior vaginal prolapse: review of anatomy and techniques of surgical repair. *Obstet Gynecol* 1997;89(2):311–318.
4. Ercoli A, Delmas V, Fanfani F, et al. Terminologia Anatomica versus unofficial descriptions and nomenclature of the fasciae and ligaments of the female pelvis: a dissection-based comparative study. *Am J Obstet Gynecol* 2005;193(4):1565–1573.

5. Yabuki Y, Sasaki H, Hatakeyama N, et al. Discrepancies between classic anatomy and modern gynecologic surgery on pelvic connective tissue structure: harmonization of those concepts by collaborative cadaver dissection. *Am J Obstet Gynecol* 2005;193(1):7–15.

6. DeLancey JO. Anatomic aspects of vaginal eversion after hysterectomy. *Am J Obstet Gynecol* 1992;166(6 Pt 1):1717–1724.

7. DeLancey JO. Anatomy and biomechanics of genital prolapse. *Clin Obstet Gynecol* 1993;36(4):897–909.

8. DeLancey JO, Starr RA. Histology of the connection between the vagina and levator ani muscles. Implications for urinary tract function. *J Reprod Med* 1990; 35(8):765–771.

9. Richardson AC, Lyon JB, Williams NL. A new look at pelvic relaxation. *Am J Obstet Gynecol* 1976;126(5): 568–573.

10. Leffler KS, Thompson JR, Cundiff GW, et al. Attachment of the rectovaginal septum to the pelvic sidewall. *Am J Obstet Gynecol* 2001;185(1):41–43.

11. Richardson AC. The rectovaginal septum revisited: its relationship to rectocele and its importance in rectocele repair. *Clin Obstet Gynecol* 1993;36(4):976–983.

12. Kleeman SD, Westermann C, Karram MM. Rectoceles and the anatomy of the posterior vaginal wall: revisited. *Am J Obstet Gynecol* 2005;193(6):2050–2055.

13. Farrell SA, Dempsey T, Geldenhuys L. Histologic examination of "fascia" used in colporrhaphy. *Obstet Gynecol* 2001;98(5 Pt 1):794–798.

14. Berglas B, Rubin IC. Histologic study of the pelvic connective tissue. *Surg Gynecol Obstet* 1953;97(3):277–289.

15. Cundiff GW, Weidner AC, Visco AG, et al. An anatomic and functional assessment of the discrete defect rectocele repair. *Am J Obstet Gynecol* 1998;179(6 Pt 1): 1451–1457.

16. Kenton K, Shott S, Brubaker L. Outcome after rectovaginal fascia reattachment for rectocele repair. *Am J Obstet Gynecol* 1999;181(6):1360–1364.

17. Berglas B, Rubin IC. Study of the supportive structures of the uterus by levator myography. *Surg Gynecol Obstet* 1953;97(6):677–692.

18. Hoyte L, Schierlitz L, Zou K, et al. Two- and 3-dimensional MRI comparison of levator ani structure, volume, and integrity in women with stress incontinence and prolapse. *Am J Obstet Gynecol* 2001;185(1):11–19.

19. Singh K, Jakab M, Reid WM, et al. Three-dimensional magnetic resonance imaging assessment of levator ani morphologic features in different grades of prolapse. *Am J Obstet Gynecol* 2003;188(4):910–915.

20. Ghetti C, Gregory WT, Edwards SR, et al. Severity of pelvic organ prolapse associated with measurements of pelvic floor function. *Int Urogynecol J Pelvic Floor Dysfunct* 2005;16(6):432–436.

21. Handa VL, Pannu HK, Siddique S, et al. Architectural differences in the bony pelvis of women with and without pelvic floor disorders. *Obstet Gynecol* 2003;102(6): 1283–1290.

22. Sze EH, Kohli N, Miklos JR, et al. Computed tomography comparison of bony pelvis dimensions between women with and without genital prolapse. *Obstet Gynecol* 1999;93(2):229–232.

23. Hendrix SL, Clark A, Nygaard I, et al. Pelvic organ prolapse in the Women's Health Initiative: gravity and gravidity. *Am J Obstet Gynecol* 2002;186(6):1160–1166.

24. Moloy HC. *Moloy's evaluation of the pelvis in obstetrics.* Philadelphia: Saunders, 1959.

25. Tegerstedt G, Maehle-Schmidt M, Nyren O, et al. Prevalence of symptomatic pelvic organ prolapse in a Swedish population. *Int Urogynecol J Pelvic Floor Dysfunct* 2005;16(6):497–503.

26. Weber AM, Richter HE. Pelvic organ prolapse. *Obstet Gynecol* 2005;106(3):615–634.

27. Falconer C, Ekman G, Malmstrom A, et al. Decreased collagen synthesis in stress-incontinent women. *Obstet Gynecol* 1994;84(4):583–586.

28. Wong MY, Harmanli OH, Agar M, et al. Collagen content of nonsupport tissue in pelvic organ prolapse and stress urinary incontinence. *Am J Obstet Gynecol* 2003; 189(6):1597–1600.

29. Norton PA. Pelvic floor disorders: the role of fascia and ligaments. *Clin Obstet Gynecol* 1993;36(4):926–938.

30. Norton PA, Baker JE, Sharp HC, et al. Genitourinary prolapse and joint hypermobility in women. *Obstet Gynecol* 1995;85(2):225–228.

31. Carley ME, Schaffer J. Urinary incontinence and pelvic organ prolapse in women with Marfan or Ehlers Danlos syndrome. *Am J Obstet Gynecol* 2000;182(5):1021–1023.

32. el-Shahaly HA, el-Sherif AK. Is the benign joint hypermobility syndrome benign? *Clin Rheumatol* 1991; 10(3):302–307.

33. Hansell NK, Dietz HP, Treloar SA, et al. Genetic covariation of pelvic organ and elbow mobility in twins and their sisters. *Twin Res* 2004;7(3):254–260.

34. Moalli PA, Shand SH, Zyczynski HM, et al. Remodeling of vaginal connective tissue in patients with prolapse. *Obstet Gynecol* 2005;106(5 Pt 1):953–963.

35. O'Boyle AL, O'Boyle JD, Calhoun B, et al. Pelvic organ support in pregnancy and postpartum. *Int Urogynecol J Pelvic Floor Dysfunct* 2005;16(1):69–72.

36. Sze EH, Sherard GB, 3rd, Dolezal JM. Pregnancy, labor, delivery, and pelvic organ prolapse. *Obstet Gynecol* 2002;100(5 Pt 1):981–986.

37. Davis GD. Uterine prolapse after laparoscopic uterosacral transection in nulliparous airborne trainees. A report of three cases. *J Reprod Med* 1996;41(4):279–282.

38. Woodman PJ, Swift SE, O'Boyle A L, et al. Prevalence of severe pelvic organ prolapse in relation to job description and socioeconomic status: a multicenter cross-sectional study. *Int Urogynecol J Pelvic Floor Dysfunct* 2006;17:340–345.

39. Larsen WI, Yavorek TA. Pelvic organ prolapse and urinary incontinence in nulliparous women at the United States Military Academy. *Int Urogynecol J Pelvic Floor Dysfunct* 2006;17:208–210.

40. DeLancey JO, Kearney R, Chou Q, et al. The appearance of levator ani muscle abnormalities in magnetic resonance images after vaginal delivery. *Obstet Gynecol* 2003;101(1):46–53.

41. Tunn R, DeLancey JO, Howard D, et al. MR imaging of levator ani muscle recovery following vaginal delivery. *Int Urogynecol J Pelvic Floor Dysfunct* 1999;10(5): 300–307.

42. Sharf B Z, Sharf M, Mitrani A. Electromyogram of pelvic floor muscles in genital prolapse. *Int J Gynaecol Obstet* 1976;14:2–4.

43. Smith AR, Hosker GL, Warrell DW. The role of partial denervation of the pelvic floor in the etiology of genitourinary prolapse and stress incontinence of urine. A neurophysiological study. *Br J Obstet Gynaecol* 1989; 96(1):24–28.

44. Weidner AC, Barber MD, Visco AG, et al. Pelvic muscle electromyography of levator ani and external anal sphincter in nulliparous women and women with pelvic floor dysfunction. *Am J Obstet Gynecol* 2000;183(6): 1390–1401.

45. Handa VL, Garrett E, Hendrix S, et al. Progression and remission of pelvic organ prolapse: a longitudinal study of menopausal women. *Am J Obstet Gynecol* 2004; 190(1):27–32.

46. Mant J, Painter R, Vessey M. Epidemiology of genital prolapse: observations from the Oxford Family Planning Association Study. *Br J Obstet Gynaecol* 1997; 104(5):579–585.

47. Swift SE, Pound T, Dias JK. Case-control study of etiologic factors in the development of severe pelvic organ prolapse. *Int Urogynecol J Pelvic Floor Dysfunct* 2001; 12(3):187–192.

48. Learman LA, Summitt RL, Jr., Varner RE, et al. A randomized comparison of total or supracervical hysterec-

tomy: surgical complications and clinical outcomes. *Obstet Gynecol* 2003;102(3):453–462.

49. Thakar R, Ayers S, Clarkson P, et al. Outcomes after total versus subtotal abdominal hysterectomy. *N Engl J Med* 2002;347(17):1318–1325.

50. Wiskind AK, Creighton SM, Stanton SL. The incidence of genital prolapse after the Burch colposuspension. *Am J Obstet Gynecol* 1992;167(2):399–404.

51. Sze EH, Miklos JR, Partoll L, et al. Sacrospinous ligament fixation with transvaginal needle suspension for advanced pelvic organ prolapse and stress incontinence. *Obstet Gynecol* 1997;89(1):94–96.

52. Arking R. *Biology of aging: observations & principles,* 2nd ed. Sunderland, MA: Sinauer Associates, 1998.

CHAPTER 25

The Clinical Evaluation of Pelvic Organ Prolapse

Geoffrey W. Cundiff

INTRODUCTION

There are several key principles that inform the clinical evaluation of pelvic organ prolapse (POP). Firstly, vaginal support defects occur with and without symptoms. Secondly, many of the symptoms attributed to POP can result from other etiologies. Consequently, the clinical evaluation focuses on eliciting the patient's complaints, defining and quantifying the location and severity of support defects, and establishing a relationship between the symptoms and the support defects, through elimination of other etiologies of pelvic floor symptomatology.

EARLY EFFORTS

The earliest attempts to quantify POP objectified the degree of bulge by comparing it to a known volume, such as a "hen's egg" (1). These descriptive systems were imprecise and were used inconsistently. The absence of a standardized objective system frustrated many surgeons, as was clearly expressed by Friedman and Little in 1961: "Specious and misleading discrepancies exist with reference to classification of the extent of descent of the uterus in disorders involving fascial relaxation" (2). Thereafter, several grading systems were introduced that helped to define the important facets of evaluating POP. Beecham recognized the importance of evaluating the vaginal apex and anterior and posterior walls independently, although his system was limited by the prescribed absence of straining by the patient during the examination (3). Baden and Walker also recommended a site-specific system initially in 1968, with later modifications that evolved into the "halfway" system (4). The system was widely used for many years. While it provided a means to quantify the amount of prolapse at six vaginal sites, it provided only an estimate and not an exact measurement of descent of the prolapsing structure relative to the hymen (Table 25.1).

In September 1993, a subcommittee of the International Continence Society (ICS) met in Rome to draft a system to enable accurate quantitative description of pelvic support findings. The subcommittee completed a final draft of their recommendations that was distributed to members of the ICS, the American Urogynecologic Society (AUGS), and the Society of Gynecologic Surgeons (SGS) in late 1994 and early 1995. This quantification system, the Pelvic Organ Prolapse Quantification (POPQ) system, was formally adopted by the ICS in October 1995, the AUGS in January 1996, and the SGS in March 1996 (5). The system is an adaptation of Baden and Walker's site-specific system that requires measuring eight sites to create a tandem vaginal profile before assigning site-specific ordinal stages.

The subcommittee report also addressed the presence of functional symptoms related to the presence of POP. Specifically, the report acknowledged four functional symptom groups, including urinary, bowel, sexual, and other local symptoms, and emphasized the importance of systematically assessing associated symptoms.

SYMPTOMS ASSOCIATED WITH PELVIC ORGAN PROLAPSE

Recent studies have sought to define the symptoms associated with POP. Ellerkmann et al investigated symptoms commonly attributed to POP, categorizing symptoms according to both prolapse severity

TABLE 25.1

Halfway System for Grading Relaxations

Urethrocele, cystocele, uterine prolapse, culdocele, or rectocele: patient strains firmly. Grade descent of desired sites. Grade posterior urethral descent, lowest part other sites.
    Grade 0: normal position *for each* respective site
    Grade 1: descent *halfway* to the hymen
    Grade 2: descent to the hymen
    Grade 3: descent *halfway past* the hymen
    Grade 4: maximum possible descent for each site
Anterior perineal laceration: grade with patient holding
    Grade 0: normal; superficial epithelial laceration
    Grade 1: laceration *halfway* to the anal sphincter
    Grade 2: laceration to the anal sphincter
    Grade 3: laceration involves anal sphincter
    Grade 4: laceration involves rectal mucosa

When choosing between two grades, use the greater grade (i.e., if there is a question as to grade 2 or 3 cystocele, use cystocele, grade 3). Grade still in doubt? Regrade with patient standing. Grade worst site, worst segment, or vaginal canal PRN. Grades are interchanged with mild to severe and degrees methods.
From Baden W, Walker T. *Surgical repair of vaginal defects.* Philadelphia: JB Lippincott, 1992:14, with permission.

and associated anatomic compartment (6). Pelvic pressure and discomfort along with visualization of prolapse were strongly associated with worsening stages of POP in all compartments. Impairment of sexual relations, including dyspareunia, and urinary incontinence associated with coitus, as well as duration of abstinence were also strongly associated with worsening POP. Defecatory dysfunction, including incomplete evacuation and digital manipulation, was weakly associated with worsening posterior POP. Similarly, in a multicenter, cross-sectional study, 1,004 women attending routine gynecologic health care underwent POPQ measurements and were surveyed regarding symptoms of disordered defecation (7). Most associations between bowel symptoms and vaginal or pelvic organ descent were weak, although after controlling for important covariates, straining at stool remained associated with anterior vaginal wall and perineal descent. Weber et al also described defecatory dysfunction in association with posterior POP (8). The majority of the sample in this study had stage I or greater posterior POP. While most (92%) reported normal stool frequency, 74% reported straining and 24% strained usually or always. Similarly, 31% required splinting of the posterior vaginal wall or digitation of the rectum during

bowel movement, and 16% reported fecal incontinence. Not surprisingly, on a 10-point "bother" scale, the impact of bowel function was 5 or more in 50% and 8 or more in 28%. While these symptoms occur with posterior POP, they also result from other forms of defecatory dysfunction.

Appropriate treatment of posterior prolapse, therefore, requires the pelvic surgeon treating posterior POP to understand and apply the differential diagnosis of defecatory dysfunction. The same is true for treatment of symptomatic POP in the apical and anterior compartments (Table 25.2). Validated condition-specific questionnaires are available that help to elicit symptoms associated with POP (9). Generally, symptoms related to protrusion are the most reliably associated with POP, while urinary, defecatory, and sexual symptoms demand a careful investigation for other possible etiologies.

ELEMENTS OF THE PELVIC EXAMINATION

The goals of the pelvic examination are to objectively define the degree of prolapse and to determine the integrity of the connective tissue and muscular support of the pelvic organs. The POPQ staging system reliably objectifies the degree of POP, while the evaluation of the integrity of the

TABLE 25.2

Differential Diagnosis for Prolapse-Associated Symptoms

Symptom Group	Symptom	Other Aspects of Differential Diagnosis
Herniation symptoms	Pelvic pressure	Rectal prolapse
	Vaginal protrusion	
Voiding symptoms	Urinary hesitancy	Detrusor dysfunction
	Incomplete emptying	Detrusor sphincter dyssynergia
	Splinting to complete urination	Behavioral voiding disorders
Lower urinary tract symptoms	Urinary frequency	Overactive bladder
	Urinary urgency	Excessive fluid intake
	Dysuria	Interstitial cystitis
		Urinary tract infection
Urinary incontinence	Urinary incontinence	Stress incontinence
		Detrusor overactivity
Defecatory dysfunction	Dyschezia	Irritable bowel syndrome
	Incomplete defecation	Colonic inertia
	Splinting to complete defecation	Anismus
Fecal incontinence	Fecal urgency	Irritable bowel syndrome
	Fecal incontinence	Diarrhea
		External anal sphincter dysfunction
Sexual dysfunction	Dyspareunia	Levator ani syndrome
	Decreased sensation	Libido dysfunction

connective tissue and muscular supports is more subjective.

While patients are generally most symptomatic when standing or sitting, the pelvic examination is usually performed in the dorsal lithotomy position, which has the potential to mask the severity of prolapse. It is, therefore, important that the patient confirms maximal protrusion at the time of examination. This may require further examination on a commode or in the standing position. Valsalva with hard straining facilitates maximal protrusion, and the patient can use a hand mirror to confirm maximal protrusion (4).

Vaginal support should be evaluated independently at all sites, including the vaginal apex, the anterior wall, and the posterior wall. After the maximal extent of POP is noted without a speculum, the support of the apex is evaluated with a bivalved speculum. Gradually removing the open speculum permits the examiner to assess apical support isolated from the anterior and posterior vaginal walls. The anterior wall is then assessed while supporting the vaginal apex and posterior wall with a Sims speculum or with a disarticulated posterior blade of a Graves speculum (Fig. 25.1). Similarly, the single speculum blade supports the

vaginal apex and anterior wall while evaluating the posterior wall (Fig. 25.2). This permits the examiner to focus on the support defects in each compartment.

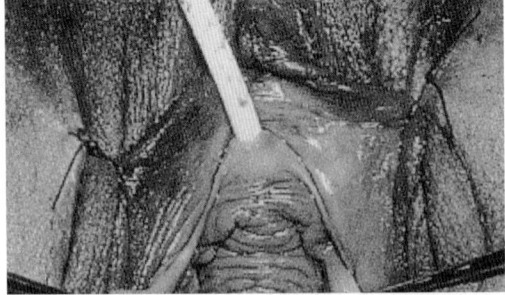

FIGURE 25.1 ● Support of the posterior vaginal wall and vaginal apex with a single-blade speculum permits an isolated evaluation of the support of the anterior vaginal wall. Note the normal rugated epithelium of the anterior vaginal wall. (From Baggish MS, Karram MM. *Atlas of pelvic anatomy and gynecologic surgery.* Singapore: WB Saunders, 2001:382, with permission.)

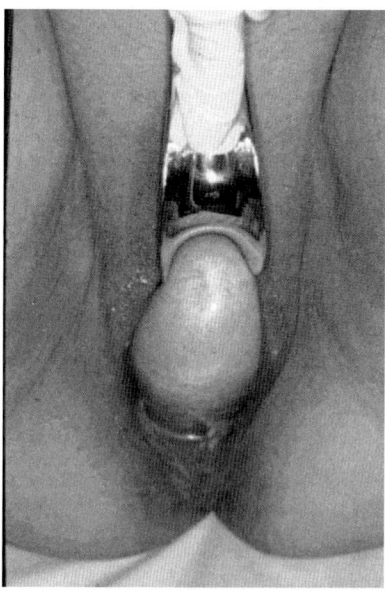

FIGURE 25.2 ● Support of the anterior vaginal wall and vaginal apex with a single-blade speculum permits an isolated evaluation of the support of the posterior vaginal wall.

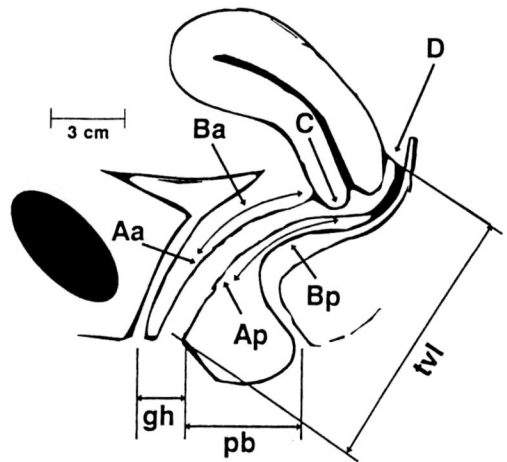

FIGURE 25.3 ● Six sites (points *Aa, Ba, C, D, Bp,* and *Ap*), genital hiatus (*gh*), perineal body (*pb*), and total vaginal length (*tvl*) used for pelvic organ support quantitation. (From Bump RC, Mattiasson A, Bø K, et al. The standardization of terminology of female pelvic organ prolapse and pelvic floor dysfunction. *Am J Obstet Gynecol* 1996;175:10–17, with permission.)

STAGING PELVIC ORGAN PROLAPSE

It is important to objectively document the extent of prolapse, both before and after interventions. There are a number of ordinal staging systems to describe the degree of descent, although the POPQ examination is the most widely accepted.

Pelvic Organ Prolapse Quantification System

This standardized system was published in the *American Journal of Obstetrics and Gynecology* in July 1996 (4). The system measures eight sites to create a tandem vaginal profile before assigning site-specific ordinal stages. Keys to this classification scheme are specifically defined points of measurement and use of a defined anatomic landmark as a fixed point of reference. The hymen is the fixed point by which measurements of six vaginal points are referenced. The report discourages the use of imprecise terms such as introitus. Points of measurement within the vaginal canal are defined for the anterior and posterior vaginal wall and vaginal apex. Anteriorly, the two points of reference include a point 3 cm proximal to the external urethral meatus (point Aa) and a point Ba that represents the most distal or dependent portion of

the anterior vaginal wall proximal to Aa (Fig. 25.3). Posteriorly, the points of reference are similar by use of a midline posterior point 3 cm proximal to the hymen (point Ap) and a point Bp that represents the most distal or dependent position of the posterior vaginal wall proximal to point Ap (see Fig. 25.3). The vaginal apex is defined by two points: the most distal edge of the cervix or vaginal cuff scar (point C) and the location of the posterior fornix or pouch of Douglas (point D; see Fig. 25.3). This last point is omitted in patients who have no cervix. Measurements of the genital hiatus, perineal body, and total vaginal length are also included in this classification scheme (see Fig. 25.3). A grid or line diagram may be used to describe normal support as well as support defects of the vaginal cuff and anterior and posterior vaginal walls (Figs. 25.4 and 25.5).

All measurements are made in centimeters and expressed as above (proximal) or below (distal) the hymen and designated negative or positive, respectively. The numbers may then be recorded as a simple line of numbers (tandem profile) or as a three-by-three grid. In addition, the report establishes an ordinal staging system to be used after the quantitative description is completed (Table 25.3).

The committee acknowledges the arbitrary nature of such a staging system but concludes that it

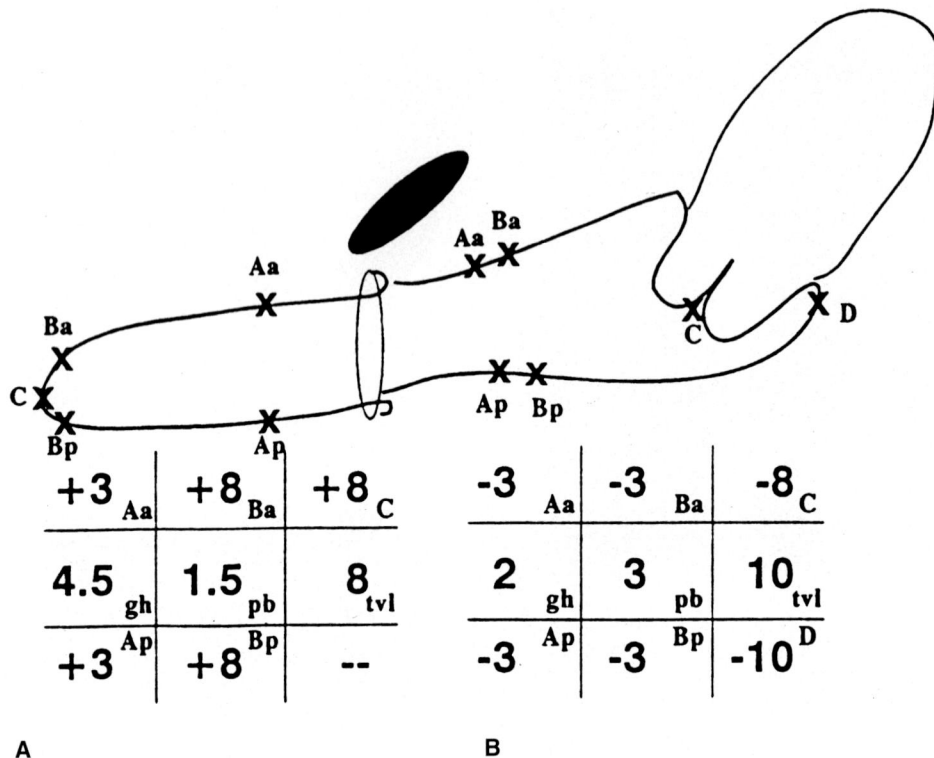

+3 $_{Aa}$	+8 $_{Ba}$	+8 $_C$
4.5 $_{gh}$	1.5 $_{pb}$	8 $_{tvl}$
+3 ^{Ap}	+8 ^{Bp}	--

-3 $_{Aa}$	-3 $_{Ba}$	-8 $_C$
2 $_{gh}$	3 $_{pb}$	10 $_{tvl}$
-3 ^{Ap}	-3 ^{Bp}	-10 ^{D}

A   B

FIGURE 25.4 ● **(A)** Grid and line diagram of complete eversion of vagina. Most distal point of anterior wall (point *Ba*), vaginal cuff scar (point *C*), and most distal point of the posterior wall (point *Bp*) are all at same position (+8), and points *Aa* and *Ap* are maximally distal (both at +3). Because total vaginal length equals maximum protrusion, this is stage IV prolapse. **(B)** Normal support. Points *Aa* and *Ba* and points *Ap* and *Bp* are all −3 because there is no anterior or posterior wall descent. Lowest point of the cervix is 8 cm above hymen (−8) and posterior fornix is 2 cm above this (−10). Vaginal length is 10 cm, and genital hiatus and perineal body measure 2 and 3 cm, respectively. This represents stage 0 support. (From Bump RC, Mattiasson A, Bø K, et al. The standardization of terminology of female pelvic organ prolapse and pelvic floor dysfunction. *Am J Obstet Gynecol* 1996;175:10–17, with permission.)

is necessary as staging allows for description and comparison of populations of patients, correlation of symptoms with severity of prolapse, and assessment of treatment outcomes. Unfortunately, the staging system does not predict women who will be symptomatic. For example, a retrospective cross-sectional study assessing prolapse in 905 women using the POPQ examination found no discrete stage that discriminated between symptomatic and nonsymptomatic prolapse (10).

The subcommittee's efforts in creating this classification scheme and incorporating objective criteria for the description of pelvic organ prolapse were a first step toward establishing a standard, reliable, and validated description of pelvic anatomy and function. They acknowledged the need for studies designed to evaluate and validate the descriptions and definitions they propose. In 1996,

Hall et al evaluated the interobserver and intraobserver reliability of the POPQ system (11). The reproducibilities of the nine site-specific measurements and the summary stage and substage were evaluated. There was substantial and highly significant correlation between measurements for both interobserver and intraobserver examinations. Although it took new POPQ examiners an average of 1.7 minutes longer than experienced POPQ examiners to complete the examination, the reliability did not vary between the groups.

Reports suggest that the degree of prolapse observed varies by patient position, with an increase in prolapse with the patient in a sitting "45% upright" position in a birthing chair as compared with the patient in a dorsal lithotomy position (11–13). This difference did not seem to be related to other patient characteristics, including age, race, parity,

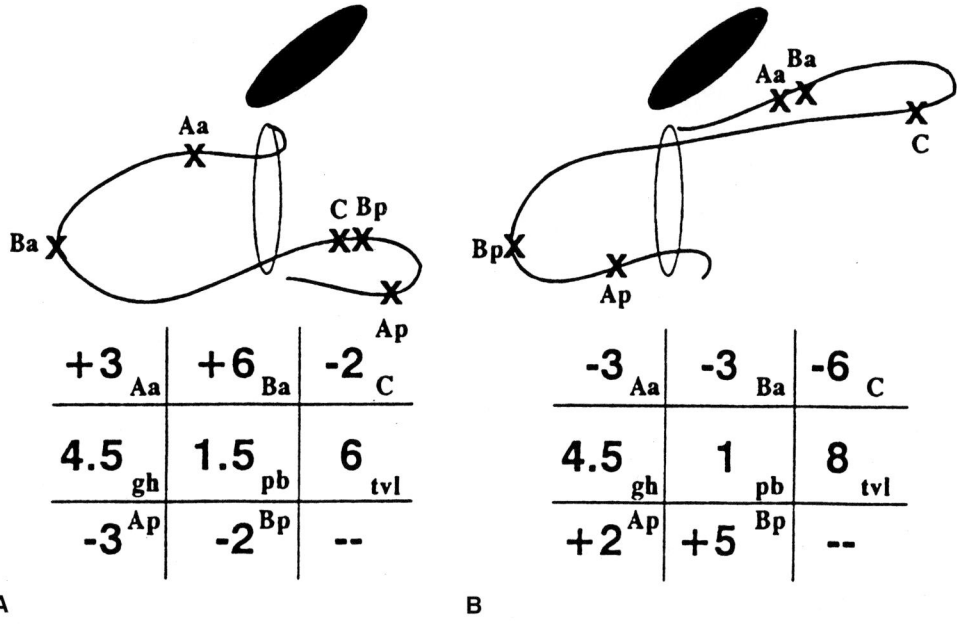

FIGURE 25.5 ● **(A)** Grid and line diagram of predominant anterior support defect. Leading point of prolapse is upper anterior vaginal wall, point *Ba* (+6). There is significant elongation of bulging anterior wall. Point *Aa* is maximally distal (+3), and vaginal cuff scar is 2 cm above hymen (*C* = −2). Cuff scar has undergone 4 cm of descent because it would be at −6 (total vaginal length) if it were perfectly supported. In this example, total vaginal length is not maximum depth of vagina with elongated anterior vaginal wall maximally reduced but rather depth of vagina at cuff, with point C reduced to its normal full extent, as specified in text. This represents state III *Ba* prolapse. **(B)** Predominant posterior support defect. Leading point of prolapse is upper posterior vaginal wall, point *Bp* (+5). Point *Ap* is 2 cm distal to hymen (+2), and vaginal cuff scar is 6 cm above hymen (−6). Cuff has undergone only 2 cm of descent distal to hymen (+2), and vaginal cuff scar is 6 cm above hymen (−6). Cuff has undergone only 2 cm of descent because it would be at −8 (total vaginal length) if it were perfectly supported. This represents stage III *Bp* prolapse. (From Bump RC, Mattiasson A, Bø K, et al. The standardization of terminology of female pelvic organ prolapse and pelvic floor dysfunction. *Am J Obstet Gynecol* 1996;175:10–17, with permission.)

weight, or the prolapse stage or genital hiatus measurement in the lithotomy position (13). POPQ measurements have also been compared by Swift and Herring in the standing and dorsal lithotomy positions (14). A high degree of correlation of measurements in the two positions was found, and it has been postulated that this was related to differences in pelvic tilt produced by standing and dorsal lithotomy positions as compared with a sitting position. As with the McRoberts maneuver, maximum hip flexion is likely to occur in the birthing chair, which results in opening of the pelvic outlet (13,14).

The immediate reaction to the POPQ system suggested that it was too complicated, confusing, and difficult to learn (15,16). An informal questionnaire distributed to a select group of the ICS showed that only 20% of the respondents were using the system, with the most commonly re-

ported reason being that the POPQ was "too difficult to learn and teach" (16). Consequently, alternative classification methods are being explored. The International Federation of Gynecologists and Obstetricians (FIGO) has expressed interest in developing a system that allows for description of common physical examination findings in women with POP, demonstrates good reproducibility, and can be easily learned by health care providers worldwide (16). The Standardization of Terminology Committee of the International Urogynecology Association is preparing an opinion regarding the current classification systems and anticipates publication of the system for worldwide adoption.

Despite reported concerns regarding the complexity of the POPQ system, Steele et al reported that the POPQ system could be effectively taught to obstetric and gynecology residents and medical

TABLE 25.3

International Continence Society Pelvic Organ Prolapse Ordinal Staging System

Stage 0	Points Aa, Ap, Ba, and Bp are all at ~3 cm and either point C or D is at no more than ~(X2) cm.
Stage I:	The criteria for stage 0 are not met and the leading edge of prolapse is less than ~1 cm.
Stage II:	Leading edge of prolapse is at least ~1 cm but no more than +1 cm.
Stage III:	Leading edge of prolapse is greater than +1 cm but less than +(X 2) cm.
Stage IV:	Leading edge of prolapse is at least +(X 2) cm.

X, total vaginal length in centimeters in stages 0, III, and IV. Stages I through IV can be subgrouped according to which portion of the lower reproductive tract is the leading edge of the prolapse using the following qualifiers: a, anterior vaginal wall; p, posterior vaginal wall; C, vaginal cuff; Cx, cervix; and Aa, Ba, Ap, Bp, and D for the defined points of measurement (e.g., IV-Cx, II-a, or III-Bp).

From Bump RC, Mattiasson A, Bø K, et al. The standardization of terminology of female pelvic organ prolapse and pelvic floor dysfunction. *Am J Obstet Gynecol* 1996;175:10–17, with permission.

students (17). Likewise, we have found that it can be readily taught to interested medical students, residents, and practicing gynecologists. It has become a useful clinical and research tool to allow for the longitudinal study of patient populations and evaluation of nonsurgical and surgical treatment outcomes.

The ICS subcommittee report on the POPQ also addressed the use of ancillary techniques for describing pelvic organ prolapse (4). It suggested that these ancillary techniques may be used to characterize further the observed prolapse; however, careful description by investigators of the technique and the methods used is essential. Ancillary techniques may include digital rectal and vaginal examination, cotton swab testing for mobility of the urethral axis, and endoscopic or imaging studies.

Evaluation of Connective Tissue Support

When encountering a visible bulge or prolapse of some portion of the vaginal wall, the quantitative description of the bulges provided by the POPQ system aids in understanding the degree of compromise to the support tissues but does not identify the underlying support defects. The nature of the support defects remains controversial. Richardson popularized the concept that POP resulted from tears in the endopelvic fascial envelope of the vagina (18). Subsequent surgical studies demonstrated discrete tears in patients with anterior vaginal prolapse and posterior vaginal prolapse (19,20), while a histological study failed to show a defect in the endopelvic fascia of three patients with enterocele (21). To some extent this contro-

versy revolves around nomenclature, as opponents of the theory correctly point out that the fibromuscular layer of the vaginal walls has smooth muscle and fibroblasts that are not typically found in "fascial" tissues. Interestingly, there are numerous studies demonstrating the efficacy of surgical procedures that are limited to the dissection and repair of isolated "fascial tears" (22–25).

The network of visceral supporting fascia within the female pelvis is continuous and interdependent from the pelvic brim to the level of the ischial spines, along the muscular pelvic sidewalls, to the pubic symphysis and perineum.

Although the current gynecologic surgical literature speaks of isolated, site-specific defects, in reality in the unoperated patient, the support defects are rarely isolated to one specific support area. The general rule of vaginal support anatomy is that support defects are not due to one visceral fascial break in one specific area but are caused by two or more fascial breaks in the same support area as well in two or more other vaginal support areas. In addition, the quantity and quality of the pelvic support connective tissues themselves are highly variable from patient to patient and are dependent on many constituent factors. Factors that affect the visceral endopelvic support tissues include mechanical, genetic, hormonal, nutritional, and environmental factors, along with the functional state of the surrounding pelvic muscular support and the somatic and visceral innervation of these tissues.

Diagnosing defects in the fibromuscular support system and judging the overall quality of the tissues demand a careful, intelligent examination, as the findings can be subtle. This art is facilitated by a full appreciation of the mobility and feel of the healthy tissues in the nonpregnant, normal nulliparous young patient. In addition, the examiner must appreciate the importance of the appearance of the vaginal epithelium itself and the presence and quality of the rugae. Vaginal rugae result from two factors. The first is the irregular surface of the vaginal epithelium owing to variations in its thickness. The second, and more important in diagnosing vaginal support defects, is the pleated rugosity of the vaginal epithelium as a result of the intact, underlying visceral connective tissue. Healthy, functional visceral fascia contains contractile smooth muscle and elastin fibers, both of which are physiologically active. These findings are best demonstrated in the well-estrogenized vagina. In the very elderly patient with marked vaginal atrophy, the prominent vaginal rugae are flattened and subtle but can still be seen by the careful observer (26).

Vaginal Apex

In a woman with normal vaginal support, when a bivalved speculum is placed into the vagina, the examiner can view the cervix, which is stabilized by the attachments of the pericervical ring to the cardinal ligament–uterosacral ligament complexes bilaterally. The cervix lies in the upper aspect of the anterior vaginal wall at the level of the ischial spines, approximately 4.5 cm medial to the ischial spine and 1 cm anterior and superior (27). It is attached to the sacrum by the uterosacral ligaments. These ligaments permit minimal downward motion limited to the upper third of the vagina. With gentle traction on the cervix, the physician can palpate the thick, firm uterosacral ligaments as they attach to the posterolateral aspects of the pericervical ring of visceral fascia. This relationship is sometimes better appreciated during a rectal examination. The attachments of the cardinal ligaments to the pericervical ring also limit the lateral motion of the cervix. The cardinal ligaments attach to the upper portion of the vagina bilaterally to help secure the lateral fornices seen within the vagina. The anterior fornix is formed by the fusion of the pubocervical fascia onto the pericervical ring anteriorly. The posterior fornix is bounded by the uterosacral ligaments inserting into the posterolateral aspects of the pericervical ring and by the rectovaginal fascia.

In patients with uterine prolapse or vaginal cuff prolapse, the examination should begin with an assessment of the integrity of the cardinal and uterosacral ligaments. The uterosacral ligament usually detaches or elongates at the pericervical ring near the level of the ischial spines. When the

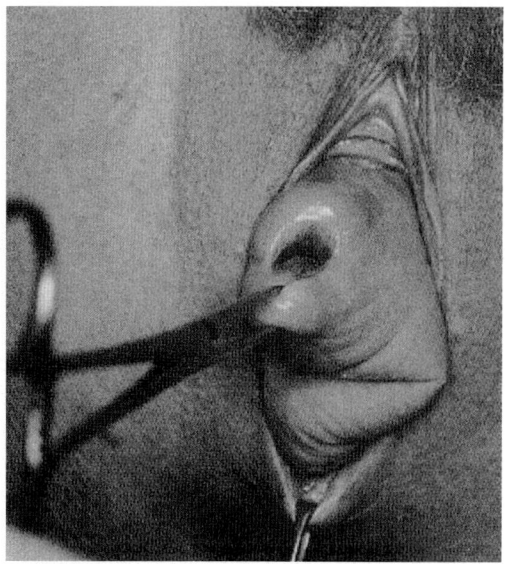

FIGURE 25.6 ● Uterine prolapse with bulging of the posterior and lateral vaginal walls and a loose introitus. (From Baggish MS, Karram MM. *Atlas of pelvic anatomy and gynecologic surgery.* Singapore: WB Saunders, 2001:402, with permission.)

patient bears down during a Valsalva maneuver, the lateral fornices of the vagina bulge down due to the detachment from the cardinal ligament sheaths. The posterior fornix also bulges significantly because of the separation of the rectovaginal fascia from the uterosacral ligaments. Because of these detachments from the cardinal

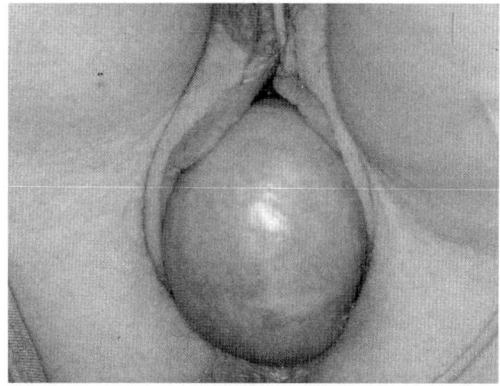

FIGURE 25.7 ● Posthysterectomy vaginal vault prolapse. This patient has lost the support of the cardinal and uterosacral ligaments and also has an apical enterocele due to discontinuity between the superior pubocervical fascia and rectovaginal fascia. Note the loss of rugation in the center of the bulge and the superior edges of the pubocervical and rectovaginal fascia beneath the vaginal epithelium.

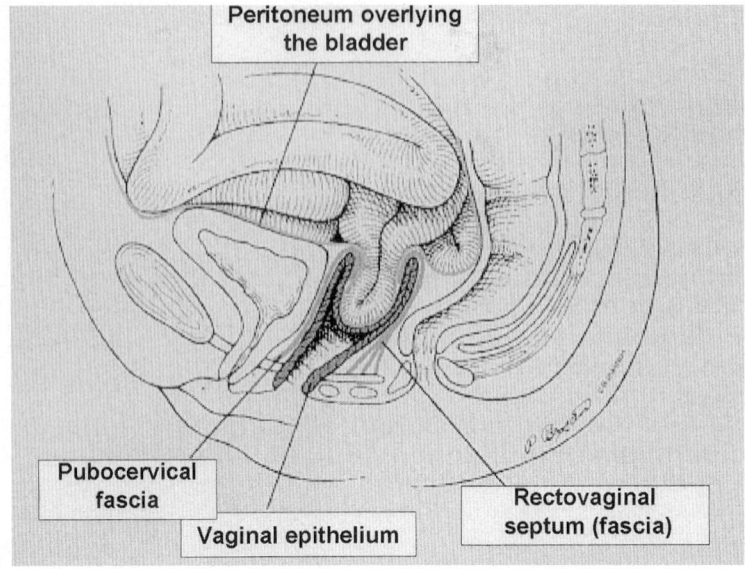

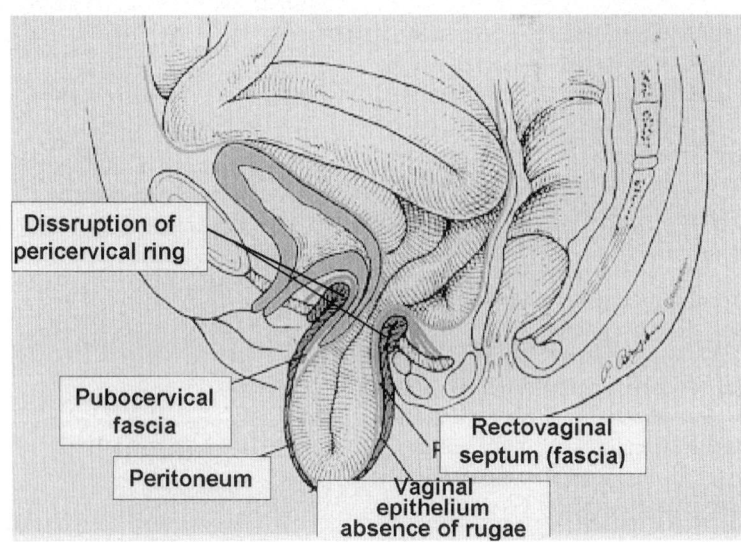

FIGURE 25.8   ●   **(A)** Beginning of apical enterocele with some separation of pubocervical and recto-vaginal fascia. **(B)** Further separation of pubocervical and rectovaginal fascia and descent of vaginal vault with accompanying cystocele and rectocele.

ligament–uterosacral ligament complexes, the cervix demonstrates wide lateral mobility (Fig. 25.6). Because cervical elongation has been observed with uterine prolapse, it is wise to estimate the length of the cervix from the external cervical os to the internal cervical os.

Prolapse of the vaginal cuff after hysterectomy frequently includes an apical enterocele, in which the superior margins of the pubocervical fascia and rectovaginal fascia are separated due to disruption

of the pericervical ring (Fig. 25.7). The underlying support feels very thin as a result of the stretching of the peritoneum, which is in direct contact with the vaginal epithelium. The overlying vaginal epithelium is stretched and very smooth, without rugae (Fig. 25.8). The downward descent of the disrupted pericervical ring is frequently associated with a lateral detachment of the pubocervical fascia and the rectovaginal fascia from the fascial white lines bilaterally.

Anterior Vaginal Wall

In a woman with normal vaginal support, the anterior vaginal wall is covered by thickened epithelium with a thickened underlying fibromuscular coat, the pubocervical fascia. The transverse rugations in the anterior vaginal wall demonstrate the well-estrogenized vaginal epithelium, but more importantly, they demonstrate the thick, intact, and healthy nature of the underlying pubocervical fascia (see Fig. 25.1). Using a Sims retractor to depress the posterior vaginal wall, the observer should be able to visualize the anterolateral sulci going from the midvagina back toward the ischial spines. Each of these anterolateral sulci represents the attachment of the pubocervical fascia along each pelvic sidewall through the fascia endopelvina to the fascial white line (arcus tendineus fasciae pelvis). The urethrovesical junction is supported by the hammock of pubocervical fascia that attaches laterally to each fascial white line. Gentle traction along the side of the urethra reveals limited lateral mobility and the pubocervical fascia prevents the fingers from reaching the superior pubic ramus because of the attachments to the fascial white lines.

Bulging of the anterior vaginal wall into the vagina beyond its normal limits, generally beyond

the midportion of the vagina, is frequently referred to as a cystocele. The term cystocele implies a defect concerning the bladder itself, although it actually results from a defect in the supporting pubocervical fascia. Consequently, the preferred terminology is anterior vaginal prolapse (28). Defects within the pubocervical fascial support system that cause anterior vaginal wall prolapse are found in the following areas: the lateral attachments of the pubocervical fascia to the fascial white lines; centrally underneath the bladder itself; transversely as the pubocervical fascia inserts into the pericervical ring and the uterosacral ligaments; and very rarely, distally, where the urethra detaches from the perineal membrane and the overlying symphysis pubis (19) (Fig. 25.9).

The detachment of the pubocervical fascia from the lateral attachments to the fascial white lines is commonly called a paravaginal defect. The paravaginal defect results from a partial or complete tearing of the fascia endopelvina and attached pubocervical fascia from one or both fascial white lines. The detachment of the pubocervical fascia may be from the fascial white line itself, with the fascial white line remaining on the levator ani muscle; or there may be a complete detachment of the pubocervical fascia and the white line from the parietal fascia of the levator ani (29). With a Sims

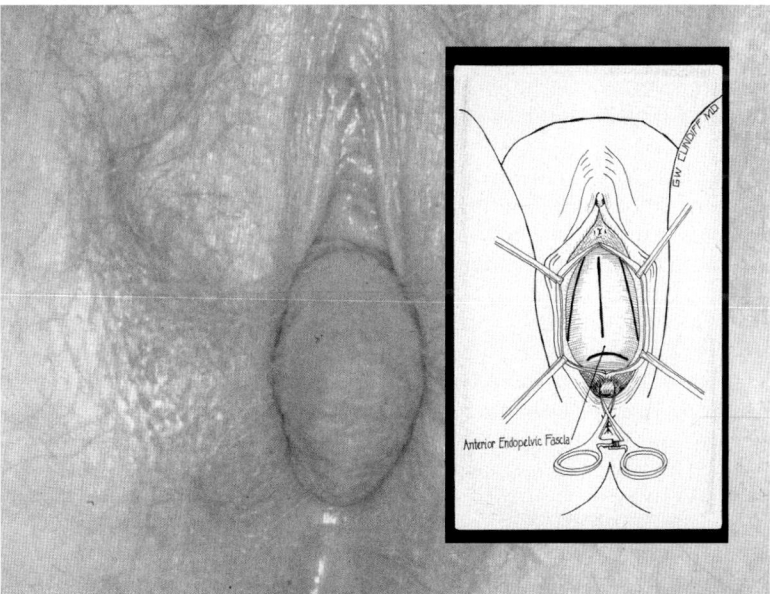

FIGURE 25.9 ● Anterior vaginal wall prolapse can occur due to tears in different parts of the pubocervical fascia. The *inset* shows the pubocervical fascia, with the epithelium dissected away. The *solid lines* indicate the common areas of defects in the pubocervical fascial support. These include lateral detachments from the arcus tendineus fascia pelvis, midline longitudinal tears, and transverse defects superiorly. (With permission from Geoffrey Cundiff, MD.)

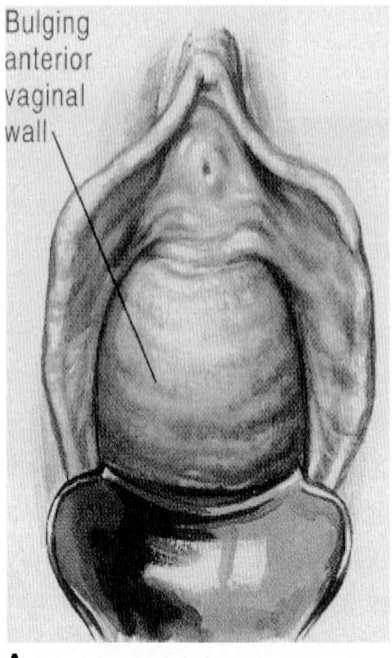 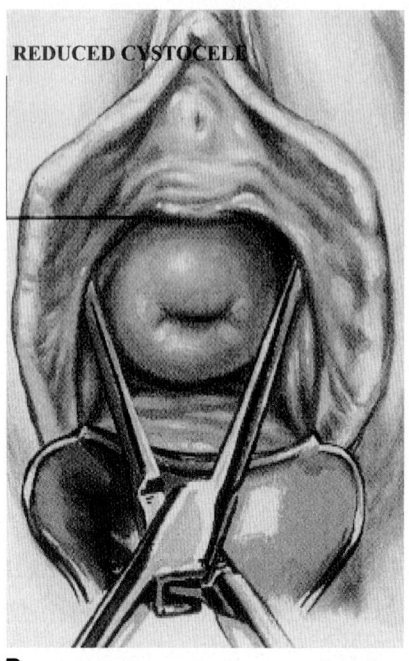

A   **B**

FIGURE 25.10 ● **(A)** Bulging anterior vaginal wall defect. **(B)** Paravaginal defect cystocele reduced with ring forceps placed laterally to elevate the pubocervical fascial detachment toward the white line. (From Retzky SS, Rogers RM. *Urinary incontinence in women.* Summit, NJ: Clinical Symposia Ciba-Geigy Corp, 1995;47(3):22, adapted from Plate 11. Copyright © 1995. ICON Learning Systems, LLC, a subsidiary of MediMedia USA Inc. Reprinted with permission from ICON Learning Systems, LLC, illustrated by John A. Craig, M.D. All rights reserved.)

retractor or the lower blade of a Graves speculum depressing the posterior vaginal wall, a paravaginal defect is diagnosed by observing the significant loss of one or both anterolateral sulci as the patient bears down (Fig. 25.10A). With a paravaginal defect in the well-estrogenized patient, excellent vaginal rugae are observable in the midline. A paravaginal defect is further substantiated by supporting the anterolateral regions of the vagina up against each fascial white line, traveling from the pubic arch back toward the ischial spines. The examiner may use a ring forceps or a Baden vaginal defect analyzer. This instrument can also be used to support the vaginal apex against each ischial spine, thus approximating the reattachment of the pericervical ring to each uterosacral ligament. If the temporary instrument support during straining by the patient eliminates the bulge of the anterior vaginal wall, then it suggests that this is the site of the support defect (see Fig. 25.10B). In a comparison of clinical findings to surgical findings, the sensitivity of a clinical assessment of paravaginal defect was high (92%), but the specificity was not (53%). In this study the prevalence of par-

avaginal defects at surgery was 47% on the right and 41% on the left (19).

The transverse tear, which may be accompanied by some degree of a paravaginal defect, can be caused by either a transverse separation of the pubocervical fascia from the anterior margin of the pericervical ring (see Fig. 25.9) or a separation of the pericervical ring with intact pubocervical fascia from the uterosacral ligaments. In the first case, a straining patient causes a distinct bulging out of the anterior vaginal fornix and a loss of thickness and strength in the underlying visceral fascia in this area. In the second case, a detachment of each uterosacral ligament to the pericervical ring results in a significant cervical descensus or vaginal vault descensus, with no thickness of uterosacral ligaments being palpated near the pericervical ring. In the transverse defect where there is a bulging out of the anterior fornix, the bulge normally has very poor rugations owing to the loss of the underlying pubocervical fascia.

Central breaks or central defects (see Fig. 25.9) in the pubocervical fascia result in a midvaginal bulge when the lateral sulci and apex of the vagina are supported by an instrument such as ring forceps or Baden vaginal analyzer. Most of these central breaks occur around the bladder neck or urethrovesical junction. The vesical neck is usually hypermobile in all directions.

A distal defect results from the distal urethra detaching from the perineal membrane and thus from the overlying symphysis. These defects are very rare. Such defects demonstrate telescoping of the urethra straight outward with straining. There is little downward motion.

Posterior Vaginal Wall

In a woman with normal posterior vaginal wall support, the vaginal epithelium has transverse rugations reflecting the underlying smooth muscle and elastin. However, the underlying fibromuscular coat, the rectovaginal fascia, is generally thinner than the anterior pubocervical fascia. Rectovaginal examination allows the examiner to appreciate the thickness and the tautness provided by the attachments of this layer. Inspection of the lateral vaginal wall reveals that the anterolateral sulcus travels toward the pubic arch, whereas the posterolateral sulcus courses down toward the perineal body. At the midvaginal area, a separation of the anterolateral sulcus from the posterolateral sulcus can be seen. This constitutes the line of attachment of the rectovaginal fascia to the parietal fascia of the levator ani muscles, the arcus tendineus fasciae rectovaginalis (30).

A bulge in the posterior vaginal wall, commonly known as a rectocele, indicates a loss in the integrity of the rectovaginal septum, also known as the rectovaginal fascia. The preferred terminology

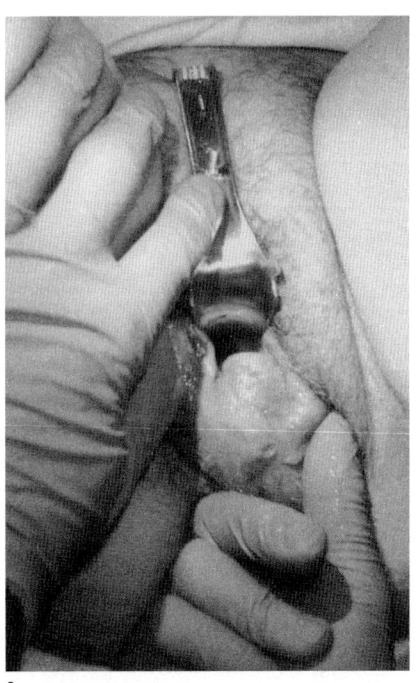

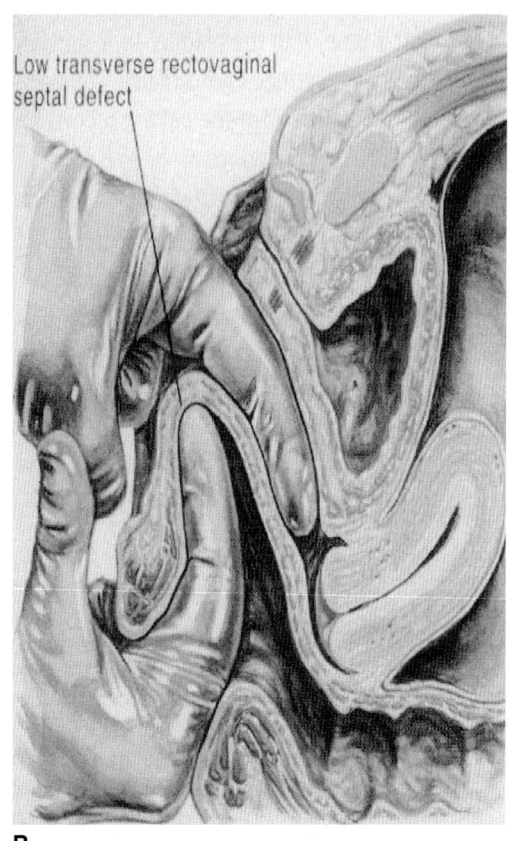

Low transverse rectovaginal septal defect

A   **B**

FIGURE 25.11 ● **(A)** Low rectocele defect demonstrated by rectal examination with retraction of the anterior vaginal wall in order to view the full length of the posterior vagina. **(B)** Demonstration of examination for low defect type of rectocele. (From Retzky SS, Rogers RM. *Urinary incontinence in women.* Summit, NJ: Clinical Symposia Ciba-Geigy Corp, 1995;47(3):23, adapted from Plate 12. Copyright © 1995. ICON Learning Systems, LLC, a subsidiary of MediMedia USA Inc. Reprinted with permission from ICON Learning Systems, LLC, illustrated by John A. Craig, M.D. All rights reserved.)

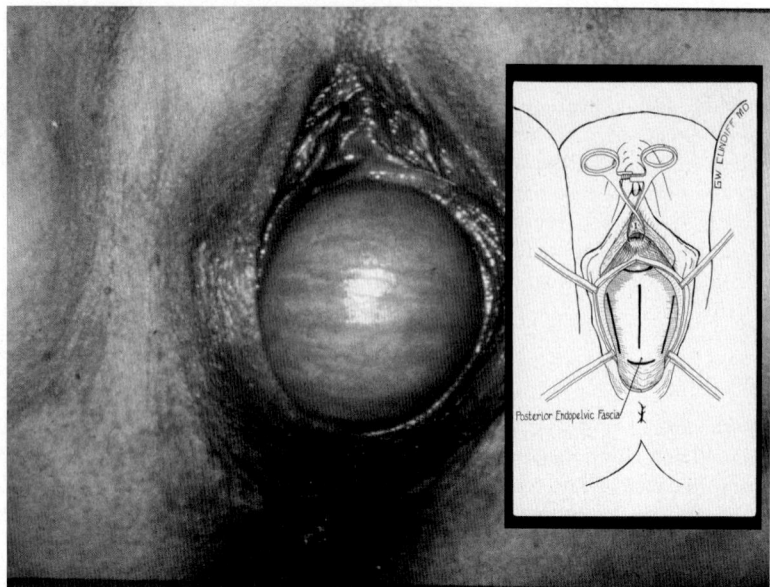

FIGURE 25.12 ● Posterior vaginal wall prolapse can occur due to tears in different parts of the rectovaginal fascia. The *inset* shows the rectovaginal fascia, with the epithelium dissected away. The *solid lines* indicate the common areas of defects in the rectovaginal fascial support. These include lateral detachments from the arcus tendineus fascia rectovaginalis, midline longitudinal tears, and transverse defects superiorly and inferiorly from the perineal body. (With permission from Geoffrey Cundiff, MD.)

is posterior vaginal prolapse (28). During a rectovaginal examination, an appreciation of the normal feel and attachments of the rectovaginal fascia allows the examiner to appreciate some of the breaks and defects in the rectovaginal fascial support system (Fig. 25.11). The breaks of the rectovaginal fascia most commonly are away from the perineal body and away from the lateral attachments to the pubococcygeus muscles of the levator hiatus, along the arcus tendineus fasciae rectovaginalis (31) (Fig. 25.12). These defects are manifested as a low rectocele or, more clinically, as a low posterior vaginal wall prolapse (see Fig. 25.11).

In the upper third of the vagina, the peritoneum covers the surface of the rectovaginal fascia, whereas in the middle third of the vagina, the rectovaginal fascia is in contact with and loosely attached just underneath the posterior vaginal wall. Posterior vaginal prolapse results from a tearing of the rectovaginal fascia that allows the rectal muscularis to push upward against the vaginal epithelium with no intervening visceral fascia. In a high rectocele (prolapse of the upper posterior wall), the break in the rectovaginal fascia allows the peri-

toneum to be pushed into contact with the vaginal epithelium of the upper third of the vagina with no intervening visceral fascia. The vaginal epithelium is smooth without rugae because there is no intervening visceral fascia (Fig. 25.13). Careful inspection in some patients with enteroceles will reveal peristaltic movements beneath the vaginal epithelium (29).

High rectoceles are associated with posterior and apical enteroceles (Fig. 25.14).These are manifested by a bulging down or prolapse of the cul-de-sac and posterolateral walls of the vagina toward the middle third of the vagina or lower. The high rectocele is a result of the separation of the rectovaginal fascia from each uterosacral ligament and from its posterior insertion onto the pericervical ring. In addition, the rectovaginal fascia has torn away from the fascial white lines near the ischial spines.

In a comparison of clinical findings to surgical findings, clinical examination findings concurred with surgical findings in 60%. The majority of patients had multiple defects, with the most common combination being left lateral and inferior (20).

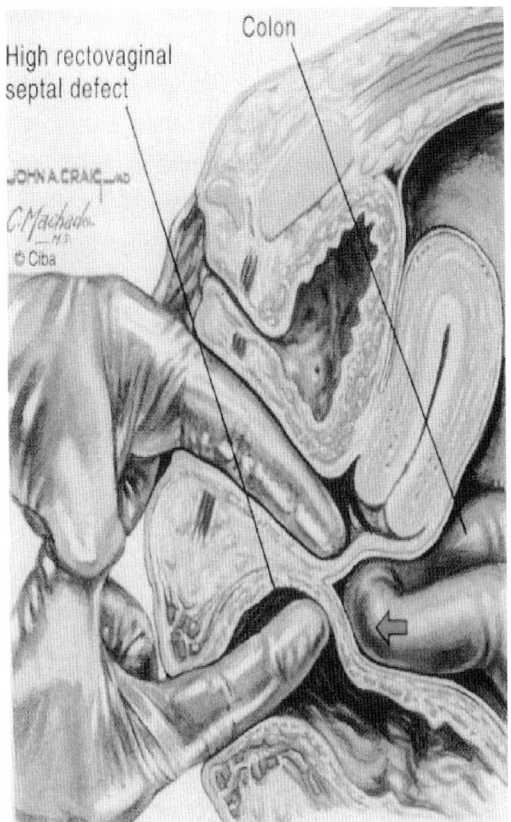

High rectovaginal septal defect

Colon

JOHN A.CRAIG—MD

C.Machado
© Ciba

FIGURE 25.13 ● Demonstration of high rectocele defect. (From Retzky SS, Rogers RM. *Urinary incontinence in women.* Summit, NJ: Clinical Symposia Ciba-Geigy Corp, 1995;47(3):23, adapted from Plate 12. Copyright © 1995. ICON Learning Systems, LLC, a subsidiary of MediMedia USA Inc. Reprinted with permission from ICON Learning Systems, LLC, illustrated by John A. Craig, M.D. All rights reserved.)

EVALUATION OF THE PERINEUM

Normally, the perineum should be located at the level of the ischial tuberosities, or within 2 cm of this landmark. A perineum below this level, either at rest or with straining, represents perineal descent. Subjective findings of perineal descent include widening of the genital hiatus and perineal body, as well as flattening of the intergluteal sulcus (Fig. 25.15). Women with perineal descent also tend to have less severe POP based on the POPQ staging system, since it measures descent from the hymenal ring, which is not a fixed point in perineal descent. One of the unique aspects of the POPQ system is the assessment of the perineum, including measurement of the length of the genital hiatus and perineal body with and without straining. An increase in these values with straining suggests perineal descent. The degree of perineal descent can also be objectively measured with a thin ruler placed in the posterior introitus at the level of the ischial tuberosities. Descent is measured as the distance the perineal body moves when the patient strains, although pelvic floor fluoroscopy is the gold standard for measuring perineal descent. We usually reserve fluoroscopy for patients with symptoms of severe defecatory dysfunction and evidence of perineal descent on pelvic examination.

Rectovaginal examination in a patient with normal support allows the examiner to appreciate the limits on downward (inferior) movement of the perineal body. The perineal body is thickened and broad between the anus and vaginal introitus. As the finger moves through the anal canal toward the rectum, the examiner should appreciate the pyramidal shape of the perineal body as the examining fingers palpate the close approximation of the rectum with the middle and upper portions of the vagina. The apex of the perineal body is found at the level of the lower third and middle third of the vagina. Because of the attachment of the rectovaginal fascia to the apex of the perineal body and then to the uterosacral ligaments at the level of the ischial spines, the downward movement of the perineal body should not be more than about 1 cm. The perineum is normally concave owing to the attachment of the rectovaginal fascia from above. In reality, the perineal body is suspended from the sacrum by the rectovaginal fascia and the uterosacral ligaments.

Normally, the perineum is concave because the intact perineal body is attached to the sacrum by the uterosacral ligaments and rectovaginal fascia. Any significant break along this continuity results in an outward bulging of the perineal body as well as its descent far below its normal position. In addition, when a straightedge is placed between the two ischial tuberosities, the anus should lie along that line but pulled 1 to 2 cm above it or superiorly toward the promontory of the sacrum. The anus is fused with the perineal body. Therefore, any descent of the perineal body, as described previously, allows the anus to descend and be deflected outward and down toward the coccyx. This results in abnormal angulation of the anal canal as indicated by a Q-tip placed in the canal. During a rectal examination, the lateral attachments, the posterior attachment, the uterosacral ligaments, and the lower attachments to the perineal body can be felt.

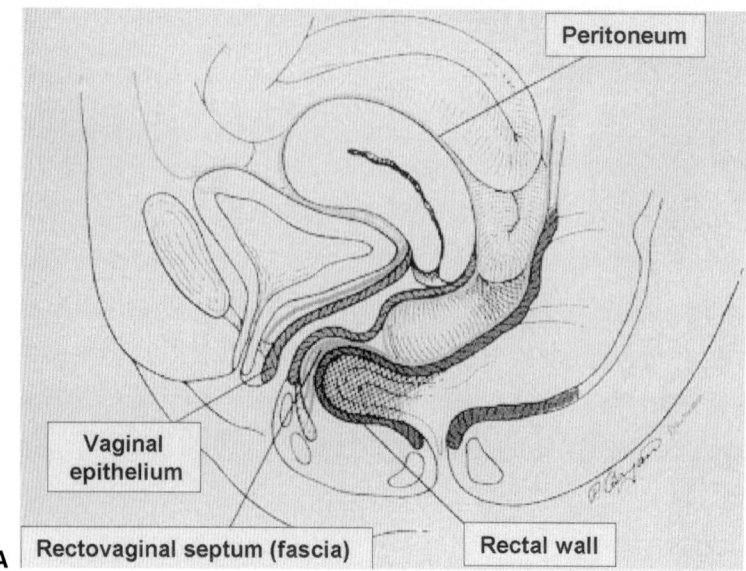

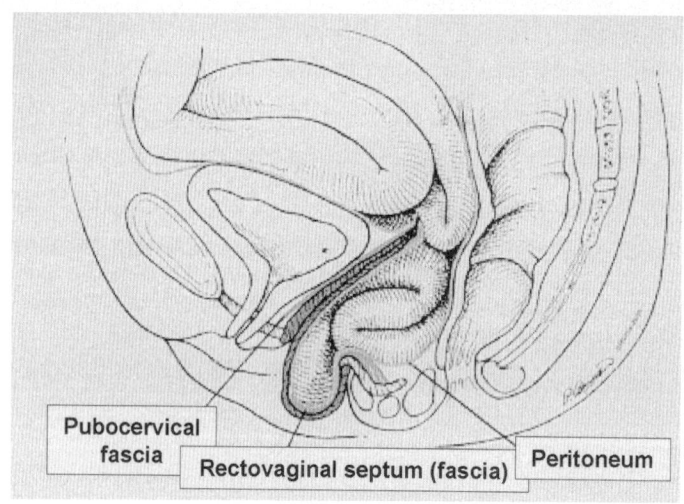

FIGURE 25.14 ● Posterior enteroceles. **(A)** The uterus is preserved, but there is a defect in the low rectovaginal fascia. **(B)** The uterus has been removed and there is good fusion of pubocervical and recto-vaginal fascia at the apex of the vagina, but there is a low defect in the rectovaginal fascia leading to both rectocele and enterocele. (From Richardson AC. The anatomic defects in rectocele and enterocele. *J Pelvic Surg* 1995;1(4):219, with permission.)

In a perineal rectocele, the rectal muscularis is in direct contact with the perineal skin, with no intervening fascia (Fig. 25.16). The underlying defect is a complete disruption of the integrity of the perineal body itself. Obviously, there has been a complete disruption of the fibrous connective tissue as well as the superficial transverse perinei muscles, the bulbocavernosus muscles in the midline, and the contributing levator ani muscles.

Physically, there is a wide area of skin between the vaginal opening and the anus. Bimanual examination of the perineum reveals the presence of only skin and rectal muscularis. With a Valsalva maneuver, the perineum demonstrates a significant bulge. The skin is stretched and smooth. Anal examination reveals a loss of the normal funneling of the anus and a marked widening above the anal sphincter in the rectum.

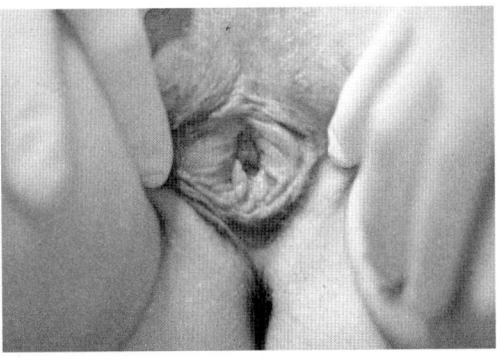 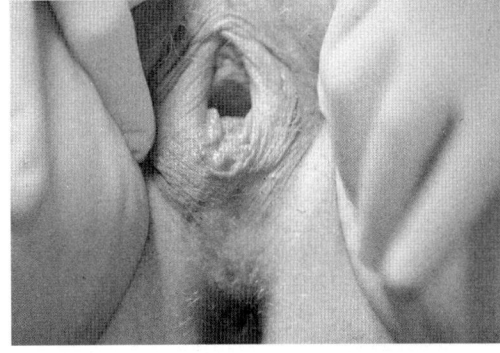

A   **B**

FIGURE 25.15 ● Perineal descent. Perineum of a patient with perineal descent at rest **(A)** and with straining **(B)**. With straining there is widening of the genital hiatus, flattening of the intergluteal sulcus, and descent of the perineal body.

EVALUATION OF MUSCULAR SUPPORT

The bimanual examination investigates the location, size, and tenderness of the bladder, uterus, cervix, and adnexa. The pelvic diaphragm should be assessed for integrity of the muscle body and insertion, as well as the strength, duration, and anterior lift of the contraction. Several standardized systems have been described to assess muscle strength objectively, but none are universally accepted (32). The integrity of the pelvic diaphragm muscles can be evaluated by observation and palpation of these structures during voluntary contraction, although clinical examination is less sensitive in demonstrating separations of the pubococcygeus muscles from the pubic rami than magnetic resonance imaging (33). The firm muscular sling of the puborectalis should be readily palpable posteriorly as it creates a 90-degree angle between the anal and rectal canals. Voluntary contraction of this muscle pulls the examining finger anteriorly towards of the muscle's insertion on the pubic rami. Neuropathy affecting the puborectalis can likewise be recognized if the anorectal angle is obtuse and if there is a palpable weakness with voluntary contraction.

As previously mentioned, a rectovaginal examination provides useful information regarding the integrity of the rectovaginal septum, and can demonstrate laxity in the support of the perineal body. The rectovaginal examination also helps in the diagnosis of a high enterocele, which can be felt filling the rectovaginal septum between the vaginal and rectal fingers during patient straining. The presence of fecal material in the anal canal may suggest fecal impaction or neuromuscular weakness of the anal continence mechanism.

SUMMARY

In evaluating POP, the first task is to determine which of the patient's symptoms can be attributed to the anatomical defects. This requires a firm understanding of the differential diagnosis of pelvic floor symptoms and a meticulous assessment for alternative etiologies. The clinical evaluation focuses on eliciting the patient's complaints, defining and quantifying the location and severity of support defects, and establishing a relationship between the symptoms and the support defects, through elimination of other etiologies of pelvic floor symptomatology. Objective evaluation of pelvic support includes staging of the anatomical defects, an assessment of the epithelial quality, and an assessment of the integrity of the connective tissue support, muscular support, and perineal support.

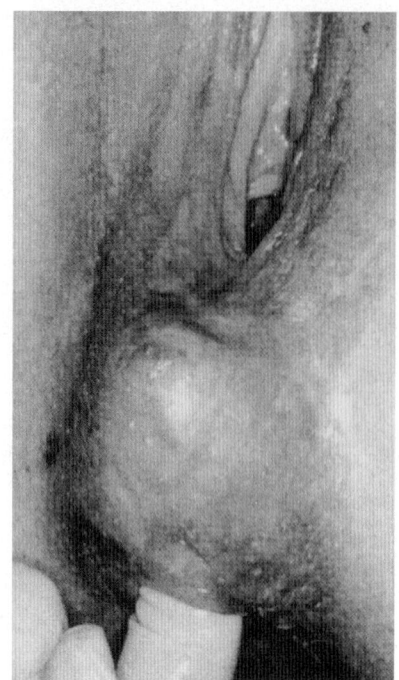

A

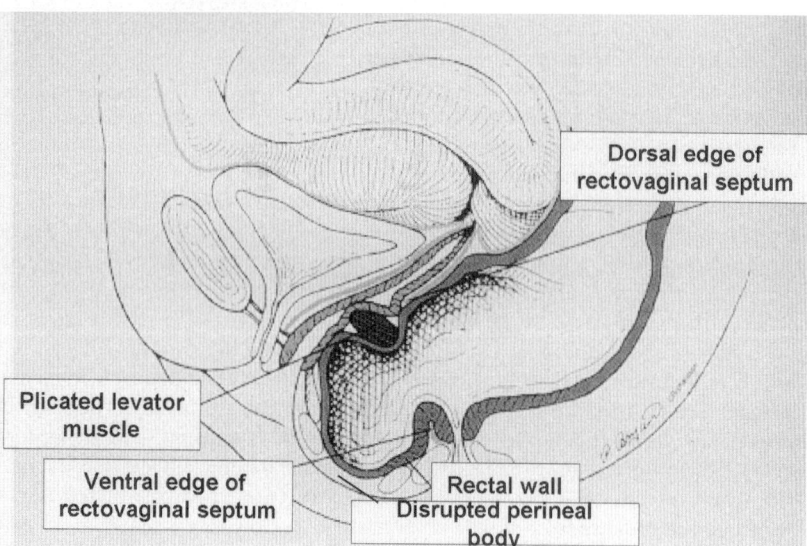

B

FIGURE 25.16 ● Perineal rectocele. **(A)** Defect demonstrated by digital rectal examination. **(B)** The break in the rectovaginal fascia brings rectal wall in contact with perineal skin. (From Richardson AC. The anatomic defects in rectocele and enterocele. *J Pelvic Surg* 1995;1(4):218, with permission.)

REFERENCES

1. Miller NF. End-results from correction of cystocele by the simple fascia pleating method. *Surg Gynecol Obstet* 1928;46:403–410.
2. Friedman EA, Little WA. The conflict in nomenclature for descensus uteri. *Am J Obstet Gynecol* 1961;81: 817–820.
3. Beecham CT. Classification of vaginal relaxation. *Am J Obstet Gynecol* 1980;136:957–958.
4. Baden W, Walker T. *Surgical repair of vaginal defects.* Philadelphia: JB Lippincott, 1992.
5. Bump RC, Bo K, Brubaker LP, et al. The standardization of terminology of female pelvic organ prolapse and pelvic floor dysfunction. *Am J Obstet Gynecol* 1996; 175(1):10–17.
6. Ellerkmann RM, Cundiff GW, Melick CF, et al. Correlation of symptoms with location and severity of pelvic organ prolapse. *Am J Obstet Gynecol* 2001;185: 1332–1338.
7. Kahn MA, Breitkopf CR, Valley MT, et al. Pelvic Organ Support Study (POSST) and bowel symptoms: straining at stool is associated with perineal and anterior vaginal descent in a general gynecologic population. *Am J Obstet Gynecol* 2005;192(5):1516–1522.
8. Weber AM, Walters MD, Ballard LA, et al. Posterior vaginal prolapse and bowel function. *Obstet Gynecol* 1998;179(6)1:1446–1449.
9. Barber MD, Kuchibhatla MN, Pieper CF, et al. Psychometric evaluation of 2 comprehensive condition-specific quality of life instruments for women with pelvic floor disorders. *Am J Obstet Gynecol* 2001;185(6): 1388–1395.
10. Ghetti C, Gregory WT, Edwards SR, et al. Pelvic organ descent and symptoms of pelvic floor disorders. *Am J Obstet Gynecol* 2005;193(1):53–57.
11. Hall AF, Theofrastous JP, Cundiff GW, et al. Interobserver and intraobserver reliability of the proposed International Continence Society, Society of Gynecologic Surgeons, and American Urogynecologic Society pelvic organ prolapse classification system. *Am J Obstet Gynecol* 1996;175:1467–1471.
12. Montella JM, Cater JR. Comparison of measurement obtained in supine and sitting position in the evaluation of pelvic organ prolapse [abstract]. *Int Urogynecol J* 1995;6:304.
13. Barber MD, Lambers AR, Visco AG, et al. Effect of patient position on clinical evaluation of pelvic organ prolapse. *Obstet Gynecol* 2000;96:18–22.
14. Swift SE, Herring M. Comparison of pelvic organ prolapse in the dorsal lithotomy compared with the standing position. *Obstet Gynecol* 1998;91:961–964.
15. Scotti RJ, Flora R, Greston WM, et al. Characterizing and reporting pelvic floor defects: the revised New York classification system. *Int Urogynecol J* 2000;11: 48–60.
16. Swift S, Freeman R, Petri E, et al. Proposal for a worldwide, user-friendly classification system for pelvic organ prolapse [abstract]. 26th annual meeting of the International Urogynecologic Association, Melbourne, Australia, December 5–7, 2001.
17. Steele A, Mallipeddi P, Welgoss J, et al. Teaching the pelvic organ prolapse quantitation system. *Am J Obstet Gynecol* 1998;179:1458–1464.
18. Richardson AC. Female pelvic floor support defects. *Int Urogynecol J Pelvic Floor Dysfunct* 1996;7(5):241.
19. Barber MD, Cundiff GW, Weidner AC, et al. Accuracy of clinical assessment of paravaginal defects in women with anterior vaginal wall prolapse. *Am J Obstet Gynecol* 1999;181:87–90.
20. Burrows LJ, Sewell C, Leffler KS, et al. The accuracy of clinical evaluation of posterior vaginal wall defects. *Int Urogynecol J Pelvic Floor Dysfunct* 2003;14:160–163.
21. Tulikangas PK, Walters MD, Brainard JA, et al. Enterocele: is there a histologic defect? *Obstet Gynecol* 2001; 98(4):634–637.
22. Shull BL, Benn SJ, Kuehl TJ. Surgical management of prolapse of the anterior vaginal segment: an analysis of support defects, operative morbidity, and anatomic outcome. Am J Obstet Gynecol 1994;171(6):1429–1439.
23. Young SB, Daman JJ, Bony LG. Vaginal paravaginal repair: one-year outcomes. *Am J Obstet Gynecol* 2001; 185:1360–1367.
24. Galvind K, Madsen H. A prospective study of the discrete fascial defect rectocele repair. *Acta Obstet Gynecol Scand* 1000;79:145–147.
25. Porter WE, Steele A, Walsh P, et al. The anatomic and functional outcomes of defect-specific rectocele repairs. *Am J Obstet Gynecol* 1999;181:1353–1359.
26. Richardson AC. Female pelvic floor support defects. *Int Urogynecol J Pelvic Floor Dysfunct* 1996;7(5):241.
27. Gutman RE, Pannu HK, Cundiff GW, et al. Anatomic relationship between the vaginal apex and the bony architecture of the pelvis: a magnetic resonance imaging evaluation. *Am J Obstet Gynecol* 2005;192(5):1544–1548.
28. Weber AM, Abrams P, Brubaker L, et al. The standardization of terminology for researchers in female pelvic floor disorders. *Int Urogyn J* 2001;12:178–186.
29. Richardson AC, Lyon JB, Williams NL. A new look at pelvic relaxation. *Am J Obstet Gynecol* 1976;126(5): 568–573.
30. Leffler KS, Thompson JR, Cundiff GW, et al. Attachment of the rectovaginal septum to the pelvic sidewall. *Am J Obstet Gynecol* 2001;185:41–43.
31. Richardson AC. The rectovaginal septum revisited: its relationship to rectocele and its importance in rectocele repair. *Clin Obstet Gynecol* 1993;36(4):976–983.
32. Brink C, Sampselle CM, Tallie ER, et al. A digital test for pelvic muscle strength in women with urinary incontinence. *Nurs Res* 1994;43:352–356.
33. Kearney R, Miller JM, Delancey JO. Interrater reliability and physical examination of the pubovisceral portion of the levator ani muscle, validity comparisons using MR imaging. *Neurourol Urodyn* 2006;25(1):50–54.

CHAPTER 26

Diagnostic Testing of Disorders of Pelvic Support

Olugbenga A. Adekanmi and Robert M. Freeman

The complex interaction between the integrated pelvic support structures making up the bony pelvis, muscles, and fascia helps to maintain normal positioning and function of the pelvic organs both at rest and during physical activity. Symptoms of female pelvic floor disorders often arise as a result of disruption of the normal interaction between these supporting structures. This chapter examines the current role of diagnostic testing for dysfunction of pelvic floor support.

INTRODUCTION

Management of female pelvic floor disorders usually relies on careful and detailed clinical assessment of the anterior, middle, and posterior compartments as an integrated functional unit. However, diagnostic testing may be necessary in order to assess complex symptoms, to plan surgical intervention, or even to determine the presence of "occult" dysfunction that might give rise to new symptoms following surgical intervention. Investigations available for the assessment of disorders of the pelvic support include imaging techniques for visualization of the supporting structures and their function and urodynamic investigations for assessing function of the "displaced" lower urinary tract.

The imaging techniques currently available for assessment of female pelvic floor support disorders include traditional radiology examinations such as abdominal radiography, colpography, cystography, and proctography. More recent techniques include magnetic resonance imaging (MRI)

and ultrasonography. Traditional conventional techniques involving x-ray imaging, although simple and relatively inexpensive, appear to have limited value in the evaluation of female pelvic floor dysfunction because they offer poor visualization of soft tissues and involve exposure of patients to irradiation. The relatively new imaging techniques of MRI and ultrasound offer more detailed visualization of the soft tissues and provide improved knowledge about the dynamic interaction between the pelvic supporting structures. However, their current role should probably be considered as that of a research tool because of a lack of internationally agreed test methodology, image analysis and interpretation, and more importantly a lack of evidence to show that application of the tests can improve clinical outcomes.

Urodynamic investigations can be useful in the evaluation of lower urinary tract symptoms associated with pelvic support defects and might help to determine or exclude the presence of occult lower urinary tract dysfunction (e.g., incontinence) that can become evident following surgical correction of pelvic organ prolapse.

CONVENTIONAL RADIOLOGY

Plain Abdominal and Pelvic X-Ray

Plain x-ray imaging offers good visualization of the bony pelvis and is valuable in the identification and location of suspected radiopaque foreign bodies. It does not show soft tissue abnormalities and is unable to demonstrate the pelvic support anatomy. For that reason plain x-ray imaging has a very limited role in investigating pelvic support disorders.

Lateral Bead Chain Cystourethrography

Cystourethrography was first applied to the investigation of female urinary disorders in 1928. Subsequently, imaging with a metallic bead chain in the urethra to aid lateral visualization of the bladder neck was included. However, it has virtually disappeared from routine clinical practice because of the lack of reproducibility and the lack of validity of the posterior vesicourethral angle as a useful marker of urodynamic stress incontinence (1).

Colpocystourethrography

Colpocystourethrography was introduced as an x-ray contrast imaging technique to outline the vagina (and rectum) in addition to the bladder. It involved the insertion of radiopaque dye into the bladder, urethra, vagina, and rectum. Dynamic imaging was performed with the patient standing, first while contracting the pelvic floor and second during Valsalva. It was used to investigate the dynamics of the pelvic organs during prolapse and also to study female urinary incontinence. It is no longer routinely performed.

Voiding Cystourethrography

Voiding cystourethrography enables visualization of the lower urinary tract during voiding, which can be difficult using other imaging techniques. It can detect diverticula of the bladder and urethra (2), urethral obstruction, vesicoureteric reflux trabeculation of the bladder (often associated with detrusor overactivity) and "occult/potential" stress incontinence associated with cystocele. It remains a useful tool in the evaluation of recurrent urinary incontinence after previous failed surgery, and with prolapse reduction in continent women with pelvic organ prolapse, combined cystometry and cystourethrography (videocystourethrography) can increase the detection rate of occult stress incontinence (3).

Defecography

Defecography is used to demonstrate the dynamics of rectal evacuation and identify support abnormalities of the posterior vaginal compartment. It involves injection of a thick barium paste into the rectum and subsequent videofluoroscopic observation at various stages of rest, Valsalva, voluntary evacuation, and recovery. The small bowel is opacified with an oral barium meal. Defecography can identify the presence of enteroceles, rectoceles

(Fig. 26.1), rectal intussusception, rectal prolapse (Fig. 26.2), and incomplete evacuation. A recent development is cystodefecoperitoneography (CDP), which involves the use of contrast medium in the urinary bladder and intraperitoneally (4,5). It allows for further assessment of peritoneoceles and enteroceles (5,6). Assessment of the anterior vaginal compartment with the simultaneous imaging of the bladder does not correlate well with clinical assessment of anterior vaginal wall descent (7).

MAGNETIC RESONANCE IMAGING (MRI)

The role of MRI in the evaluation of pelvic support anatomy has increased in popularity since its introduction in 1990 by Klutke et al (8). At present the use of MRI should be limited to clinical research because of the need for improved understanding of its role in the management of pelvic organ prolapse, the current lack of standardized techniques, and the relatively high costs. Nevertheless, MRI has been used for grading pelvic organ descent, and it appears to be a valuable tool in the evaluation of anatomic defects associated with prolapse. It has the *potential* for being the "gold standard" test for pelvic support imaging because it is easily reproducible and provides a permanent visual record of the bony, soft tissue, fascial connections, and musculature of the pelvic support structures.

MRI allows evaluation of tissue states, function, and motion dynamics and has many advantages over traditional imaging techniques, including its excellent tissue contrast, noninvasive nature, and the absence of ionizing radiation. It produces relatively easily recognizable images. MRI works on the principle that every tissue contains hydrogen nuclei that have a constant magnetic spin, and the MRI scanner utilizes an extremely powerful magnet with a field strength of approximately 0.3 to 2.0 Tesla (i.e., the unit of magnetic field strength; in comparison, a refrigerator magnet has a field strength of 0.01 T; the earth's magnetic field is 0.00003 to 0.00007 T).

Three commonly used imaging sequences help to distinguish tissues from one another. The T1-weighted sequence provides good spatial resolution (detail) and is useful for visualizing anatomy. Fat appears bright and water appears dark. The T2-weighted sequence is sensitive to local edema and is useful for identifying pathology. Fat appears bright but less than on T1-weighted images. Water also appears bright. In proton density images, fat

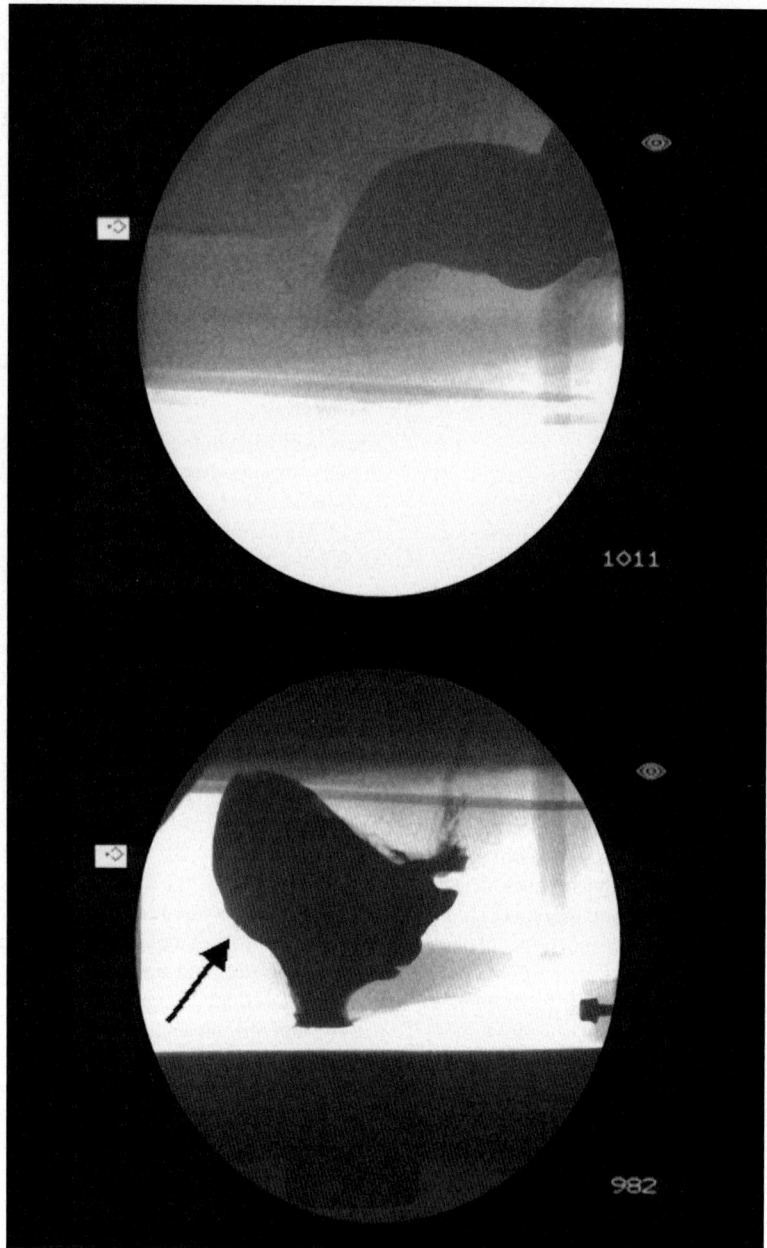

FIGURE 26.1 ● Defecography in a patient with defecatory symptoms but no obvious prolapse on clinical examination. Image below shows an anterior rectocele with incomplete bowel emptying on evacuation.

appears bright and water/simple fluid dark. For all the sequences, cortical bone and air appear black (9).

Visibility of Vaginal Compartments on MRI

Although sagittal pelvic MRI allows simultaneous visualization of all vaginal compartments, en-abling an accurate determination of the relationship of the contents to each other (Figs. 26.3 and 26.4), there has been concern about its ability to adequately visualize the posterior compartment. Healy et al (10) found that there was poor agreement between MRI and evacuation proctography for the measurement of anorectal junction descent and anorectal angle. Also, MRI detected fewer rectoceles, possibly because it was performed in

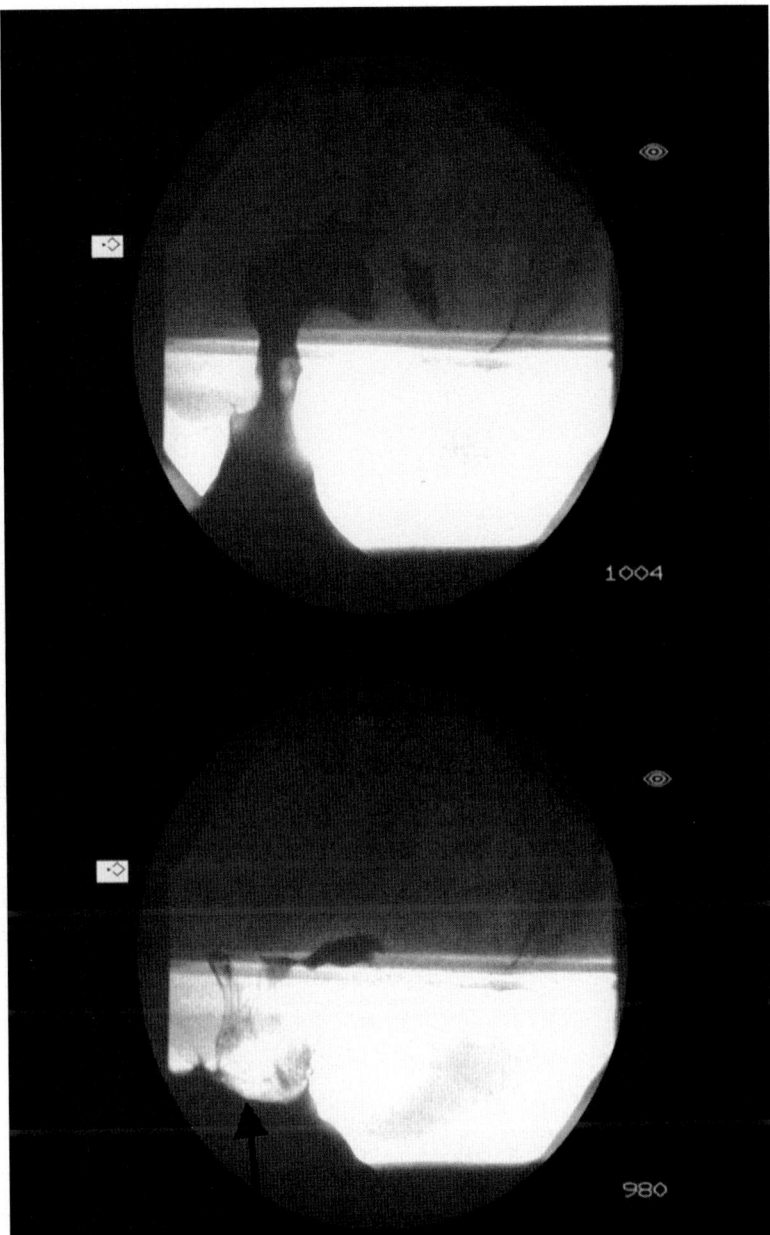

FIGURE 26.2 ● Defecography in a woman with rectal mucosal prolapse, showing images at rest (*above*) and on straining (*below*). The image below shows anterior rectal mucosal prolapse on straining to evacuate the rectum.

the supine position, thus excluding the effects of "gravity" and downward pressure. Techniques to improve visualization of the posterior compartment, including filling the rectum with 100 mL aqueous sonographic gel (11) and use of open configuration MRI scanning that allows imaging in the sitting position, have been undertaken to improve assessment of pelvic organ prolapse (12,13).

MR Quantification (Grading) of Pelvic Organ Prolapse

The use of MRI to quantify pelvic descent in all three vaginal compartments was first described by Yang et al (14), who analyzed sagittal images of 26 symptomatic and 16 control women. They evaluated pelvic descent using the pubococcygeal line (PCL) (Fig. 26.5) as the internal reference from

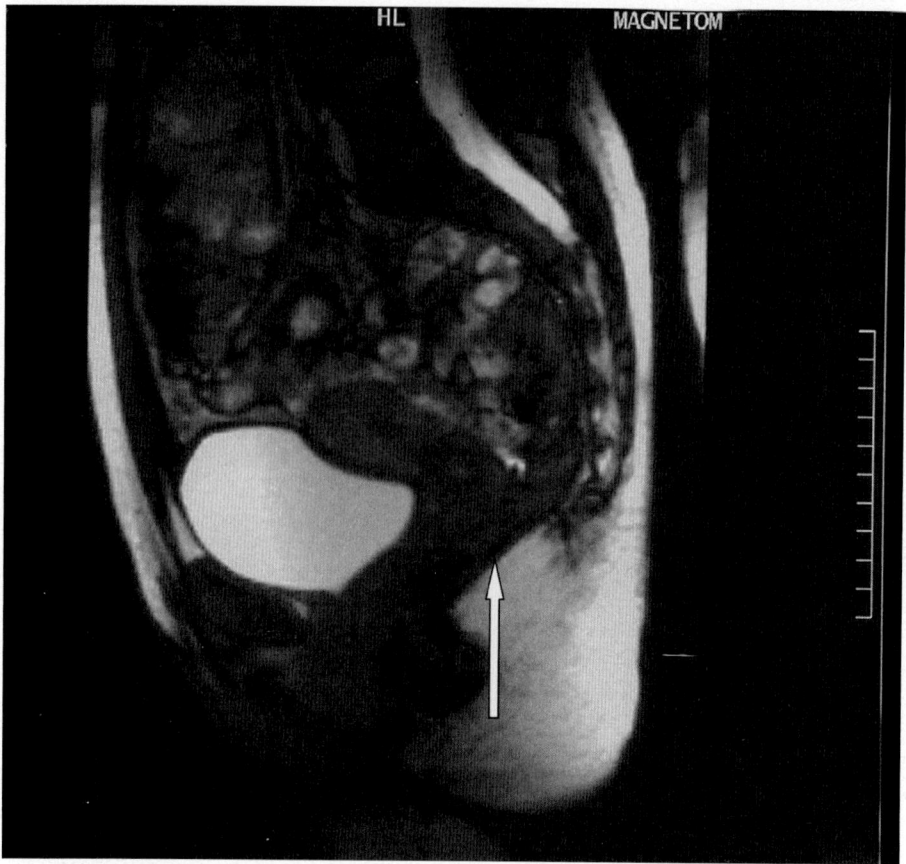

FIGURE 26.3 ● Midline sagittal T2-weighted pelvic MRI image of a normal nulliparous woman, showing well-supported pelvic organs while straining. The *arrow* indicates an intact levator plate offering support to the pelvic organs.

which measurements are made. The PCL was defined as a line extending from the most inferior portion of the symphysis pubis to the tangent of the last coccygeal joint. Normal reference limits were determined and it was established that the bladder base should not descend more than 1 cm below, the cervix or vaginal cuff should remain at least 1 cm above, and the rectum no more than 2.5 cm below the PCL. They also demonstrated that other measurements, such as the thickness of levator ani muscles, length of the urethral, and periurethral muscle ring, can be obtained on MRI (14). The PCL has subsequently been used by other investigators (11,12,15–23). Hodroff et al (24) found that MRI grading of prolapse differentiated between those without prolapse and those with prolapse of the anterior vaginal wall (i.e., Pelvic

Organ Prolapse Quantification [POPQ] grade 0 from grades I and II) but it did not differentiate between the International Continence Society (ICS) POPQ grades of prolapse (i.e., ICS POPQ [25] grades I and II).

A slight variation of the PCL referred to as the sacrococcygeal inferior pubic point (SCIPP) line has also been used for grading of pelvic descent on MRI (26). This line extends from the inferior border of the pubic symphysis to the sacrococcygeal joint.

Recently, a new reference line, the midpubic line (MPL) (see Fig. 26.5), was described as a line drawn through the longitudinal axis of the pubic bone, passing through its midequatorial point (27). It corresponds to the level of the hymenal ring, the reference point used in the POPQ system (25).

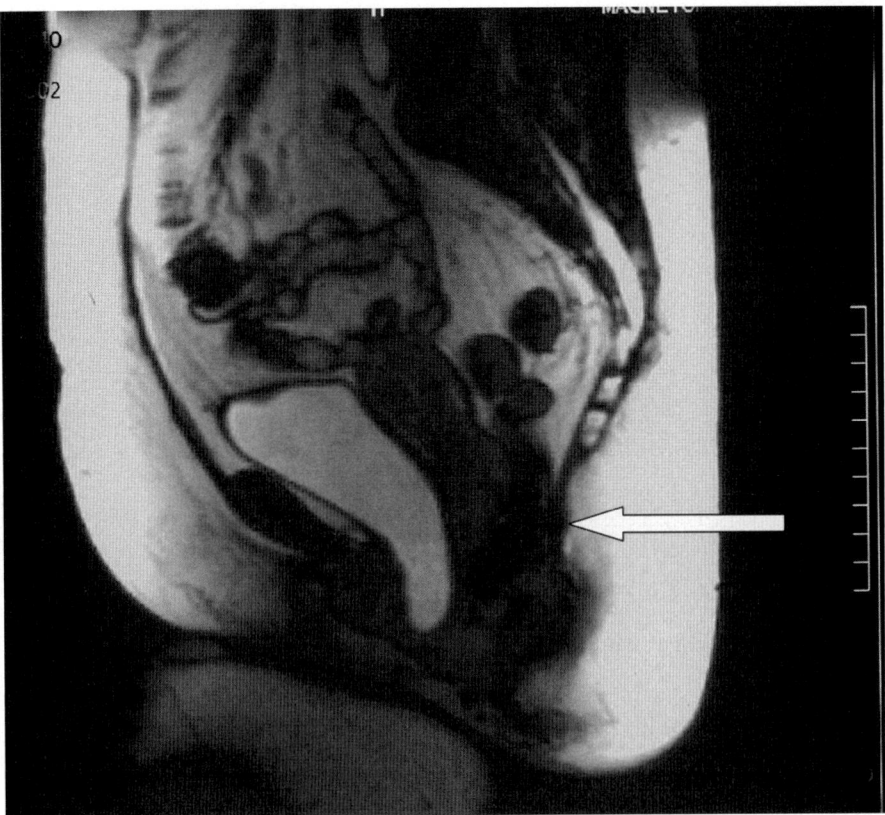

FIGURE 26.4 ● Midline sagittal T2-weighted pelvic MRI image of a parous woman with symptomatic pelvic organ prolapse, showing descent of the pelvic organs while straining. The *arrow* shows a disrupted levator plate.

MRI grading of pelvic organ prolapse using this method was shown to have a good agreement with ICS POPQ clinical staging.

MR Imaging of Pelvic Support Anatomy

The role of MRI in the evaluation of female paraurethral and bladder neck anatomy was first demonstrated by Klutke et al (8) in a study involving a female cadaver with no known history of urinary incontinence, and 50 (5 continent, 45 incontinent) patients between the ages of 30 and 73 years. It was seen on MRI that levator muscle fibers support the pelvic organs like a hammock. They found medial extensions from the levator muscles to the bladder neck and proximal urethra, which they referred to as the urethropelvic ligaments. On axial MRI of the lower third of the vagina (vaginal support level III [28]), the anterior vaginal wall conforms to and reflects the well-supported bladder neck and proximal urethral area; the normal H configuration on cross-sections of the vagina is easily visualized on MRI (8) (Fig. 26.6). Based on deviation from the normal anatomical appear-

ances, it is possible to demonstrate paravaginal defects (Fig. 26.7) on MRI at the three vaginal levels (8,28,29). The appearances on MRI of anterior vaginal compartment central endopelvic fascial defects have also been described (30) (Fig. 26.8). However, this still requires validation.

At vaginal support level I, the fibers within the uterosacral ligaments are seen in their entirety on axial images (31). At level II, the more direct relationship between the pelvic side wall is seen and the endopelvic fascial attachments (a combination of vessels and connective tissue) of the vagina to the inner surfaces of the levator ani muscle can be seen. The position of the arcus tendineus levator ani can be inferred from the angle formed between the levator ani and the surface of the internal obturator muscles. At level II, the concave forward configuration of the vagina is well defined; the periurethral sulci and attachments of the levator ani are present. The thick pubovisceral parts of the levator ani are seen (31). A structured system with good inter- and intra-observer agreement for the evaluation of urethral support anatomy has been developed (32).

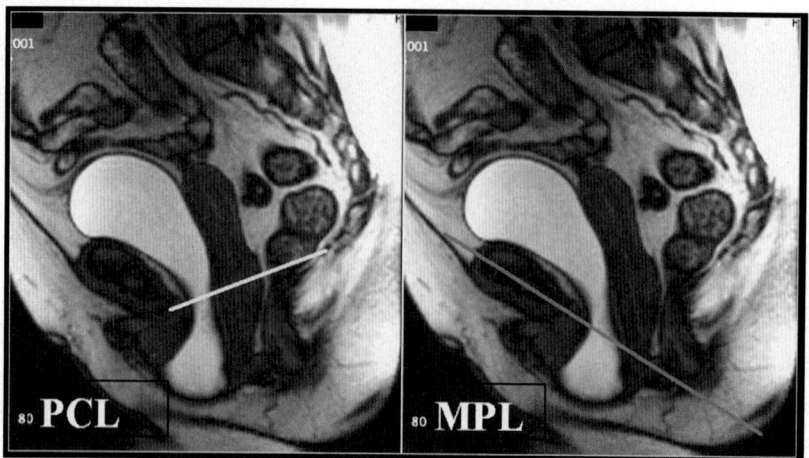

FIGURE 26.5 ● Midsagittal MRI images of a female pelvis with pelvic organ prolapse, demonstrating the pubococcygeal line (PCL) and the midpubic line (MPL).

MRI Appearances of Pelvic Floor Muscles

The levator ani muscle complex can be seen in its entirety from origins to attachments (33). Serial MRI has been used to assess changes in the levator ani muscles after vaginal delivery (34,35). The iliococcygeus muscle on MRI appears as a thin muscle with apparent gaps in the muscle at the site of its origin from the obturator fascia, whereas the pubococcygeus/pubovisceral muscle on MRI appears as a thicker muscle arising from the lower lateral border of the pubic symphysis (36). Women with symptomatic pelvic organ prolapse have a higher prevalence of pubococcygeus muscle attach-ment defects, especially on the right side, in comparison to normal nulliparous asymptomatic women (37) (Fig. 26.7).

The levator hiatus morphology can be assessed on MRI, including the length of the urogenital hiatus, the distance from the pubic bone to the anterior rectal wall; the width of the urogenital and levator hiatus (Fig. 26.9), the maximal distance between the medial margins of the right and left pubococcygeus muscles; the length of the levator hiatus, the distance from the pubic bone to the posterior rectal wall; and the pubococcygeus muscle thickness, the

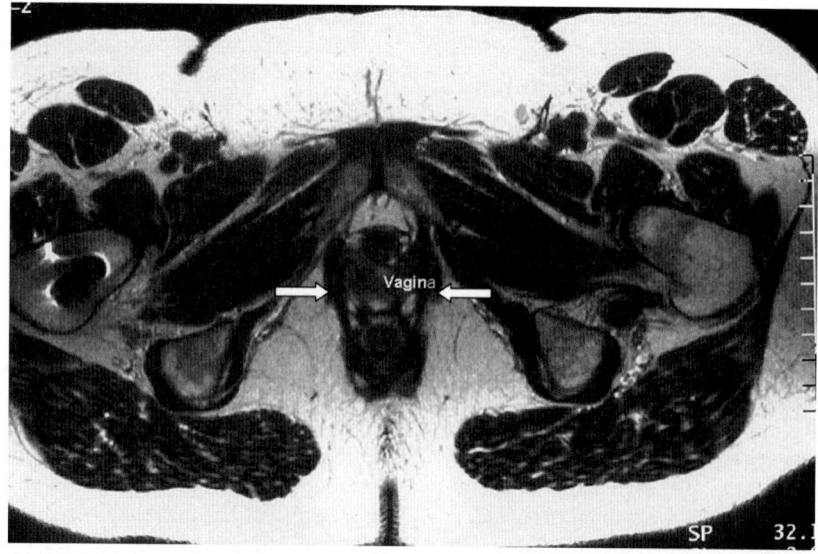

FIGURE 26.6 ● Axial T2-weighted pelvic MRI image of vaginal support level III (lower third) in a normal nulliparous woman, showing bilaterally intact pubococcygeal muscles (*arrows*) and normal butterfly-shaped "H" vaginal configuration.

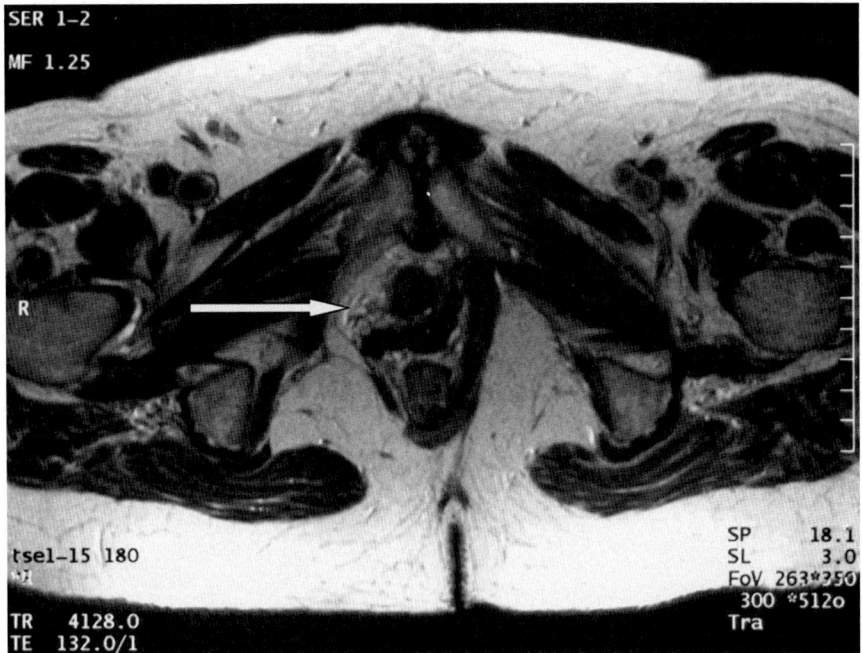

FIGURE 26.7 ● Axial T2-weighted pelvic MRI image of vaginal support level III (lower third) in a parous woman with symptomatic prolapse, showing detached right pubococcygeal muscle attachment and an associated right-sided paravaginal defect with loss of muscle and the normal vaginal configuration on the right side.

maximal transverse thickness of the pubococcygeus muscles (35).

Recent improvements in the MRI evaluation of pelvic floor muscles include the use of three-dimensional modeling (38,39), which enables quantification of levator muscle volume and is potentially a tool for analysis of the complex anatomical and functional relationships between pelvic support structures and the pelvic organs (40–42).

While MRI provides better images and potentially is the gold standard, it cannot be used as an office-based imaging tool. The knowledge from MRI imaging studies of pelvic support defects, however, could be correlated with the findings on ultrasound imaging (Fig. 26.10).

ULTRASONOGRAPHY

Ultrasound imaging has been used in the assessment of pelvic floor support defects. However, unlike MRI, the technique and imaging is operator-dependent.

Ultrasonography and Pelvic Support Defects

The use of ultrasound in the assessment and diagnosis of pelvic support defects is relatively new and includes transabdominal, transvaginal, introital, transperineal/translabial, and transrectal approaches.

Ultrasonography and Fascial Defects

Use of contrast transabdominal ultrasonography to diagnose paravaginal defects in women with urinary incontinence was reported in 1997 (43). In an attempt to standardize technique and evaluate qualitatively and quantitatively the effects of bladder and vaginal volumes on the transabdominal ultrasound diagnosis of paravaginal defects, Nguyen et al (44) found that the sonographic paravaginal defects were artificially created by ventral displacement of the bladder base (in 15 women with ICS POPQ stage IV and 15 normal asymptomatic controls). They concluded that transabdominal ultrasound (2D) was not useful in detecting paravaginal defects.

More recently 3D ultrasound technology for imaging pelvic floor structure and function has been described. The potential advantage of 3D ultrasound pelvic floor imaging over other imaging techniques is that it offers the opportunity for office-based dynamic assessment of pelvic support defects and functional anatomy (45). Translabial 3D ultrasound findings do not appear to correlate

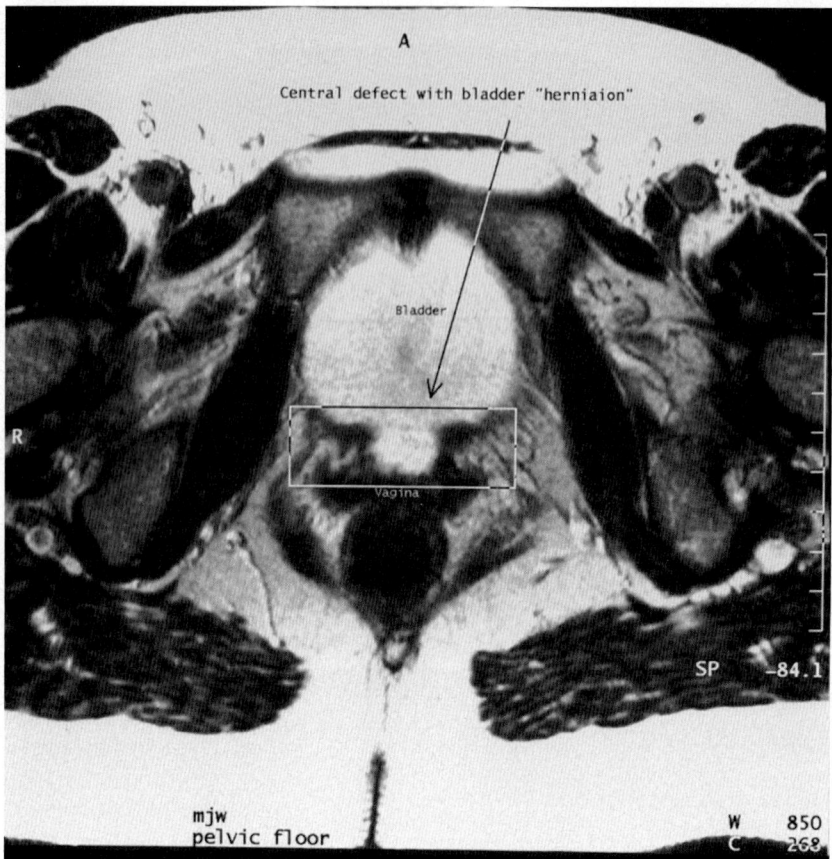

FIGURE 26.8 ● Axial pelvic MRI image of vaginal support level II (middle third), showing central fascial defect associated with symptomatic cystocele.

well with clinical assessment for paravaginal defects (46). It does, however, appear useful in the identification of rectovaginal septal defects associated with rectoceles (47) and has been used to measure urethral sphincter volume and the surface area of the levator hiatus (Fig. 26.11) (48). The urethral sphincter volume appears increased in women with obstructive voiding and abnormal sphincter electromyographic (EMG) activity (49) and correlates with urethral pressure profilometry (UPP) in nulliparous women (50). Similarly, in women with urodynamic stress incontinence, increased resting levator hiatus dimensions on sonographic imaging imply anterior vaginal wall prolapse and are associated with functional impairment of urethral closure (51).

Ultrasound Assessment of Bladder Neck Mobility and Function

Various techniques to locate the bladder neck on ultrasound have been described. These include transrectal, transvaginal (52), perineal (53), and in-

troital (54) sonography. The most commonly used, however, is the transperineal approach involving measurements using a system of coordinates (55). The ventral point of the urethral wall at the immediate transition into the bladder is identified as the bladder neck, and two distances are measured: Dx, which is the distance between the bladder neck and the Y axis, and Dy, which is the distance between the bladder neck and the X axis. The X axis is constructed by drawing a line between the superior and inferior borders of the symphysis pubis, and the Y axis is perpendicular to the X axis at the inferior symphysis border (Fig 26.12). This method of assessment has been shown to have good interexaminer agreement (55), and normal values of urethral, bladder, cervical, and rectal descent on Valsalva have been reported (56,57).

Antenatal bladder neck mobility on ultrasound scanning is increased in asymptomatic pregnant nulliparous women who develop postpartum urinary incontinence in comparison to those who remain continent irrespective of the delivery variables (58). Ultrasound assessment of bladder

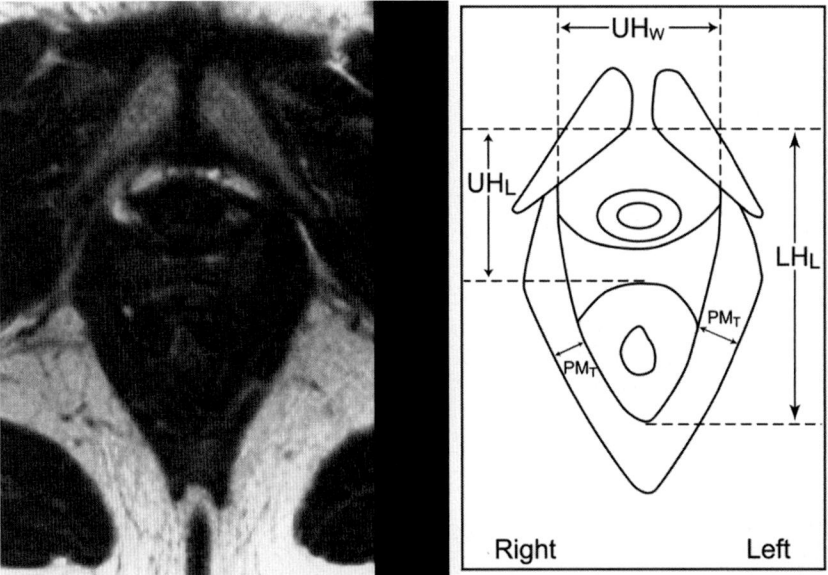

FIGURE 26.9 ● Axial MRI image and schematic diagram of the levator hiatus in a normal asymptomatic nulliparous volunteer. The diagram shows measured dimensions of the levator hiatus. LH_L = length of the levator hiatus, UH_L = length of the urogenital hiatus, UH_W = width of the urogenital hiatus, PM_T = pubococcygeal muscle thickness.

neck mobility therefore may be clinically useful in assessing and predicting the risk of women developing postpartum stress urinary incontinence.

In addition to assessing bladder neck mobility and stress urinary incontinence, ultrasound scanning can aid in the diagnosis of detrusor overactivity. Transvaginal ultrasound imaging of empty bladder wall thickness using a cutoff value of 6 mm appears to be a sensitive screening tool for detrusor overactivity in symptomatic women (59–61).

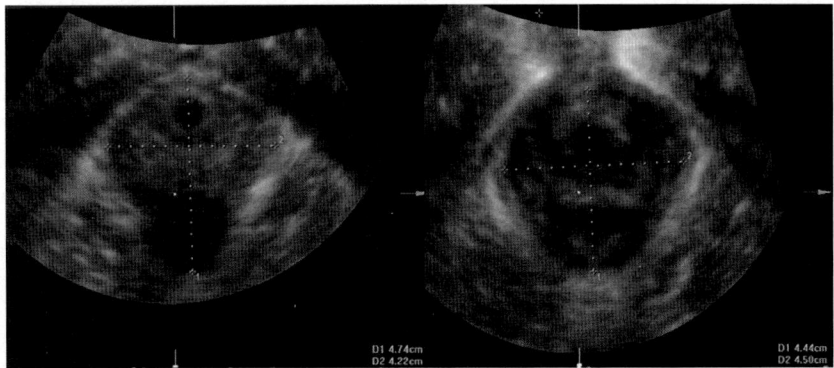

FIGURE 26.10 ● Three-dimensional ultrasound image of the levator hiatus in a young asymptomatic, nulliparous woman at rest and on Valsalva. The *dotted lines* indicate the length and width of the levator hiatus. (Image courtesy of Dr. H.P. Dietz, Sydney, Australia.) Compare to MRI image of Figure 26.9.

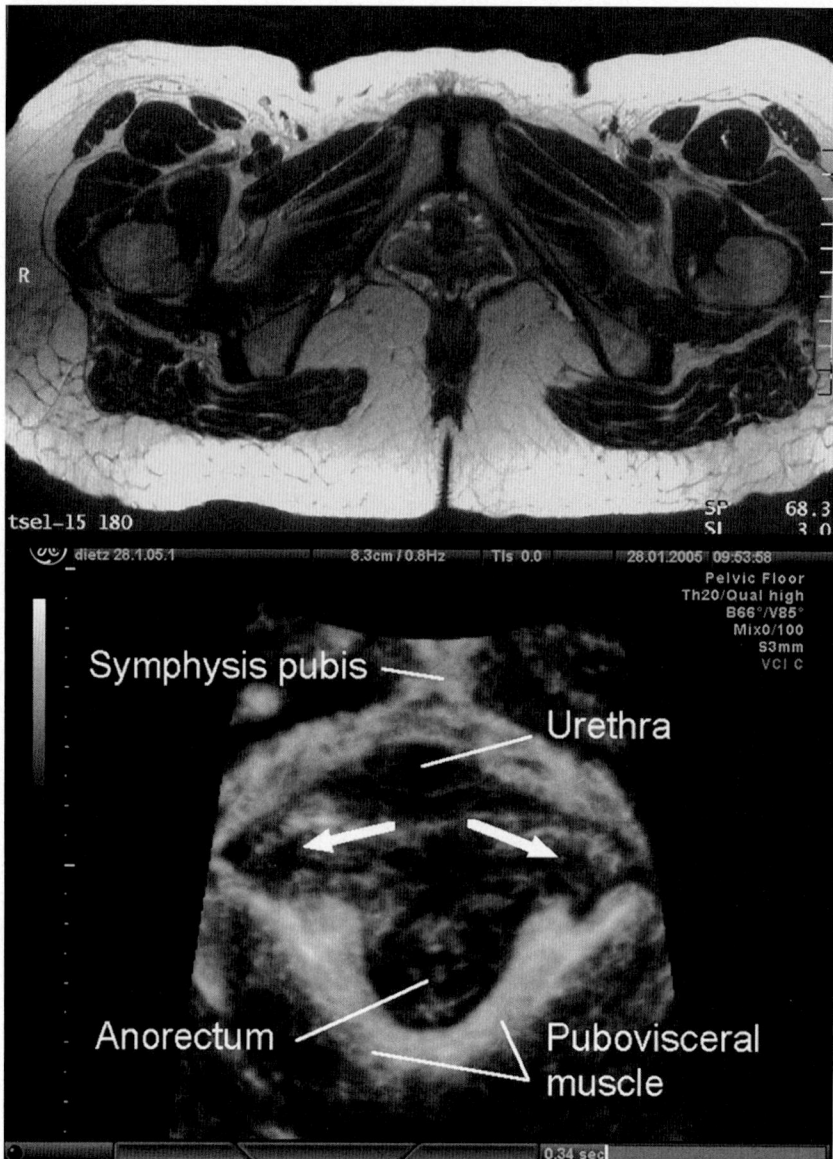

FIGURE 26.11 ● Axial pelvic MRI image (*above*) and 3D ultrasound image (*below*) of vaginal support level III (lower third) from two symptomatic women each demonstrating bilateral loss of anterior vaginal attachment to the pubic bone. (Three-dimensional ultrasound image courtesy of Dr. H.P. Dietz, Sydney, Australia.)

URODYNAMICS

The role of urodynamic testing in the assessment of female pelvic support defects includes assessment and diagnosis of associated conditions and assessment of the effects of prolapse reduction on bladder and urethral function.

Conventional Urodynamic Testing with Prolapse Reduction

It is widely recognized that severe female pelvic organ prolapse can mask symptoms of stress urinary incontinence in some women. This "occult/potential" incontinence may be revealed in up to 83% of women with severe prolapse following reduction of the prolapse during conventional

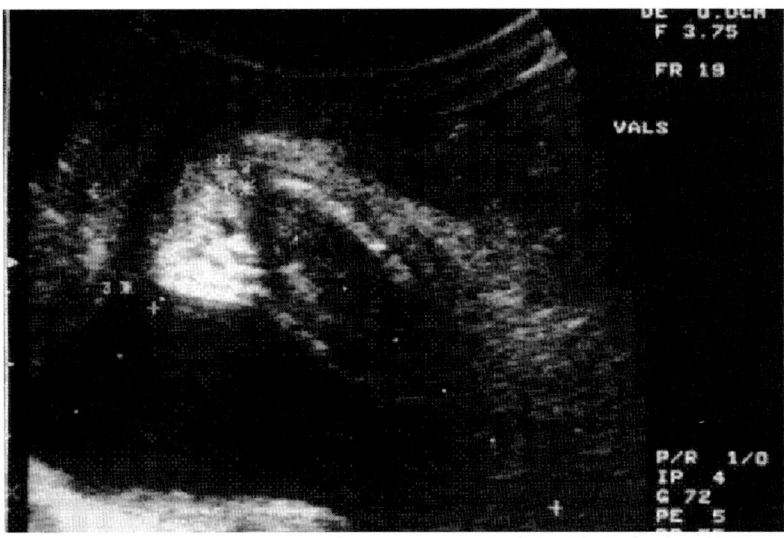

FIGURE 26.12 • Transperineal 2D ultrasound scan image of bladder neck position at rest. Measurement of bladder neck position in relation to the pubic bone is obtained using the X and Y coordinates (*dotted lines*).

urodynamic investigations by the insertion of a vaginal pessary (62–64) or, to the distress of the patient and physician, following surgical repair of the pelvic organ prolapse in up to 28% of previously continent women (65,66).

Performing urodynamic investigations with and without pelvic organ prolapse reduction using vaginal pessaries might help to identify women at risk of "occult/potential" stress urinary incontinence following pelvic organ prolapse surgery. Conversely, resolution of detrusor overactivity following reduction of prolapse can be demonstrated in some women.

Although the reliability of this urodynamic testing with prolapse reduction is uncertain due to the unknown effects of different barrier pessaries currently used for the test, it appears to overestimate the risk of developing new symptoms of stress urinary incontinence following prolapse surgery. That notwithstanding, it helps to provide information for preoperative counseling of patients about the likely effects of corrective prolapse surgery on lower urinary tract function. There is a need for further research work in order to identify the ideal prolapse reduction test.

Video Urodynamics/Videocystourethrography

The combination of conventional dual-channel cystometry using radiological contrast media with the simultaneous radiological observations of cystourethrography is generally considered the "gold standard" investigation for urinary incontinence. It is particularly useful in patients presenting with complex lower urinary tract symptoms, but not for the routine investigation. It might help demonstrate urethral obstruction associated with pelvic support defects and the effects of prolapse reduction on the obstruction (64,67). It remains a useful tool in the evaluation of complex urinary incontinence in tertiary referral centers.

CONCLUSIONS

Imaging of pelvic support defects has evolved over the past century. A number of radiological tests once considered the ultimate gold standard are now regarded as obsolete because of poor reproducibility and limited clinical application. While the newer and more attractive imaging technique of pelvic MRI and 3D ultrasound scanning have contributed to improving knowledge of the pelvic support anatomy, they should still be considered research tools because of a lack of standardized imaging and interpretation techniques, and a current lack of evidence of a positive influence on clinical management and outcomes. It is hoped that further research into the use of these new imaging modalities will extend their current role into routine clinical use. Potentially these investigations will be valuable tools in preoperative identification of the fascial and muscular defects underlying pelvic organ prolapse in individual patients, thus enabling targeted site-specific repair with improved surgical outcomes.

CHAPTER 27

Overview of Treatment

Joseph Schaffer, David D. Rahn, and Cecilia K. Wieslander

INTRODUCTION

Disorders of pelvic support affect quality of life but are generally not life-threatening. Most patients with pelvic organ prolapse (POP) are candidates for nonsurgical or surgical therapy, as well as expectant management for those who are asymptomatic or mildly symptomatic. The choice of treatment depends on the type and severity of symptoms, age and medical comorbidities, desire for future sexual function and/or fertility, and risk factors for recurrence. The goal of treatment is always to provide as much relief of symptoms as possible, and the benefits of treatment should always outweigh the risks. In this chapter we will discuss how patient symptoms, history, and physical findings are used to formulate a specific treatment plan and provide an overview of the different types of treatment.

SYMPTOMS ASSOCIATED WITH DISORDERS OF PELVIC SUPPORT

POP involves multiple systems and is commonly associated with genitourinary, gastrointestinal, and musculoskeletal symptoms. Treatment planning involves a full assessment of all symptoms, which should be characterized with regard to how bothersome they are and how much they affect quality of life. A plan should be developed for each complaint. To address all symptoms, the overall treatment approach may need to include both nonsurgical and surgical therapy.

Vaginal Bulge/Pelvic Pressure

Two of the most common symptoms associated with prolapse are vaginal bulge and pelvic pressure. Patients with these symptoms often complain of feeling a ball in the vagina, sitting on a weight, or a bulge rubbing on their clothes. If bulge symptoms are the primary complaint, successful replace-

ment of the prolapse with nonsurgical or surgical therapy will usually provide adequate treatment.

Urinary Symptoms

Patients with POP often have concurrent urinary symptoms, including stress urinary incontinence, urge urinary incontinence, frequency, urgency, urinary retention, recurrent urinary tract infection, or voiding dysfunction. Although some of these symptoms may be caused or exacerbated by the prolapse, it should not be assumed that surgical correction will be curative. For example, irritative bladder symptoms (frequency, urgency, urge urinary incontinence) may or may not improve with replacement of prolapse and sometimes worsen after surgical management. Therefore, urodynamic testing should be performed in women with urinary symptoms who are undergoing surgical correction of prolapse. This testing attempts to reflect the relationship of urinary symptoms to the prolapse. Additionally, consideration may also be given to temporarily placing a pessary prior to surgery to determine if urinary symptoms improve, thereby predicting whether surgical reduction of prolapse will be beneficial.

Gastrointestinal Symptoms

Constipation is often present in women with POP; however, replacement of the bulge either by surgical repair or with a pessary does not consistently cure this symptom and may actually worsen it. In one study of defect-directed posterior repair, constipation resolved postoperatively in 72% (1) of patients, while another study noted resolution in only 43% (2). Similarly, one study of posterior colporrhaphy reported a 28% reduction in constipation (3), while another reported a 50% increase (4). These seemingly contradictory data reflect that constipation frequently has different definitions, and more importantly, has multiple causes besides POP. Therefore, if a patient's primary symptom is constipation, surgical repair may not be indicated without a complete evaluation to address the other etiologies in its differential diagnosis.

Digital decompression of the posterior vaginal wall, the perineal body, or the distal rectum itself to defecate is often associated with prolapse. Surgical approaches to this problem are relatively ineffective, with symptom resolution as low as 36% (2).

Anal incontinence of flatus or liquid or solid stool may be seen in conjunction with POP. If this disorder is present, a full anorectal evaluation should be performed. On occasion, prolapse may lead to stool trapping in the distal rectum with subsequent leaking of liquid stool around trapped stool. However, most types of anal incontinence would not be expected to improve with surgical repair of prolapse. If evaluation reveals an anal sphincter defect as the cause of anal incontinence, anal sphincteroplasty may be performed in conjunction with prolapse repair.

Sexual Dysfunction

Sexual dysfunction is often seen in women with POP. The etiology of this symptom is frequently multifactorial. However, an obstructing bulge can be part of the problem, and therapy that reduces the bulge may be beneficial. Some prolapse procedures, such as posterior repair with levator plication, are believed to contribute to postoperative dyspareunia, and care should be taken in planning appropriate surgical procedures for patients with concomitant sexual dysfunction.

Pelvic and Back Pain

Anecdotal experience suggests that POP is associated with pelvic and low back pain. This pain may not necessarily be caused by the bulge itself but may be due to altered body mechanics that result from prolapse. However, a cross-sectional study of 152 consecutive patients with POP did not find an association between pelvic or low back pain and prolapse after controlling for age and prior surgery (5). If the primary complaint is back pain, referral for back evaluation is indicated. Additionally in this situation, temporary pessary placement is often beneficial to determine whether prolapse reduction will improve pain symptoms.

Asymptomatic

Mild to advanced prolapse may also be present without bothersome symptoms. In this situation, the risk/benefit ratio must be evaluated prior to proceeding with surgical treatment. Because the natural history of prolapse is unknown, it is difficult to predict if the condition will worsen or if symptoms will develop. Therefore, in the absence of other factors, it is prudent to avoid invasive therapy in an asymptomatic patient.

Comparing Symptoms to Degree and Location of Prolapse

Although POP has been associated with several different types of symptoms, the presence and severity of symptoms does not correlate well with advancing stages of prolapse. In addition, many common symptoms do not differentiate between compartments. Several studies have shown a poor predictive value between symptoms or the degree of their severity and the degree of prolapse in a particular vaginal compartment. Ellerkmann et al found that degree of prolapse in all vaginal compartments—anterior, posterior, and apical—correlated globally only with complaints of pelvic discomfort and visualization of a "bulge or protrusion" (6). The degree of posterior compartment prolapse only weakly correlated with complaints of incomplete evacuation and digital manipulation for bowel movements. Weber also found that with respect to stage of posterior compartment prolapse, there was no clinically significant correlation to symptoms of bowel dysfunction (7). The Pelvic Organ Support Study (POSST) found only weak associations between bowel symptoms and pelvic organ descent (8), and constipation has not been found to relate to the stage of prolapse (9).

Sexual dysfunction has been attributed to prolapse. One study has shown that increasing degree of prolapse did predict interference with sexual activity, but it did not affect the description of satisfaction with the sexual relationship or the frequency of intercourse (10). Ellerkmann et al found a moderate correlation between impairment of sexual activity and worsening prolapse in all three compartments (6). After surgery for incontinence or prolapse, Helstrom et al found no improvement in sexual function (11).

Urinary incontinence and hesitancy, as well as prolonged and intermittent micturition, correlate with worsening prolapse, but in all vaginal compartments. In contrast, there is a weak inverse relationship between worsening anterior compartment prolapse and stress incontinence. This improvement may result from mechanical kinking or obstruction of the urethra (6).

When planning surgical or nonsurgical therapy, realistic expectations should be set with regard to relief of symptoms. A patient must be made aware that some symptoms cannot reliably be expected to improve.

IMPACT OF AGE AND MEDICAL COMORBIDITIES

Symptomatic POP develops across the age spectrum. Factors related to age and function have a strong impact on the choice of treatment. Younger women with a long lifespan often opt for a definitive surgery that has the greatest chance of fixing the problem permanently. These women may find long-term pessary treatment unacceptable. In addition, younger women may be more sexually active and require a functional vagina.

Elderly women are candidates for nonsurgical or surgical therapy. Age alone should not be a contraindication to surgery, particularly if a patient is healthy. For example, investigators evaluated 54 women aged 70 to 85 years who underwent major gynecologic surgery in which 92.6% included indications of prolapse and urinary incontinence. This retrospective study showed that elderly women can undergo elective gynecologic surgery with an acceptable rate of complications (12). All serious complications occurred in patients who were classified as ASA class II (presence of mild systemic disease, but no functional limitations) and ASA class III (presence of severe systemic disease that limits activity but that is not incapacitating). Elderly patients do have decreased reserve, even if apparently healthy. Thus, if significant medical comorbidities such as cardiovascular disease and diabetes exist, surgical risk increases and nonsurgical management should be considered.

Elderly women may also have different needs with respect to sexual function. In the sexually active older woman, a careful discussion of sexual function should take place prior to surgical treatment. Some procedures may decrease vaginal caliber and introital dimensions and could possibly prohibit sexual intercourse if her partner has decreased erectile function. In older women who are not sexually active, obliterative procedures may be considered.

DESIRE FOR FUTURE FERTILITY

Treatment planning is challenging for a symptomatic woman who wants to maintain future fertility or retain her uterus. The patient's wishes should always be respected. This may entail pessary use until menopause or performing a prolapse procedure that avoids hysterectomy. Patients must be cautioned that future pregnancy and delivery could compromise the effectiveness of a repair.

RISK FACTORS FOR PROLAPSE AND RECURRENCE

Results from several large epidemiologic studies show that age, Hispanic and Caucasian ethnicity, increasing parity, and obesity increase the risk of POP. Similarly, women with connective tissue disorders are also at higher risk. Other suspected risk factors include chronically increased intra-abdominal pressure, smoking, pulmonary disease, and chronic constipation. Risk factors that contributed to the development of POP usually persist after therapy. Recurrence rates of prolapse after reconstructive surgery have been estimated to range from 30% to 58% (13,14). Accordingly, the process of treatment selection requires consideration of risk factors and potential for recurrence (15–21). For example, a patient with numerous risk factors might be expected to be at higher risk for recurrence and therefore would merit the most durable repair.

EXPECTANT MANAGEMENT

Expectant management is an option in women who are asymptomatic or mildly symptomatic or who decline treatment. Severity of prolapse does not always positively correlate with symptom severity, and prolapse, even beyond the hymeneal ring, does not require treatment in an asymptomatic patient.

Although asymptomatic patients often request surgery for fear that prolapse will worsen, delaying surgery should be considered in the absence of symptoms. The natural history of prolapse is unknown and disease progress is unpredictable. An exception may be a woman who cannot effectively empty her bladder secondary to prolapse. Long term, this patient may be at risk for upper tract genitourinary disease, and therefore a pessary or surgery should be strongly considered.

Expectant management consists of regular evaluation with objective assessment of symptoms and anatomy over time. Patients are assessed every 6 months to 1 year and are carefully questioned about urinary, bowel, or bulge-related symptoms as well as pain and sexual function and the impact on their quality of life. A prolapse examination is performed at each visit with use of the Pelvic Organ Prolapse Quantification (POPQ) scale to objectively follow the progression of descent. If symptoms and amount of descent worsen, patients can be triaged into nonsurgical or surgical management.

PESSARY USE IN PELVIC ORGAN PROLAPSE

In patients for whom expectant management is not desired, pessaries are the standard nonsurgical treatment. Throughout history, various vaginal devices and materials for prolapse have been described, including cloth, wood, wax, metal, ivory, bone, sponge, and cork. Today's pessaries are usually made of silicone or inert plastic, and they are safe and simple to manage. Despite a long history of use, literature describing their efficacy, indications, the selection of pessary type, and the management of a pessary and its complications is often anecdotal or contradictory.

Indications for Use

POP is still the most common indication for vaginal pessary use. Traditionally, pessaries have been reserved for women either unfit or unwilling to undergo surgery. A survey of the membership of the American Urogynecologic Society confirmed this sentiment among gynecologists with greater than 20 years in practice (22). However, the same survey showed that younger gynecologists, particularly those who described themselves as urogynecologists, used pessaries as a first-line therapy before recommending surgery. Women who have undergone at least one previous attempt at surgical management without relief may often choose a pessary over additional surgery.

Pessaries have also been used for treatment of stress incontinence. Although generally not used as first-line therapy, some studies have demonstrated the usefulness of specially modified pessaries that compress the bladder neck (23,24). In addition, pessary use in conjunction with other nonsurgical means such as periurethral collagen injections has been shown to be effective (25).

Pessaries may also be used diagnostically. As previously discussed, symptoms may not correlate with the type or severity of prolapse. Discerning to what degree prolapse is contributing to symptoms is important before embarking on difficult surgeries with possibly prolonged recovery. Short-term pessary use may be a helpful tool in this process. Even if a patient declines long-term pessary use, she may agree to a short trial to determine if her chief complaint is improved or resolved. A pessary may also be placed diagnostically to identify which patients are at risk for urinary incontinence after prolapse-correcting surgery (26–28).

A recent multicenter randomized cross-over trial compared two pessary types for relief of prolapse symptoms and also examined treatment of urinary complaints using the urinary scale of the Pelvic Floor Distress Inventory (PFDI) and the Urinary Distress Inventory. This study demonstrated that pessaries provide a modest improvement in urinary obstructive, irritative, and stress symptoms (29).

Certain pessaries have been used in pregnant women with a history of cervical incompetence in prior pregnancy to prevent premature cervical dilation. These devices may also be used during pregnancy for patients who develop symptomatic uterine and cervical prolapse. Generally, as the uterus rises out of the pelvis during the second trimester, a pessary is no longer necessary.

Types of Pessaries

Two broad categories of pessaries exist: support and space-filling pessaries (Fig. 27.1). Support pessaries are defined as those that use a spring mechanism that rests in the posterior fornix and against the posterior aspect of the symphysis pubis. With support pessaries, such as the ring, vaginal support results from elevation of the superior vagina by the spring, which is supported by the symphysis pubis. Space-filling pessaries are defined as those that maintain their position by creating suction between the pessary and vaginal walls (cube), by providing a diameter larger than the genital hiatus (donut), or by both mechanisms (Gellhorn). The two most commonly used and studied devices are the ring pessary and Gellhorn.

The ring pessary is marketed as a simple circular ring or as a ring with a diaphragm or support that appears like a large contraceptive diaphragm. These are effective in women with first- and second-degree prolapse, and the support diaphragm is especially useful in women with accompanying cystocele. When properly fitted, the device should lie behind the pubic symphysis anteriorly and behind the cervix posteriorly.

The Gellhorn is often used for moderate to severe prolapse and for complete procidentia. It contains a concave disk that fits against the cervix or vaginal cuff and has a stem that is positioned just posterior to the introitus. The concave disk supports the vaginal apex by creating suction; the stem is useful for device removal.

Patient Evaluation and Pessary Placement

A patient must be an active participant in the treatment decision to use a pessary, as its success will

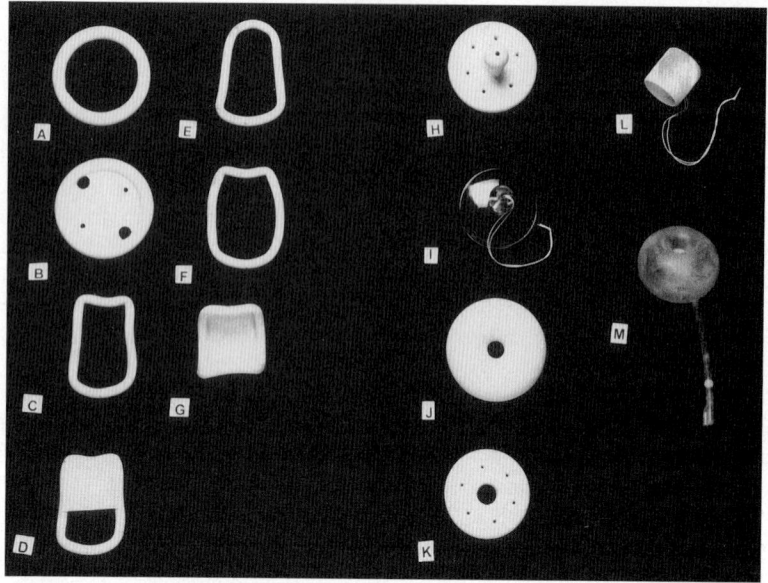

FIGURE 27.1 ● Pessary types. Support pessaries (columns 1 and 2 from left) and space-filling pessaries (columns 3 and 4 from left). (From Cundiff GW, Weidner AC, Visco AG, et al. A survey of pessary use by the membership of the American Urogynecologic Society. *Obstet Gynecol* 2000;95:931–935.)

depend upon her ability to care for the pessary—either alone or with the assistance of a caretaker—and her willingness and availability to come for follow-up evaluations. Vaginal atrophy should be treated before or concomitantly with pessary initiation. Besides choosing a support versus space-filling pessary, the type of device selected may be affected by patient factors such as hormonal status, sexual activity, prior hysterectomy, and stage and site of POP. After an appropriate type of pessary is selected, she should be fitted with the largest size that can be comfortably worn. If a pessary is ideally fitted, a patient is not aware of its presence. As a woman ages and gains or loses weight, the size may need to be adjusted.

Generally, a patient is fitted with a pessary while in the lithotomy position after she has emptied both her bladder and rectum. A digital examination is performed to assess vaginal depth and width and an initial estimation of pessary size is made. To introduce a ring pessary, the device is held in one's dominant hand in the folded position. Lubricant is placed on either the vaginal introitus or the pessary's leading edge. While holding the labia apart, the pessary is inserted by pushing in an inferior direction against the posterior vaginal wall. Next, the index finger of the right hand is directed into the posterior vaginal fornix to ensure that the cervix is resting above the pessary. The examiner's finger should be able to just barely slide between the lateral edges of the ring pessary and the vaginal side wall.

Following pessary placement, the patient is instructed to Valsalva and perform other various maneuvers that might dislodge an improperly fitted pessary. She should be able to stand, walk, cough, and urinate without difficulty or discomfort. The patient or her caregiver is then taught to remove and replace the device. To remove a ring pessary, an index finger is inserted into the vagina to hook the ring's leading edge. Traction is applied along the vaginal axis to bring the ring toward the introitus, where it may be grasped by the thumb and index finger of the dominant hand and removed.

Ideally, a pessary is removed nightly to weekly, washed in soap and water, and replaced the next morning. Patients are sent home from their initial fitting session with instructions describing the management of commonly encountered problems (Table 27.1). After initial placement, the first return visit may be in a few days to a week. For patients comfortable with their pessary management, return visits may be semiannually. For patients unable or unwilling to remove and replace a device themselves, a pessary may be removed and the patient's vagina inspected at the physician's office every 3 months. The scheduling of subsequent visits will be tailored to each patient.

Complications

Serious complications such as erosions into adjacent organs are rare with proper use of pessaries and usually occur only after years of neglect. At

TABLE 27.1

Guidelines for Pessary Care

Pessary type_____
size_____

1. After your initial pessary fitting is successful, you will be asked to return for a follow-up appointment in about 2 weeks. The purpose of this visit is to check the pessary and examine the vagina to ensure that it is healthy. Follow-up appointments will follow this schedule:

   1st year—every 3 to 6 months
   2nd year and beyond—every 6 months

   You may learn to care for the pessary yourself. For those patients who can remove and insert the pessary themselves, we recommend weekly overnight removal and cleansing of the pessary with soap and warm water. These patients should see the doctor at least once per year.

2. The following is a list of problems you may encounter with the pessary and our recommendations for the management.

Problem	Management
a. The pessary falls out.	Keep the pessary and notify your doctor's office. An appointment will be made. It may be possible that a change in the size or the type of pessary is needed.
b. You experience pelvic pain.	Notify your doctor's office. If the pessary has slipped and you can remove it, do so. Otherwise, have your doctor remove the pessary. A change in pessary size or type may be needed.
c. Vaginal discharge and odor	You can douche with warm water and you may want to try using Trimo-San vaginal gel 1 to 3 times a week.
d. Vaginal bleeding	Vaginal bleeding may be a sign that the pessary is irritating the lining of the vagina. Call your doctor's office and arrange an appointment.
e. Leaking from the bladder	Sometimes the support provided by the pessary will cause leaking from the bladder. Notify your doctor and discuss this problem.

From Farrell SA. Practical advice for ring pessary fitting and management. *J SOGC* 1997;19:632, with permission.

each return visit, the pessary is removed and the vagina is inspected for erosions, abrasions, ulcerations, or granulation tissue. Pessary ulcers or abrasions are treated by changing the pessary type or size to alleviate pressure points, or by removing the pessary completely until healing occurs. Treatment of vaginal atrophy with local or systemic estrogen is commonly required. Alternatively, water-based lubricants may help prevent these complications.

Pelvic pain with pessaries is not normal. This usually indicates that the size is too large and is an indication for substituting a smaller-sized pessary. Vaginal bleeding usually results from superficial abrasions, which with time can progress to frank erosions. Thus, this symptom cannot be ignored. All pessaries tend to trap vaginal secretions and obstruct normal drainage to some degree. The resultant odor may be managed by encouraging more frequent nighttime device removal, washing, and reinsertion the next day. Alternatively, a patient may use Trimo-San gel (Milex Products, Inc., Chicago, IL) one or two times weekly or douche with warm water.

Conclusions

Although many patients with POP opt for surgical management, the pessary is an excellent alternative for patients unwilling or unable to undergo surgery. It is a useful tool to define the relationship of symptoms to prolapse, for relief of symptoms while awaiting surgery, and as a diagnostic device for identifying patients whose surgeries are likely to unmask urinary incontinence. The pessary may also serve as a treatment for common irritative urinary symptoms. Thus, the pessary is an indispensable part of the gynecologist's armamentarium.

PELVIC FLOOR REHABILITATION

Nonsurgical management of prolapse may include a trial of pelvic floor rehabilitation (30,31). Current theories regarding the development of prolapse suggest that it may arise from the compromised ability of the pelvic floor muscles to support the pelvic organs. This may develop as a consequence of mechanical injury (a stretching or widening of the genital hiatus) or as a result of denervation and subsequent muscle atrophy. Although pelvic floor rehabilitation as a treatment for prolapse is unproven, if it results in the recovery of some muscle function, it may have some value in the reversal of minor degrees of pelvic prolapse and in the prevention of progression to more severe degrees of pelvic prolapse. In an asymptomatic, mildly symptomatic, or postsurgical patient, a regular program of pelvic floor exercise has potential to be beneficial, with little associated risk.

SURGERY

The two approaches to POP repair are reconstructive and obliterative. Reconstructive surgery attempts to restore normal anatomy and function and to relieve symptoms. Reconstructive surgery is therefore appropriate for a woman who is sexually active or may be in the future and needs to maintain a functional vagina. However, reconstructive surgery has a significant recurrence rate, approximating 30%.

The obliterative approach also aims to relieve symptoms, but it does so by closing the vagina. Normal anatomy and function are lost. Obliterative surgery (partial or complete colpocleisis) is very successful in reducing prolapse and resolving symptoms, and prolapse recurrence is rare. However, sexual intercourse is not possible after obliteration. Thus, the procedure should never be performed in a woman who is sexually active or has the desire to be so in the future. For this reason, a patient's partner should be involved in the informed consent process, as the decision to close the vagina will affect him also.

Obliterative procedures can be performed in less time than reconstructive procedures and may be done under regional or local anesthesia. Thus, in an elderly woman in poor medical condition, obliteration should be considered.

Reconstructive Surgery

Reconstructive surgery may be performed by the vaginal, abdominal, or laparoscopic route. The best approach is not known. There are very few randomized controlled surgical trials, and therefore the decision must be individualized. Surgeons should make an effort to objectively evaluate their own surgical results and provide information to the patient regarding the procedures that they believe they can do most successfully. Likewise, a patient's specific risk factors and symptoms should be assessed and a procedure should be designed specifically for the unique situation.

With an estimated 30% recurrence rate after reconstructive surgery, patients should have realistic expectations. Certain prolapse-related symptoms such as stress urinary incontinence can be successfully repaired, but other associated symptoms, such as constipation, cannot reliably be repaired. A symptom-specific discussion should be part of the informed consent process.

Preoperative prolapse evaluation always includes an assessment of all compartments and an attempt to identify all defects. However, it is not known whether all defects require repair. Compensatory defects may develop after prolapse repair. For instance, after an apical suspension and anterior wall repair, a small asymptomatic posterior wall prolapse may develop into a large prolapse. But the decision to repair a small posterior wall defect in this context must be weighed against the possibility that dyspareunia or other complications could develop. Surgeons must again individualize therapy based on the patient's specific symptoms and risk factors as well as their own experience. When considering site-specific repair, a surgeon can also counsel a woman that some sites are corrected with a higher success rate than others. A variety of apical suspension procedures have success rates that approximate 90% (32,33) and stress incontinence procedures have rates ranging near 85% (34,35). However, procedures for anterior vaginal wall prolapse have been found in some studies to be corrective less than 50% of the time (36). Anatomic cure rates for posterior vaginal wall prolapse range from 70% to 90% (37).

The recent Colpopexy and Urinary Reduction Efforts (CARE) trial has provided valuable information regarding whether potential stress incontinence should be repaired at the time of prolapse surgery (38). In this trial, to prevent the development of de novo postoperative stress incontinence, continent women with anterior wall prolapse undergoing sacrocolpopexy were randomly assigned to undergo Burch colposuspension or not. It was found that 44% of women who did not receive this additional procedure developed stress incontinence versus 24% who had the anti-incontinence surgery performed. Moreover, the subjects in the Burch arm had no difference in the prevalence of postoperative urge incontinence or voiding dysfunction. Although data from this trial cannot automatically be extrapolated to other apical suspension and anti-incontinence procedures, it certainly suggests that it is prudent to consider an anti-incontinence procedure in a patient with anterior wall prolapse who is undergoing an apical suspension. The CARE trial provides information for preoperative discussion with the patient. If a woman chooses not to undergo an anti-incontinence procedure, she is aware that one might be necessary at a later date.

The use of synthetic mesh and biomaterials in prolapse continues to be controversial. A discussion of the issues related to mesh and materials is beyond the scope of this chapter. Suffice it to say that definitive data do not exist regarding the safety or effectiveness of these materials, and caution must be exercised in their use.

CONCLUSIONS

POP is a complex condition that presents with a multitude of anatomic variants and a wide spectrum of symptoms. Each patient has unique physical findings and symptoms. Before treatment is begun, all symptoms and all systems should be considered. Therapy must focus first on alleviating symptoms. Most patients can be offered expectant management or nonsurgical or surgical treatment. In many patients, a combination of nonsurgical and surgical therapies will be effective.

REFERENCES

1. Cundiff GW, Weidner AC, Visco AG, et al. An anatomic and functional assessment of the discrete defect rectocele repair. *Am J Obstet Gynecol* 1998;179: 1451–1457.
2. Kenton K, Shott S, Brubaker L. Outcomes after rectovaginal fascia reattachment for rectocele repair. *Am J Obstet Gynecol* 1999;181(6):1360–1364.
3. Mellgren A, Anzen B, Nilsson BY, et al. Results of rectocele repair: a prospective study. *Dis Colon Rectum* 1995;38:7–13.
4. Kahn MA, Stanton SL. Posterior colporrhaphy: its effects on bowel and sexual function. *Br J Obstet Gynaecol* 1997;104:82–86.
5. Heit M, Culligan P, Rosenquist C, et al. Is pelvic organ prolapse a cause of pelvic or low back pain? *Obstet Gynecol* 2002;99:23–28.
6. Ellerkmann RM, Cundiff GW, Melick CF, et al. Correlation of symptoms with location and severity of pelvic organ prolapse. *Am J Obstet Gynecol* 2001;185: 1332–1338.
7. Weber AM, Walters MD, Ballard LA, et al. Posterior vaginal wall prolapse and bowel function. *Obstet Gynecol* 1998;179:1446–1449.
8. Kahn MA, Breitkopf CR, Valley MT, et al. Pelvic Organ Support Study (POSST) and bowel symptoms: Straining at stool is associated with perineal and anterior vaginal descent in a general gynecologic population. *Am J Obstet Gynecol* 2005;192:1516–1522.
9. Jelovsek JE, Barber MD, Paraiso MFR, et al. Functional bowel and anorectal disorders in patients with pelvic organ prolapse and incontinence. *Am J Obstet Gynecol* 2005;193:2105–2111.
10. Weber AM, Walters MD, Schover LR. Sexual function in women with uterovaginal prolapse and urinary incontinence. *Obstet Gynecol* 1995;85:483–487.
11. Helstrom L, Nilsson B. Impact of vaginal surgery on sexuality and quality of life in women with urinary incontinence or genital decensus. *Acta Obstet Gynecol Scand* 2005;84:79–84.
12. Toglia MR, Nolan TE. Morbidity and mortality rates of elective gynecologic surgery in elderly women. *Am J Obstet Gynecol* 2003;189:1584–1589.
13. Luber KM, Boero S, Choe JY. The demographics of pelvic floor disorders: current observations and future projections. *Am J Obstet Gynecol* 2001;184:1496–1501.
14. Whiteside JL, Weber AM, Meyn LA, et al. Risk factors for prolapse recurrence after vaginal repair. *Am J Obstet Gynecol* 2004;191:1533–1538.
15. Olsen AL, Smith VJ, Bergstrom JO, et al. Epidemiology of surgically managed pelvic organ prolapse and urinary incontinence. *Obstet Gynecol* 1997;89(4):501–506.
16. Mant J, Painter R, Vessey M. Epidemiology of genital prolapse: observations from the Oxford Family Planning Association Study. *Br J Obstet Gynaecol* 1997;104(5):579–585.
17. Hendrix S, Clark A, Nygaard I, et al. Pelvic organ prolapse in the Women's Health Initiative: Gravity and gravidity. *Am J Obstet Gynecol* 2002;186(6):1160–1166.
18. Swift S, Woodman P, O'Boyle A, et al. Pelvic Organ Support Study (POSST): The distribution, clinical definition, and epidemiologic condition of pelvic organ support defects. *Am J Obstet Gynecol* 2005;192:795–806.
19. Lukacz ES, Lawrence JM, Contreras R, et al. Parity, mode of delivery, and pelvic floor disorders. *Obstet Gynecol* 2006;107:1253–1260.
20. Norton PA, Baker JE, Sharp HC, et al. Genitourinary prolapse and joint hypermobility in women. *Obstet Gynecol* 1995;85(2):225–228.
21. Erata YE, Kilic B, Saygili U, et al. Risk factors for pelvic surgery. *Arch Gynecol Obstet* 2002;267(1):14–18.
22. Cundiff GW, Weidner AC, Visco AG, et al. A survey of pessary use by the membership of the American Urogynecologic Society. *Obstet Gynecol* 2000;95: 931–935.
23. Kondo A, Yokoyama E, Koshiba K, et al. Bladder neck support prosthesis: a nonoperative treatment for stress or mixed urinary incontinence. *J Urol* 1997;157:824–827.

24. Davila GW, Neal D, Horbach N, et al. A bladder-neck support prosthesis for women with stress and mixed incontinence. *Obstet Gynecol* 1999;96:938–942.

25. Walters MD, Iannetta LT. Combination of pessary and periurethral collagen injections for nonsurgical treatment of uterovaginal prolapse and genuine stress urinary incontinence. *Obstet Gynecol* 1997;90:691–692.

26. Chaikin DC, Groutz A, Blaivas JG. Predicting the need for anti-incontinence surgery in continent women undergoing repair of severe urogenital prolapse. *J Urol* 2000;163:531–534.

27. Liang CC, Chang YL, Chang SD, et al. Pessary test to predict postoperative urinary incontinence in women undergoing hysterectomy for prolapse. *Obstet Gynecol* 2004;104:795–800.

28. Klutke JJ, Ramos S. Urodynamic outcome after surgery for severe prolapse and potential stress incontinence. *Am J Obstet Gynecol* 2000;182:1378–1380.

29. Schaffer JI, Cundiff GW, Amundsen CL, et al. Do pessaries improve lower urinary tract symptoms? *J Pelvic Med Surg* 2006;12:72–73.

30. Kegel AH. Progressive resistance exercises in the functional restoration of the perineal muscles. *Am J Obstet Gynecol* 1948;56:238–248.

31. Greenhill JP. The nonsurgical management of vaginal relaxation. *Clin Obstet Gynecol* 1972;15:1083–1097.

32. Sze EH, Miklos JR, Partoll L, et al. Sacrospinous ligament fixation with transvaginal needle suspension for advanced pelvic organ prolapse and stress incontinence. *Obstet Gynecol* 1997;89(1):94–96.

33. Nygaard IE, McCreery R, Brubaker L, et al. Pelvic Floor Disorders Network. Abdominal sacrocolpopexy: a comprehensive review. *Obstet Gynecol* 2004;104(4): 805–823.

34. Nilsson GC, Falconer C, Rezapour M. Seven-year follow-up of the tension-free vaginal tape procedure for treatment of urinary incontinence. *Obstet Gynecol* 2004;104:1259–1262.

35. Leach GE, Dmochowski RR, Appell RA, et al. Female stress urinary incontinence clinical guidelines panel summary report on surgical management of female stress urinary incontinence. *J Urol* 1997;158:875–880.

36. Weber AM, Walters MD, Piedmont MR, et al. Anterior colporrhaphy: a randomized trial of three surgical techniques. *Am J Obstet Gynecol* 2001;185(6):1299–1304.

37. Cundiff GW, Fenner D. Evaluation and treatment of women with rectocele: focus on associated defecatory and sexual dysfunction. *Obstet Gynecol* 2004;104(6): 1403–1421.

38. Brubaker L, Cundiff GW, Fine P, et al. Pelvic Floor Disorders Network. Abdominal sacrocolpopexy with Burch colposuspension to reduce urinary stress incontinence. *N Engl J Med* 2006;354(15):1557–1566.

CHAPTER 28

Anterior Wall Support Defects

Stephen B. Young and Scott M. Kambiss

ANATOMY

For many years gynecologists have debated the composition and nature of vaginal tissues in relation to the urinary bladder. There are two distinct schools of thought: one group believes that between the bladder and the vagina there exists a fascial layer, and the other group does not. The "fascialists" have termed this layer the pubocervical fascia in the anterior compartment—one part of a total supportive pelvic skeleton, the "endopelvic fascia." To further understand the vaginal anatomy as it relates to the urinary bladder, histologic studies have been performed to determine the true composition of these tissues. Weber and Walters reported their results of microscopic examination of full-thickness sections of the vagina and urinary bladder taken from autopsy specimens (1). Weber and Boreham et al separately found that the anterior vaginal wall was composed of three layers: epithelium, muscularis, and adventitia. Immediately deep to the vaginal adventitia is bladder adventitia. Deep to that is detrusor muscle and finally bladder mucosa. They found no fascia (Fig. 28.1) (1,2).

Laterally, the anterior vaginal walls are attached by fibrous connections (endopelvic fascia) to the levator ani at the arcus tendineus fascia pelvis (ATFP) or the "white line." The ATFP extends from the underside of the pubic symphysis and inferolateral pubic bone to the ischial spine bilaterally (3). In addition, the cardinal and uterosacral ligament complex helps support the upper vagina with its attachments to the sacrum and lateral pelvic walls.

Progress has occurred during the past 15 years in our understanding of anterior pelvic floor support and prolapse with research utilizing anatomic dissection and histologic/histochemical microstudy, a variety of magnetic resonance imaging (MRI) techniques with computer applications, and other basic science work (e.g., biomechanics and muscle physiology). John DeLancey has brought us an evolution in pelvic floor anatomic understanding from his elegant cadaver dissection work (4). He has used MRI studies to help resolve long-contentious issues over the presence or absence of fascia, the constituents of the pelvic floor support "ligaments," the great importance of the levator ani muscles, and the entire panoply of pelvic floor support (5,6). He and biomechanical engineer John Ashton Miller have increased our knowledge of pelvic function. MRI also allows for specific measurements to be made within the anterior compartment. In 1995, Aronson et al clearly demonstrated normal and abnormal pelvic anatomy utilizing continent and incontinent women including paravaginal defects (7). There is a great deal more that MRI and other research tools will teach us about pelvic floor anatomy, function, and pathophysiology.

PATHOPHYSIOLOGY: TYPES OF DESCENT

Prolapse of the anterior vaginal wall is the most common single site of pelvic organ prolapse (POP), with an overall prevalence of 33.8% (8). It may occur alone or more commonly along with other pelvic defects. Early grades may be asymptomatic, yet more advanced anterior prolapse may cause multiple mechanical and functional symptoms. In the early 20th century, George White described anterior pelvic floor descent as being due to overstretching and thinning out of the anterior vaginal wall and other supports of the bladder to descend in the form of a hernia (8,9).

The anterior vaginal wall is lined on the vaginal lumen side by a nonkeratinizing squamous epithe-

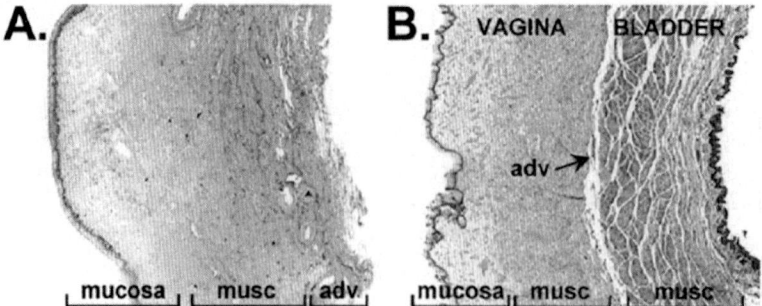

FIGURE 28.1 ● Anatomic/histologic layers of vagina and bladder. Both **(A)** and **(B)** are full-thickness, cross-sectional anterior vaginal wall specimens. **(A)** taken at hysterectomy, **(B)** cadaveric and containing bladder wall. Both show vagina contains squamous epithelium, muscularis (musc), and adventitia (adv). Deep to this is only bladder muscularis and bladder mucosa. No fascia is seen. (From Boreham MK, Wai CY, Miller RT, et al. Morphometric analysis of smooth muscle in the anterior vaginal wall of women with pelvic organ prolapse. *Am J Obstet Gynecol* 2002;187(1):56–63, Fig. 2, with permission.)

lial lining that ends at the lamina propria. The muscular layer lies beneath the lamina propria and consists of mostly smooth muscle fibers along with small amounts of a collagen and elastin connective tissue (1). When this muscularis is surgically dissected from the epithelium during a split-thickness anterior colporrhaphy dissection, it is often referred to as "pubocervical fascia" (10). The third layer is known as the adventitia. It is loose areolar tissue and is shared by the bladder. Boreham et al compared specimens taken from the anterior vaginal cuff in both normal subjects and those with prolapse (2). Following immunohistologic review it was noted that women with prolapse had a significantly reduced fraction of smooth muscle, disorganized smooth muscle bundles, and decreased alpha-actin staining in the muscularis as well as dilated venules in the lamina propria of the anterior wall compared to control subjects (2).

The International Continence Society defines anterior vaginal wall prolapse as "descent of the anterior vagina so that the urethrovesical junction (a point 3 cm proximal to the external urinary meatus) or any anterior point proximal to this is less than 3 cm above the plane of the hymen" (11). The cause of anterior prolapse, while not fully understood, is clearly multifactorial. Largely, the acute traumatic events—vaginal birth and pelvic surgery—are etiologically coupled with our lifelong "slings and arrows" of hard work: raising a family, gaining weight, aging, menopause, and the many problems "flesh is heir to." Parity and obesity are strongly associated with increased risk for anterior compartment prolapse (8). Neurologic pelvic floor injury and underlying connective tissue disorders have been implicated (12,13). Physical work demands (14) and previous pelvic floor surgery (15) have also been shown to confer increased risk. The

Pelvic Organ Support Study (POSST) demonstrated that straining at stool is also associated with anterior vaginal wall descent (16).

The key to anterior vaginal support is an interaction between the pelvic musculature, in which the anterior compartment sits, and the connective tissue attachments, which keep it stabilized. Any damage to either the pelvic muscular lift or the connective tissue stabilization, such as those that occur with parturition, can lead to a pathologic loss of support or destabilization (14,17). This is the excellent "boat in dry dock" analogy (18).

Nichols and Randall (19) describe two distinct types of anterior vaginal prolapse: distention and displacement (Fig. 28.2). These defects may occur individually or together. A distention cystocele is the result of attenuation of the midline anterior vaginal wall, usually secondary to overdistention at vaginal delivery. A Nichols distention cystocele is basically equivalent to a Richardson central defect. It may remain asymptomatic until menopause, when estrogen-related elastic tissue and smooth muscle are lost. The vaginal walls in these patients appear thin, with a loss of rugal folds. Since the epithelium is separated from the muscularis, it is stretched and the rugae are lost as the epithelium becomes smooth. The displacement cystocele is the other major type. It results from tearing of lateral vaginal fibroelastic cells from one or both arcus tendineii, either apically or completely (20). This is also known as a paravaginal defect (PVD). Pure PVD will spare rugae.

George White was first to describe the PVD and its vaginal repair from 1909 to 1911 (8,21). A. Cullen Richardson in the 1970s, 1980s, and 1990s (22) and then John DeLancey in the 1980s to the present (4) have advanced our understanding of female pelvic floor anatomy. Through their cadaver work we have learned the integral importance of

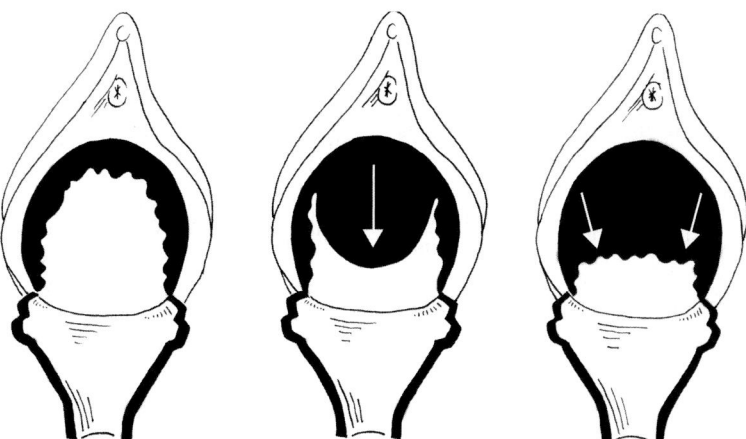

FIGURE 28.2 ● Two types of cystocele. **(A)** Well-supported: all areas of support are intact. **(B)** Distention: midline or central loss of support. **(C)** Displacement: lateral or paravaginal separation.

the ATFP (white line) and lateral attachments along with the arcus tendineus levator ani in anterior vaginal support. They have taught us well the lesson that we must carefully observe the anterior lateral sulci, in our clinic and operating rooms, given the limitations of each examination, regardless of Valsalva effort and with as much uprightness as possible, so as to not miss the PVD, complete or apical, unilateral or bilateral, when present.

Richardson et al described a transverse defect (TD) occurring as a result of separation of the anterior compartment muscular/connective tissue from its attachment to the pericervical ring of fibromuscular tissue as well as from the cardinal and uterosacral ligament complex. This defect results in a large cystocele with a bladder neck that is otherwise well supported (20).

The least common defect of anterior vaginal wall support is the distal defect, in which the distal portion of the urethra is separated from its attachment at the urogenital diaphragm/perineal membrane near the symphysis pubis. This defect is evident as an outward projection of the external urethral meatus (20).

EVALUATION

History

It is essential to quality care that the physician carefully evaluate all aspects of pelvic support and whether or not a patient has coexisting defects or problems such as urinary incontinence. Many patients who present with anterior vaginal prolapse will complain of symptoms directly associated with the protrusion of the vaginal wall as well as symptoms of voiding difficulty or urinary incontinence (22,23). Symptoms directly related to the prolapse include pelvic pressure, sensation of a vaginal bulge, vaginal fullness, low back pain, difficulty sitting, spotting, and dyspareunia. Urinary symptoms such as voiding difficulty or stress urinary incontinence commonly occur in patients with anterior vaginal prolapse (24). Many women report the need to manipulate the prolapse or use abdominal or vaginal pressure in order to facilitate voiding. Often patients report a feeling of incomplete emptying of the bladder. As the prolapse advances, many women with prior urinary incontinence will report an improvement of this condition. This is due to a kinking-type mechanism between the urethra and the advancing anterior vagina, which results in an obstruction to normal urinary flow (23). This condition could place the patient at greater risk for urinary tract infections.

Other important medical considerations include the presence of urinary urgency or frequency and past history of significant diseases, surgeries, medications, and allergies. If the patient has undergone prior pelvic operations, particularly for incontinence or prolapse, we find it very important to review these operative notes. There are sometimes important technical lessons to be learned from them, and this is preferable to learning them intraoperatively. Occasionally, such notes may guide the surgeon to alter the surgical recommendation. At the very least, the operative details, if thoroughly dictated, will add preincision knowledge and confidence to the surgical team.

Immediately after a definite plane is established (white, hypovascular, shiny), the flexed dominant index fingertip is inserted into that plane to that point where the plane ends and is extended against the vaginal undersurface. This will deepen and enlarge the dissected plane. This act is in complete counterdistinction to wrapping a Ray-tec sponge around one's index finger and, with or worse without an open plane, bluntly pulling the vaginal muscularis or bladder off the epithelium; such a rough, blunt dissection act ought to be avoided.

Although many vaginal surgeons cease the dissection more medially (31), we prefer to carry sharp dissection laterally out to the level of the medial aspect of the ischiopubic rami, apically to the anterior fornix or cuff, and distally to the periurethral connective tissue. The distal dissection limit must often be modified if a concomitant anti-incontinence procedure is to be performed. Similarly, one may not wish to disturb a well-supported anterior vault. There is at least a theoretical issue over performing a central repair, especially apically, when a PVD may have been missed. The anterior colporrhaphy may be seen to aggravate an ongoing lateral defect. Could this be one of the many possible factors responsible for the high (29%) rate of recurrent prolapse surgery (40)? There exists, therefore, an ethical and clinical imperative to get the site or sites of anterior wall defect on clinical examination and EUA "right the first time."

Venous bleeding can be encountered anywhere during anterior compartment dissection but can be most troublesome lateral to the urethrovesical junction. The minor vessels of the incision or the more apical dissection can be fully controlled with cautery or hemostat/forceps and cautery. However, the larger paraurethral venous sinuses, especially those proximate to the anterior aspect of the inferior pubic ramus, require more attention. Figure-of-eight sutures may effectively surround these low-pressure complexes, and the knots are brought down gently. We use 3-0 polyglactin on a UR-6 (5/8-circle urologic) needle passed on a Heaney needle driver in this tight place to surround the bleeding sinus while making the acute curve complete short of the bone.

Repair

Regardless of the depth of dissection and repair about to be performed, exposure in the VVS allows optional plication and imbrication of a large prolapsing bladder and its adventitia. This reduces the width of the VVS but adds little strength to the repair. It may be first plicated with a purse-string or other type of running 2-0 polyglactin or polyglycolic acid suture and imbricated with an inter-rupted or running second and sometimes third layer of the same material. The strength of the repair comes from the next layer. In the Goff full-thickness repair, the weakened distended excess medial vaginal wall is excised. Then, the repair's strength comes from suturing the undersurface of the more lateral full-thickness anterior vaginal wall where the muscular-adventitial tissue has been left connected to the epithelium. Using Bullard's split-thickness technique, the dissected muscular-adventitial vaginal layer over the bladder is carefully examined. Generally poor tissue and specific tears related to pathophysiology or dissection are noted and strategies for correction developed. Individual, site-specific tears are repaired with interrupted 2-0 polydiaxanone. The entire dissected layer can be brought together and reinforced in the midline using one or two layers of interrupted or running 2-0 polydiaxanone. The edges of the vaginal epithelium are then brought together comfortably with running 2-0 or 3-0 polyglactin after the excess is trimmed.

Regardless of dissection depth choice, one must beware of the ureter: it is closer in anterior repair than in any other gynecologic surgery (41). After initially establishing ureteral location and course during total vaginal hysterectomy anterior cul-de-sac entry, one ought to palpate it again prior to placing the first anterior colporrhaphy suture and at any point during the entire surgery where one may be within proximity to it. Figure 28.4 depicts a ureteral palpation technique. Gynecologists are concerned about avoiding the ureter near the uterine vessels during vaginal hysterectomy. A site where it is even in closer proximity to operative maneuvers is at the initial suturing of an anterior colporrhaphy, where it may be within 0.9 cm (41).

Paravaginal Repair

As George White published in 1909 (9) and Cullen Richardson in 1976 (22), a major aspect of vaginal support consists of lateral connective tissue attachments from the lateral sulcus of the anterior vaginal wall to the ATFP. Disruptions of these attachments can be corrected with high success rates utilizing the paravaginal repair, be it via vaginal (1,37), abdominal (20,34), or laparoscopic approaches (42,43).

Vaginal Paravaginal Repair

The vaginal paravaginal repair involves thorough anatomic placement of permanent sutures around the ATFP, under direct observation within the retropubic space/paravesical space by careful dis-

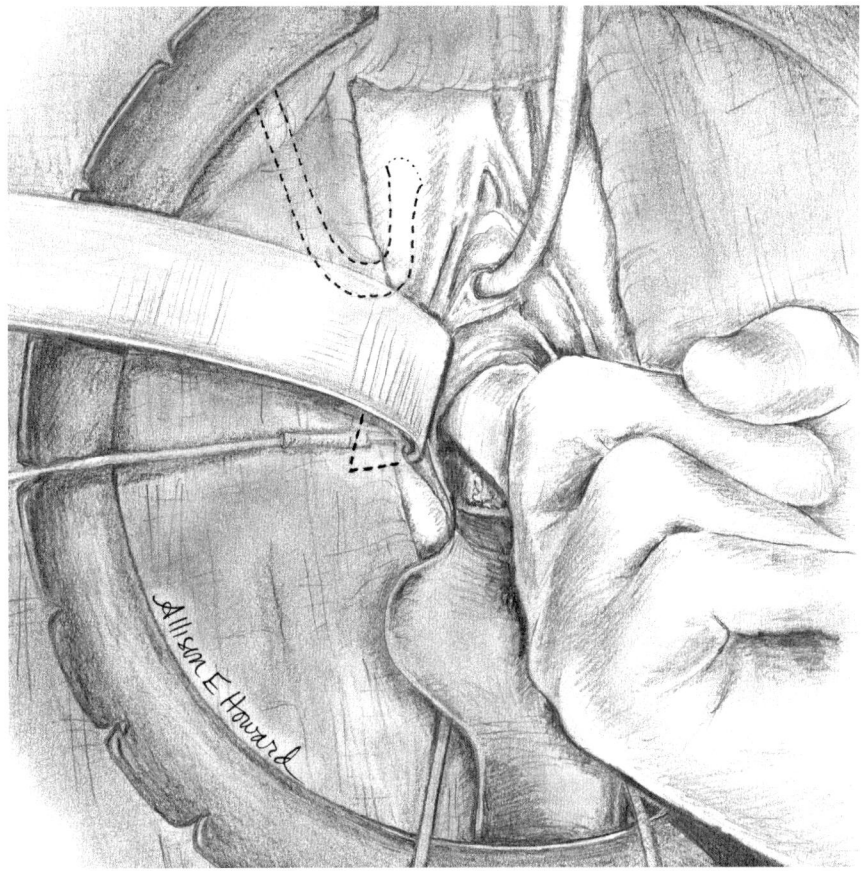

FIGURE 28.4 ● Ureteral palpation technique during vaginal surgery. One method is to begin identification from within or just outside of the anterior cul-de-sac. The dominant index fingertip begins just lateral to the tractioned Foley balloon (urethrovesical junction). It moves 3 to 4 cm cephalad and lateral, at a 30-degree angle toward the same shoulder, to the area of the ipsilateral ureterovesical junction. The ureter is felt by gentle index fingertip palpation as its volar aspect slides down in an arc posterior and lateral from 10:30 o'clock on the right side, slowly toward a vaginal Deaver tip at 9 o'clock. One often senses one's fingertip run over the ureter as a nonpulsatile, somewhat mobile, cylindrical tube, quite akin to a cooked spaghetti strand, as it approaches the Deaver. Alternatively, it may snap at the edge of the Deaver tip or just over its anterior surface. It is generally felt 2 to 4 cm away from the vaginal incision.

section from the VVS. Therefore, maximum exposure and lighting are critical. Use of the Lone Star retractor with yellow and blue hooks, a laparoscopy drape with two Velcro straps on the medial thighs, a catheterized bladder, an empty rectum, and a weighted speculum are all important. Additional lighting instruments that we use include the Vital Vue Gyn-tip and the Miyazaki lighted retractor.

The lateral limit of the anterior colporrhaphy dissection, the ischiopubic ramus, is the beginning of the paravaginal dissection. First the ischial spine is palpated laterally under the apical end of the ramus. Naturally, its anterior facet feels different than it usually does from a posterior perspective. Running one's dominant index finger medially, anterior, and cephalad, the operator comes to

the inferolateral pubic bone. It is not quite as distinct as the anterior aspect of the spine and feels like a rough corner. These two points are critical because they mark the boundaries of the linear ATFP to which one will reattach the vaginal anterior lateral sulcus.

At 1 to 2 cm anterior to the spine, exerting slight lateral, perpendicular pressure on a closed curved Mayo scissor, just under the ramus and over the volar aspect of the nondominant index fingertip, very gently opens a small window into the retropubic space. This window is enlarged minimally with cautious scissor and fingertip dissection before placing serially sized Breisky or Deaver retractors anteriorly and a Miyazaki (Miya) lighted retractor medially, all very deliberately just within the window. Proof that the dissection is correctly in the RPS is obtained by demonstrating the pelvic side wall, retropubic fat, and the fatty cylindrical obturator neurovascular bundle descending at the far limit of the exposure. The ATFP is prepared for suturing by carefully retracting the bladder medially with the Miya lighted retractor and the ureter and anterior abdominal wall anteriorly with a Deaver. A posterior Breisky is optional. The operator is anxious to obtain optimal exposure prior to placing arcus sutures. Nevertheless, one must be extremely cautious with forward movement of the retractor tips. If the long retractor tips are adjusted forward without direct observation by the surgeon, they are at high risk of endangering large veins.

Damaged paravaginal attachments result in an ATFP that is quite variable to palpation and appearance. Palpating between the two landmark limits of the arcus will show whether it is present or has been torn away from the side wall. In the latter case, we suture in the same manner as if it were present. The line (arcus) that is or was between the two bony prominences serves as a series of points 1 cm apart. Each point marks the center of a circle around which a 0-grade permanent suture is sewn, having a diameter of 2 cm, and is passed perpendicular to the ATFP. The CT-1 type of needle pass may begin with a 1-cm 90-degree curve on either the obturator internus or levator ani side, turning widely around the real or surmised arcus and turning back 90 degrees widely to include a 1-cm pass through the other muscle. We begin suturing 1.5 cm anterior to the spine (Fig. 28.5) and move up 1 cm apart toward the pubic bone with each successive vaginal paravaginal repair stitch. Usually four to six sutures are placed

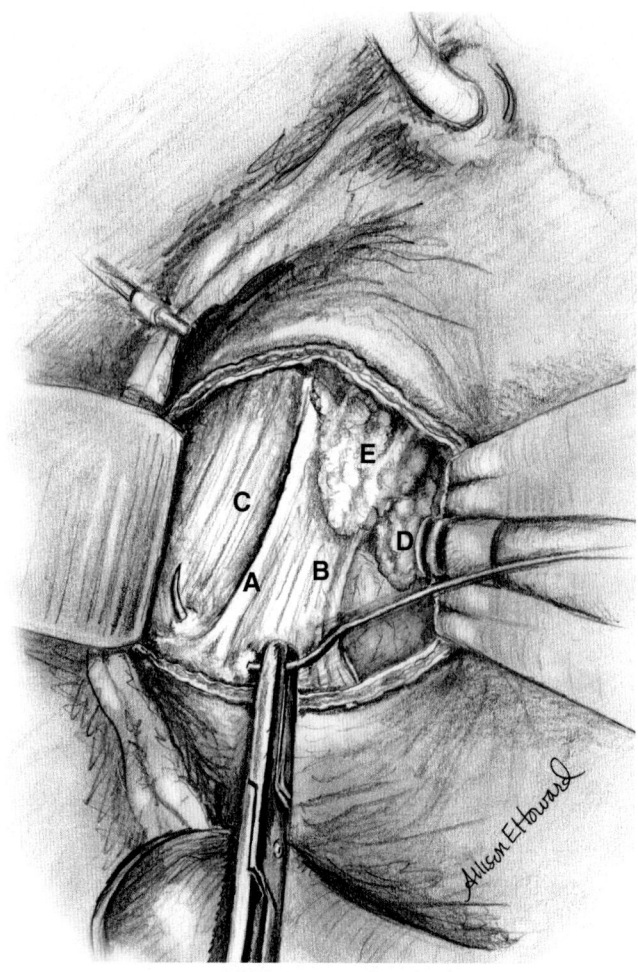

FIGURE 28.5 ● Vaginal paravaginal repair: first suture. A = arcus tendineus fascia pelvis (ATFP), B = obturator internus muscle, C = levator ani muscle, D = obturator neurovascular bundle, E = retropubic fat.

on each side in a complete bilateral paravaginal defect. We prefer the heavy-jawed 14-inch Nolan needle driver, not so much for its extreme length as for its jaw's steadiness and the instrument's overall ease and security in obtaining the important paravaginal wide bites. A long straight needle driver facilitates needle retrieval. Alternatively, some prefer the Capio Suture Capturing Device (Boston Scientific, Natick, MA). Gentle traction in the opposite direction on the arcus suture should give the sense of a secure purchase. Any doubt mandates a second slightly deeper throw while placing mild traction on the first throw. The ATFP sutures must be kept parallel. The Velcro straps that come with the double-aperture laparoscopy drape with cystoscopy drainage bag work very well for this. Before sewing the arcus sutures to the vagina and bladder, we perform the anterior muscularis plication and other anterior compartment procedures as indicated.

The ATFP sutures are then sewn to the connective tissue layers of the bladder and the vagina at matching levels. For each of these two points, we locate halfway between the ramus and the midline. Sewing the vagina and bladder to the ATFP at points too lateral results in an inadequate lift. Choosing points too medial yields a very dramatic anterolateral elevation of a vagina that one cannot close. In contrast, sewing and tying at the midpoints yields dramatic anterolateral lift and tension-free skin closure. Any remaining slight excess epithelium is trimmed and the vagina closed with running, 2-0 polyglycolic acid or polyglactin suture.

Transverse Defect Repair

Following vaginal hysterectomy, the anterior vaginal wall is shorter than the posterior wall due to cervical excision. The connective tissue supports of the proximal anterior vagina will also be weakened if there is a transverse defect. This leaves a large anterior apical gap and an even larger area without a muscular-adventitial layer. Repair of the TD is performed as part of the culdeplasty. When supporting the apex and orienting the vault more horizontally over the levator plate with the high (or deep) uterosacral ligament vaginal vault suspension (HUS), one must remember the importance of lifting the anterior as well as the posterior vault. It is important to repair a transverse defect and cervical gap as well as to support the proximal anterior wall. Many techniques accomplish this (44,45). Is the inclusion of the anterior apical skin in the HUS adequate to close the cervical gap and repair the transverse defect? Do we not often leave a signifi-

cant anterior apical gap in women suffering from transverse defect?

The technique that follows is one possible method to repair a TD, close the cervical gap, and help suspend the anterior apex. 0 polypropyl or polydiaxanone sutures support, close, and elevate the anterior and posterior lateral apices to the midcardinal ligament bilaterally, while a midline suture connects both anterior and posterior apices, right and left sides. During a preliminary vaginal hysterectomy, the cardinal ligament pedicle must be taken in a manner similar to preparing the uterosacral ligaments for HUS. Essentially, this means palpation and pedicle preparation such that the cardinal ligament pedicle will be free of vessels yet its support value maximized. After completion of the anterior repair, a running suture is used to close the anterior wall. The bilateral and midline TD repair sutures are placed as described in Figure 28.6. It is always wise to repalpate the ureter before suturing the cardinal ligament. The HUS, with or without wedge excision, may have already been performed and wedge closure completed. This should not compromise TD repair exposure and will facilitate its posterior apical suture site choice. Even in the absence of a transverse defect, these three sutures help support the apex and close the anterior apical gap left from cervical excision.

Once the surgeon is satisfied with all support and anterior work, the sutures are tied and held to facilitate removal should cystoscopy reveal a problem. Thorough intravesical evaluation for sutures and ureteral patency via IV indigo carmine is essential following every major anterior and/or apical operation. Failure to see projectile blue dye from one or both ureteral orifices mandates investigation.

To our knowledge this is a new modification for anterior apical support and TD repair. We have found no studies of any kind either describing this technique or quantifying its results in the literature since 1966. We have not yet studied this technique, as we have begun using it only in January 2006.

Pubourethral Ligament Plication

When performing an anterior colporrhaphy, what is the surgeon to do when the patient complains of stress urinary incontinence and demonstrates urethral hypermobility but has no urodynamic stress incontinence on urodynamic evaluation? One can repeat the cough stress test. If it remains negative, one may feel hard-pressed to perform a definitive antiincontinence procedure. This is a good opportunity to perform the single-suture pubourethral ligament plication (PULP), which should decrease urethral hypermobility and may eliminate stress urinary in-

all; its appearance is quite variable depending upon the nature of the PVD. Having found the two bony landmarks, we take large sutures around the line connecting the two points. Although the ATFP's condition in PVD is quite variable, the sharp angle seen where the vertical obturator internus meets the horizontal lateral vagina clarifies any ATFP suture placement dilemma. Naturally, the junction of vertical and horizontal is often separated; this is the defect. To repair the defect one should continue to use the junction line between the two bony points as a series of suture centers for large (2-cm diameter) permanent stitches reattaching the lateral vaginal sulcus to the obturator internus, trying to include both ATFP and superior levator ani.

The vaginal vault is the keystone of pelvic support and we must focus on it during every reconstructive operation. When PVDs are partial, the defect occurs first at the apical end; therefore, we feel it most important to primarily sew the apex of the defect. The index and middle fingers of the nondominant hand intravaginally elevate the apical anterior sulcus. This will further help delineate both anatomy and defect. The intravaginal finger will aid in judging the depth of the needle to spare the vaginal lumen, while obtaining a wide 1-cm-long bite. If the suture is thin and short, it will increase the risk of tear-out when exposed to impact activities.

After sewing the vaginal apical sulcus, the needle is passed widely around the inferior aspect of the obturator internus fascia, 1.5 cm anterior to the ischial spine. Continuing toward the pubis, 2-cm-diameter sutures are placed reattaching the lateral vagina to the pelvic side wall, 1 to 1.5 cm apart. If bleeding occurs on suturing, tying them will usually stop it. They are otherwise held parallel. After all sutures are placed, the knots are tied, again from spine towards the pubis.

Laparoscopic Paravaginal Repair

The goal of laparoscopic pelvic reconstruction is to accomplish the same type of pelvic repair that would otherwise be done through an open incision. Miklos et al (43) describe their laparoscopic repair as follows. Utilizing an infraumbilical open laparoscopy technique and three ancillary ports, the peritoneal cavity is entered and the superior bladder border identified with retrograde fill. Transperitoneal entry into the RPS above the bladder reflection is confirmed by the presence of loose areolar tissue. From this point and following bladder drainage, RPS exposure, identification of landmarks, and visualization of RP anatomy follows just as it did during the open abdominal and vaginal approaches. Again, an intravaginal finger may aid in demonstrating the location and extent of the PVD on either side. The first stitch is near the vaginal apex and then the obturator internus muscle and fascia, with the ATFP if present, all within 1 to 2 cm of the ischial spine. This may be secured with extracorporeal knot tying. Four or five similar sutures are placed between the ischial spine and the midurethra and repeated on both sides for the very common bilateral defects.

Augmented Repairs

Long-term cystocele cure rates vary widely in the recent literature, more likely due to evolving patient-centered outcome measures than to different procedures utilized or surgeons performing them. Reliable authors have reached long-term success rates between 40% and 97% (see Table 28.1). The pelvic connective tissues have been weakened and/or torn. The muscles and nerves are often damaged. Although we may reattach connective tissue to strong locations, the tissue we are using is weak. Therefore, might it be worthwhile to replace or reinforce badly damaged or absent muscular-connective tissue with biologic graft or synthetic mesh? The ideal mesh would be permanently strong, made of monofilament single inert fibers that are not woven but form a very large pore. The vaginal bacterial flora should find the pores too large for colonization, yet they should allow the body's defensive and connective tissue cells access to get through and do their work. Polypropylene has been rated a type I mesh in anterior compartment prolapse erosion risk (the least likely to cause erosion). Erosion is a localized denudation of vaginal epithelium that can leave granulation, usually in the form of a small circle (up to 1×1 cm) in the midincision line. This may be asymptomatic (exposure) or cause mucosanguinous discharge. Further discussion of vaginal mesh is in a dedicated chapter. Unfortunately, up until 2006, there has been a good deal of "heat" from both the pro- and anti-mesh and graft sides, without benefit of real light in the form of high-level clinical research from either.

COMMENTS

The body of this chapter is meant to demonstrate how we have begun to finally put an end to Ahlfelt's admonition. The long-term success of anterior compartment prolapse surgery, based on high-quality objective and subjective outcome measures, patient-centered goals, and quality-of-life instruments, will improve during the next two decades. Why? Our subspecialty is rapidly growing. The number of fellowship-trained urogynecologists, both in academic and private practice, has enlarged greatly during the past decade as our American Urogynecologic Society has similarly shown dramatic growth. Our better pelvic floor research is both of high quality and creative. Newer imaging, epidemiologic, biomechanical, risk assessment, and basic science studies will possibly lead us all the way to effective preventive strategies to help avoid a significant percentage of anterior compartment and other forms of prolapse. John DeLancey, during his SGS presidential address at the First Joint AUGS/SGS Meeting in 2004, set for us a goal of "25% prevention and 25% treatment improvement achieved by 2025" (46). Therapeutically, reconstructive pelvic surgeons' techniques, experience, and instrumentation are becoming more often expert as their training and understanding continue to rapidly grow and evolve.

As the newest therapeutic wave to hit the clinical shore, synthetic meshes and organic grafts should be evaluated via type I evidence-based research. They ought to be studied in randomized clinical trials, controlled against today's best reconstructive operations without augmentation. If, for example, an anterior colporrhaphy with polypropylene mesh, properly anchored, albeit tension-free, demonstrates a higher 2-year or better 5-year success rate without an increased complication rate than the standard repair, then the mesh anterior colporrhaphy ought to gain broad credibility and general acceptance.

Whether the mesh and/or graft wave proves a success and eventually covers most recurrent prolapses or ends as so many other failed waves have is a story soon to be told. With or without meshes and grafts, this extraordinarily common and troubling problem of anterior prolapse is gradually responding better to our newer reconstructive pelvic surgical procedures. As the beautifully intricate three-dimensional anatomy, pathophysiology, and surgery of anterior pelvic floor prolapse reach a deeper clarity to all of us, who now constitute a critical mass of fully trained subspecialty gynecologic surgeons, we can truly expect to see continued improvements in all aspects of reconstructive surgical outcomes. Also, using public awareness programs to transmit lessons learned from our epidemiologic and other research colleagues who are defining prolapse risk factors, a new generation of women may learn how to minimize their potential for pelvic floor prolapse. In the anterior prolapse category of pelvic floor dysfunction, an increase in both prevention and surgical efficacy will mean a great deal to our patients, where the prevalence is now 34% and the problem so often becomes a major disturbance to a woman's life.

REFERENCES

1. Weber AM, Walter MD. Anterior vaginal prolapse: Review of anatomy and techniques of surgical repair. *Obstet Gynecol* 1997;89:311–318.
2. Boreham MK, Wai CY, Miller RT, et al. Morphometric analysis of smooth muscle in the anterior vaginal wall of women with pelvic organ prolapse. *Am J Obstet Gynecol* 2002;187(1):56–63.
3. Albright TS, Gehrich AP, Davis GD, et al. Arcus tendineus fascia pelvis: A further understanding. *Am J Obstet Gynecol* 2005;193:677–681.
4. DeLancey JOL. Anatomic aspects of vaginal eversion after hysterectomy. *Am J Obstet Gynecol* 1992;166:1717–1728.
5. Tunn R, DeLancey JOL, Quint EE. Visibility of pelvic organ support system structures in magnetic resonance images without an endovaginal coil. *Am J Obstet Gynecol* 2001;184:1156–1163.
6. DeLancey JO, Kearney R, Chou Q, et al. The appearance of levator ani muscle abnormalities in magnetic resonance images after vaginal delivery. *Obstet Gynecol* 2003;101(1):46–53.
7. Aronson MP, Bates SM, Jacoby AF. Periurethral and paravaginal anatomy: an endovaginal magnetic resonance imaging study. *Am J Obstet Gynecol* 1995;173(6):1702–1708.
8. Hendrix SL, Clark A, Nygaard I, et al. Pelvic organ prolapse in the Women's Health Initiative: Gravity and gravidity. *Am J Obstet Gynecol* 2002;186:1160–1166.
9. White GR. Cystocele, a radical cure by suturing lateral sulci of vagina to white line of pelvic fascia. *JAMA* 1909;21:1707–1710.
10. Leffler KS, Thompson JR, Cundiff GW, et al. Attachment of the rectovaginal septum to the pelvic sidewall. *Am J Obstet Gynecol* 2001;185(1):41–43.
11. Abrams P, Cardozo L, Fall M, et al. Standardization Subcommittee of the International Continence Society. The standardization of terminology in lower urinary tract function. *Urology* 2003;61(1):37–49.
12. Smith AR, Hosker GL, Warrell DW. The role of pudendal nerve damage in the etiology of genuine stress incontinence in women. *Br J Obstet Gynaecol* 1989;96:29–32.
13. Norton PA, Baker JE, Sharp HC, et al. Genitourinary prolapse and joint hypermobility in women. *Obstet Gynecol* 1995;85:225–228.
14. Chiaffarino F, Chatenoud L, Dindelli M, et al. Reproductive factors, family history, occupation, and risk of urogenital prolapse. *Eur J Obstet Gynecol Reprod Biol* 1999;82(1):63–67.
15. Swift SE, Pound T, Dias JK. Case-control study of etiologic factors in the development of severe pelvic organ prolapse. *Int Urogynecol J* 2001;12(3):187–192.
16. Kahn MA, Radecki Breitkopf C, Valley MT, et al. Pelvic Organ Support Study (POSST) and bowel symptoms: Straining at stool is associated with perineal and anterior vaginal descent in a general gynecologic population. *Am J Obstet Gynecol* 2005;192(5):1516–1522.
17. Schaffer JI, Wai CY, Boreham MK. Etiology of pelvic organ prolapse. *Clin Obstet Gynecol* 2005;48(3):639–647.

18. Norton PA. Pelvic floor disorders: the role of fascia and ligaments. *Clin Obstet Gynecol* 1993;36(4):926–938.

19. Nichols DH, Randall CL, eds. *Vaginal surgery*, 4th ed. Baltimore: Williams & Wilkins, 1996.

20. Richardson AC. Paravaginal repair. In: Hurt WG, ed. *Urogynecologic surgery*. Maryland: Ashland Publishers, 1992;5-3:73–80.

21. White GR. *An anatomical operation for the cure of cystocele*. Read before the 24th annual Meeting of the American Association of Obstetricians/Gynecologists, Louisville, KY, September 1911.

22. Richardson AC, Lyons JB, Williams NL. A new look at pelvic relaxation. *Am J Obstet Gynecol* 1976;126: 568–573.

23. Romanzi LJ, Chaikin DC, Blaivas JG. The effect of genital prolapse on voiding. *J Urol* 1999;161(2): 581–586.

24. Bump RC, Fantl JA, Hurt WG. The mechanism of urinary incontinence in women with severe uterovaginal prolapse: results of barrier studies. *Obstet Gynecol* 1988; 72(3 pt 1):291–295.

25. Bump RC, Mattiasson A, Bo K, et al. The standardization of terminology of female pelvic organ prolapse and pelvic floor dysfunction. *Am J Obstet Gynecol* 1996; 175(1):10–17.

26. Whiteside JL, Barber MD, Paraiso MF, et al. Clinical evaluation of anterior vaginal wall support defects: interexaminer and intraexaminer reliability. *Am J Obstet Gynecol* 2004;191(1):100–104.

27. Baden WF, Walker TA. Statistical evaluation of vaginal relaxation. *Clin Obstet Gynecol* 1972;15:1070–1072.

28. Bhatia NN, Bergman A. Pessary test in women with urinary incontinence. *Obstet Gynecol* 1985;65(2):220–226.

29. Porges RF, Smilen SW. Long-term analysis of the surgical management of pelvic support defects. *Am J Obstet Gynecol* 1994;171:1518–1528.

30. Colombo M, Vitobello D, Proietti F, et al. Randomized comparison of Burch colposuspension versus anterior colporrhaphy in women with stress urinary incontinence and anterior vaginal wall prolapse. *Br J Obstet Gynaecol* 2000;107(4):544–551.

31. Weber AM, Walter MD, Piedmonte MR, et al. Anterior colporrhaphy: A randomized trial of three surgical techniques. *Am J Obstet Gynecol* 2001;185:1299–1306.

32. Korshunov MY, Sergeeva IV, Zhivov AV, et al. *Prospective randomized controlled trial of polypropylene mesh to prevent recurrence of anterior vaginal prolapse*. Oral Poster Presentation, AUGS/SGS Joint Scientific Meeting, San Diego, CA, August 2004.

33. Gandhi S, Goldberg RP, Kwon C, et al. A prospective randomized trial using solvent dehydrated fascia lata for the prevention of recurrent anterior vaginal wall prolapse. *Am J Obstet Gynecol* 2005;192:1649–1654.

34. Richardson AC, Edmonds PB, Williams NL. Treatment of stress urinary incontinence due to paravaginal fascial defect. *Obstet Gynecol* 1981;57:357–362.

35. Shull BL, Baden WF. A six-year experience with paravaginal defect repair for stress urinary incontinence. *Am J Obstet Gynecol* 1989;160:1432–1440.

36. Shull BL, Benn SJ, Kuehl TJ. Surgical management of prolapse of the anterior vaginal segment: an analysis of support defects, operative morbidity, and anatomic outcome. *Am J Obstet Gynecol* 1994;171(6):1429–1439.

37. Young SB, Daman JJ, Bony LG. Vaginal paravaginal repair: One-year outcomes. *Am J Obstet Gynecol* 2001; 185:1360–1367.

38. Barber MD, Cundiff GW, Weidner AC, et al. Accuracy of clinical assessment of paravaginal defects in women with anterior vaginal wall prolapse. *Am J Obstet Gynecol* 1999;181(1):87–90.

39. Segal JL, Vassallo BJ, Kleeman SD, et al. Paravaginal defects: prevalence and accuracy of preoperative detection. *Int Urogynecol J* 2004;15(6):378–383.

40. Olsen AL, Smith VJ, Bergstrom JO, et al. Epidemiology of surgically managed pelvic organ prolapse and urinary incontinence. *Obstet Gynecol* 1997;89(4):501–506.

41. Hofmeister FJ. "Cinefluorography" video. Marquette University Medical School, Milwaukee Hospital, Milwaukee County Hospital.

42. Weber AM. New approaches to surgery for urinary incontinence and pelvic organ prolapse from the laparoscopic perspective. *Clin Obstet Gynecol* 2003;46(1):44–60.

43. Miklos JR, Moore RD, Kohli N. Laparoscopic pelvic floor repair. *Obstet Gynecol Clin North Am* 2004;31(3): 551–565.

44. Cruikshank SH, Kovac SR. Anterior vaginal wall culdeplasty at vaginal hysterectomy to prevent posthysterectomy anterior vaginal wall prolapse. *Am J Obstet Gynecol* 1996;174(6):1863–1872.

45. Shull BL, Bachofen C, Coates KW, et al. A transvaginal approach to repair of apical and other associated sites of pelvic organ prolapse with uterosacral ligaments. *Am J Obstet Gynecol* 2000;183:1365–1374.

46. DeLancey JOL. The hidden epidemic of pelvic floor dysfunction: achievable goals for improved prevention and treatment. *Am J Obstet Gynecol* 2005;192(5):1488–1495.

CHAPTER 29

Apical Support Defects

Robert E. Gutman

INTRODUCTION

Pelvic organ prolapse (POP) is a common condition, with an estimated 225,964 surgical procedures performed in 1997, according to the National Hospital Discharge Survey (1). There is an 11% lifetime risk of surgery for prolapse and urinary incontinence, with a reoperation rate of about 30% (2). The annual cost for treating POP has been estimated to be $1 billion (3). Prolapse treatment options include observation without intervention, pessary fitting, or surgery, as previously discussed in Chapter 27. This chapter provides a comprehensive review of surgical management of apical support defects and a decision analysis for choosing an appropriate procedure.

Anatomical studies of vaginal support have demonstrated different levels of support, and POP in any given patient is usually a combination of support defects. The uterosacral and cardinal ligaments provide level I support of the vaginal apex; the lateral attachments of the endopelvic fascia and vagina to the arcus tendineus fascia pelvis contribute level II support of the anterior and posterior vaginal walls; and the perineal membrane and perineal body ensure level III support of the distal vagina and surrounding structures (urethrovesical junction and perineum) (4). The muscular integrity and neurological function of the levator ani also play a critical role in the support mechanism. Proper surgical correction requires identification of the anatomical defects, which can be present at the vaginal apex, rectovaginal fascia, and pubocervical fascia. Recent studies displayed a high correlation of apical descensus with anterior vaginal wall prolapse (5,6). While this seems relatively intuitive, it emphasizes the need for appropriate apical suspension to adequately correct anterior vaginal wall prolapse. Posterior vaginal wall prolapse may also be correlated with apical support, although the degree of correlation seems less than that of the anterior wall. Surgical repair frequently combines repairs of the anterior vaginal wall, posterior vaginal wall, and vaginal apex, depending on the specific support defects present. Consequently, proper identification of all support defects is essential, and correction of apical support is frequently the cornerstone of many prolapse surgeries.

Prolapse surgery should strive to alleviate symptoms related to pelvic support, restore normal anatomical relationships, optimize bladder, bowel, and coital function, and correct coexisting pelvic pathology using a durable repair with low morbidity. In choosing the best procedure for a patient, surgery should be individualized taking into account patient factors, surgeon factors, as well as patient preferences and expectations. Patient factors include those that potentially increase the risk of recurrent prolapse (prior prolapse surgery, severity of prolapse [7], young age [7], wide genital hiatus [8], levator weakness, and increased intra-abdominal pressures from occupation/recreation involving heavy lifting, continual cough from tobacco use, obesity, and chronic constipation) and those that may favor one approach over another due to morbidity and effect on vaginal dimensions (comorbid conditions, obesity, shortened vaginal length). Surgeon factors that influence selection of a specific procedure include the surgeon's repertoire, specific surgical expertise, concomitant procedures planned (hysterectomy, incontinence surgery, cystocele repair, rectocele repair), and existing biases. These factors are all greatly influenced by residency and/or fellowship training.

SURGICAL PROCEDURES FOR APICAL SUPPORT

Apical support procedures can be divided into three groups: restorative procedures that use native support structures; compensatory procedures that add a graft for increased strength; and obliterative procedures that close the vaginal lumen. Sacral colpopexy is the most commonly utilized compensatory repair. While typically performed through a laparotomy, it can also be accomplished laparoscopically. It is widely considered to be the most durable surgical procedure for anatomical support of the vaginal apex, with the lowest rate of recurrent vault prolapse (9–12). There are several restorative procedures, which are usually vaginal repairs, including uterosacral ligament suspension, sacrospinous ligament fixation, iliococcygeus suspension, and McCall culdoplasty. Obliterative procedures such as the LeFort colpocleisis or total colpocleisis/colpectomy are less invasive and offer success rates similar to sacral colpopexy, with low complication rates. Although these are apical support procedures, they are covered in detail in Chapter 31. This chapter will concentrate on restorative and compensatory procedures that maintain vaginal integrity.

There is a wide variety of opinion regarding the optimal vaginal procedure, and there are no prospective comparative studies. There are retrospective and prospective trials comparing sacral colpopexy to sacrospinous ligament fixation, with conflicting results. Sacral colpopexy appears to have less recurrent apical prolapse, but there may be advantages of the vaginal approach such as decreased morbidity, less postoperative pain, and quicker return to activities of daily living. There may not be an advantage for either approach when considering symptomatic improvement or overall patient satisfaction. Alternatively, one approach may have benefits for certain patient populations. Therefore, surgeons must decipher the literature to determine the best approach for a particular patient. The choice of procedure also depends on the surgeon's comfort with a procedure and his or her ability to perform a variety of different operations for apical prolapse.

The purpose of the following sections is to provide an in-depth analysis of the most commonly used restorative and compensatory repairs. Surgical technique will be discussed with specific attention paid to key steps in the procedures. Anatomical outcomes, symptomatic improvement, and complication rates will be reviewed based on the available literature. After this has been outlined for each individual surgery, the results of comparative studies, both prospective and retrospective, will be appraised.

Restorative Procedures

McCall Culdoplasty

Surgical Technique

McCall was the first to publish a technique known by many as the "New Orleans culdoplasty" that used the uterosacral ligaments for support and treatment of enterocele. While he named the technique the "posterior culdeplasty," the technique became known as the McCall culdoplasty (13). Though described initially as a primary apical support procedure at the time of vaginal hysterectomy, many utilize the McCall culdoplasty prophylactically to prevent enteroceles. Apical descensus permitting vaginal hysterectomy suggests the need for an apical support procedure to prevent development of vaginal vault prolapse.

The McCall culdoplasty has been modified over the years, but the basic principles remain unchanged. McCall recommended placement of internal nonabsorbable sutures and external absorbable sutures. He advocated at least three internal nonabsorbable sutures, with the first suture placed approximately 2 cm above the cut edge of the uterosacral ligament. After stitching the uterosacral ligament, several bites of peritoneum overlying the rectum, including the redundant enterocele sac, are taken at 1- to 2-cm intervals until the contralateral uterosacral ligament is reached and stitched. While the ends of the first suture are held, additional internal sutures are placed proximal to the first. The number of internal sutures depends on the size of the enterocele. Next, the external absorbable sutures are placed just lateral to the midline, near the vaginal cuff, through the proximal posterior vaginal wall and peritoneum. The posteromedial aspect of the ipsilateral ligament is then sutured, followed by the contralateral ligament, and finally the suture exits the peritoneum and proximal posterior vaginal wall close to the cuff just lateral to the midline at the level of insertion. McCall recommended three external sutures, placed at intervals between the internal stitches, with the highest suture placed at the top of the newly supported vagina. Internal sutures are tied first, followed by external sutures, plicating the uterosacral ligaments to the posterior vaginal cuff and obliterating the cul-de-sac.

Modifications of this technique have subsequently been developed, including the Mayo, Mayo-McCall, modified, and high McCall culdoplasty. These variations differ with respect to the number of internal and external sutures, shortening of the uterosacral ligaments, and external sutures that incorporate the cul-de-sac peritoneum. When performing this procedure, we typically use one or two nonabsorbable internal sutures followed by a single absorbable external suture, all of which incorporate cul-de-sac peritoneum. The external McCall suture is normally tied after cuff closure by pushing the cuff cephalad toward the sacrum. Cuff closure can be considerably more challenging after these sutures have already been tied into place (Fig. 29.1).

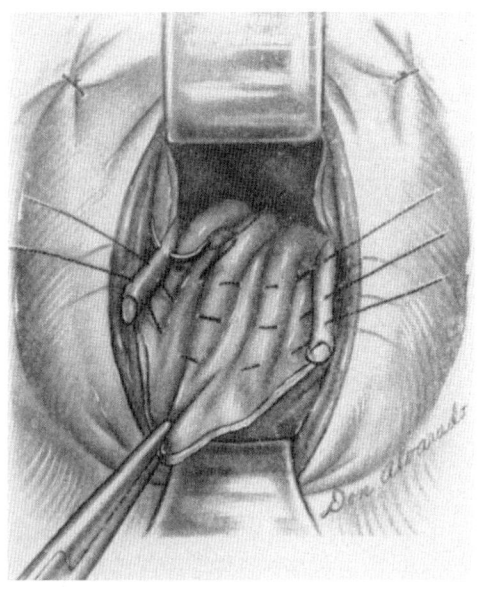
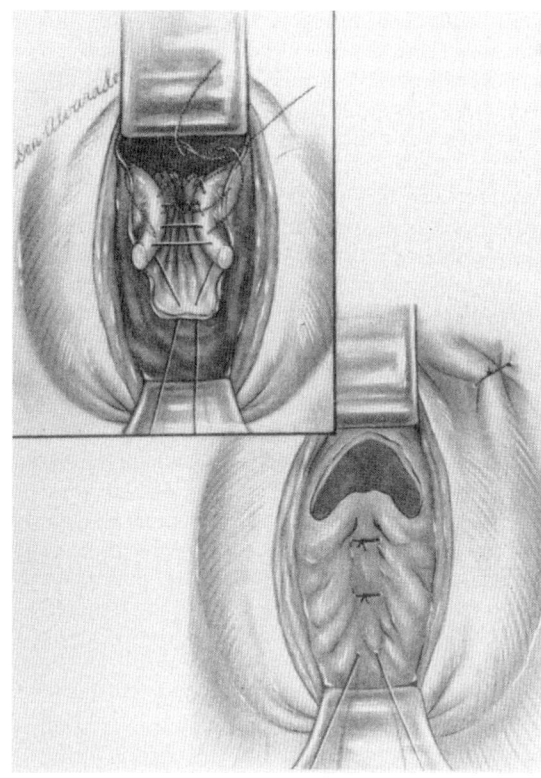

A   B

FIGURE 29.1 • McCall culdoplasty. **(A)** The three internal stitches have been placed from one uterosacral ligament to the other, incorporating peritoneum in between. **(B)** In the upper frame, the internal stitches are tied down, plicating the uterosacral ligaments in the midline. In the lower frame, the external stitches are tied down, suspending the vaginal cuff to the uterosacral ligaments.

Surgical Outcomes

McCall (13) reported on a series of 45 patients undergoing posterior culdeplasty. All but two procedures were done at the time of vaginal hysterectomy. Follow-up ranged from 3 months to 3 years, and there had been no known cases of recurrent enterocele formation or vault prolapse. The procedure was found to restore vaginal length without shortening.

Symmonds et al (14) evaluated the results of 180 patients undergoing a Mayo culdoplasty for grade III or IV vault prolapse. Successful repair based on anatomical assessment, and overall patient satisfaction was accomplished in 142 (89%) of the 160 patients available for follow-up between 1 and 12 years postoperatively. Nine (5.5%) women had "fair" results, all of whom had adequate apical support but required reoperation for recurrent anterior or posterior wall prolapse. Seven (4%) of the nine who had "poor" results required reoperation to obtain a "good" result. Among the other two patients with a "poor" result, one had recurrent vault prolapse and the other died postoper-

atively from a myocardial infarction. Other serious complications were rare.

Webb et al (15) reported on 660 women undergoing Mayo culdoplasty for primary repair of post-hysterectomy vault prolapse. Subjective outcomes of mailed and telephone questionnaires revealed an absence of prolapse symptoms, overall satisfaction, and a low reoperation rate for the majority of respondents. Low intraoperative and perioperative complication rates were observed: 2.3% cystotomy or proctotomy repaired immediately without sequelae, 1.3% vault hematoma, 0.6% cuff cellulitis or abscess, and 2.2% blood transfusions.

Karram et al (16) performed a large retrospective case series of high uterosacral ligament suspension with plication, a similar but modified McCall culdoplasty. The uterosacral ligaments and intervening peritoneum were plicated with nonabsorbable sutures and the superior aspects of the pubocervical and rectovaginal fascia were then anchored to the ligaments on each side using delayed absorbable sutures. Of the 168 women available for follow-up, 150 (89%) were "happy" or "satisfied" with their results at an average of 21.6 months. There were two (1%) apical recurrences and a 5.5% overall reoperation rate, with an additional 5% having at least grade 2 recurrent prolapse that was either asymptomatic or did not require further treatment. There was also one small bowel injury that required laparotomy and one postoperative ileus from a pelvic abscess that required delayed laparotomy, abscess draining, and colonic diversion.

Colombo and Milani (17) retrospectively evaluated 62 women undergoing a modified McCall culdoplasty for grade 2 or 3 uterine prolapse using a series of three absorbable sutures. Over a median follow-up of 3 years, 15% had recurrent prolapse, but only 5% had recurrences that involved the vaginal apex. There were no major complications.

A major concern in surgeries that require suture placement through the uterosacral ligament is ureteral injury. McCall culdoplasty procedures have low rates of ureteral injury, ranging from 0% to 3%. Colombo (17) and Symmonds (14) did not observe any ureteral injuries in their series. This is in contrast to the larger Webb et al (15) series of 660, with four (0.6%) ureteral injuries: 1 patient developed a ureterovaginal fistula requiring ureteroneocystotomy; 1 injury resolved with observation; 1 patient required stent placement; and 1 patient needed laparotomy with removal of the modified McCall sutures. Most likely these four cases present only the symptomatic postoperative ureteral obstructions. The true ureteral injury rate may be higher with potentially asymptomatic undiagnosed cases in the absence of routine intraoperative cystoscopy. Using universal intraoperative cystoscopy, Karram et al (16) had five (3%) ureteral injuries: four involved ureteral kinking, which resolved after releasing the sutures, and one ureterotomy requiring ureteral reimplantation. Aronson et al (18) more recently reported only three (0.7%) ureteral injuries in 411 consecutive cases using intraoperative cystoscopy with intravenous indigo carmine, with only one (0.24%) attributable to a Mayo-McCall uterosacral ligament suspension.

While the above procedures document success rates for McCall culdoplasty as an apical support procedure, many consider it primarily for prevention and treatment of enteroceles. Cruikshank and Kovak (19) performed a randomized control trial comparing three different surgical treatments to prevent enterocele formation at the time of vaginal hysterectomy. At 3 years, the modified McCall culdoplasty had fewer stage I and stage II posterior superior vaginal segment (enterocele) recurrences (2/33 vs. 10/33 and 13/33 in the other two groups,

$p = 0.004$). Thus, McCall culdoplasty is useful for prevention and treatment of enteroceles as well as apical support.

Uterosacral Ligament Suspension

Surgical Technique

The uterosacral ligaments have been utilized in vaginal reconstructions as early as 1927, when Miller (20) described bilateral suspension of the vaginal vault to the uterosacral ligaments. Techniques have evolved over time with modifications to the attachment sites, plication methods, and cul-de-sac closure. More recently there has been a trend to leave the uterosacral ligaments in a more physiologic position without midline plication. We believe this to be the major distinction between the McCall culdoplasty techniques listed above and uterosacral ligament suspensions.

Following vaginal hysterectomy or posthysterectomy cuff colpotomy, the patient is placed in Trendelenburg position and the small bowel is packed away using a moistened 6-inch Kerlix sponge. Breisky-Navratil retractors help deflect the rectum medially and the bowel and surgical pack cephalad. The remnants of the distal uterosacral ligaments are identified and grasped. Caudal traction on the distal uterosacral ligament along with the use of a headlamp facilitates visualization of the fanlike projection toward the sacrum. The first nonabsorbable suture of at least 2-0 gauge is placed at the level of the ischial spine, with care taken to avoid locations within 1 cm of the anterior edge of the uterosacral ligament, where the ureter is more vulnerable. Traction on this first suture assists placement of a second more proximal suture approximately 1 cm craniosacral to the ischial spine. One end of each suture is then secured to the pubocervical fascia and anterior vaginal wall excluding the epithelium and the other to the rectovaginal fascia and posterior vaginal wall excluding the epithelium. If using two sutures on each side, the proximal uterosacral suture is placed approximately 1 cm medial to the distal uterosacral suture, which is secured near the angle of the vaginal cuff. Some authors have advocated placing up to three sutures on each side; however, we have concerns about increased risk of sacral trunk nerve injury (especially S2 and S3) with a third suture placed closer to the sacrum as well as with deep suture placement. An additional nonabsorbable mattress suture approximates the midline pubocervical and rectovaginal fascia, preventing enterocele formation. Next the sutures are tied into place and the long ends held until cystoscopy confirms ureteral patency. The sutures are then trimmed and the cuff is closed (Fig. 29.2). Stent

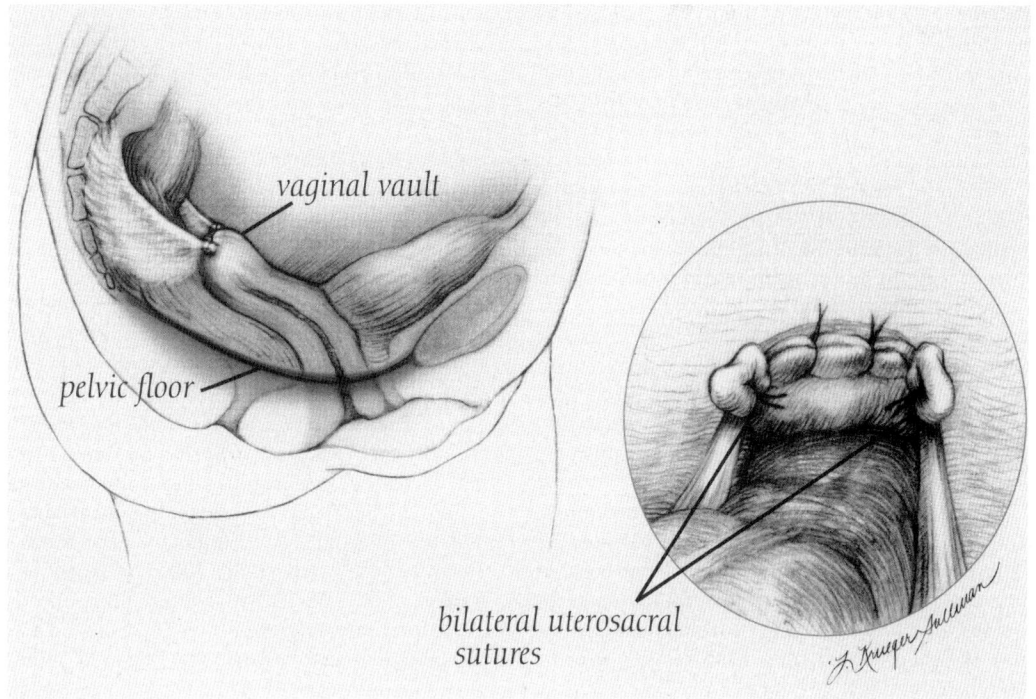

FIGURE 29.2 ● Uterosacral ligament suspension. After one arm of each uterosacral suture has been passed through the pubocervical fascia and the other through the rectovaginal fascia on each side, they are tied down, anchoring the vaginal cuff to the proximal uterosacral ligaments. Additional sutures are placed in the midline, approximating the anterior and posterior fascia in the middle. The end result is a normal vaginal axis and length.

placement may be attempted in the absence of ureteral flow. Usually, release of the distal uterosacral suture alleviates the obstruction caused by kinking of the ureter. Direct ureteral injury requiring reimplantation is rare. Nevertheless, postoperative cystoscopy is essential for a safe repair.

Buller et al (21) performed suture pullout studies on cadavers and concluded that the intermediate segment of the uterosacral ligament was the optimal site when balancing strength and safety in vaginal reconstruction. The ischial spine was found to be a good marker of this intermediate segment, which has good strength with fewer vital, subjacent structures, including vasculature and nerves. The course of the ureter and uterosacral ligament diverges with less tension transmitted to the ureter as we proceed from the cervical portion toward the sacrum.

This procedure can also be performed abdominally during laparotomy or laparoscopy. It may be useful for cases of mild vault laxity or as a temporary measure without hysterectomy for women with more severe uterine prolapse planning future childbearing. Although the operative technique is altered by the approach, the critical landmarks and

uterosacral ligament suture location remain unchanged. Results from small case series with short-term follow-up indicate similar success for laparoscopic uterosacral hysteropexy (22,23).

Surgical Outcomes

Several retrospective case series report excellent subjective and objective outcomes ranging from 80% to 100% with low morbidity and mortality during uterosacral ligament suspension (24–27). In the largest of these series, Shull et al (26) discovered a high objective success rate using the Baden-Walker halfway scoring system. Of the 302 consecutive cases, 289 (96%) patients returned for at least one follow-up visit and 251 (87%) had completely normal support. Recurrent prolapse at any site was found in 13%, but only 5% had grade 2 or more prolapse. There were no apical recurrences at the initial postoperative visit and only four (1%) apical recurrences up to 3 years postoperatively. The cuff and cul-de-sac displayed the most durable support, followed by the posterior compartment and then the anterior compartment. There were four (1%) ureteral injuries: two required removal and replacement of suspensory sutures, one sustained a needle-stick injury, and one required ureteroneocystotomy for an injury occurring during multiple vaginal repairs of all compartments. Only three (1%) patients needed transfusions, and there was one death shortly after release from the hospital. Shull et al's series did not address symptom resolution.

Similarly, Jenkins (27) performed retrospective chart reviews on 50 women undergoing uterosacral ligament suspension focusing on anatomical outcomes. Initially he used permanent monofilament sutures but later changed to delayed absorbable sutures secondary to three cases of suture erosion. Follow-up ranged from 6 to 48 months, and there were no cases of recurrent apical prolapse. Two cystotomies occurred during entry in posthysterectomy patients, and there were no transfusions, ureteral injuries, or bowel injuries.

Several studies address subjective outcomes. Amundsen et al (24) retrospectively evaluated 33 patients undergoing uterosacral vault suspension with absorbable sutures at a mean follow-up of 28 months. Eighty-two percent of women had resolution of prolapse symptoms with overall support less than or equal to stage I on Pelvic Organ Prolapse Quantification (POPQ) examination. Recurrences were seen at the posterior wall in 12% and the apex in 6%. Vaginal length decreased by 0.9 cm, which was statistically but not clinically significant. The only complications consisted of one (3%) case of ureteral kinking, which resolved with suture removal, and one patient who required transfusion.

Wheeler et al (28) discovered similarly high patient satisfaction (84%) with apical support stage I or greater on POPQ examinations for women undergoing uterosacral suspension combined with cystocele repair augmented by porcine dermis graft. Unfortunately, there was a high rate of at least stage II recurrent anterior wall prolapse (50%).

Barber et al (25) retrospectively reported on 46 women at a mean follow-up of 15.5 months after uterosacral ligament vaginal vault suspension performed with permanent and delayed absorbable sutures. Symptomatic and anatomical improvement occurred in 90% of women, with two (5%) cases of recurrent stage III apical prolapse. Only 67% had anatomical support for all compartments less than or equal to stage I based on the POPQ system; however, apical support was better, with 82% at stage 0 and 13% at stage 1. This series had the highest rate of ureteral injury, seen in five (11%) subjects. Three resolved with suture removal and two required reimplantation. Other complications included one transfusion, one case of cuff cellulitis, and one myocardial infarction resulting in cardiogenic shock and death in a patient with known preoperative coronary artery disease. Vaginal shortening of 0.75 cm was observed, with 36/41 (88%) having a total vaginal length of at least 7 cm. Thus, uterosacral ligament suspension appears to consistently decrease the vaginal length approximately 1 cm and may not be appropriate in sexually active women with shortened vaginal length preoperatively.

It is difficult to clearly distinguish the uterosacral ligament suspensions described above from the high uterosacral ligament plications found in the McCall culdoplasty section. All use the proximal uterosacral ligaments for support, but they differ with respect to midline plication of these ligaments. The distinction becomes blurred when we consider that Jenkins and Barber performed separate McCall culdeplasty-like procedures with plication of the distal uterosacral ligaments in the majority of women to treat enteroceles. Rates of ureteral injuries were similar, with the exception of Barber's study. We tend to avoid midline plication of the uterosacral ligaments, which results in a less physiologic repair; however, the impact of midline plication on vaginal length, vaginal caliber, and sexual function remains unclear.

More recently neuropathic pain has been associated with uterosacral ligament suspension. We believe that this is an underreported phenomenon that has been largely ignored and falsely attributed to surgical positioning. Based on recent anatomical evaluation, we consider this pain to result from entrapment of or direct injury to the sacral nerve roots, primarily S2 and S3, which are more vulnerable with deep suture placement at proximal uterosacral ligament sites closer to the sacrum (29,30). The majority of this pain is self-limited and will resolve over time, but there have been reported cases of rapid resolution with suture removal (31).

Iliococcygeus Suspension

Surgical Technique

Originally described by Inmon in 1963 (32), this procedure is indicated for patients in whom the "uterosacral ligaments can not be identified or may be deemed insufficient to support the vaginal cuff." This may also be performed when entry into the peritoneal cavity cannot be accomplished due to adhesions obliterating the cul-de-sac. Inmon described bilateral placement of a suture through the fascia overlying the iliococcygeus muscle just caudal to the ischial spine. The sutures are then anchored into the angles of the vaginal cuff, including the pubocervical and rectovaginal fascia. He emphasized the importance of reapproximating the superior aspects of the pubocervical fascia and rectovaginal septum to prevent enterocele formation. Iliococcygeus suspension is infrequently necessary but provides a good option for vaginal reconstruction in the absence of adequate uterosacral ligaments. The vaginal axis is similar to uterosacral ligament suspension, and both are more physiologic than the extreme posterior deflection seen with sacrospinous ligament fixation. Due to the location of apical support, there is an inherent risk of vaginal shortening, which would be slightly worse than with uterosacral ligament suspension (Fig. 29.3).

One advantage of this procedure is the avoidance of critical structures, thereby decreasing rates of nerve and ureteral injury that may occur during the other restorative surgeries. However, the nerve innervating the levator ani, which runs along the anterior surface of the muscle (33), could potentially be injured, as well as sacral nerves posterior to the iliococcygeus muscle, which may be damaged or entrapped with deep suture placement. The risk of sacral nerve root injury with iliococcygeus suspension should be lower than during uterosacral ligament suspension because suture placement is more caudal.

Surgical Outcomes

Inmon (32) performed the first three iliococcygeus suspension procedures between 1959 and 1961. At the time of the publication in 1963, all three patients had a well-supported vaginal cuff without "descensus on straining or coughing." Since then there have been two larger case series. Shull et al (34) and Meeks et al (35) reported on 42 and 110 women respectively who had undergone iliococcygeus suspension with concomitant repairs.

Thirteen (8%) of the 152 women developed recurrent prolapse. Only two (1%) prolapses recurred at the vaginal vault, while eight (5%) involved the anterior wall and three (2%) occurred at the posterior wall. All of Meeks' subjects had at least 3 years of follow-up, while Shull's ranged from 6 weeks to 5 years. In the larger series, there were two patients who required transfusion, one bowel injury, and one bladder injury, and 41/110 (37%) had a postoperative complication. Maher et al (36) retrospectively analyzed 36 women undergoing iliococcygeus suspension. At a mean follow-up of 21 months, subjective success was 91%, objective success was 53%, and overall patient satisfaction on a visual analog scale was 78 of 100. Eight percent had recurrent vault prolapse (at least grade II), 33% had recurrent cystocele, and 11% had recurrent rectocele. There was a surprisingly high rate of buttock pain and sciatica in 19% that resolved spontaneously within 3 months, and only one patient needed a transfusion. A more recent retrospective series evaluated 24 patients undergoing a combined modified McCall culdoplasty with an iliococcygeus suspension (37). They found one case of recurrent vault prolapse, one anterior vaginal wall prolapse, and one posterior vaginal wall prolapse over a mean follow-up of 24.4 months.

Sacrospinous Ligament Fixation

Surgical Technique

Sacrospinous ligament fixation was developed in Germany by Amreich and Richter in 1951 (38) and gained popularity in the United States through the work of Randall and Nichols (39,40). This vaginal

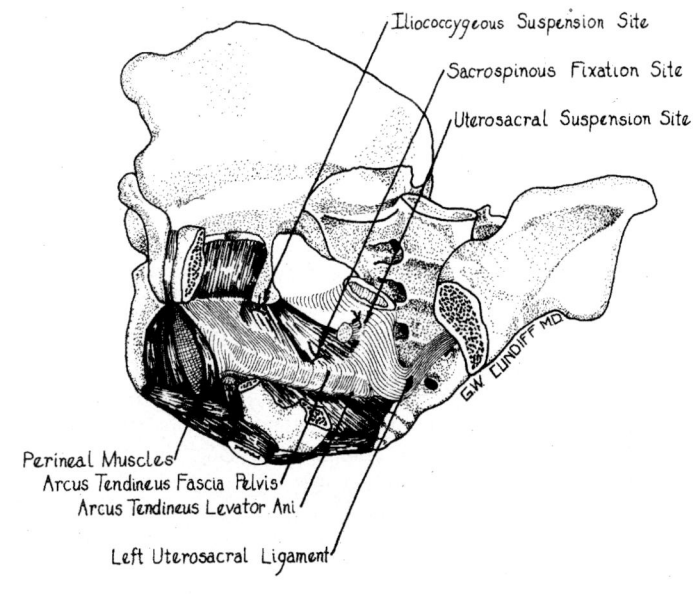

FIGURE 29.3 ● Oblique view of pelvis to demonstrate three different sites of attachment for vaginal vault suspensions. A window is viewed in the vaginal vault to permit viewing of these anchorage sites. The iliococcygeus suspension is in the normal vaginal axis but falls short of the normal vaginal length. The sacrospinous ligament is deflected posteriorly. The uterosacral ligaments are in the normal vaginal axis and do not compromise vaginal length.

Iliococcygeous Suspension Site
Sacrospinous Fixation Site
Uterosacral Suspension Site

Perineal Muscles
Arcus Tendineus Fascia Pelvis
Arcus Tendineus Levator Ani

Left Uterosacral Ligament

G.W. CUNDIFF MD

reconstructive surgery fixes the apex unilaterally or bilaterally to the sacrospinous ligament(s). The posterior vaginal wall is opened and the pararectal space is entered by penetrating the rectal pillar bluntly or sharply near the ischial spine. Straight retractors such as Breisky-Navratil retractors are inserted, deflecting the rectum medially and the bladder and ureter anteriorly. The course of the sacrospinous ligament is identified as the aponeurosis located within the substance of the coccygeus muscle running from the ischial spine toward the lower sacrum. One or two nonabsorbable sutures of at least 2-0 gauge are placed through the ligament 1.5 to 2 fingerbreadths medial to the ischial spine to avoid injury to the pudendal nerve and artery that pass just posterior to the ischial spine as they enter Alcock's canal. Several devices have been developed to facilitate passage of the sutures through the ligament, including the Miya hook, Deschamps ligature carrier, Laurus needle driver, Nichols-Veronikis ligature carrier, and Shutt suture punch. The sutures are then anchored to the vaginal apex, including the superior aspect of the pubocervical and rectovaginal fascia. Most commonly a nonabsorbable suture excluding the vaginal epithelium is used with a pulley stitch; however, full-thickness vaginal wall delayed absorbable sutures have also been described. The sutures are then tied so that the apex of the vagina is approximated to the sacrospinous ligament without an intervening suture bridge. This procedure has also been described with uterine conservation for women wishing to preserve fertility.

Surgical Outcomes

Sze and Karram reviewed 22 retrospective case series with 1,229 vault suspensions, of which 1,062 (86%) were available for follow-up. Duration of follow-up varied from 1 month to 11 years in 726 patients and unspecified duration in the remaining 336 subjects. There were 193 (18%) recurrences, including 81 (8%) at the anterior vaginal wall, 32 (3%) at the vault, 24 (2%) at the posterior wall, and 56 (5%) at unspecified or multiple sites. The severity of these recurrences was poorly documented and many did not require reoperation. Among the studies included in this review with over 80 subjects, success rates ranged between 65% and 97% (40–45). Most were objective outcomes alone; however, some involved combined objective and subjective measures, while others were unspecified. Serious complications rarely occurred, with the most common complication being hemorrhage. The transfusion rate was 2%, and three patients suffered life-threatening hemorrhages. There were only four cystotomies and five proctotomies, which were repaired immediately

without further sequelae. Nerve injuries occurred in 4%, and 3% complained of gluteal pain that was localized to the side of the sacrospinous suture. There was one death from coronary thrombosis and another from vaginal evisceration. Only a handful of studies evaluated sexual function, discovering a small percentage of vaginal shortening, vaginal stenosis, and apareunia.

A more recent large retrospective case series of almost 700 patients showed high success rates for support of the vaginal apex, from 87% to 99% (46). They evaluated three groups that differed as their techniques evolved. Earlier surgeries that focused solely on apical support had the lowest success rates, while later surgeries that addressed support defects at all sites had higher success rates. David-Montefiore et al (47) compared complication rates from a retrospective series of 195 patients to other case series containing at least 50 subjects. They found similar high complication rates of 41%, with the majority of these being minor complications (29%). There are three classifications of major complications specifically associated with this procedure: rectal injury, hemorrhage from vascular injury, and neurological injury. Vascular injuries are the most serious and can involve the hypogastric plexus, pudendal vessels, or perirectal and presacral vessels. Repair may require suturing or clipping of vessels, vaginal packing, embolization, and reoperation to control bleeding or drain a hematoma. The ischiorectal fossa is the most common site for hematoma formation, and cases of perirectal abscess have been reported. Neurological injury associated with buttock pain typically resolves by 6 weeks; however, pain that radiates down the posterior thigh suggests sacral trunk injury and should prompt rapid suture removal.

Colombo and Milani (17) displayed successful outcomes for apical support in 92% and overall support in 83%. Maher et al (36) found a 67% objective success rate and 94% subjective success rate at 19 months. Fourteen percent of patients encountered buttock pain that resolved by 3 months and did not require suture removal. Both of these retrospective comparative trials will be discussed later in the section on vaginal comparative procedures.

The only prospective trials for sacrospinous ligament fixation are studies comparing vaginal and abdominal approaches. Benson et al (12) found the lowest success rates using combined objective and subjective criteria. Optimal effectiveness was present in 29%, satisfactory outcomes in 38%, and unsatisfactory in 33%. Most of the recurrences occurred at the anterior wall (25%), but there were over 10% apical recurrences as well. This trial used a bilateral sacrospinous fixation technique. Lo and Wang (48) displayed an optimal success rate of 80% but did not comment on the location of vaginal recurrences. The most disturbing finding was that 7 of 18 sexually active patients had dyspareunia and 4 were sexually inactive because of the dyspareunia. Maher et al (49) had high subjective success (91%) and mean patient satisfaction (81%), with an objective success rate of 69% over 22 months. These randomized trials will be reviewed in greater detail toward the end of this chapter.

Compensatory Repairs

Sacral Colpopexy

Surgical Technique

Sacral hysteropexy was first described in 1957 (50). Since then, technique has been modified and evolved with the use of an intervening graft, performance of hysterectomy, and fixation to the anterior longitudinal ligament at various locations ranging from the sacral promontory to the S4 vertebra. Most surgeons currently use the S1 to S2 level to avoid life-threatening hemorrhages, which are more likely to occur at lower levels from injury to the middle sacral artery (51). Modern sacral colpopexy involves attachment of a graft to the anterior and posterior vaginal walls at the vaginal cuff. We use a two-strap technique (52), which permits differential tensioning of the anterior and posterior grafts (Fig. 29.4).

After laparotomy and possible hysterectomy, a large obturator, such as an EEA sizer, is placed vaginally, elevating the cuff and facilitating dissection. The vesicovaginal space is entered and the bladder dissected off the anterior vaginal wall and pubocervical fascia either sharply or with electrocautery. An adequate area is developed for attachment of the anterior graft (usually at least 3 cm distal to the vaginal apex and 3 to 5 cm wide). Similarly, the rectovaginal space is entered and the rectum dissected off the posterior vaginal wall and rectovaginal septum until the superior aspect of the rectovaginal septum can be identified. Identification is confirmed by placement of an Allis clamp on the superior aspect of the rectovaginal septum. If there is continuity of the rectovaginal septum, traction on the Allis clamp results in lifting of the perineal body. During this dissection, it is critical to recognize the direction of the vaginal axis to avoid injury to the rectum. Next, the grafts are fashioned appropriately to fit the attachment sites. A variety of grafts have been employed, including synthetic, allogenic, xenograft, and au-

tologous materials, which will subsequently be discussed with surgical outcomes. The grafts are secured anteriorly and posteriorly using broad attachments with multiple sutures (usually nonabsorbable) to distribute tensile forces and minimize the risk of avulsion of the graft from the vaginal apex. It is also important to avoid bunching the graft material and tying the sutures too tightly, which may predispose to necrosis and mesh erosion (53).

The presacral space is entered after the right ureter, iliac vessels, and aortic bifurcation have been identified. The sigmoid colon is retracted laterally and the peritoneum overlying the S1 to S3 vertebra is carefully grasped, elevated anteriorly, and incised with electrocautery, exposing underlying loose areolar tissue. The space is further explored and the anterior longitudinal ligament exposed using a combination of blunt dissection, sharp dissection, and electrocautery, with care taken to identify and avoid the superior hypogastric nerve plexus and middle sacral vessels. Next, two or three nonabsorbable sutures of at least 2-0 gauge are placed through the anterior longitudinal ligament at the level of the distal S1 and proximal S2 vertebra. It is helpful to use a needle with a 5/8-circle curve to place these sutures. Depending on the location of the middle sacral vessels, it may be helpful to encircle the vessels; in the event of bleeding, these sutures can be tied to aid in hemostasis. If large bleeding persists, additional sutures can be placed, packing may be necessary, and sterile tacks are often required.

If a culdoplasty is to be performed, it must be done prior to attaching the grafts to the sacrum. A Halban culdoplasty avoids injury to the ureter, obliterates the cul-de-sac, and may prevent enterocele formation. Attaching the culdoplasty sutures into the posterior graft may also provide additional anterior rectal wall support (53). Each presacral suture is then passed through the anterior and posterior grafts at the appropriate level and then tied down, approximating the grafts directly to the sacrum. With proper positioning, the vaginal apex is lifted without undue tension. The anterior strap is usually tensioned looser than the posterior graft to decrease the risk of potential urinary incontinence from excessive straightening of the urethrovesical junction. Finally, the peritoneum is closed over the mesh to prevent small bowel adhesions to the mesh (Fig. 29.4).

More recently, several reconstructive pelvic surgeons have begun to perform this procedure laparoscopically. A minimum of four ports are placed: infraumbilical, right lower quadrant, left lower quadrant, and left midabdomen (lateral to

cells, especially macrophages and neutrophils, seems to decrease the potential for chronic infection. Chronic infections may be more likely to occur with the use of multifilament sutures to attach the mesh. The only disadvantages of the macroporous meshes are that they are more likely to form intestinal adhesions, erosions, and even fistula when in direct contact with bowel (65,66).

Autologous grafts such as fascia lata or rectus fascia should provide durable repairs with minimal risk of graft erosion, inflammation, or infection. However, harvesting of the graft adds operative time, cost, and possible complications, including incisional hernia (with rectus fascia harvest), pain at the operative site, hematoma formation, and change in leg contour (with fascia lata harvest). Allogenic grafts, most commonly fascia lata and dermis, have been used in an effort to minimize synthetic graft-related complications and the need for autologous harvesting. A recent randomized control trial provides level I evidence that allogenic fascia lata is inferior to synthetic mesh (68% versus 91% respectively at 1 year) for sacral colpopexy (67). These results confirm data from retrospective prolapse and incontinence studies evaluating allogenic fascia lata. Xenografts have also been utilized in prolapse and incontinence surgery, with level I evidence displaying similar results for suburethral slings performed with porcine dermal grafts and polypropylene mesh (68,69). A recent retrospective cohort compared the use of porcine dermal graft to polypropylene and polytetrafluoroethylene for sacral colpopexy (70). Of the 52 subjects included, they found similar high rates of recurrent stage II vault prolapse (29% xenograft group and 24% synthetic mesh group) at a mean short-term follow-up of 7 months using the Baden Walker system. Complications were similar among groups, with the exception of postoperative fever persisting more than 3 days in the xenograft group. This may indicate more of an inflammatory reaction with the porcine dermal graft. There were no differences in subjective outcomes at longer-term follow-up (mean 2.5 years xenograft group and 4.3 years synthetic mesh group), and none of the subjects had undergone repeat sacral colpopexy. Objective outcome measures were not documented at the long-term follow-up. To date, there are no randomized control trials comparing xenograft to synthetic mesh for sacral colpopexy.

Effect of Hysterectomy on Erosion Rates

The effect of hysterectomy on erosion rates remains controversial. Placement of synthetic mesh over a healing sutured incision plus exposure to vaginal microbes theoretically increases the risk of graft erosion when hysterectomy is performed at the time of sacral colpopexy. Culligan et al (58) discovered 3 of 11 (27%) erosions with hysterectomy compared with 3 of 234 (1.3%) without hysterectomy. The number of hysterectomy patients was very low but the difference was still statistically significant ($p < 0.001$). On the other hand, Brizzolara and Pillai-Allen (57) saw no erosions in 60 subjects with concurrent hysterectomy and one erosion among the 64 without hysterectomy. Wu et al (71) performed a large retrospective cohort study confirming the lack of a significant difference in erosion rates with concomitant hysterectomy. The erosion rates for the 101 (32.3%) concurrent hysterectomy subjects and 212 (67.7%) prior hysterectomy subjects were similar at 6.9% and 4.7% respectively ($p = 0.42$). Some have suggested that supracervical hysterectomy with sacral colpocervicopexy may decrease erosion rates. While the cervix may serve as a potential barrier, there are no published studies to substantiate this claim. The cervical os may serve as a channel for ascending infection and mesh erosion, while the presence of the cervix may complicate treatment of mesh erosions. Also, those with a long intravaginal cervix may be at higher risk for recurrent prolapse with only minor apical descent. Sacral colpohysteropexy with uterine preservation also has the potential to decrease erosion rate, but this may be at the expense of anterior vaginal wall support.

Abdominal Sacral Colpoperineopexy

Sacral colpoperineopexy is a modification of sacral colpopexy aimed at correcting a combination of conditions, including apical prolapse, rectocele, and perineal descent (72). Excessive perineal descent, as described by Parks and Hardcastle (73,74), occurs due to inferior detachment of the rectovaginal septum from the perineal body. Perineal descent has been associated with a variety of defecatory disorders, and with progressive descent, stretch injury can occur to the pudendal nerve, resulting in neuropathy. During sacral colpoperineopexy, a continuous graft is placed from the anterior longitudinal ligament to the perineal body. This can be accomplished either through a total abdominal approach or a combined abdominal and vaginal procedure. With the total abdominal approach, the rectovaginal space is opened similar to sacral colpopexy; however, the dissection is carried down further toward the perineal body. The graft is then sutured to the perineal body or as close to it as possible. A rectovaginal examination with the surgeon's nondominant hand facilitates this attachment by supporting the perineal body. The graft is secured to additional points along the posterior vaginal wall and apex, and sacral colpopexy is completed in the usual fashion.

With the combined abdominal and vaginal approach, the posterior vaginal wall is opened and a rectocele repair is performed. Sacral colpopexy is accomplished in the usual fashion except that a window is made connecting the abdominal and vaginal dissections in the rectovaginal space. The graft can then be passed down from the abdominal field to the vaginal field and anchored inferiorly to the perineal body and laterally to the arcus tendineus fascia rectovaginalis. Alternatively, perineal body stitches can be placed vaginally, retrieved abdominally upon entering the rectovaginal space, and incorporated into the caudal portion of the graft. The latter technique minimizes graft exposure to vaginal microbes, which may theoretically decrease erosion rates (see Fig. 29.5).

Cundiff et al (72) displayed good anatomical support of the vaginal apex, posterior wall, and perineum over short-term follow-up for 19 women undergoing sacral colpoperineopexy. Defecatory dysfunction symptoms completely resolved in 66% of patients. Sullivan et al (75) reported outcomes for a slightly different variation of sacral colpoperineopexy involving attachment of Marlex mesh to the perineal body using a needle carrier. The failure

rate was 25% and the mesh erosion rate was 5% for 205 patients with up to 10-year follow-up. Visco et al (76) reported Mersilene mesh erosion rates of 3.2% for sacral colpopexy, 4.5% for sacral colpoperineopexy with the total abdominal approach, 16% for sacral colpoperineopexy with vaginal suture placement, and 40% for sacral colpoperineopexy with vaginal mesh placement. High erosion rates with the combined abdominal and vaginal approaches have compelled us to select nonsynthetic grafts such as xenograft for the combined vaginal and abdominal approach. Use of xenografts may decrease vaginal erosion rates and reoperation rates to treat erosions since they tend to resolve spontaneously. However, the role of nonsynthetic grafts for apical support is still in question, as previously discussed. We have also modified our technique by placing a nonsynthetic graft vaginally and a synthetic graft abdominally so that the two grafts are connected by nonabsorbable sutures without being in direct contact with each other. This may decrease vaginal contamination of the abdominal field, potentially decreasing mesh erosion rates. Sacral colpoperineopexy appears to have value for a select group of patients, but larger

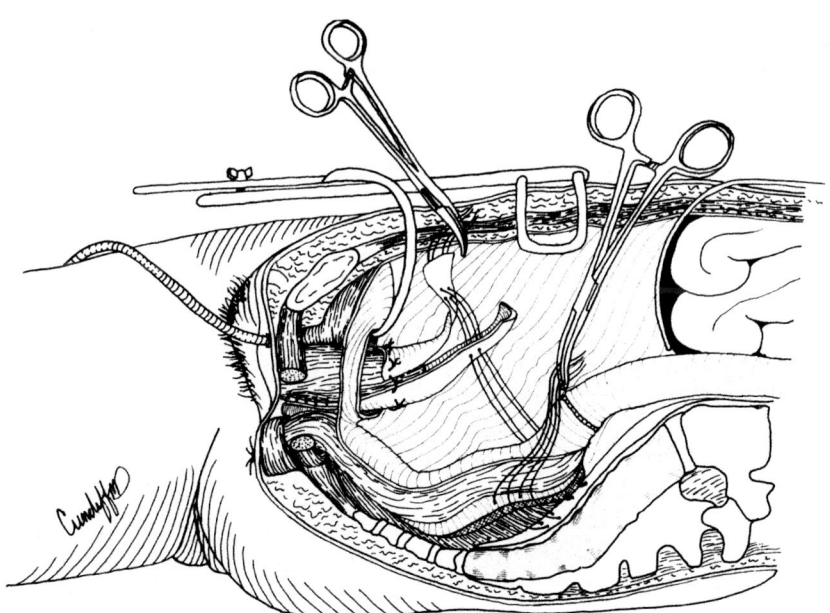

FIGURE 29.5 ● Sacral colpoperineopexy. Grafts have been attached to the posterior vaginal vault and anterior vaginal vault. The posterior graft is attached to the perineal body and brought through the rectovaginal space into the abdominal field. On the patient's left, rectopexy sutures are placed through the longitudinal sacral ligament and the lateral ligaments of the rectum and are untied. On the patient's right, rectopexy sutures are placed through the longitudinal sacral ligament, the lateral ligaments of the rectum, and the anterior and posterior vaginal grafts and are untied.

prospective series with long-term anatomical and symptomatic outcomes are necessary to evaluate the durability of this procedure.

Comparative Outcomes Among Vaginal Procedures

At present there are no prospective trials comparing vaginal apical support procedures, so we must rely on a small number of retrospective studies to determine the relative merits of the vaginal suspension previously reviewed.

Colombo and Milani (17) performed a retrospective case-control study using 62 cases of sacrospinous ligament fixation and 62 matched controls undergoing modified McCall culdoplasty. Controls were matching for grade of prolapse, age, parity, macrosomia or operative delivery, menopause, body mass index, prior vaginal surgery for prolapse, heavy work, constipation, and chronic cough. There were no statistically significant differences in postoperative objective support, even for women with procidentia. Seventeen (27%) overall recurrences and five (8%) vault recurrences were observed in the sacrospinous group compared to nine (15%) overall and three (5%) vault recurrences in the McCall group. There was a higher rate of recurrent anterior vaginal wall prolapse in the sacrospinous group (13 [21%] vs. 4 [6%], OR 4.1, $p = 0.04$). This is due to the greater posterior deflection of the vaginal axis resulting in increased intra-abdominal pressure on the anterior vaginal wall, which has been confirmed by other authors. There was a longer duration of surgery and greater blood loss associated with sacrospinous ligament fixation. Vaginal length was slightly longer in the sacrospinous group (8.4 ± 1.5 cm vs. 7.6 ± 1.4 cm), which was statistically but not clinically significant. The authors concluded that McCall culdoplasty was equally efficacious as sacrospinous ligament suspension with less morbidity, and sacrospinous suspension should no longer be considered as a treatment in patients with uterovaginal prolapse.

Maher et al (36) performed a case-control study of 36 iliococcygeus suspensions and 36 sacrospinous fixations. Patients were matched to similar characteristics as the Colombo and Milani study (17). Subjective success rates (91% vs. 94% respectively) and objective success rates (53% vs. 67% respectively) were similar for iliococcygeus suspension and sacrospinous fixation at a mean follow-up of 21 and 19 months respectively. They observed similar recurrence locations, with the most common site being the anterior wall (33% vs. 25% respectively) and fewer recurrences at the

apex (8% vs. 3% respectively). The lack of increased anterior wall recurrences in the sacrospinous group is surprising and contradicts the findings of most other studies. Overall patient satisfaction on a visual analog scale was higher for the sacrospinous group (78 of 100 vs. 91of 100, $p = 0.01$). The most frequent complication encountered by each group was buttock pain and sciatica (19% vs. 14% respectively) that resolved spontaneously by 3 months postoperatively. The authors suggest that the gluteal pain may have been due to muscular ischemia rather than neurologic injury.

Koyama et al (37) retrospectively compared 24 patients undergoing modified McCall culdoplasty with iliococcygeus suspension to 21 patients undergoing McCall culdoplasty alone. The McCall-only group had milder prolapse with fewer apical support defects and lack of enteroceles. At a mean follow-up of 24.4 months, there were similar rates of recurrent vault prolapse (1 in each group) but higher rates of recurrent anterior wall prolapse (4 vs. 1) and reoperation (for cystocele and stress incontinence) in the group that did not have an iliococcygeus suspension. It is unclear whether the improved outcomes for urinary incontinence and anterior wall support were due to the addition of an iliococcygeus suspension or the result of selection bias.

At present there are no retrospective or prospective studies comparing sacrospinous ligament fixation to uterosacral ligament suspension. All of the vaginal restorative procedures appear to provide substantial apical support with an increased risk of anterior wall recurrences that vary by procedure. Numerous studies indicate greater anterior compartment failures with sacrospinous ligament fixation balanced by an increased risk of ureteral injury with uterosacral ligament suspension. Assuming routine intraoperative cystoscopy is performed, the more physiologic position of the vaginal axis with uterosacral sususpension supports its use over sacrospinous fixation. A survey of AUGS and SGS members confirmed this contention, showing uterosacral ligament suspension to be the preferred vaginal procedure for apical pelvic organ prolapse (77). A randomized controlled trial is necessary to validate these beliefs.

Comparative Outcomes Between Vaginal and Abdominal Procedures

In addition to a handful of retrospective studies, there are currently only four prospective randomized controlled trials comparing abdominal and vaginal approaches for the treatment of apical prolapse (Table 29.1). Three of the four studies compare abdominal sacral colpopexy to sacrospinous

TABLE 29.1

Abdominal Versus Vaginal Randomized Controlled Trials for Apical Prolapse

Study	Procedures	n	Follow-up	Outcomes	Complications
Benson et al, 1996 (12)	**Abdominal** ASC, TAH, Burch or SUS, CUL, ANT, POS	40	Mean 2.5 years (range 1–5.5 years)	Combined subj and obj Optimal 22 (58%) Satisfactory 10 (26%) Unsatisfactory 6 (16%)	Similar complication rates, more severe in abdominal group Reoperation 6 Cystocele (4), vault prolapse (1), rectocele (2), incontinence (1)
	Vaginal Bilateral SSF, PVR, TVH, needle susp or SUS, CUL, ANT, POS	48		Optimal 12 (29%) Satisfactory 16 (38%) Unsatisfactory 14 (33%)	Reoperation 14 Cystocele (12), vault prolapse (5), rectocele (1), incontinence (5)
Lo and Wang, 1998 (48)	**Abdominal** ASC, TAH, POS	52	Mean 2.1 years (range 1–5.2 years)	Obj success 49/52 (94%)	Reoperation 4/52 (8%) Dyspareunia 1 Apareunia 0
	Vaginal Unilateral SSF, TVH, ANT, POS	66		Obj success 53/66 (80%)	Reoperation 7/66 (11%) More sexual dysfunction Dyspareunia 7 Apareunia 4
Maher et al, 2004 (49)	**Abdominal** ASC, Burch, PVR, CUL, POS	47	Mean 24 months (range 6–60 months)	Subj success 43/46 (94%) Satisfaction 39/46 (85%) Obj success 35/46 (76%)	Similar complication rates Reoperation 6 Incisional hernia (2), TVT (2), Vaginal removal infected mesh (1), POS (1)
	Vaginal Unilateral SSF, Enterocele repair, Burch, ANT, POS	48	Mean 22 months (range 6–58 months)	Subj success 39/43 (91%) Satisfaction 35/43 (81%) Obj success 29/42 (69%)	Reoperation 7 TVT (2), periurethral injection (1), Fenton repair for dyspareunia (2), ANT (1), AFR (1), POS (1)
Roovers et al, 2002 (78)	**Abdominal** ASC (uterine preservation), Cul, Burch	41	1 year	Subj UDI improved Vault prolapse 5% Cystocele 36% Rectocele 5%	Similar complication rates Reoperation for: Cystocele 5 Uterine prolapse 4
	Vaginal TVH, USLF, ANT, POS, needle susp	41		Subj UDI more improved Uterine prolapse 5% Cystocele 39% Rectocele 15%	Reoperation for: Vault prolapse 1

ASC, sacral colpopexy; TAH, total abdominal hysterectomy; TVH, total vaginal hysterectomy; CUL, culdoplasty; ANT, anterior colporrhaphy; POS, posterior colporrhaphy; SSF, sacrospinous ligament fixation; PVR, paravaginal repair; SUS, suburethral sling, needle susp, needle suspension; TVT, tension-free vaginal tape sling; AFR, anterior fascial replacement with mesh; USLF, uterosacral ligament fixation.

ligament fixation. The other study compares sacral colpohysteropexy to uterosacral-cardinal ligament fixation at the vaginal cuff.

Benson et al (12) performed the first prospective randomized control trial comparing bilateral sacrospinous ligament fixation to abdominal sacral colpopexy. Subjects with urodynamic stress incontinence were treated with needle urethropexy in the vaginal arm and retropubic urethropexy in the abdominal arm. Outcomes were considered optimal when women were prolapse symptom-free with the vaginal apex supported above the levator plate without protrusion of any vaginal tissue beyond the hymen. Outcomes were considered unsatisfactory when there was symptomatic descent of the vaginal apex more than 50% of its length or vaginal wall protrusion beyond the hymen. There was a two-fold increase in optimal effectiveness (58% vs. 29%) and a two-fold decrease in unsatisfactory outcome (16% vs. 33%) with a sacral colpopexy. The majority of vaginal failures occurred in the anterior compartment. There was no statistical difference in the overall number of complications; however, they seemed to be more severe in the abdominal group. The external validity of this study is compromised by the recognition that the sacrospinous group patients underwent an inferior incontinence surgery, predisposing them to a higher reoperation rate for stress incontinence. As a result, reoperation for urinary incontinence significantly affected the overall surgical failure rate in the vaginal arm.

Lo and Wang (48) randomized women with at least stage III apical support defects to either abdominal sacral colpopexy or sacrospinous ligament fixation. Optimal surgical effectiveness required absence of stage II prolapse at any site. They discovered greater success with less complications in the sacral colpopexy group. Sacral colpopexy was optimally effective in 49 (94%) compared to 53 (80%) in the sacrospinous group ($p = 0.029$). Of the three failures in the sacral colpopexy group, only one (2%) occurred at the apex and the other two (4%) involved the anterior wall. There were no recurrent rectoceles despite the fact that only 37% underwent posterior colporrhaphy in the abdominal group while almost all underwent this procedure in the vaginal group. Unfortunately, the authors did not comment on the location of failures in the sacrospinous group, so we are unable to determine how many involved the vaginal apex. There were no differences in the complication rates requiring reoperation. Incontinence surgery was not performed in this study and only a few subjects developed postoperative urinary incontinence (2 sacral colpopexy vs.

1 sacrospinous fixation). The abdominal group had three cases of ileus managed conservatively, while the vaginal group was more likely to have dyspareunia (7 vs. 1) and apareunia (4 vs. 0). There was greater blood loss, length of hospitalization, and prolonged catherization in the sacrospinous group.

Maher et al (49) randomized women with at least stage II post-hysterectomy vault prolapse to abdominal sacral colpopexy or unilateral sacrospinous colpopexy. They excluded those who had undergone a previous sacral colpopexy or had a significantly foreshortened vagina. Women with urodynamic stress incontinence underwent Burch urethropexy with stratification to ensure equal representation in each group. Objective success was defined as no vault prolapse beyond the halfway point of the vagina with Valsalva and no prolapse grade II or more at any vaginal site. Subjective success involved no symptoms of prolapse. The objective success rate was 76% in the abdominal group and 69% in the vaginal group at approximately 2 years ($p = 0.46$). Sample size calculation based on Benson's study caused them to be underpowered to detect an anatomical difference in their primary outcome. When these failures were broken down into compartments, there was a higher rate of anterior wall prolapse (14% vs. 7%, $p = 0.19$) and vault prolapse (19% vs. 4%, p not calculated) in the vaginal group, and a higher rate of posterior wall prolapse in the abdominal group (17% vs. 7%, $p = 0.19$). The discrepancy in posterior wall prolapse may be attributed to the fact that only a quarter of the sacral colpopexy group underwent posterior colporrhaphy as opposed to almost all of the sacrospinous group. There were no detectable differences in subjective success rates (94% vs. 91%), mean patient satisfaction (85% vs. 81%), efficacy of colposuspension (79% vs. 87%), quality of life measures, or complication rates between the abdominal and vaginal groups respectively. Operative time (+30 minutes) and surgical costs (+$1,875) were higher in the abdominal group, and the vaginal group had quicker return to activities of daily living (–8 days). While the authors concluded that the two procedures are equally effective, sacral colpopexy may confer better support to the vaginal apex and anterior wall. Also, use of colposuspension during vaginal surgery decreases generalizability and may protect the anterior wall support, which would not necessarily be present with midurethral slings.

Roovers et al (78) performed the remaining prospective randomized controlled trial of abominal and vaginal approaches for women with at least stage II uterine prolapse. Subjects underwent either a vaginal hysterectomy, possible anterior and posterior colporrhaphy, fixation of the vault to the uterosacral-cardinal ligaments with absorbable suture, and possible needle suspension or a sacral colpopexy with preservation of the uterus, culdoplasty, and possible Burch colposuspension. It is unclear if the vaginal group had a true apical suspension procedure using the uterosacral ligaments or if the distal ligaments were simply transfixed to the vaginal cuff. For their primary outcome, both groups had reduction in Urogenital Distress Inventory scores (Dutch version) with maximal reduction in the prolapse domain. However, the vaginal group had a greater reduction of score even after controlling for preoperative differences. There were no differences in duration of surgery, blood loss, hospital stay, or number of complications. Anatomical outcomes were similar at 1 year, with a 5% stage II or greater apical recurrence rate for each group. Nevertheless, patients who underwent sacral colpohysteropexy were more likely to have subsequent surgery for recurrent anterior wall (n = 5) or uterine (n = 4) prolapse compared to only one reoperation for vault prolapse in the vaginal group. Uterine preservation in the abdominal group decreases the generalizability of sacral colpopexy, reduces uniformity among approaches, and potentially affects subjective and objective outcomes, including the need for reoperation. There was also an inferior stress incontinence surgery performed in the vaginal arm, which will likely affect long-term outcomes.

Each of these studies overstate their conclusions, allowing their biases to be revealed. One could easily argue for a different conclusion based on the data presented. They conflict with respect to their recommendation for an abdominal or vaginal approach as the ideal treatment of apical prolapse. They also differ with respect to primary outcome, which varies between anatomy, symptomatology, or a combination of the two. Sacral colpopexy appears to provide more durable support of the vaginal apex and anterior vaginal wall with potentially greater complications compared to sacrospinous ligament fixation. At present there are no studies comparing uterosacral ligament suspension to sacral colpopexy (without uterine preservation) despite the fact that uterosacral suspension is the preferred vaginal apical support procedure among AUGS and SGS members (77). A well-done prospective randomized study would help to define the relative balance between morbidity, anatomical support, and symptomatic improvement. It is unlikely that study results would show one approach to have lower morbidity with better anatomical and symptomatic outcomes. Rather, we would anticipate better anatomical outcomes with

higher morbidity for more invasive abdominal procedures. We do not know if symptomatic outcomes correlate with anatomical outcomes and the relative importance of each of these on overall patient satisfaction. Nevertheless, this type of information would be invaluable for surgical planning and informed consent.

Choice of Surgical Procedure

There are generally two schools of thought with respect to restoring apical support. The first is a commonly held belief that initial repairs of primary apical support defects (uterine prolapse and posthysterectomy vault prolapse without a prior apical support procedure) should always be attempted vaginally. In cases of uterine prolapse, the repair usually involves hysterectomy for anterior wall support purposes. Assuming success rates are as high as previously discussed for vaginal apical support procedures, the small percentage of recurrences at the vaginal apex should be treated with sacral colpopexy. The second philosophy is to choose vaginal restorative procedures for women with lower risks of recurrent prolapse and abdominal compensatory repairs for those with high risks of recurrence. While the data are limited, some potential risk factors for recurrence include prior prolapse surgery, severity of prolapse (7), young age (7), wide genital hiatus (8), levator weakness, and increased intra-abdominal pressures from occupation/recreation involving heavy lifting, continual cough from tobacco use, obesity, and chronic constipation.

There is no evidence that one philosophy is superior to the other. The first approach may predispose to a higher rate of recurrent prolapse, especially at the anterior wall due to the posterior deflection of the apex and axis with vaginal reconstructions. Recurrent anterior wall prolapse has been a common problem with vaginal repairs, and most attribute this to midline defects or paravaginal defects. We would argue that this is due to inadequate support of the upper anterior vaginal wall, which can be better corrected by placing an anterior graft during sacral colpopexy. The second philosophy places the woman at increased risk of undergoing a potentially unnecessary and more invasive procedure that may be associated with increased morbidity. Laparoscopic sacral colpopexy is an attempt to make sacral colpopexy less invasive with a quicker recovery, similar to vaginal surgery. Unfortunately, this procedure often requires two experienced laparoscopic surgeons and takes more time than an open abdominal approach, with only small decreases in the length of hospitalization. Complication rates, operative time, duration of hospitalization, recovery time, postoperative recovery, and cost have not been prospectively compared for laparoscopic and open sacral colpopexy. The ideal surgery would be a vaginal compensatory repair that is as durable as sacral colpopexy for supporting the vaginal apex and upper anterior and posterior walls, while providing the benefits of vaginal surgery for postoperative pain, morbidity, and ease of recovery.

Emerging Technologies

Numerous surgical devices under development and in use offer minimally invasive approaches for treating POP and urinary incontinence. This important innovation is being driven by industry. The Food & Drug Administration approves medical devices more quickly and easily with less rigorous testing required than pharmaceuticals. Companies must only prove product safety and are not required to document efficacy. Therefore, the surgeon is left with the difficult task of determining how to incorporate these new technologies into his or her practice. Many of the products are later withdrawn for safety or efficacy concerns; an example of this is the posterior intravaginal slingplasty (Posterior IVS Tyco/US Surgical, Norwalk, CT). However, some of these products revolutionize the field and rapidly replace standard operations. The classic example of this is the tension-free midurethral suprapubic sling originally developed by Ulmsten et al (79). This procedure has become the gold standard primary operation for stress urinary incontinence. Since its inception there have been many variations, including the most recent transobturator approach.

Recently, there has been an influx of devices for the treatment of POP. The most promising systems are vaginal compensatory repairs using polypropylene mesh that rely on the sacrospinous ligament for posterior apical support and the arcus tendineus fascia pelvis and levator ani attachments near the ischial spine for anterior apical support. The repairs differ from conventional repairs through the tension-free placement of mesh without suturing, use of the obturator space, and recommendation to leave the uterus in place. Although these devices have only recently been approved for use in the United States, they have been employed in Europe for several years. Recent short-term safety data for cystocele repair with tension-free polypropylene (Gynemesh) application were published, indicating a high mesh erosion rate of 20% and a 10% de novo dyspareunia rate (80). Most of the erosions required further treatment. Collinet et al (81) evaluated short-term

complications and mesh erosion rate for the transvaginal mesh procedure. Erosions occurred in 34 (12.3%) of the 277 patients, with 25 (9%) requiring reoperation to treat the erosion and the others resolving with medical management. The majority resolved after one reoperation; however, five patients required multiple surgeries and one of these was complicated by a vesicovaginal fistula. Erosions were more common when concomitant hysterectomy was performed or an inverted-T colpotomy incision was used for vault prolapse, and all but one were localized to the anterior colpotomy site. Other perioperative complications included one rectal injury, four bladder injuries, and one hematoma. While data regarding efficacy are sparse, there are several prospective studies underway to analyze these new vaginal compensatory procedures. Use of these devices is appealing because they potentially offer all the benefits of the ideal prolapse surgery previously mentioned— namely, they are quick and minimally invasive, with low postoperative pain and an easier recovery. There is still a need to prove equal or greater anatomical and subjective outcomes with low morbidity. We must be cautious in our adoption of these devices, especially in young women where procedure- or graft-related complications could potentially leave them with permanent sexual dysfunction or intractable pelvic pain. Further studies are necessary to evaluate postoperative sexual function as well as anatomical studies to determine proximity of critical nerves and blood vessels, especially during passage of the posterior trocar through the ischiorectal fossa and sacrospinous ligament. Proper informed consent is critical when performing these procedures, since they should still be considered investigational.

REFERENCES

1. Brown JS, Waetjen LE, Subak LL, et al. Pelvic organ prolapse surgery in the United States, 1997. *Am J Obstet Gynecol* 2002;186:712–716.
2. Olsen AL, Smith VJ, Bergstrom JO, et al. Epidemiology of surgically managed pelvic organ prolapse and urinary incontinence. *Obstet Gynecol* 1997;89:501–506.
3. Subak LL, Waetjen LE, van den Eeden S, et al. Cost of pelvic organ prolapse surgery in the United States. *Obstet Gynecol* 2001;98:646–651.
4. DeLancey JO. Anatomic aspects of vaginal eversion after hysterectomy. *Am J Obstet Gynecol* 1992;166:1717–28.
5. Summers A, Winkel LA, Hussain HK, et al. The relationship between anterior and apical compartment support. *Am J Obstet Gynecol* 2006;194:1438–1443.
6. Rooney K, Mueller ER, Kenton K, et al. Can advanced stages of anterior or posterior vaginal wall prolapse occur without apical involvement? Abstract, 32nd Annual Society of Gynecologic Surgeons Meeting, Tucson, AZ, April 3–5, 2006.

7. Whiteside JL, Weber AM, Meyn LA, et al. Risk factors for prolapse recurrence after vaginal repair. *Am J Obstet Gynecol* 2004;191:1533–1538.

8. Delancey JO, Hurd WW. Size of the urogenital hiatus in the levator ani muscles in normal women and women with pelvic organ prolapse. *Obstet Gynecol* 1998;91:364–368.

9. Beer M, Kuhn A. Surgical techniques for vault prolapse: A review of the literature. *Eur J Obstet Gynecol Reprod Biol* 2005;119:144–155.

10. Maher C, Baessler K, Glazener CM, et al. Surgical management of pelvic organ prolapse in women. *Cochrane Database Syst Rev* 2004;(4):CD004014.

11. Weber AM, Richter HE. Pelvic organ prolapse. *Obstet Gynecol* 2005;106:615–634.

12. Benson JT, Lucente V, McClellan E. Vaginal versus abdominal reconstructive surgery for the treatment of pelvic support defects: A prospective randomized study with long-term outcome evaluation. *Am J Obstet Gynecol* 1996;175:1418–1422.

13. McCall ML. Posterior culdeplasty; surgical correction of enterocele during vaginal hysterectomy; a preliminary report. *Obstet Gynecol* 1957;10:595–602.

14. Symmonds RE, Williams TJ, Lee RA, et al. Posthysterectomy enterocele and vaginal vault prolapse. *Am J Obstet Gynecol* 1981;140:852–859.

15. Webb MJ, Aronson MP, Ferguson LK, et al. Posthysterectomy vaginal vault prolapse: Primary repair in 693 patients. *Obstet Gynecol* 1998;92:281–285.

16. Karram M, Goldwasser S, Kleeman S, et al. High uterosacral vaginal vault suspension with fascial reconstruction for vaginal repair of enterocele and vaginal vault prolapse. *Am J Obstet Gynecol* 2001;185:1339–1343.

17. Colombo M, Milani R. Sacrospinous ligament fixation and modified McCall culdoplasty during vaginal hysterectomy for advanced uterovaginal prolapse. *Am J Obstet Gynecol* 1998;179:13–20.

18. Aronson MP, Aronson PK, Howard AE, et al. Low risk of ureteral obstruction with "deep" (dorsal/posterior) uterosacral ligament suture placement for transvaginal apical suspension. *Am J Obstet Gynecol* 2005;192:1530–1536.

19. Cruikshank SH, Kovac SR. Randomized comparison of three surgical methods used at the time of vaginal hysterectomy to prevent posterior enterocele. *Am J Obstet Gynecol* 1999;180:859–865.

20. Miller N. A new method of correcting complete inversion of the vagina: With or without complete prolapse; report of two cases. *Surg Gynecol Obstet* 1927:550–555.

21. Buller JL, Thompson JR, Cundiff GW, et al. Uterosacral ligament: Description of anatomic relationships to optimize surgical safety. *Obstet Gynecol* 2001;97:873–879.

22. Maher CF, Carey MP, Murray CJ. Laparoscopic suture hysteropexy for uterine prolapse. *Obstet Gynecol* 2001; 97:1010–1014.

23. Diwan A, Rardin CR, Strohsnitter WC, et al. Laparoscopic uterosacral ligament uterine suspension compared with vaginal hysterectomy with vaginal vault suspension for uterovaginal prolapse. *Int Urogynecol J Pelvic Floor Dysfunct* 2006;17:79–83.

24. Amundsen CL, Flynn BJ, Webster GD. Anatomical correction of vaginal vault prolapse by uterosacral ligament fixation in women who also require a pubovaginal sling. *J Urol* 2003;169:1770–1774.

25. Barber MD, Visco AG, Weidner AC, et al. Bilateral uterosacral ligament vaginal vault suspension with site-specific endopelvic fascia defect repair for treatment of pelvic organ prolapse. *Am J Obstet Gynecol* 2000;183:1402–1411.

26. Shull BL, Bachofen C, Coates KW, et al. A transvaginal approach to repair of apical and other associated sites of pelvic organ prolapse with uterosacral ligaments. *Am J Obstet Gynecol* 2000;183:1365–1374.

27. Jenkins VR 2nd. Uterosacral ligament fixation for vaginal vault suspension in uterine and vaginal vault prolapse. *Am J Obstet Gynecol* 1997;177:1337–1344.

28. Wheeler TL 2nd, Richter HE, Duke AG, et al. Outcomes with porcine graft placement in the anterior vaginal compartment in patients who undergo high vaginal uterosacral suspension and cystocele repair. *Am J Obstet Gynecol* 2006;194:1486–1491.

29. Siddique SA, Gutman RE, Schon Ybarra MA, et al. Relationship of the uterosacral ligament to the sacral plexus and to the pudendal nerve. *Int Urogynecol J Pelvic Floor Dysfunct* 2006;17:642–645.

30. Flynn M, Amundsen C, Weidner A. Sensory nerve injury after uterosacral ligament suspension. Abstract, 32nd Annual Society of Gynecologic Surgeons Meeting, Tucson, AZ, April 3–5, 2006.

31. Lowenstein L, Dooley Y, Kenton K, et al. Neural pain after uterosacral ligament vaginal suspension. *Int Urogynecol J Pelvic Floor Dysfunct* 2007;18:109–110.

32. Inmon WB. Pelvic relaxation and repair including prolapse of vagina following hysterectomy. *South Med J* 1963;56:577–582.

33. Barber MD, Bremer RE, Thor KB, et al. Innervation of the female levator ani muscles. *Am J Obstet Gynecol* 2002;187:64–71.

34. Shull BL, Capen CV, Riggs MW, et al. Bilateral attachment of the vaginal cuff to iliococcygeus fascia: An effective method of cuff suspension. *Am J Obstet Gynecol.* 1993;168:1669–1677.

35. Meeks GR, Washburne JF, McGehee RP, et al. Repair of vaginal vault prolapse by suspension of the vagina to iliococcygeus (prespinous) fascia. *Am J Obstet Gynecol* 1994;171:1444–1454.

36. Maher CF, Murray CJ, Carey MP, et al. Iliococcygeus or sacrospinous fixation for vaginal vault prolapse. *Obstet Gynecol* 2001;98:40–44.

37. Koyama M, Yoshida S, Koyama S, et al. Surgical reinforcement of support for the vagina in pelvic organ prolapse: Concurrent iliococcygeus fascia colpopexy (Inmon technique). *Int Urogynecol J Pelvic Floor Dysfunct* 2005;16:197–202.

38. Amreich J. Etiology and surgery of vaginal stump prolapses. *Wien Klin Wochenschr* 1951;63:74–77.

39. Randall CL, Nichols DH. Surgical treatment of vaginal inversion. *Obstet Gynecol* 1971;38:327–332.

40. Nichols DH. Sacrospinous fixation for massive eversion of the vagina. *Am J Obstet Gynecol* 1982;142:901–904.

41. Richter K, Albrich W. Long-term results following fixation of the vagina on the sacrospinal ligament by the vaginal route (vaginae fixatio sacrospinalis vaginalis). *Am J Obstet Gynecol* 1981;141:811–816.

42. Richter K. Massive eversion of the vagina: Pathogenesis, diagnosis, and therapy of the "true" prolapse of the vaginal stump. *Clin Obstet Gynecol* 1982;25:897–912.

43. Morley GW, DeLancey JO. Sacrospinous ligament fixation for eversion of the vagina. *Am J Obstet Gynecol* 1988;158:872–881.

44. Imparato E, Aspesi G, Rovetta E, et al. Surgical management and prevention of vaginal vault prolapse. *Surg Gynecol Obstet* 1992;175:233–237.

45. Shull BL, Capen CV, Riggs MW, et al. Preoperative and postoperative analysis of site-specific pelvic support defects in 81 women treated with sacrospinous ligament

plex. Laterally it attaches to the pelvic sidewall (Fig. 30.1) via the arcus tendineus fascia pelvis and arcus tendineus fascia rectovaginalis (4). Inferiorly, the rectovaginal septum fuses with the perineal body (DeLancey level III). The lateral attachment (DeLancey level II) prevents ventral movement of the posterior vaginal wall. Through its attachment to the cardinal and uterosacral ligaments, the rectovaginal septum stabilizes the perineal body. Due to the support of the rectovaginal septum and pelvic diaphragm, there is limited downward mobility of the perineal body, which normally lies within 2 cm of an imaginary line between the ischial tuberosities.

Through his work on cadavers, Richardson hypothesized that most rectoceles were the result of discrete tears in the rectovaginal septum (5). Surgically tears have been shown to occur within the rectovaginal septum itself as well as at the lateral, superior, and inferior attachments (6). Perineal descent results from detachment of the rectovaginal septum from the perineal body. This was first described by Parks et al in 1966 (7). Since then, others have shown an association between perineal descent and defecatory dysfunction, including constipation, incomplete emptying, tenesmus, and the need to splint or use digital manipulation for defecation.

POSTERIOR COLPORRHAPHY

Posterior colporrhaphy was first described in the early 19th century. The procedure was originally designed to deal with obstetrical perineal tears by narrowing the caliber of the vagina, creating a perineal shelf, and partially closing the genital hiatus (8). A tight perineorrhaphy was also used to improve the patient's ability to hold a pessary in place and was thought to prevent the progressions of upper genital prolapse. The original description included plication of the pubococcygeus muscles and posterior vaginal wall (colporrhaphy) and reconstruction of the perineal body (perineorrhaphy). Although developed without any real understanding of uterine and vaginal supports, transvaginal colporrhaphies have been the most commonly used surgical procedure for rectocele repair among gynecologic surgeons for over 100 years.

A posterior colporrhaphy begins with a perineal skin incision (Fig. 30.2). The perineal incision may be horizontal, triangular, or diamond-shaped, depending on the degree of perineal relaxation present. If the introitus needs to be narrowed with a perineorrhaphy, a triangular or diamond-shaped incision is made. The posterior vaginal epithelium is then opened in the midline to the apex of the vagina or to the cephalad border of the rectocele. The rectovaginal septum is then carefully dissected off the vaginal epithelium and plicated in the midline with continuous or interrupted delayed absorbable sutures. Some authors advocate a more aggressive plication of the levator ani muscles in the midline as well. Excess vaginal epithelium is trimmed and the vaginal epithelium is closed with a running or interrupted absorbable suture. If a perineorrhaphy is to be performed, the superficial perineal muscles and the bulbocavernosus muscles are brought to the midline using fine absorbable suture. The perineal epithelium is then closed with a subcuticular absorbable suture.

Despite its long history, the anatomic and functional success of posterior colporrhaphy was not studied until recently. Table 30.1 summarizes the recent literature on posterior colporrhaphy with and without levator plications. Anatomic cure rates range from 76% to 96% whether levator plication is performed or not. Functional outcomes have

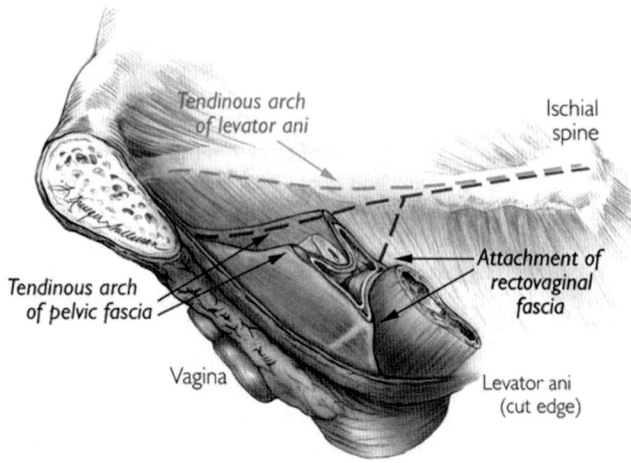

Tendinous arch of levator ani

Tendinous arch of pelvic fascia

Vagina

Ischial spine

Attachment of rectovaginal fascia

Levator ani (cut edge)

FIGURE 30.1 ● Oblique view of the anatomy of the rectovaginal septum's attachments to the perineal body and pelvic side wall. In its distal half the lateral rectovaginal septum attaches to the inner (superior) surface of the levator ani muscles, while it coalesces with the fascial layer of the anterior vaginal wall at the tendinous arch of the pelvic fascia in its upper half. (From Cundiff GW, Fenner D. The management of rectocele and defecatory dysfunction. *Obstet Gynecol* 2004;104(6):1403–1421. Courtesy of Lianne Sullivan.)

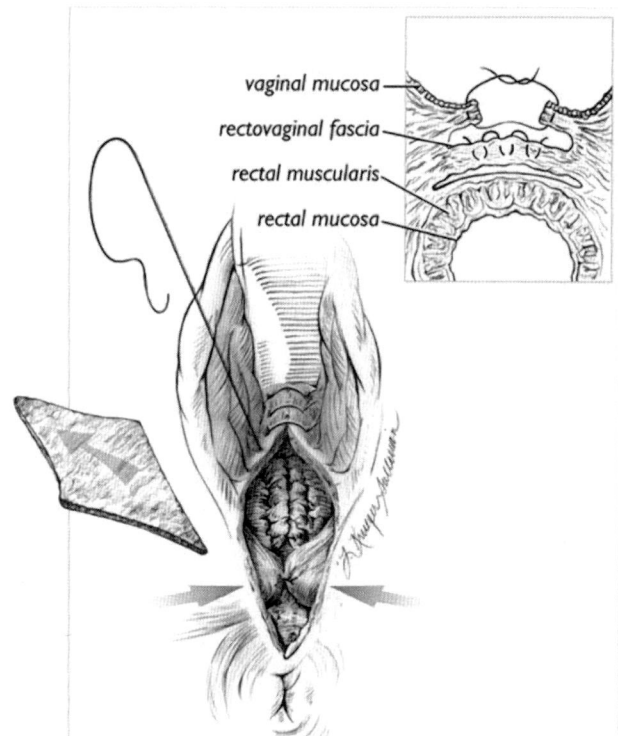

vaginal mucosa
rectovaginal fascia
rectal muscularis
rectal mucosa

FIGURE 30.2 ● Surgical view of the posterior colporrhaphy. A diamond-shaped piece of skin overlying the perineum is removed. The rectovaginal septum is plicated as shown in the oblique view in the inset. The trimmed skin edges are then reapproximated. (From Cundiff GW, Fenner D. The management of rectocele and defecatory dysfunction. *Obstet Gynecol* 2004;104(6):1403–1421. Courtesy of Lianne Sullivan.)

more variable results. Kahn and Stanton (14) reported on a large retrospective series of 171 patients who underwent posterior colporrhaphy with levator plication. Constipation increased from 22% preoperatively to 33% postoperatively and fecal incontinence increased from 4% preoperatively to 11% postoperatively. In the only prospective study addressing functional outcome, Maher et al (9) reported a decrease in constipation from 76% preoperatively to 24% postoperatively.

Francis and Jeffcoate first described an association between dyspareunia and posterior repair in 1961 (15). Recent studies report de novo dyspareunia rates between 8% and 26%. Although thought to be related to levator plication, de novo dyspareunia occurs in posterior colporrhaphy without levator plication as well. Weber et al (10) prospectively followed 81 women with pelvic organ prolapse and urinary incontinence before and after surgery for sexual function and vaginal anatomy. Dyspareunia occurred in 14 (25%) women after posterior colporrhaphy ($p = 0.01$) and in 8 (38%) of 21 women who had Burch colposuspension and posterior colporrhaphy performed together ($p = 0.01$). The postoperative introital caliber was not different when comparing the women with and without dyspareunia.

In summary, the traditional transvaginal colpoperineorrhaphy provides good anatomic sup-

port with potential relief of functional symptoms and a high rate of de novo dyspareunia.

DEFECT-DIRECTED REPAIR

The defect-directed repair is based on the work of Richardson. As mentioned above, Richardson hypothesized that most rectoceles are the result of discrete tears in the rectovaginal septum. These tears may occur in the fascia itself or at the superior, lateral, or inferior attachment sites. The defect-directed repair aims to fix rectoceles by identifying and closing these discrete tears. By restoring normal anatomy, advocates suggest that the defect-directed method may offer the advantage of better functional outcomes and less dyspareunia.

The posterior vaginal epithelium is opened in the midline and the epithelium is separated from the underlying rectovaginal septum as described in the posterior colporrhaphy section (Fig. 30.3). A finger from the surgeon's nondominant hand is placed in the rectum, allowing identification of the fascial defects. The defects are repaired with interrupted delayed absorbable sutures. Perineorrhaphy is performed as needed. The vaginal epithelium is closed so as not to constrict the vagina.

Table 30.2 summarizes the available data on defect-directed repairs. Several retrospective reviews

TABLE 30.1

Posterior Colporrhaphy

Study	n	Mean Follow-Up (mo)	Levator Plication	Anatomic Cure (%)	Constipation	Fecal Incontinence	De Novo Dyspareunia in Sexually Active Patients
Maher (9)							
Preop	38	12.5	No		76%		37%
Postop				95%	24%		5%
Weber (10)							
Preop	53	12	No				
Postop	53						26%
Sand (11)							
Preop	70	12	No				
Postop	67			90%			
Arnold (12)							
Preop	29		Yes				
Postop	24			80%		36%	23%
Mellegren (13)							
Preop	25	12	Yes		100%	8%	
Postop	25			96%	88%	8%	8%
Kahn (14)							
Preop	231	42	Yes		22%	4%	
Postop	171			76%	33%	11%	16%
Paraiso (22)							
Preop	37	16	No				
Postop	33			91%			

have shown anatomic cure rates of 82% to 100% with improvement in dyspareunia. Cundiff et al (16) reported on 69 women who underwent the defect-directed repair over a 3-year time period. They showed improvement in constipation, difficult evacuation, fecal incontinence, and dyspareunia while maintaining an 82% cure rate. Kenton et al (18) showed a similar cure rate and improvement in dyspareunia, but only about 50% of patients with constipation and difficult evacuation improved.

Abramov et al (21) published the first comparative study between traditional colporrhaphy and defect-directed repair. In this retrospective study, 124 patients underwent defect-directed repair and 183 patients underwent standard posterior colporrhaphy without levator plication. The procedures were not randomized as the choice of procedure was based on the operative findings—that is, if discrete defects were found, a defect-directed repair was performed, and if no discrete defects were

found, a traditional posterior colporrhaphy was performed. Rates of recurrence of rectocele beyond the midvaginal plane (33% vs. 14%, $p = 0.001$) and beyond the hymenal ring (11% vs. 4%, $p = 0.02$) and recurrence of a symptomatic bulge (11% vs. 4%, $p = 0.02$) were significantly higher after the site-specific rectocele repair. Rates of postoperative dyspareunia, constipation, and fecal incontinence were not significantly different between the two groups. The authors comment on the fact that the patients were not randomly assigned to the surgical procedure, so selection bias may affect the results. Paraiso et al presented the first prospective randomized trial in 2006 (22). Anatomic failure was noted in 13.5% of the site-specific group and 9% of the posterior colporrhaphy group. There was no difference between groups in functional outcome or dyspareunia.

In summary, studies to date on the defect-directed repair show low dyspareunia rates with good

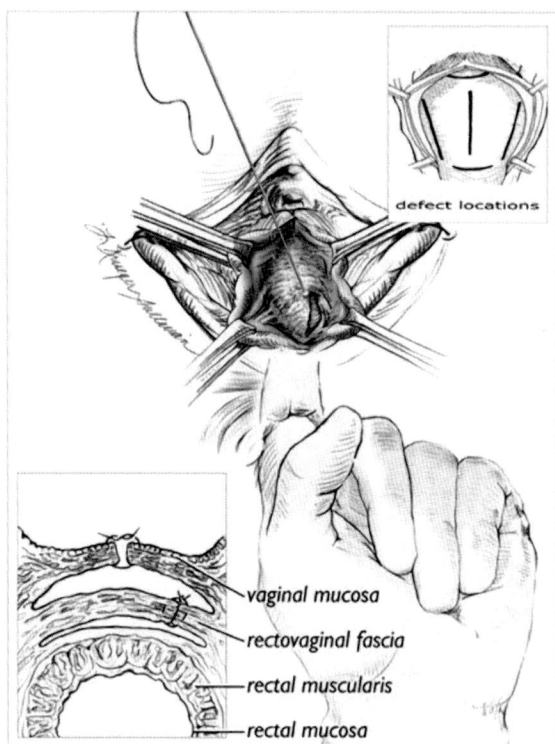

defect locations

vaginal mucosa

rectovaginal fascia

rectal muscularis

rectal mucosa

FIGURE 30.3 • Surgical view showing the defect-directed rectocele repair. The upper inset (cross-section) delineates surgical layers, while the lower inset demonstrates the potential locations for tears in the recto-vaginal septum. (From Cundiff GW, Fenner D. The management of rectocele and defecatory dysfunction. *Obstet Gynecol* 2004;104(6): 1403–1421. Courtesy of Lianne Sullivan.)

functional and anatomic results. Larger prospective randomized trials between traditional colporrhaphy and defect-directed repairs are needed to further assess the question of anatomic cure and durability of the repairs.

TRANSANAL REPAIR

Transanal repair of a rectocele was first advocated by Marks, a colorectal surgeon, in the 1960s (23). He noted that many women had continued difficulties with rectal evacuation after transvaginal rectocele repair. He also noted that many women diagnosed with a rectocele had thinning of the anterior rectal wall and an enlarged rectal ampulla. The aim of the procedure is to remove or plicate the redundant rectal mucosa and plicate the anterior rectal wall musculature.

A U-shaped or T incision is made transanally above the dentate line with the patient in the prone jackknife position (Fig 30.4). A flap of rectal mucosa is separated from the underlying rectovaginal septum and excised. The rectovaginal septum is then plicated from the rectal side. The rectal mucosa and submucosa are closed in a separate layer.

The transanal approach allows repair of other anorectal pathology, such as hemorrhoids or anterior rectal wall prolapse, at the same time. Repair of high rectoceles, perineal relaxation, and other vaginal prolapse is more difficult. Complications such as infection (6%) and rectovaginal fistula (3%) are rare.

Arnold et al (24) retrospectively reported on 64 nonrandomized patients who underwent rectocele repair for defecatory dysfunction based on symptoms only. Thirty-five of the women underwent transanal repair and 29 underwent transvaginal repair. Forty-six of the 64 women were available for follow-up at a minimum of 2 years postoperatively. At follow-up there was no difference in constipation, anal incontinence, sexual dysfunction, dyspareunia, or patient satisfaction between groups. More patients in the transvaginal group complained of postoperative pain (32% vs. 4%). In addition, 38% of patients developed fecal incontinence after transanal repair. Fecal incontinence may result from an occult sphincter laceration that becomes symptomatic with aging or as a result of the anal dilation and stretching during the rectocele repair (25).

Two randomized controlled trials comparing transvaginal and transanal approaches to rectocele have been reported. Nieminen et al (26) randomized 30 women, 15 to each arm. Patients were assessed by interview, examination, defecography, colon transit study, and anorectal manometry be-

TABLE 30.2

Defect-Directed Posterior Repair

Study	n	Mean Follow-Up (mo)	Anatomic Cure	Constipation	Difficult Evacuation	Fecal Incontinence	Dyspareunia
Cundiff (16)							
Preop	69			46%	32%	13%	29%
Postop	61	12	82%	13%	15%	8%	19%
Porter (17)							
Preop	125			60%	61%	24%	67%
Postop	72	6	82%	50%	44%	21%	46%
Kenton (18)							
Preop	66			46%	52%	30%	28%
Postop	46	12	90%	20%	30%		8%
Singh (19)							
Preop	42				57%	9%	31%
Postop	33	18	92%		27%	5%	15%
Glavind (20)							
Preop	67				40%		12%
Postop	67	3	100%		4%		3%
Abramov (21)							
Preop	124			31%		17%	8%
Postop	124	12.2	77%	37%		19%	16%
Paraiso (22)							
Preop	37	16					48%
Postop	37		86.5%				no change

fore randomization and at 12 months postoperatively. Ninety-three percent of patients in the transvaginal group and 77% of patients in the transanal group reported symptomatic improvement ($p = 0.08$). Recurrence rate of rectocele and/or enterocele was higher in the transanal group (66% vs. 7%, $p = 0.01$). The vaginal approach was associated with a higher blood loss (120 ± 90 mL vs. 60 ± 40 mL, $p = 0.03$). No patients reported de novo dyspareunia. Kahn et al (27) randomly assigned 57 women with symptomatic rectoceles to transanal (n = 33) or transvaginal (n = 24) repair with a mean follow-up of 2 years. Thirty percent of patients in the transanal group required further surgery for rectoceles or enteroceles compared to 13% in the transvaginal group ($p = 0.10$). De novo dyspareunia was reported in one patient in the transvaginal group. The Cochrane Database Review (28) concluded that the results for posterior vaginal wall repair were better than for transanal repair in terms of subjective (RR 0.36, 95% CI 0.13 to 1) and objective (RR 0.24, 95% CI 0.09 to 0.64) cure. In summary, level 1 evidence shows that the vaginal approach to rectocele repair is superior to the transanal approach.

POSTERIOR FASCIAL REPLACEMENT

A variety of graft materials and meshes have been used in recent years to augment posterior repairs. Augmentation is done to improve anatomic outcome, decrease the risk of rectocele recurrence, and cure or improve defecatory difficulties while maintaining normal sexual and vaginal function. The purpose of the graft is either to replace the fascia as a permanent barrier to herniation or to act as an absorbable scaffold for fibroblast infiltration and scar formation. The ideal graft for posterior compartment defects should have a low rejection rate, be relatively inexpensive, decrease recurrence rates, and cause no harm with respect to bowel and sexual function. Grafts may be allografts (human donor), autografts (self donor), xenograft (animal donor), or synthetic materials. Examples include autologous fascia, allograft fascia lata, dura mater, autologous muscle,

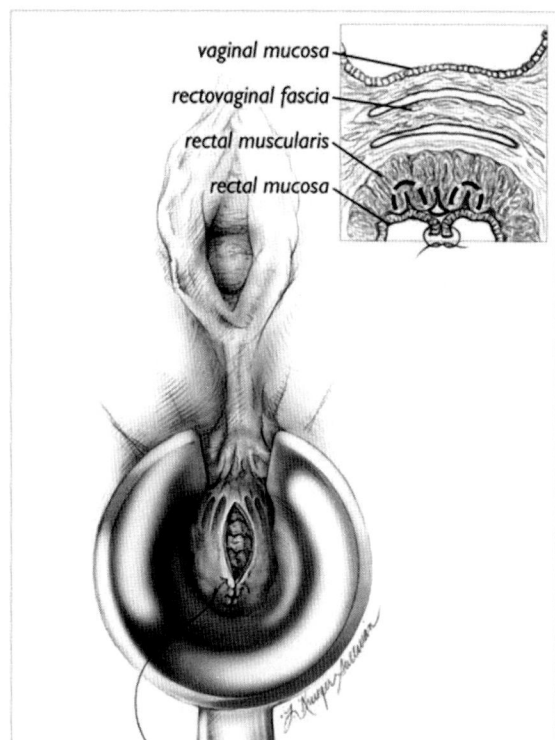

vaginal mucosa

rectovaginal fascia

rectal muscularis

rectal mucosa

FIGURE 30.4 ● Surgical view showing the transanal rectocele repair. The cross-section inset delineates surgical layers. (From Cundiff GW, Fenner D. The management of rectocele and defecatory dysfunction. *Obstet Gynecol* 2004;104(6):1403–1421. Courtesy of Lianne Sullivan.)

porcine dermal collagen, allograft dermis, and polypropylene.

The technique for graft placement is as varied as the types of grafts available. Some authors advocate placing the graft over the rectocele repair whether that repair be a traditional posterior colporrhaphy or a defect-directed repair (Fig. 30.5). The graft is attached superiorly, laterally, and inferiorly to the perineal body. Others recommend replacing the rectovaginal septum with the graft (i.e., not repairing the native fascia first). Still others incorporate pieces of the graft into the imbricating folds of a traditional posterior colporrhaphy (11).

Grafts have been used in other surgical procedures, such as abdominal hernia repair, for decades. Concern about mesh erosion and fistula formation has limited the use of grafts in vaginal reconstructive surgery for some time. Newer graft choices with the potential for fewer complications as well as the high recurrence rates of traditional repairs have increased the interest and use of grafts in vaginal reconstructive surgery. An expanding volume of literature on the use of grafts in rectocele repairs is beginning to develop. Two reviews on the topic have recently been published (29,30).

Biologic Grafts

Table 30.3 summarizes the data on biologic implants used in posterior fascial replacements. Oster and Austrup (31) first looked at using autologous dermal grafts in posterior repairs in 1981. A 100% anatomic cure rate was noted in 15 patients at a mean follow-up of 30 months. Other prospective cohort studies have shown similar high anatomic cure rates with biologic grafts. Although not reported in many studies, defecatory dysfunction seems to improve and de novo dyspareunia rates are relatively low. A randomized controlled trial compared posterior colporrhaphy alone and augmented with a 2×4 patch of allograft fascia lata (36). In a preliminary report at 1 year, the success rate for posterior colporrhaphy alone was 89% (59 of 66) compared to 76% (48 of 56) in the graft group ($p = 0.54$). Similarly, the only prospective, randomized trial to date (22) reported on traditional posterior colporrhaphy versus site-specific repair augmented with a porcine small intestinal submucosa bioengineered collagen matrix (Fortagen). Subjects who received the site-specific repair with graft augmentation had a significantly

Posterior Facial Replacement

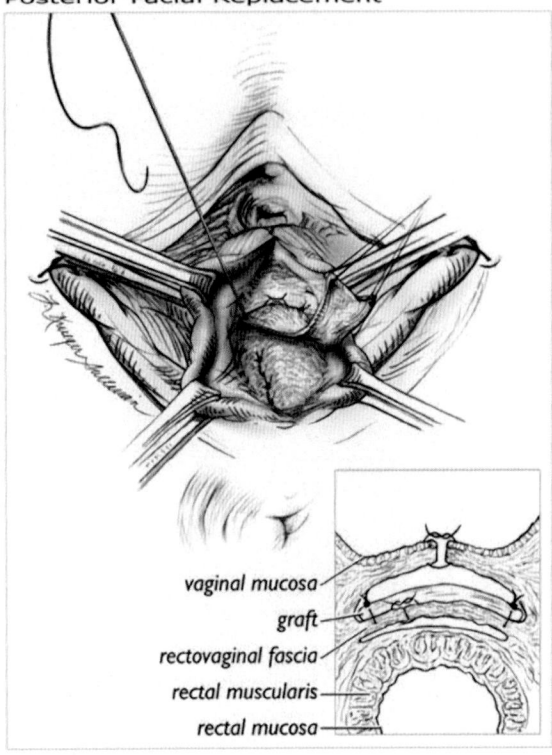

vaginal mucosa

graft

rectovaginal fascia

rectal muscularis

rectal mucosa

FIGURE 30.5 ● Surgical view showing the posterior fascial replacement. The graft is connected superiorly but has not yet been attached laterally or inferiorly, permitting visualization of the defect-directed rectocele repair beneath the graft. The cross-section inset delineates surgical layers. (From Cundiff GW, Fenner D. The management of rectocele and defecatory dysfunction. *Obstet Gynecol* 2004;104(6):1403–1421. Courtesy of Lianne Sullivan.)

greater anatomic failure rate (9/27, 33%) than those who received a site-specific repair alone (5/37, 13.5%) or a traditional posterior colporrhaphy (3/33, 9%; p = 0.035). There was no difference in functional outcome or rates of dyspareunia between the three groups. The only graft complication noted in the above studies was vaginal wound separation in 3 of 62 patients (35), which healed spontaneously.

Synthetic Grafts

Table 30.4 summarizes the data on synthetic implants used in posterior fascial replacement. A number of case series using synthetic grafts show a high anatomic cure rate. The functional cure rate has not been as well studied. Two studies have shown a 50% improvement in difficult evacuation (38,39). Lim showed in improvement in dyspareunia (39% preoperatively, 10% postoperatively), whereas Mercer-Jones showed an increase (4% preoperatively, 8% postoperatively). Sand et al (11) presented the only prospective randomized trial. One hundred forty-three women were randomized to traditional posterior colporrhaphy versus traditional colporrhaphy with incorporation of strips of polyglactin 910 into the imbricated folds of the repair. No difference in anatomic cure rates

was noted. Functional outcome and dyspareunia were not studied.

Several complications have been reported with synthetic mesh use. Lim found a 12.9% mesh erosion rate; however, all but one resolved with a simple office procedure. In a series of 43 women, Goh et al (40) reported three mesh erosions and one rectovaginal fistula. In a series of 26 patients, de Tayrac et al (41) reported three erosions, two of which required mesh removal in the operating room. They also reported one patient with de novo dyspareunia, which resolved after mesh removal. Although rare, the complications may be quite serious.

In summary, the literature on the use of grafts in the repair of posterior compartment defects is expanding; however, most reports are case series and vary widely with regards to type of grafts and specific procedure used. Although the anatomic success rates look promising, functional outcomes are not well studied and serious complications such as mesh erosions and rectovaginal fistulas have been reported. The only randomized controlled trial comparing posterior colporrhaphy with and without a biologic graft showed a higher success rate for posterior colporrhaphy alone. The only prospective randomized trial comparing posterior colporrhaphy with and without a synthetic mesh

TABLE 30.3

Biologic Grafts in Posterior Compartment Defect Repairs

Study	n	Graft Material	Mean Follow-Up (mo)	Anatomic Cure	Constipation	Difficult Evacuation	Dyspareunia
Oster (31)							
Preop	15	Autologous				37%	
Postop	15	dermis	30	100%	33%	0%	20%
Kohli (32)	43	Allograft dermis	12	93%			
Dell (33)							
Preop	35	Xenograft					
Postop	35	porcine	12	93%			
Altman (34)							
Preop	32	Xenograft				100%	84%
Postop	29	porcine	12	62%		55%	86%
Kobashi (35)							
Preop	73	Allograft					
Postop	62	fascia lata	13.72	93%			35.9% 23.1% (10% de novo)
Gandhi (36)							
Preop		Allograft					
Postop	56	fascia lata	12	76%			
Paraiso (22)							
Preop	37	Xenograft					48%
Postop	37	porcine	16	67%			no change

showed no difference in anatomic outcomes. Further prospective randomized studies are warranted before the routine use of grafts can be recommended.

ABDOMINAL APPROACH

An abdominal approach to repair of rectocele may be appropriate when a woman has an associated apical defect such as enterocele, uterine prolapse, or vaginal vault prolapse. If an abdominal procedure such as an abdominosacrocolpopexy is planned, a superior posterior compartment defect can be repaired through the cul-de-sac via the laparotomy incision. The posterior graft used for the abdominosacrocolpopexy can be extended down the posterior wall of the vagina. Perez et al (42) and Villet et al (43) both described extending the posterior mesh down to the levator ani muscle. Villet et al reported an 86% anatomic cure rate and

a 70% functional cure rate in their series of 56 women.

An abdominosacral colpoperineopexy has been described to treat a combination of apical and posterior wall prolapse as well as perineal descent (44). In this procedure, a graft is used to replace the rectovaginal septum along its entire length — that is, from the sacrum to the perineal body. The peritoneum covering the posterior and apical vagina is opened and the rectovaginal space is developed. Sutures are placed along the entire length of the rectovaginal septum down to the perineal body. With the nondominant hand, the surgeon elevates the perineal body vaginally so sutures can be placed transabdominally into the perineal body. The graft is attached to the sutures. The procedure concludes with attachment of the apex of the graft to the longitudinal anterior sacral ligament. As an alternative, a combination vaginal and abdominal approach may be used. The posterior vaginal ep-

TABLE 30.4

Synthetic Grafts in Posterior Compartment Defect Repairs

Study	n	Graft Material	Mean Follow-Up (mo)	Anatomic Cure	Difficult Evacuation	Dyspareunia	Graft Complications
Watson (37)							
Preop	9	Polypropylene					none
Postop	9	transperineal	29	88%			
Sand (11)							
Mesh	73	Polyglactin 910		92%			none
No mesh	70	transvaginal	12	90%			
Mercer-Jones (38)							
Preop	22	Polypropylene (14)			100%	4%	none
Postop	22	Polyvinyl chloride (8) transperineal	12.5	95%	50%	8%	
Lim (39)							
Preop	90	Polyglactin			55%	39%	12.9% erosion
Postop	31	910 polypropylene	6	87.5%	21%	10%	
Goh (40)							
Preop	43	Polypropylene					3 erosions
Postop	43	Transvaginal	12.9	100%			1 rectovaginal fistula
de Tayrac (41)							
Preop	26	Polypropylene			20%		3 erosions
Postop	25	transvaginal	22.7	92.3%	16%	7.7% de novo	1 dyspareunia

ithelium is opened as for a traditional posterior repair. The dissection is carried cephalad until the cul-de-sac is entered. The graft is then passed from the abdominal field to the vaginal field. The graft is attached to the perineal body and arcus tendineus fascia rectovaginalis through the vaginal incision.

Sullivan et al (45) reported on 205 women who had a sacral colpoperineopexy using Marlex mesh for a combination of apical prolapse, rectocele, and enterocele. No vaginal incisions were made. He reported a 25% failure rate and 5% mesh erosion rate. Ten percent of patients required further surgery for complications specific to the repair. Cundiff et al (44) reported on 19 women who underwent a sacral colpoperineopexy for apical prolapse and perineal descent. At short-term follow-up between 3 and 7 months, 63% of patients had no prolapse, 21% had stage 1, and 16% had stage 2. Defecatory dysfunction resolved in 66% of patients. Visco et al (46) reported follow-up on 88 colpoperineopexies using Mersilene mesh. Thirty of the 88 patients had a

vaginal incision. The mesh erosion rate for those without a vaginal incision was 4.5% compared to 40% for those with mesh placed transvaginally. Use of a dermal allograft has been shown to decrease the erosion rate (44). While this approach appears to have good functional results, further evaluation is needed to determine the best approach and type of mesh to use to treat patients with a combination of apical prolapse and perineal descent.

REFERENCES

1. Olsen AL, Smith VJ, Bergstrom JO, et al. Epidemiology of surgically managed pelvic organ prolapse and urinary incontinence. *Obstet Gynecol* 1997;89:501–506.
2. Skomorowska E, Hegedus V, Christiansen J. Evaluation of perineal descent by defaecography. *Int J Colorectal Dis* 1998;3:191–194.
3. DeLancey JOL. Structural anatomy of the posterior pelvic compartment as it relates to rectocele. *Am J Obstet Gynecol* 1999;180:815–823.
4. Leffler KS, Thompson JR, Cundiff GW, et al. Attachment of the rectovaginal septum to the pelvic sidewall. *Am J Obstet Gynecol* 2001;185:41–43.

5. Richardson AC. The rectovaginal septum revisited: its relationship to rectocele and its importance in rectocele repair. *Clin Obstet Gynecol* 1993;36:976–983.

6. Burrows LJ, Sewell C, Leffler KS, et al. The accuracy of clinical evaluation of posterior vaginal wall defects. *Int Urogynecol J* 2003;14:160–163.

7. Parks AG, Porter NH, Hardcastle J. The syndrome of the descending perineum. *Proc R Soc Med* 1966;59:477–482.

8. Jeffcoate TN. Posterior colpoperineorrhaphy. *Am J Obstet Gynecol* 1959;77:490–502.

9. Maher CF, Qatawneh AM, Baessler K, et al. Midline rectovaginal plication for repair of rectocele and obstructed defecation. *Obstet Gynecol* 2004;104:685–689.

10. Weber AM, Walters MD, Piedmonte MR. Sexual function and vaginal anatomy in women before and after surgery for pelvic organ prolapse and urinary incontinence. *Am J Obstet Gynecol* 2000;182:1610–1615.

11. Sand PK, Koduri S, Lobel RW, et al. Prospective randomized trial of polyglactin 910 mesh to prevent recurrence of cystoceles and rectoceles. *Am J Obstet Gynecol* 2001;184:1357–1364.

12. Arnold MW, Stewart WRC, Agiolar PS. Rectocele repair: four years' experience. *Dis Colon Rectum* 1990;33:684–687.

13. Mellegren A, Anzen B, Nilsson B, et al. Results of rectocele repair. *Dis Colon Rectum* 1995;38:7–13.

14. Kahn MA, Stanton SL. Posterior colporrhaphy: its effects on bowel and sexual function. *Br J Obstet Gynaecol* 1997;104:82–86.

15. Francis WJA, Jeffcoate TNA. Dyspareunia following vaginal operations. *J Opt Soc Am* 1961;68:1–10.

16. Cundiff GW, Weidner AC, Visco AG, et al. An anatomic and functional assessment of the discrete defect rectocele repair. *Am J Obstet Gynecol* 1998;179:1451–1457.

17. Porter WE, Steele A, Walsh P, et al. The anatomic and functional outcomes of defect-specific rectocele repairs. *Am J Obstet Gynecol* 1999;181:1353–1359.

18. Kenton K, Shott S, Brubaker L. Outcome after rectovaginal fascia reattachment for rectocele repair. *Am J Obstet Gynecol* 1999;181:1360–1364.

19. Singh K, Cortes E, Reid WM. Evaluation of the fascial technique for surgical repair of isolated posterior vaginal wall prolapse. *Obstet Gynecol* 2003;101:320–324.

20. Galvind K, Madsen H. A prospective study of the discrete fascial defect rectocele repair. *Acta Obstet Gynecol Scand* 1000;79:145–147.

21. Abramov Y, Gandhi S, Goldberg RP, et al. Site-specific rectocele repair compared with standard posterior colporrhaphy. *Obstet Gynecol* 2005;105:314–318.

22. Paraiso M, Barber M, Muir T, et al. Rectocele repair: a randomized trial of three surgical techniques including graft augmentation. *J Pelvic Surg Med* 2006;12(2):69.

23. Marks MM. The rectal side of the rectocele. *Dis Colon Rectum* 1967;10:387–388.

24. Arnold MW, Stewart WR, Aguilar PS. Rectocele repair. Four years' experience. *Dis Colon Rectum* 1990;33:684–687.

25. van Dam JH, Huisman WM, Hop WCJ, et al. Fecal continence after rectocele repair: a prospective study. *Int J Colorectal Dis* 2000;15:54–57.

26. Nieminen K, Hiltunen K, Laitinen J, et al. Transanal or vaginal approach to rectocele repair: results of a prospective randomized study. *Neurourol Urodyn* 2003;22:547–548.

27. Kahn MA, Stanton SL, Kumar D, et al. Posterior colporrhaphy is superior to the transanal repair for treatment of posterior vaginal wall prolapse. *Neurourol Urodyn* 1999;18:70–71.

28. Maher C, Baessler K, Glazener C, et al. Surgical management of pelvic organ prolapse in women. *The Cochrane Collaboration,* Volume (4), 2005.

29. Altman D, Mellgren A, Zetterstrom J. Rectocele repair using biomaterial augmentation: current documentation and clinical experience. *Obstet Gynecol Surv* 2005; 60(11):753–760.

30. Cundiff GW, Fenner D. Evaluation and treatment of women with rectocele: focus on associated defecatory and sexual dysfunction. *Obstet Gynecol* 2004;104:1403–1421.

31. Oster S, Astrup A. A new vaginal operation for recurrent and large rectocele using dermis transplant. *Acta Obstet Gynecol Scand* 1981;60:493–495.

32. Kohli N, Miklos JR. Dermal graft-augmented rectocele repair. *Int Urogynecol J Pelvic Floor Dysfunct* 2003;14:146–149.

33. Dell J, Kelley K. PelviSoft biomesh augmentation of rectocele repair: the initial clinical experience in 35 patients. *Int Urogynecol J* 2004;16:44–47.

34. Altman D, Zetterstrom J, Lopez A, et al. Functional and anatomic outcome after transvaginal rectocele repair using collagen mesh: a prospective study. *Dis Colon Rectum* 2005;48:1233–1242.

35. Kobashi KC, Leach GE, Frederick R, et al. Initial experience with rectocele repair using nonfrozen cadaveric fascia lata interposition. *Urology* 2005;66:1203–1208.

36. Gandhi S, Kwon C, Goldberg R, et al. Does fascia lata graft decrease recurrent posterior vaginal wall prolapse? (abstract 86). In: Proceedings 28th International Urogynecology Meeting, Buenos Aires. *Int Urogynecol J Pelvic Floor Dysfunction* 2003;14;Suppl 1:86

37. Watson SJ, Loder PB, Halligan S, et al. Transperineal repair of symptomatic rectocele with Marlex mesh: a clinical, physiological, and radiologic assessment of treatment. *J Am Coll Surg* 1996;183:257–261.

38. Mercer-Jones MA, Sprowson A, Varma J. Outcome after transperineal mesh repair of rectocele: a case series. *Dis Colon Rectum* 2004;47:864–868.

39. Lim Y, Rane A, Muller R. An ambispective observational study in the safety and efficacy of posterior colporrhaphy with composite Vicryl-Prolene mesh. *Int Urogynecol J* 2005;16:126–131.

40. Goh JTW, Dwyer PL. Effectiveness and safety of polypropylene mesh in vaginal prolapse surgery. *Int Urogynecol J* 2001;12:S90.

41. de Tayrac R, Picone O, Chauveaud-Lambling A, et al. A 2-year anatomical and functional assessment of transvaginal rectocele repair using a polypropylene mesh. *Int Urogynecol J* 2006;17:100–105.

42. Perez M, Lefranc JP, Blondon. Rectoceles et troubles fonctionnels rectaux après traitement chirurgical d'un prolapsus genital. *J Chir (Paris)* 1991;128:465–469.

43. Villet R, Morice P, Bech A, et al. Approache abdominale des rectoceles et des elytroceles. *Ann Chir* 1993; 47:626–630.

44. Cundiff GW, Harris RL, Coates K, et al. Abdominal sacral colpoperineopexy: a new approach for correction of posterior compartment defects and perineal descent associated with vaginal vault prolapse. *Am J Obstet Gynecol* 1997;177:1345–1355.

45. Sullivan ES, Longaker CJ, Lee PY. Total pelvic mesh repair: a ten-year experience. *Dis Colon Rectum* 2001; 44:857–863.

46. Visco AG, Weidner AC, Barber MD, et al. Vaginal mesh erosion after abdominal sacral colpopexy. *Am J Obstet Gynecol* 2001;184:297–302.

SUGGESTED READING

Cundiff GW, Fenner D. Evaluation and treatment of women with rectocele: focus on associated defecatory and sexual dysfunction. *Obstet Gynecol* 2004;104:1403–1421.

Maher C, Baessler K. Surgical management of posterior vaginal wall prolapse: an evidence-based literature review. *Int Urogynecol J* 2006;17(1):84–88.

CHAPTER 31

Obliterative Procedures

Thomas L. Wheeler II and Holly E. Richter

INTRODUCTION

The elderly population, especially 85 years or older, is experiencing an increasing rate of growth (1). As a result, the number of patients presenting for treatment of pelvic organ prolapse, including those who do not desire to maintain sexual function, is also increasing (2,3). Many of these patients will not be sexually active for a variety of reasons and restorative reconstructive surgery may not be desired. For these patients, the pelvic reconstructive surgeon should be comfortable discussing the option of obliterative vaginal procedures. Shorter operative time and less surgical risk are the advantages of this approach over traditional vaginal reconstructive procedures (4). The obliterative procedures for severe prolapse are total colpocleisis (i.e., colpectomy) and partial colpocleisis, with or without levator myorrhaphy and high perineorrhaphy. When a colpocleisis is not technically feasible, a constricting anterior and posterior colporrhaphy with levator myorrhaphy and high perineorrhaphy may be considered.

Partial colpocleisis approximates denuded portions of the anterior and posterior vagina; therefore, the uterus may be left in place as lateral channels are formed from which cervical drainage or blood can escape. Since a total colpocleisis involves complete denudation and does not leave drainage channels, concurrent or previous hysterectomy is necessary. Either way, potential colpocleisis candidates should be counseled regarding the loss of a sexually functioning vagina.

HISTORY

Throughout history, women have endured severe pelvic organ prolapse. Ineffective methods of correction that were attempted included vaginal packing, crude pessaries, and instillation of caustic materials. Some women were even hung up-

side down to invert the prolapse back into the pelvis (5). Initial attempts at surgical management involved amputation of the prolapsing segments or closure of the vaginal introitus (6), with unsatisfactory results.

The idea to surgically obliterate severe prolapse is credited to Gerardin, who suggested suturing surgically denuded anterior and posterior vaginal walls together (7). Even though he wrote about this technique in 1823, he never attempted the procedure. Subsequently, the first known procedure was performed in 1867 by Neugebauer, who waited until 1881 to publish his technique (8). Neugebauer obliterated the vagina by denuding 6 × 3-cm anterior and posterior areas near the introitus and suturing them together. Leon Le Fort's technique was actually published first in 1877 (9). Le Fort's modifications differed in that longer and narrower areas of denudation were performed and that a colpoperineoplasty was performed 8 days after the colpocleisis to address the widened genital hiatus. In general, a partial colpocleisis is referred to as a Le Fort colpocleisis, but a less common eponym is the Neugebauer-Le Fort procedure. Edebohls, in 1901, was the first to report performing a total colpocleisis with levator myorrhaphy following hysterectomy (i.e., panhysterocolpectomy) (10,11). His report was followed by several case series that had comparable results to the partial colpocleisis-type procedures (12). Even though adoption of the colpocleisis procedure was slow in the United States, in 1880, Berlin reported three cases (one of which failed) to the New England Hospital (13). This failure was blamed on lack of a concurrent perineorrhaphy being performed.

In the attempt to make colpocleisis more acceptable, early modifications were directed at reducing the risk of recurrence or the incidence of postoperative urinary incontinence, which was as high as 25% (14) and attributed to scarring from a distal dissection and pulling down of the bladder neck. An early example to increase the robustness of the repair was creating a wider septum, as reported by Wyatt in 1912 (15). Other authors addressed postoperative urinary incontinence by sparing the distal vagina near the urethra or by supporting the bladder neck with a high perineorrhaphy (6,15–19). Goodall and Power in 1937 tried to preserve sexual function by creating a triangular septum higher in the vagina that would allow for intercourse and potentially less stress urinary incontinence (20).

PATIENT SELECTION AND CONSIDERATIONS

The classic example of a candidate for colpocleisis is an older, sexually inactive patient who has medical comorbidities that make a quick and relatively noninvasive procedure attractive. Further, she has either declined pessary or had unsatisfactory results. Sometimes this description includes patients who may have a spouse. Therefore, the patient and her partner need to be counseled that intercourse is not possible after colpocleisis, even if her quality of life improves. Candidates should also be counseled that reported satisfaction rates are greater than 85% and regret rates are less than 11% (19,21–24).

Urinary Incontinence

Another consideration when evaluating potential candidates for an obliterative procedure is postoperative urinary incontinence. Initially, the occurrence of postoperative urinary incontinence, up to 25% (14), was probably the biggest deterrent against the performance of the procedure. In fact, early in the development of colpocleisis, some surgeons did not address urinary incontinence if it existed preoperatively. De novo stress incontinence has been attributed to (a) distal vaginal dissection with scarring and resultant downward traction on the urethra and (b) unmasking of occult stress urinary incontinence by reducing the prolapse, which previously had "kinked" the bladder neck.

To minimize this problem, contemporary colpocleisis techniques avoid distal dissections that predispose to downward traction on the urethra and include incontinence procedures for appropriately selected patients (14,16,17,25).

The decision to perform an incontinence procedure in these patients is difficult and should be individualized. Patients should be evaluated for urinary incontinence and bladder function because the morbidity of postoperative stress incontinence

against the possibility of urinary retention must be considered. Unfortunately, there are mixed results on the impact of colpocleisis on bladder emptying (14,26). If no voiding dysfunction is suspected, candidates should be evaluated at least with simple cystometrics with reduction of the prolapse and measurement of a postvoid residual. Otherwise, urodynamic evaluation is warranted, even though complex urodynamics have not been shown to be sensitive in distinguishing if the cause of poor bladder emptying is due to, for instance, severe prolapse or detrusor motor impairment.

In addition to bladder testing, the surgeon must also judge the patient's ability to perform self-catheterization, because decreased manual dexterity is common in these patients. All patients, whether or not an incontinence procedure is performed, should be counseled on the possible need for prolonged bladder drainage with indwelling Foley or intermittent catheterization. As a compromise between highly effective stress incontinence procedures that may increase urinary retention rates versus no procedure, a Kelly plication procedure can be considered.

Management of the Geriatric Patient

Advanced age alone is not a contraindication to any type of surgery, including colpocleisis. However, surgeons who perform colpocleisis need to be adept at surgical care of the geriatric patient.

In addition to open communication with the anesthesiologist regarding the optimal method of anesthesia, cardiac, pulmonary, nutritional, cognitive, and functional status may need to be accounted for preoperatively. The goal is to minimize risk factors for the occurrence of complications. From a cardiac standpoint, a diastolic blood pressure greater than 110 mm Hg should postpone surgery. Many antihypertensives should be given the day of surgery and restarted immediately after surgery, as the risk of severe hypertension greatly outweighs the risk posed by giving medicine prior to anesthesia induction. Consultation with an internist or cardiologist should be considered for patients on multiple classes of antihypertensive medications. Poor functional status, as shown by decreased activities of daily living (ADL), is predictive of pulmonary complications and should prompt a rigorous preoperative assessment (27).

Postoperative delirium may be seen in up to 10% of older surgical patients and is often misdiagnosed, leading to longer hospital stays, nursing home admits, and morbidity. Baseline dementia increases the incidence of acute postoperative delirium and adverse outcomes. A basic check of cognitive function should be performed in older surgical candidates, and if cognitive processes are impaired, consultation with an internist, geriatrician, neurologist, or other individual skilled in dementia management should be considered perioperatively to reduce the risk of postoperative delirium. Poor nutrition inhibits wound healing, and a serum albumin may be checked to assess preoperative nutritional status (27). A history of alcohol abuse should be elicited, and smoking should be stopped. Routine laboratory studies include hematocrit, electrolytes, blood urea nitrogen, and creatinine, while other studies to be considered are complete blood cell count, platelets, arterial blood gases, and prothrombin time and partial thromboplastin time (27).

Perioperative and postoperative care are tailored for a speedy recovery and avoidance of a decline in functional status. After colpocleisis, early ambulation is vital. Hypertensive episodes can be managed by identifying an underlying cause such as pain or lack of medications. Potent direct vasodilators are contraindicated because of the potential exacerbation of diastolic dysfunction commonly found in the elderly; therefore, volume overload should be avoided. Adequate pain control must be ensured, along with avoidance of common drug–drug interactions in this population. Atelectasis is a common postoperative occurrence; therefore, incentive spirometry should be initiated immediately after surgery with turning, coughing, and deep breathing to prevent increased respiratory compromise. Delirium occurrence is reduced by improving orientation, decreasing sensory overload or deprivation, and providing reassurance. Prophylaxis should also be employed against deep venous thrombosis, infection, and constipation (27).

Concurrent Hysterectomy

In general, hysterectomy should be reserved for pathologic indications or if a total colpocleisis is planned. The main benefit of routine hysterectomy would be the prevention of endometrial or cervical cancer, in addition to the rare event of pyometra after partial colpocleisis secondary to blocked lateral channels (28). The main argument against routine hysterectomy is that the advantages of less operative time and a less invasive technique with partial colpocleisis are compromised. Two observational studies showed longer operating times, with one of these studies showing increased blood loss and a longer hospital stay (22,26). Von Pechmann reported two cases of conversion to exploratory laparotomy in the hysterectomy group

(22). If hysterectomy is not performed, a Pap smear, if indicated, and endometrial assessment with ultrasound or sampling should be considered. A dilatation and curettage may be performed as clinically indicated.

Perineorrhaphy and Levator Myorrhaphy

The rationale behind performing this concurrent procedure is to narrow the introitus and create a platform whereby less gravitational tension is placed on the colpocleisis procedure. In theory, this platform may reduce the risk of anatomical failure and downward tension on the urethra, a proposed etiology of postoperative stress incontinence. This procedure is encouraged, especially for candidates who are physically active. Formal study of the role of perineorrhaphy and levator myorrhaphy is probably unlikely due to the high success noted with this concurrent procedure.

TECHNIQUES

Partial Colpocleisis

The cervix or vaginal vault is grasped and brought out through the introitus. A marking pen is used to outline two rectangular areas on the vaginal wall for incision, one on the anterior vaginal wall and one on the posterior wall (Fig. 31.1). When the cervix is present, the incision borders closest to the cervix are demarcated approximately 0.5 cm from the cervical vaginal reflection. The border of the rectangle closest to the bladder neck is placed approximately 2 cm from the urethrovesical junction in order to allow for minimal traction on the bladder neck area. The sides of the rectangle are demarcated lateral to any cystocele defect that is present. In cases of vaginal vault prolapse, the rectangles begin approximately 1 cm anterior and posterior to the cuff. The inferior border of the posterior rectangle is at least 2 cm inside the hymenal ring. The lateral lines should leave approximately 2 cm between the anterior rectangle and posterior rectangle.

The outlined epithelium can be infiltrated with saline or vasoconstrictor of choice. It is then incised and removed off the underlying rectum and enterocele posteriorly and bladder anteriorly. Sharp dissection is performed to leave as much musculoconnective tissue overlying these structures as is possible while maintaining an avascular plane of dissection (Fig. 31.2). The enterocele is not entered. This dissection can be performed with electrocautery, which may decrease blood loss.

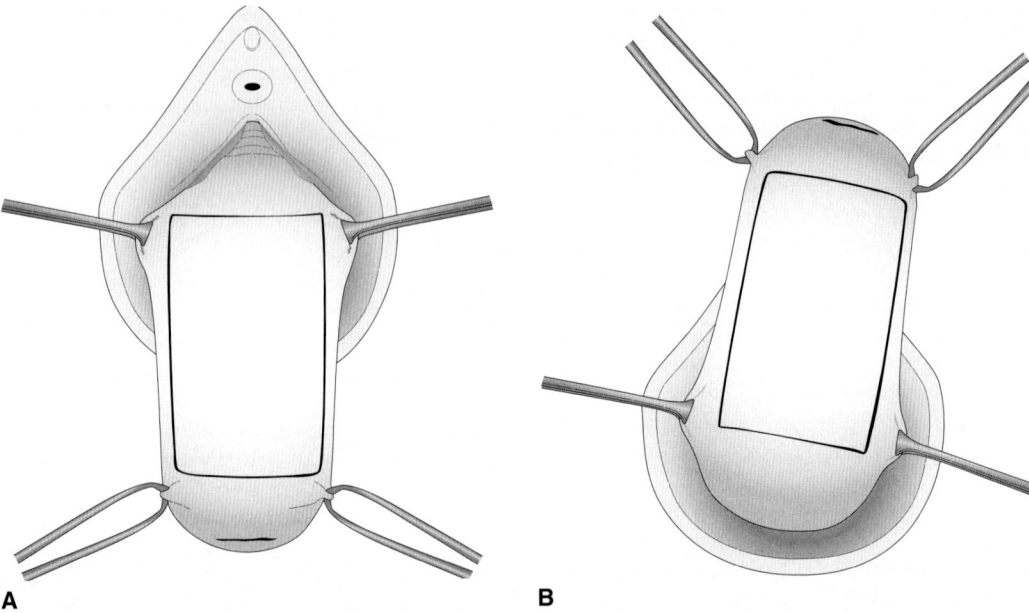

A   **B**

FIGURE 31.1 ● **Partial colpocleisis**. Rectangular portions of the anterior and posterior vaginal walls are demarcated. A 2-cm space between the rectangles is left to allow for creation of drainage tunnels. Care is taken to be distal to the urethrovesical junction.

The vaginal epithelial edges of the respective anterior and posterior rectangles are then approximated together with running delayed absorbable or nonabsorbable sutures. This epithelial approximation can be started with two side-by-side sutures that are placed anterior to the cervix or vaginal

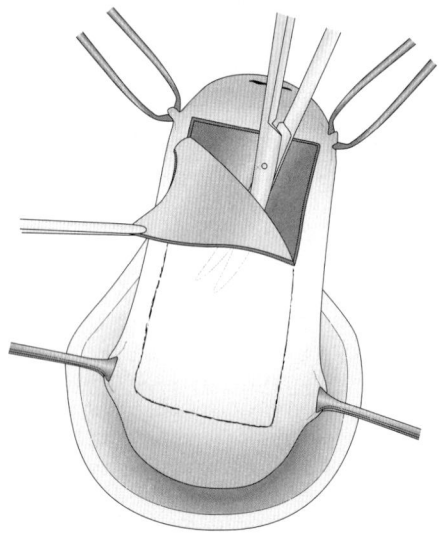

FIGURE 31.2 ● Sharp dissection is performed to remove the vaginal epithelium, leaving musculoconnective tissue on the bladder and rectum. The enterocele is not entered.

cuff and then brought across the cervix or cuff to the corresponding edge of the posterior rectangle. When these two sutures are tied, the cervix or vaginal cuff is thereby pushed cephalad. These two sutures are then run in opposite directions using a locking technique connecting the borders of the anterior rectangle to the posterior rectangle (Fig. 31.3). Before the lateral edges of the epithelium are approximated, three or four sutures are sagittally placed in the connective tissue underlying the bladder and brought to that overlying the rectum, thus approximating these (Fig. 31.4). Continuation of the running sutures to approximate the lateral anterior and posterior epithelium creates the lateral canals for drainage. The running sutures are individually tied, and the last anterior and posterior epithelial borders are closed with absorbable suture (Fig. 31.5). Vaginal depth is typically 3 to 4 cm. Cystoscopy may be performed to assess for ureteral patency.

Total Colpocleisis

For patients without a uterus, there is no need to leave lateral drainage channels and a total colpocleisis can be performed. The vaginal epithelium can be divided into four quadrants or removed en bloc. If desired, the subepithelium can be infiltrated with saline or vasoconstrictor. The dissection starts with a circumferential incision

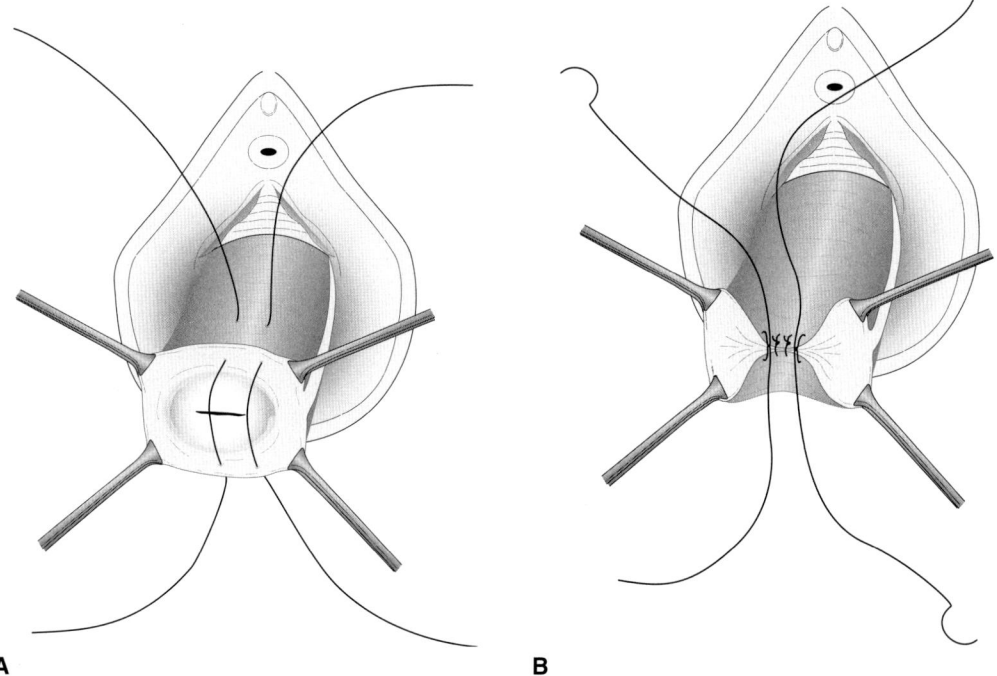

A **B**

FIGURE 31.3 ● Two delayed absorbable sutures are used to start the locking closure. The closure starts over the midline of the cervix or cuff and is run in opposite directions.

just outside of the hymenal ring (Fig. 31.6). As in the partial colpocleisis, the dissection is kept 2 cm away from the urethrovesical junction.

Again, the epithelium is dissected sharply in order to leave as much connective tissue as possible overlying the bladder, enterocele, and rectum (Fig. 31.7). Placing Allis clamps on the edge of the

epithelium being removed will aid in the dissection. Also, the operator's finger can "hook" this epithelium for countertraction. The enterocele is not entered. The vaginal tube is then obliterated with sequential purse-string sutures (or interrupted sutures) through the musculoconnective tissue, and the vaginal epithelium is closed (Fig. 31.8).

FIGURE 31.4 ● Three or four absorbable sutures are sagittally placed in the musculo-connective tissue underlying the bladder and brought to that overlying the rectum to approx-imate the middle portions of the rectangles. *Inset:* The lock-ing closure is continued to cre-ate the lateral drainage chan-nels. The *x*'s represent appropriate needle placement, paying attention to stay near the epithelial edge.

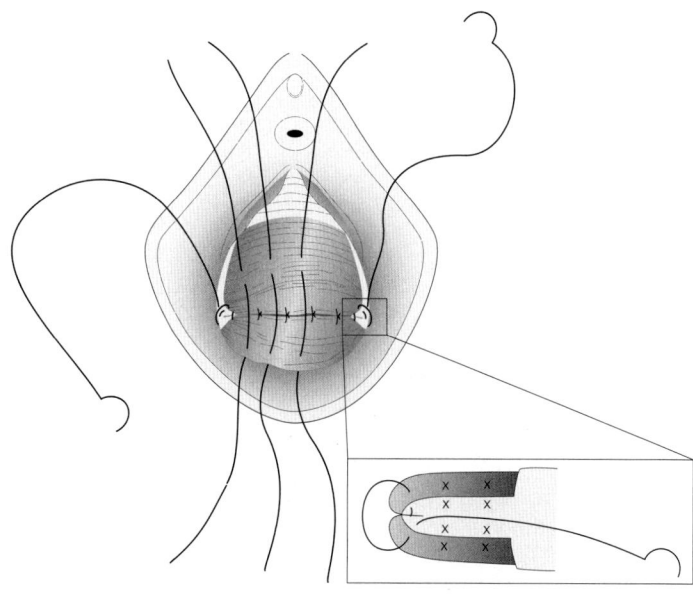

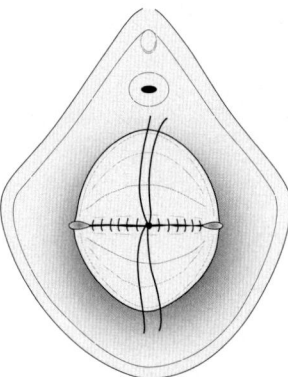

FIGURE 31.5   ●   After the prolapse is reduced, the final edges of the rectangles are closed either with a separate suture or from continuation of the running stitch. The lateral drainage channels are shown.

Incontinence Procedure

If an incontinence procedure is to be performed, it typically consists of a midurethral or pubovaginal sling or Kelly plication type of procedure. The pubovaginal sling and pubourethral ligament or Kelly plication procedure are typically performed prior to closure of the anterior and posterior vaginal epithelial edges by means of a separate midline central incision. A midurethral sling procedure can

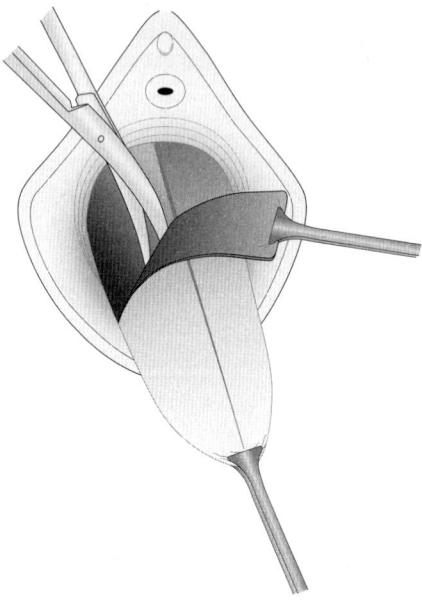

FIGURE 31.6   ●   **Total colpocleisis**. The prolapse is divided into four quadrants. A circumferential incision at the base of the prolapse starts the dissection.

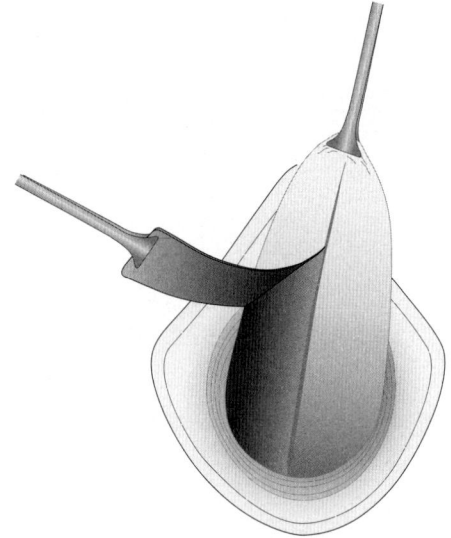

FIGURE 31.7   ●   The entire overlying vaginal epithelium is removed a quadrant at a time, leaving as much connective tissue as possible on the bladder and rectum.

be performed prior to the levator myorrhaphy/high perineorrhaphy.

Levator Myorrhaphy and High Perineorrhaphy

Two Allis clamps are placed opposite each other at the level of the hymenal ring or slightly distal to that at approximately 4 and 8 o'clock. A horizontal incision is made between the clamps just outside the hymenal ring inside the perineal body. This incision is then carried cephalad to the distal edge of the colpocleisis so that a triangular wedge of vaginal epithelium is demarcated. Dissection is then carried out in the rectovaginal space and the wedge is excised (Fig. 31.9). Dissection is also carried out laterally to free the vaginal wall from the fascia of the puborectalis and bulbocavernous muscles and from whatever perineal membrane is present (Figs. 31.10 and 31.11). Closure of the vaginal epithelium may be started with absorbable suture as long as exposure to the puborectalis muscle is not compromised. Nonabsorbable sutures are then placed through a puborectalis muscle or its fascial covering at least 3 cm posterior to its attachment to the pubic rami and then brought across to the same area of the contralateral muscle. The muscles are then plicated across the midline posterior to the vaginal wall (Fig. 31.12). The bulbocavernosus muscles are likewise plicated across the

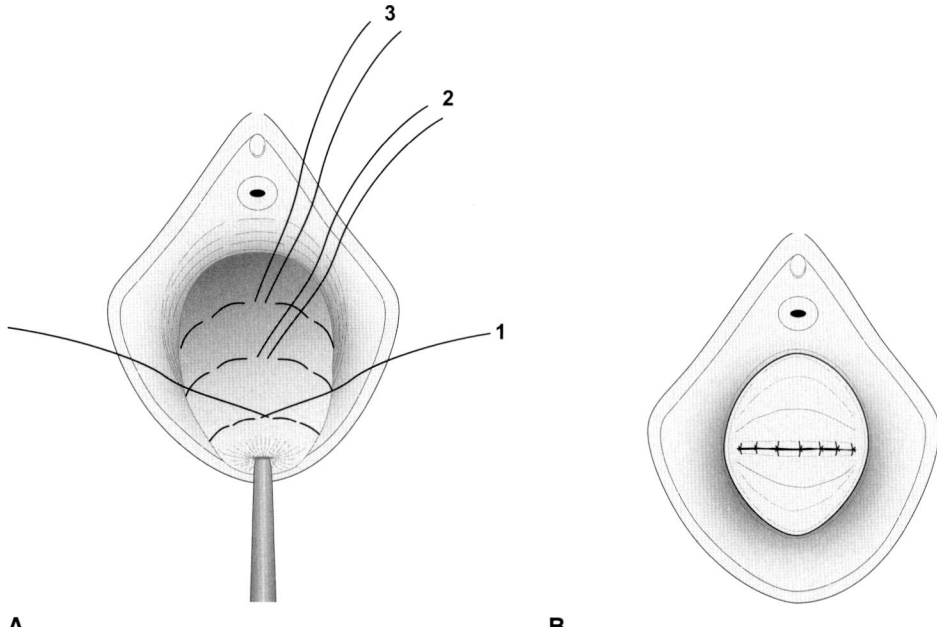

A   **B**

FIGURE 31.8 ● **(A)** Sequential purse-string delayed absorbable sutures are placed into the connective tissue. The prolapse is reduced and the purse-string sutures are tied in the order shown (here, 1 through 3). **(B)** The vaginal epithelium is then closed.

midline in the same space utilizing two plication stitches, one anterior to the other (Fig. 31.13). Lastly the perineal body is approximated (Fig. 31.14). After reconstitution of the perineal body, closure of the vaginal wall, down to the introitus, is completed with the running absorbable suture. The genital hiatus should be 1 to 2 cm (Fig. 31.15).

Constricting Colporrhaphy

For some patients who are, by history, good candidates for an obliterative procedure, there may not be enough apical descensus, or a large enough cystocele or rectocele, to make colpocleisis feasible. For these patients, constricting anterior and poste-

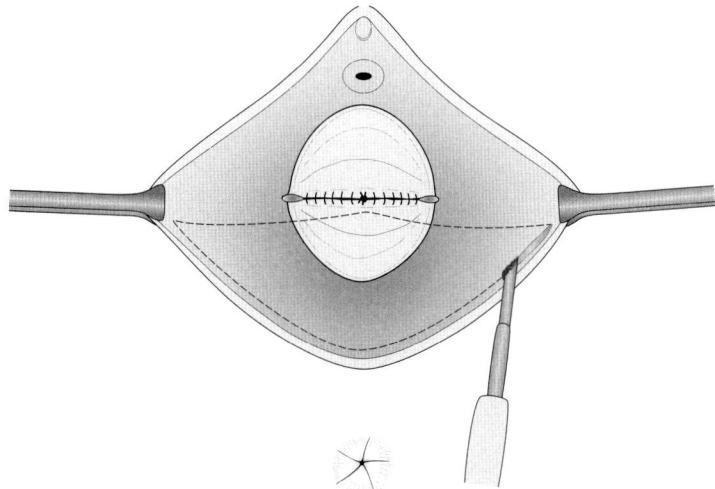

FIGURE 31.9 ● **Levator myorrhaphy and high perineorrhaphy**. Two Allis clamps are placed opposite each other at the level of the hymenal ring or slightly distal to that at approximately 4 and 8 o'clock. A horizontal incision is made between the clamps.

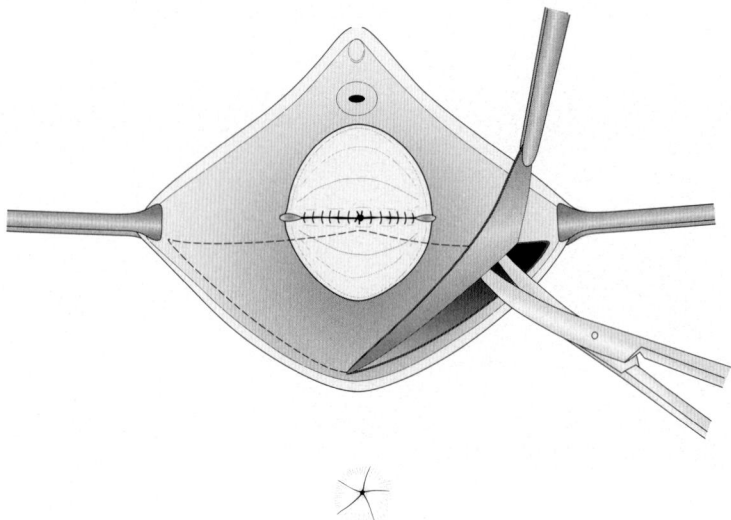

FIGURE 31.10 ● This incision is then carried cephalad to the distal edge of the colpocleisis in order to dissect free the wedge to be removed (*hash marks*).

rior colporrhaphies can be performed. The authors also recommend that a concurrent levator myorrhaphy and high perineorrhaphy be performed. The surgeon's preference for dissecting out the cystocele or rectocele is acceptable, as long as care is taken in narrowing the vaginal tube with closure of the defect.

Otherwise, a recommended technique is to use Allis clamps to grasp the cystocele, and the entire defect is demarcated with a marking pen. The subepithelium can be infiltrated with saline or vasoconstrictor of choice. The epithelium is in-

cised, and the Allis clamps are then placed on the edge of the epithelium being removed for countertraction. The demarcated epithelium is removed with sharp dissection. Dissection under the remaining epithelium is then carried out laterally to expose paravaginal connective tissue. Delayed absorbable suture, which incorporates the lateral connective tissue and overlying lateral vaginal wall epithelium, is plicated across the midline, which greatly reduces the caliber of the vaginal tube. In order to facilitate lateral exposure, if necessary, absorbable suture can be placed to reduce

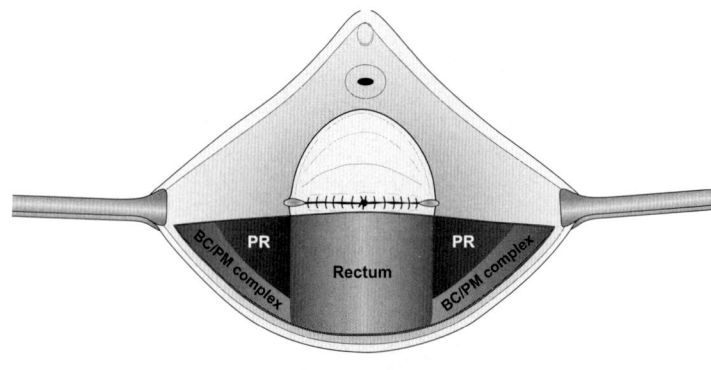

FIGURE 31.11 ● The vaginal wall is freed from the fascia of the puborectalis and bulbocavernosus muscles and from whatever perineal membrane is present.

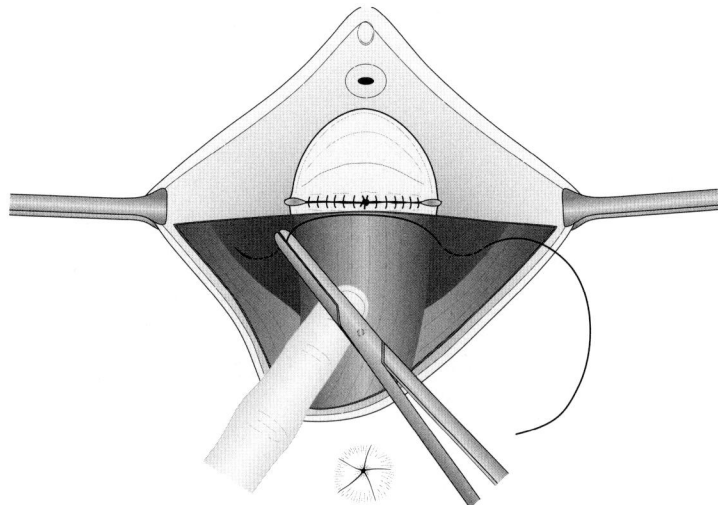

FIGURE 31.12 ● Nonabsorbable sutures are then placed through a puborectalis (PR) muscle or its fascial covering approximately 3 cm posterior to its attachment to the pubic rami and then brought across to the same area of the contralateral muscle.

the midline portion of the defect prior to plicating the lateral aspects of the anterior vaginal wall. Any excess epithelium is trimmed, and the incision is closed with absorbable suture.

The posterior compartment should be approached as described above for performing a levator myorrhaphy and high perineorrhaphy. If a rectocele is present, the lateral dissection should be

continued cephalad to expose perilevator and perirectal connective tissue lateral to the rectocele defect. Care should be taken not to enter the rectum or enterocele, if present. The operator's finger is then used to reduce the rectocele in the midline while the perilevator and perirectal fascia and the overlying lateral vaginal wall epithelium are plicated across the midline with delayed absorbable

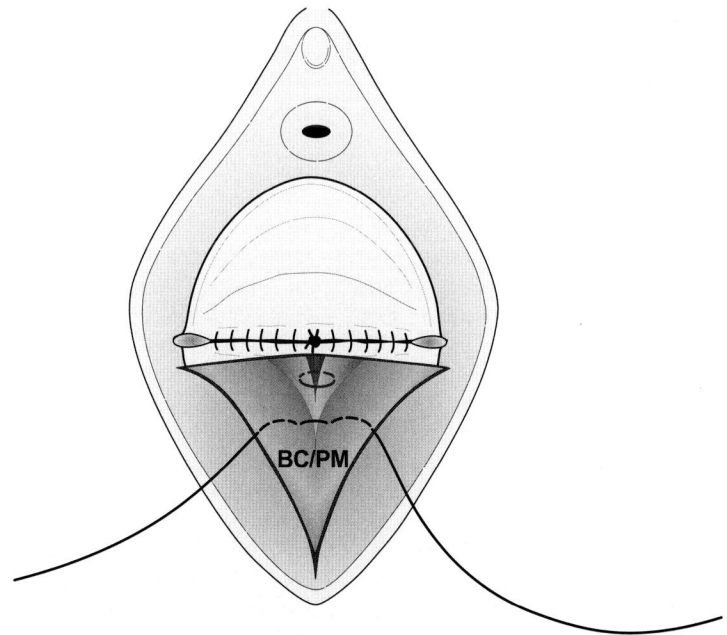

FIGURE 31.13 ● The bulbocavernosus muscles, which are not dissected from the perineal membrane, are plicated across the midline (BC/BM complex).

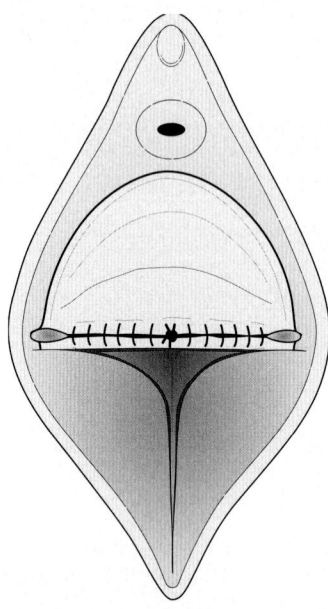

FIGURE 31.14 • The perineal membrane (BC/PM complex) is plicated.

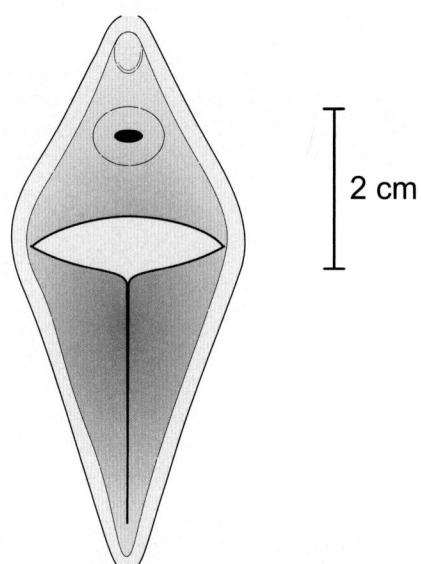

FIGURE 31.15 • Closure of the vaginal wall, down to the introitus, is completed with the running absorbable suture. The genital hiatus should be 1 to 2 cm.

suture. This plication narrows the posterior portion of the vaginal tube. Attention should be paid to not plicate too far distally before the levator myorrhaphy is performed. Once the levator myorrhaphy, bulbocavernosus myorrhaphy, and rebuilding of the perineal membrane are finished, the constricting posterior colporrhaphy can be incorporated into the rebuilt perineal membrane or be tied down separately. The rest of the procedure is completed as described in the levator myorrhaphy and high perineorrhaphy section.

RESULTS

An anatomical success rate of 100% for colpocleisis was first reported by Edebohls in 1901 for a series of four patients who underwent total colpocleisis (10). Since then, case series reports for total colpocleisis have ranged between 89% and 100%, with the majority close to or at 100% (5,12,22–24,26,29–38). Likewise, anatomical success rates for partial colpocleisis are based on case series, starting with Wyatt's report of 83% success on eight patients in 1912, and range between 75% and 100% (4,6,15–19,39–46). Case series reporting both techniques report anatomical success rates between 90% and 100% (14,25,47–49). The inherent outcome bias associated with case series reports limits comparison of the techniques.

Recurrence, satisfaction, and incontinence after colpocleisis for published results since 1972 are listed in Table 31.1. A comprehensive review has been published in the urogynecology literature (50).

Reports of satisfaction are high (86% to 100%) and regret low (0% to 13%) after colpocleisis, but these outcomes are sporadically reported. Following partial colpocleisis Ubachs reported a 10.7% regret rate, and Wheeler reported 9.3%; none cited regret over the loss of sexual function. For total colpocleisis, Harmanli had no reports of regret. As far as losing sexual function after total colpocleisis, Von Pechmann reported that 12.9% were at least somewhat regretful, while DeLancey reported that 1 patient out of 33 had remorse.

A lack of formal studies addressing urinary incontinence and postoperative bladder function in this patient cohort has created a dilemma in interpreting the impact of colpocleisis on urinary incontinence. Table 31.1 illustrates the mix of results that can occur. Until formal studies have been performed addressing this issue, counseling should be individualized with respect to performing an incontinence procedure, with consideration of the patient's activity level, the patient's subjective complaints of urinary incontinence, and the findings of objective testing. It is important to balance the risk of continued incontinence or new-onset incontinence with urinary retention.

TABLE 31.1

Results After Colpocleisis Reported Since 1972

Procedure	Author Year	n	Duration of Follow-Up	Recurrence, %	Incontinence	Colpocleisis-Related Complications	Satisfaction
Partial	Wheeler 2005	32	27.5 months	7.4%	Significant improvements on UDI-6 and IIQ-7 for both patients who did have and did not have an incontinence procedure		9.3% regret rate 86% satisfied
Both	Glavind 2005	42	46 months	0	11/29 incontinent	1 postop bleed	90% satisfied
Both	Fitzgerald 2003	64	12 weeks	3	18/21 continent after sling; 8/30 new-onset SUI	2 vaginal hematomas	
Total	Harmanli 2003	41	28.7 months	0	53.1% cure of SUI; 22.2% new-onset SUI	1 vesical injury 4 late rectal bleeding	High satisfaction and no regret
Total	Von Pechmann 2003	92	12 months (24 months for phone survey)	2.2	6/46 (13.0%) recurrent SUI; no new-onset SUI	4 ureteral occlusion; 1 proctotomy; 2 rectal prolapse; 2 laparotomies with TVH; 20 transfusions	90.3% (56/62) satisfaction; 12.9% (8/62) regret over loss of coital ability
Total	Hoffman 2003	54	22 months	0	22/33 improvement in bladder or bowel symptoms; 2 new-onset mixed UI; 4 new-onset SUI	1 CVA 1 pulmonary edema 1 A-fib	
Both	Moore 2003	30	19.1 months	10	94% cure of SUI with TVT	1 TVT release (continence maintained); 1 MI	No regret
Modified (total compartments individually constricted with extensive perineoplasty)	Cespedes 2001	38	24 months	0	3 persistent SUI	1 urethrolysis after sling	100% satisfaction No regret
Total	DeLancey 1997	33	7.7 months (34.6 months for phone survey)	1	100% cure SUI; no new-onset SUI; 2 cured, 1 improved, and 3 no change out of 8 with preoperative UUI	2 CHF; 1 pneumonia	1/22 remorse over loss of sexual function
Partial	Denehy 1995	21	25 months	5		1 arrhythmia; 3 UTI	

(continued)

TABLE 31.1 *(Continued)*

Procedure	Author Year	N	Duration of Follow-Up	Recurrence, %	Incontinence	Colpocleisis-Related Complications	Satisfaction
Partial	Ahranjani 1992	38	30/38 patients followed "long term"	0		2 transfusions; 30% minor complication rate (11 respiratory; 2 cardiac; 5 urinary)	
Both	Langmade 1986	102	35 months	0	No new-onset SUI; 2 persistent SUI; 15/20 persistent UUI	1 pyelonephritis	"No patient changed their mind in regard to (surgery) or sexual intercourse after surgery"
Partial	Goldman 1981	118	First postop exam (90 followed 1–15 years)	8.3	SUI cured in 5/6	1 pulmonary embolism 17 UTI; 6 wound infections; 3 thrombophlebitis; 1 TAH for bleeding	
Partial	Ubachs 1972	93	≥3 years	8.6	SUI cured in 23/30, UUI cured in 2/3; 3/47 new-onset SUI and 3/47 new-onset UUI	8 UTI; 2 hemorrhage; 1 PTE;1 thrombophlebitis; 10 complications of wound healing (dehiscence or putrid secretion)	84/93 satisfied; 9/93 regret
Partial	Ridley 1972	58		5			

FUTURE STUDIES

In addition to addressing the perioperative management of urinary incontinence, well-designed studies using validated instruments to better characterize patients' perceived outcomes of regret, satisfaction, quality of life, and impact on bowel function are needed. In general, these studies will help us in better counseling our patients about the risks and benefits of their surgical treatment for severe prolapse.

REFERENCES

1. Statistical abstract of the United States. In *The National Data Book*. U.S. Department of Commerce, 1998.
2. Boyles SH, Weber AM, Meyn L. Procedures for pelvic organ prolapse in the United States, 1979–97. *Am J Obstet Gynecol* 2003;188:108–115.
3. Olsen AL, Smith VJ, Bergstrom JO, et al. Epidemiology of surgically managed pelvic organ prolapse and urinary incontinence. *Obstet Gynecol* 1997;89:501–506.
4. Denehy TR, Choe JY, Gregori CA, et al. Modified Le Fort partial colpocleisis with Kelly urethral plication and posterior colpoperineoplasty in the medically compromised elderly: a comparison with vaginal hysterectomy, anterior colporrhaphy, and posterior colpoperineoplasty. *Am J Obstet Gynecol* 1995;173:1697–1702.
5. Bradbury WC. Subtotal vaginectomy. *Am J Obstet Gynecol* 1963;86:663–671.
6. Adair FL, DaSef L. The Le Fort colpocleisis. *Am J Obstet Gynecol* 1936;32:218–226.
7. Gerardin R. Memoire presente a la Societe Medicale de Metz en 1823. *Arch Gen Med* 1825;8:1825.

8. Neugebauer JA. Einige worte uber die mediane vaginal-naht als mittel zur beseitgung des gebarmuttervorfalls. *Zentralbl Gynaekol* 1881;5:3–8.

9. Le Fort L. Nouveau procede pour la guerison du prolap-sus uterin. *Bull Gen Therap* 1877;92:337–346.

10. Edebohls GM. Panhysterokolpectomy: a new prolapsus operation. *Med Rec NY* 1901;60:561–564.

11. Edebohls GM. Panhysterokolpectomy: a new prolapsus operation. *Trans Am Gynecol Soc* 1901;26:150–162.

12. Hayden RC, Levinson JM. Total vaginectomy, vaginal hysterectomy, and colpocleisis for advanced prociden-tia. *Obstet Gynecol* 1960;16:564–566.

13. Berlin F. Three cases of complete prolapus uteri oper-ated upon according to the method of Leon Le Fort. *Am J Obstet Gynecol* 1881;14:866.

14. Fitzgerald MP. Colpocleisis and urinary incontinence. *Am J Obstet Gynecol* 2003;189:1241–1244.

15. Wyatt J. LeFort's operation for prolapse, with an ac-count of eight cases. *J Obstet Gynaecol Brit Emp* 1912;22:266–269.

16. Mazer C. Israel SL. The Le Fort colpocleisis: an analysis of 43 operations. *Am J Obstet Gynecol* 1948;56:944–949.

17. Falk H, Kaufman S. Partial colpocleisis: the Le Fort procedure (analysis of 100 cases). *Obstet Gynecol* 1955;5:617.

18. Hanson GE, Keettel WC. The Neugebauer Le Fort op-eration (a review of 288 colpocleisis). *Obstet Gynecol* 1969;34:352–357.

19. Ubachs JM, van Sante TJ, Schellekens LA. Partial colpocleisis by a modification of Le Fort's operation. *Obstet Gynecol* 1973;42:415–420.

20. Goodall JR, Power RMH. A modification of the Le Fort operation for increasing its scope. *Am J Obstet Gynecol* 1937;34:968–976.

21. Wheeler TL Richter HE, Varner RE, et al. Regret, satis-faction, and symptom improvement: analysis of the im-pact of partial colpocleisis for the management of severe pelvic organ prolapse. *Am J Obstet Gynecol* 2005;193:2067–2070.

22. Von Pechmann WS, Mutone M, Fyffe J, et al. Total colpocleisis with high levator plication for the treatment of advanced pelvic organ prolapse. *Am J Obstet Gynecol* 2003;189:121–126.

23. Harmanli OH, Dandolu V, Chatwani AJ, et al. Total colpocleisis for severe pelvic organ prolapse. *J Reprod Med* 2003;48:703–706.

24. DeLancey JO, Morley GW. Total colpocleisis for vaginal eversion. *Am J Obstet Gynecol* 1997;176:1228–1235.

25. Moore RD. Colpocleisis and tension-free vaginal tape sling for severe uterine and vaginal prolapse and stress urinary incontinence under local anesthesia. *J Am Assoc Gynecol Laparoscopists* 2003;10:276–280.

26. Hoffman MS, Cardosi RJ, Lockhart J, et al. Vaginectomy with pelvic herniorrhaphy for prolapse. *Am J Obstet Gynecol* 2003;189:364–371.

27. Katz PR, Grossberg GT, Potter JF, et al. *Geriatric syl-labus for specialists.* American Geriatrics Society, 2002.

28. Kohli N, Sze E, Karram M. Pyometra following Le Fort colpocleisis. *Intl Urogynecol J* 1996;7:264–266.

29. Masson JC, Knepper PA. Vaginectomy. *Am J Obstet Gynecol* 1938;36:94–99.

30. Williams JT. Vaginal hysterectomy and colpectomy for prolapse of the uterus and bladder. *Am J Obstet Gynecol* 1950;59:365–370.

31. Phaneuf LE. Formulation of principles of treatment in uterine prolapse. *Am J Obstet Gynecol* 1954;68:446–449.

32. Symmonds RE, Williams TJ, Lee RA, et al. Post-hysterectomy enterocele and vaginal vault prolapse. *Am J Obstet Gynecol* 1981;140:852–859.

33. Cox KE, Lamar RF. Colpocleisis. *Am J Obstet Gynecol* 1952;65:583–591.

34. Adams HD. Total colpocleisis for pelvic eventration. *Surg Gynecol Obstet* 1951;92:321–324.

35. Anderson GV, Deasy PP. Hysterocolpectomy. *Obstet Gynecol* 1960;16:344–349.

36. Percy NM, Perl JI. Total colpectomy. *Surg Gynecol Obstet* 1961;113:174–184.

37. Thompson HG, Murphy CJ Jr, Picot H. Hysterocol-pectomy for the treatment of uterine procidentia. *Am J Obstet Gynecol* 1961;82:748–751.

38. Johnson CG. Vaginal hysterectomy and vaginectomy in personal retrospect. *Am J Obstet Gynecol* 1969;105:14–19.

39. Baer JL, Reis RA. Immediate and remote results in two hundred twelve cases of prolapse of the uterus. *Am J Obstet Gynecol* 1928;16:646–655.

40. Collins CG, Lock FR. The Le Fort colpocleisis. *Am J Surg* 1941;53:202.

41. Wolf W. The Le Fort operation. *Am J Obstet Gynecol* 1952;63:1346–1348.

42. Massoudnia N. Kahr colpocleisis. *Intl Surg* 1974;59:45–46.

43. Ardekany MS, Rafee R. A new modification of colpocleisis for treatment of total procidentia in old age. *Intl J Gynaecol Obstet* 1978;25:358–360.

44. Ahranjani M, Nora E 2nd, Rezai P, et al. Neugebauer–Le Fort operation for vaginal prolapse. *J Reprod Med* 1992;37:959–964.

45. Ridley JH. Evaluation of the colpocleisis operation: a report of fifty-eight cases. *Am J Obstet Gynecol* 1972;113:1114–1119.

46. Goldman J, Ovadia J, Feldberg D, The Neugebauer–Le Fort operation: A review of 118 partial colpocleisis. *Euro J Obstet Gynecol Reprod Biol* 1981;12:31–35

47. Phaneuf LE. The place of colpectomy in the treatment of uterine and vaginal prolapse. *Trans Am Gynecol Soc* 1935;60:143–156.

48. Rubovitz W, Litt S. Colpocleisis in the treatment of uter-ine and vaginal prolapse. *Am J Obstet Gynecol* 1935;29:222–230.

49. Langmade CF, Oliver JA Jr. Partial colpocleisis. *Am J Obstet Gynecol* 1986;154:1200–1205.

50. Fitzpatrick MP, Richter NE, Siddique S, et al. Colpociesis: a review. *Int Urogynecol J* 2006;17:261–271.

CHAPTER 32

Sutures and Grafts in Pelvic Reconstructive Surgery

Marjorie Jean-Michel and G. Willy Davila

INTRODUCTION

Surgeons require tools to accomplish their art. Despite our recent attempts at standardization of surgical techniques, reconstructive surgery is still an art. Besides surgical instruments, sutures, grafts, and other implants are required to complete a surgical procedure. Grafts have recently been widely promoted for use in vaginal surgery with only limited supportive evidence. Surgeons should familiarize themselves with the various available suture and graft types, as well as their indications and biologic behavior, in order to optimize surgical outcomes.

SUTURES

The surgeon's most indispensable tool is the suture. It is meant to augment the patient's own ability to re-establish normal anatomy. Sutures are available in many varieties and are categorized as permanent or absorbable, natural or synthetic, braided or nonbraided, and coated or uncoated. Suture selection depends greatly upon the tissue involved, the anticipated duration of wound closure, the healing environment, and the surgeon's preference.

The ideal suture may have the following characteristics (1):

1. Easy to manipulate
2. Does not readily tear tissue
3. Has enduring tensile strength
4. Maintains knots securely
5. Is nonallergenic
6. Resists infection
7. Changes in a predictable fashion over time

The unfortunate reality is that the ideal suture does not exist. In fact, sutures may carry several of the different properties, but not all of them. When selecting a suture, the surgeon must determine which properties can and cannot be compromised in that particular setting. Table 32.1 summarizes the various suture materials (1).

Absorbable Sutures

Natural Materials

Plain catgut is not derived from feline tissue, but from the jejunum and ileum of sheep. It is shaped into longitudinal strips and treated with formaldehyde, which confers resistance to enzymatic degradation. These strips are joined, desiccated, cut, and sterilized with cobalt 60 irradiation. This foreign body elicits a pronounced tissue response and is rapidly metabolized by immune cell proteases. Tensile strength is maintained for approximately 5 days only, and the suture is completely absorbed after 14 days.

Catgut treated with chromium salts gives rise to the chromic suture, a new and stronger material. Its tensile strength is 4-fold greater than plain catgut. It is enzymatically lysed fairly quickly, maintaining its tensile strength for 14 to 21 days. After 14 days, 34% of its original strength is retained. It is used on serosa, viscera, and the vagina, as these tissues heal within this period of time.

Synthetic Materials

Polyfilaments are thin filaments braided into various sutures. Polyglycolic acid (Dexon™) is a copolymer of glycolic acid (hydroacetic acid) that is transformed into a linear chain polymer. It is then converted into long filaments that are braided into different sizes. Polyglactin (Vicryl) is a copolymer of lactic acid and glycolic acid that is also braided. Unlike catgut, both are slowly hydrolyzed, resulting in less inflammation. Absorption occurs in a pre-

TABLE 32.1

Types of Suture

Type	Generic Name	Raw Material	Trade Name
Natural collagen	Plain catgut	Submucosa of sheep intestines	---
	Chromic catgut	Catgut & buffered chromicizing	---
Synthetic			
	Polyglycolic acid	Homoploymer of glycolide, w/ & w/o poloxamer 188 coating	Dexon, Dexon-S Dexon-Plus
	Polyglactin	Copolymer lactic & glycolic acid, w/ & w/o calcium stearate coating	Vicryl Coated vicryl
	Polydioxanone	Monofilamentous homopolymer of paradioxanone	PDS
	Polyglyconate	Monofilamentous copolymer of glycolic acid & trimethylene carbonate	Maxon
Natural fiber	Surgical cotton	Twisted natural cotton	---
	Surgical silk	Braided protein naturally spun by silkworms	Sofsilk
Synthetic	Polyamide (Nylon)	Monofilament	Dermalon, Ethilon
		Multifilament	Neurolon
		Multifilament silicone-treated	Surgilon
	Polypropylene	Monofilamentous polymer of polypropylene	Surgilene, Prolene
	Polybutester	Monofilament	Novafil
	Polyethylene	Thermoplastic synthetic resin	Dermalene
	Polyester	Multifilament of polyethylene terephthalate	
		Braided, plain	Dacron, Mersilene
		Braided, silicone-treated	Ti-Cron
		Braided, polybutilate-coated	Ethibond
		Braided, PTFE (Teflon)-coated	Polydek, Ethiflex
		Braided, heavily PTFE-impregnated	Tevdek
	Polytetrafluoroethylene (PTFE)	Multifilament	Gore-Tex
		Monofilament	Teflon
Metal	Stainless steel wire	Twisted multistrand	Flexon
		Monofilament strand	Steel

dictable fashion: it begins in 10 to 15 days and is completed in 28 to 70 days. By 21 days, 40% to 50% of its original tensile strength is maintained. These synthetic materials are more difficult to handle and more prone to knot slippage than natural materials. Coated forms of these sutures, such as Dexon-Plus and Coated Vicryl, were constructed to minimize these shortcomings. Dexon-S is composed of thinner filaments intertwined into a structure that is easier to handle, but with less knot security.

Monofilaments are single-stranded synthetic sutures, including PDS (polydioxanone) and

Maxon (polyglyconate). Tensile strength, inflammatory reaction, and knot security are similar to those of polyfilaments. The level of inflammation, however, is less marked. The lack of interstices confers an increased resistance to bacterial infection. By postoperative day 28, Maxon retains 40% its original tensile strength, while PDS retains 50% of its original tensile strength. This feature is desired in patients with delayed wound healing, as in immunosuppressed individuals. In fact, Maxon and PDS are favored sutures in vaginal and pelvic surgery. Their monofilamentous composition serves as both an advantage and a disadvantage. They are more difficult to handle and make knot tying more challenging. Aggressive suture handling with instruments can readily damage and weaken the suture, resulting in compromised wound healing.

Nonabsorbable Sutures

Natural Materials

Cotton is a naturally occurring absorbable suture that is no longer popular. It handles well but is comparatively weaker than silk. Similarly, it causes significant inflammation.

Surgical silk is also considered nonabsorbable, although it retains 50% of its tensile strength after 1 year, with minimal loss after 2 years. It is easily handled and offers good knot security secondary to its low memory. It elicits a significant immune response, which deters its use by many surgeons.

Synthetic Materials

Nylon is composed of synthetic fiber polymers. It can be manufactured as monofilaments, or twisted into polyfilament constructs. Unlike natural products, it produces less inflammation, making it a favorable option in skin closure. Twenty percent of its original tensile strength is lost by hydrolysis after the first year. It remains unchanged thereafter. Nylon is easy to handle but is more prone to knot unraveling and slipping. Good surgical technique is critical.

Polypropylene is a monofilamentous synthetic polymer of propylene [poly (1-methylethylene)]. Its structural makeup does not allow for easy handling or knot security, as it is quite stiff and has very high memory. It has low tensile strength compared to other nonabsorbable synthetic materials. Polypropylene has the advantage of low tissue reactivity and very slow absorption, which makes it useful in anchoring permanent materials, such as grafts, or in areas of slow wound healing.

Polyester sutures (Ethibond) are multifilament materials that exist in several forms. They can be noncoated or coated, with various agents: silicone, polybutilate, or polytetrafluoroethylene (PTFE or Teflon). The uncoated versions offer improved knot security, while the coated versions are easier to handle. Specifically, silicone coating improves suture manageability, at the expense of increased knot slippage and inflammation. Polybutilate coating causes less inflammation and is easy to handle, while PTFE coating simply facilitates handling. The common disadvantage of all these braided materials is they must be completely excised from tissue if infected.

Gore-Tex is a nonabsorbable suture composed of expanded PTFE, an inert compound. It therefore elicits minimal inflammatory reaction. PTFE is "expanded" to produce a material that is porous, with an air volume of approximately 50%. It was originally designed for cardiovascular anastomotic procedures. Its low immune response results in decreased adhesion formation. By the same token, infiltration of leukocytes and fibroblasts may be hindered, resulting in less tissue ingrowth. This feature is not necessarily favorable in its larger mesh form and may be associated with a heightened susceptibility to infection. As a consequence, its use in pelvic reconstructive surgery is becoming less common.

The metal suture material available is stainless steel wire, created from a metal alloy. It provides the best tensile strength and knot security of any of the suture materials previously mentioned. It produces less of an immune response than the other nonabsorbable materials. In exchange, it is very difficult to handle and deforms quite easily. An attempt to overcome this feature has been made by twisting the material into multistrands. This new, thicker construct must be managed with great care, as it can unintentionally penetrate gloves quite readily.

Suture Sizes

Sutures exist not only in different types, but also in different diameters. The standard classification system of suture sizes was introduced by the United States Pharmacopeia in 1937. This metric value designates numerical whole values for large sizes and multiple zeroes for smaller sizes. For example, 2-0 (or 00) is larger than 3-0 (000), which is larger than 4-0 (0000).

Needles

The suture unit is completed by its attachment to a sterile, stainless steel needle. The needle is composed of a distal point, a middle body, and a proximal swage. The point is designed to penetrate the tissue with little resistance. It exists as a cutting point, which facilitates entry into dense tissues; a taper point, which enters by way of stretching, thus minimizing tissue shearing and injury; and a blunt point, which does not cut tissue but dissects it. The body is the anchoring structure upon which the needle driver is placed. It, too, varies in conformation. The body of the needle can be straight and easily controlled by the hand for skin closure, such as the Keith needle; curved for use in smaller spaces; and compound curved, which has two different angulations (80 degrees proximally and 45 degrees distally), and is primarily used in microvascular and ophthalmic surgery. The shape of the curved needle ranges in fractions of an inch, from 1/4, 3/8, 1/2, 5/8. The greater the curvature, the more wrist rotation required to deliver the needle through tissue. The swage, which directly attaches to the suture, can be shaped as an eyelet or flattened onto the suture itself. Each of these features affects the degree of tissue trauma made upon entry and the durability of the suture being introduced. (See Lai SY, Becker DG. Suture and needles. 2004. http://www.emedicine.com.)

Clinical Applications

The choice of a particular suture for a surgical purpose is based traditionally on previous experience and more recently on scientific rationale. As such, catgut suture is rarely used in reconstructive surgery, although it may be used for tubal ligations and abdominal hysterectomies. Most hysterectomies are performed utilizing polyglactin sutures, which may also be used for anterior and posterior colporrhaphies and closure of the vaginal epithelium. These sutures are typically in place for 4 to 6 weeks, allowing for significant healing time of the vaginal epithelium as well as connective tissue and fascia.

Fascial defect repairs as well as suspensory procedures are typically performed utilizing synthetic, nonabsorbable, or delayed absorbable sutures. As such, polypropylene sutures are commonly used for paravaginal repairs, Burch colposuspensions, and abdominal sacrocolpopexies. The principal benefit of a synthetic monofilament suture such as polypropylene is that there is minimal tissue reaction, such that if the sutures are placed through the vaginal epithelium inadvertently, no significant inflammatory response occurs and the suture typically becomes buried spontaneously. This is in comparison to multifilament sutures such as Gore-Tex, which have been used for Burch colposuspensions and sacrocolpopexies, and are associated with some, albeit low, risk of suture infection and/or rejection. Multifilament sutures such as polyester (Ethibond) and silk are utilized in situations where permanent suspension or attachment is necessary. However, their multifilament nature may lead to a significant reaction and possibly infection, resulting in the formation of granulation tissue and the need to remove the suture. This has led to a decreased use of both of these suture materials.

As such, most pelvic surgeons' preferences are limited to the use of polyglactin (i.e., Vicryl),

polydioxanone (i.e., PDS), and polypropylene (i.e., Prolene) sutures. Development of healing abnormalities due to reactions to sutures and grafts has lead to reduced experimentation with suture materials and adherence to traditional suture materials of known reactivity.

GRAFTS

The use of artificial implanted materials to enhance tissue repair has long been a hallmark of general surgery. Based on previous data collected from hernia medicine, the use of grafts in pelvic reconstructive surgery has increased over the past 10 years. Today, abdominal herniorrhaphies are usually performed with graft augmentation, resulting in improved outcomes; the recurrence risk of abdominal incisional hernias has been shown to be reduced by half (2). Intuitively, grafts have also been used to enhance treatment of vaginal prolapse, often considered "hernias of the vagina." This makes sense, due to the relatively high recurrence rate of prolapse surgeries. The popularization of fascial defects and tears as a primary etiology for the development of genital prolapse has lead to increased graft utilization to augment fascial strength in an attempt to promote repair longevity and permanence.

Grafts serve to strengthen attenuated tissue and enhance healing in areas with compromised tissue integrity. They are available in biologic and synthetic forms. Regardless of origin, the properties of the ideal graft are similar to that of the ideal suture. They are:

1. Noncarcinogenic
2. Durable and able to withstand physical pressures
3. Chemically inert or have a predictable tissue response
4. Nontoxic to the host
5. Easily manufactured, widely available
6. Resistant to infection
7. Affordable

The absence of an ideal graft, as seen with sutures, is a common theme, as they vary greatly in physical composition and tissue response.

Synthetic Grafts

Grafts woven from synthetic material strands vary greatly in their composition and pore size, and they exist as monofilament or multifilament structures. Table 32.2 reviews the various synthetic graft materials in use (3). Due to the recent marked expansion in graft marketing, this table is not fully

TABLE 32.2

Biocompatible Synthetic Materials in Gynecologic Surgery

Clinical Component	Trade Name	Type
Polypropylene	Marlex (CR Bard)	Monofilament
	Prolene (Ethicon)	Monofilament
	Atrium (Atrium Medical)	Monofilament
Polytetrafluoroethylene (PTFE)	Teflon (CR Bard)	Multifilament
Expanded PTFE	Gore-Tex (WL Gore)	Multifilament
Polyethylene tetraphthalate	Mersilene (Ethicon)	Multifilament
Polyglycolic acid	Dexon absorbable (Davis + Geck)	Multifilament
Polyglactin 910	Vicryl absorbable (Ethicon)	Multifilament

inclusive of newly used materials and new manufacturers.

Mersilene is a polyester material composed of polyethylene terephthalate that is thin (0.23 mm) and light (43 g/m^2). Fibers are interlocked into multifilaments that are resistant to irradiation and temperatures of 120°C. Its length increases with application of increasing stress, sustaining a maximum of 76.6 N.

Marlex is composed of polypropylene fibers of 0.65 mm diameter and 152 g/m^2. These monofilament fibers are woven into constructs with a pore size of 170 μm. Similar to Mersilene, it maintains its chemical properties despite substantial heat, as in sterilization processes. However, after irradiation, small cracks are appreciated under ultramicroscopy. It is unable to sustain stresses of greater than 55.3 N.

Polypropylene is an attractive material for use in pelvic reconstructive grafts. Polypropylene grafts have greatly increased in popularity recently due to their rather inert behavior and ability to be woven into various configurations. There is thus significant variability in fiber thickness, weave, pore size, and weight. The original polypropylene mesh for hernia repair augmentation was quite heavy. In reconstructive surgery, it accomplished the goal of restoring anatomic support but was associated with problematic healing, especially when used along the anterior vaginal wall (4). A softer mesh composed of inert polypropylene fibers was thus required in order to reduce the incidence of dyspareunia and improved healing. Development of the tension-free vaginal tape (TVT) sling procedure increased the popularity of polypropylene mesh significantly. Surgeons became increasingly familiar with its inert nature and thus low risk of infection, erosion, or other healing abnormalities. This polypropylene weave was an improvement over previous weaves when used as an adjunct for correction of genital prolapse. However, it was still suboptimal for prolapse repairs. More recently, soft weave polypropylene mesh has become available, which is made from thinner polypropylene fibers. In addition, the original polypropylene mesh materials were directional, requiring precise implantation. Currently available softer polypropylene mesh is less directional and thus less apt to distort after implantation. Surgeons must thus be aware that not all polypropylene meshes are the same (Fig. 32.1). Monofilament large-pore meshes (see Fig. 32.1A) are best tolerated. Multifilament polypropylene meshes (see Fig. 32.1C) can be associated with significant healing abnormalities, as has been recently reported with the IVS tunneler tape (5). It is likely that further variations in the weave and composition of polypropylene meshes will be available in the future for use in pelvic surgery.

Teflon (see Table 32.2) is a polytetrafluoroethylene material that is 0.68 mm and weighs 316 g/m^2. It is composed of 52 homogeneous filaments with a pore size of 26 μm. Its ultimate tensile strength prior to breakage is 107.2 N. With added stress, the mesh as a whole elongates first, followed by stretch of its individual filaments.

Gore-Tex is a microporous polytetrafluoroethylene compound that is significantly thicker (1 mm) and heavier (923 g/m^2) than the previously discussed materials. Multiple modifications, including a lighter weave and antibacterial coating, have been available over the past years. It is composed of solid PTFE nodes and longitudinally extended fibrils. This makes up 20% of its total volume, the remainder of which is filled with air. It sustains heat conditions of up to 300°C. Its ultra-

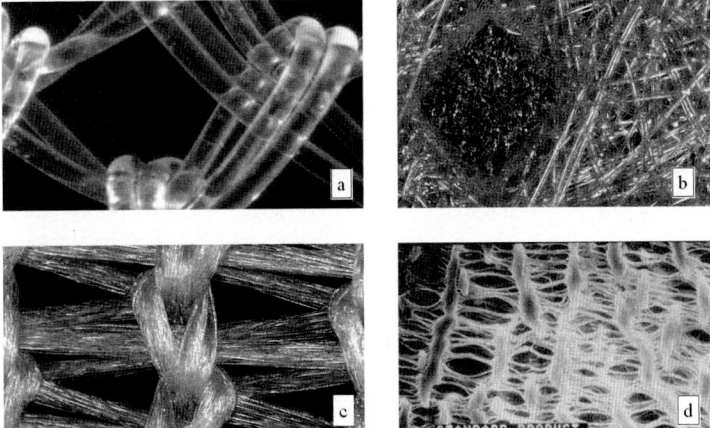

FIGURE 32.1 ● Microscopic view of synthetic mesh materials demonstrating significant differences in weave, porosity, and fiber type. **(A)** Macroporous, monofilament polypropylene (Sparc tape, AMS). **(B)** Composite microporous mesh (ObTape, Mentor). **(C)** Macroporous, multifilament polypropylene (IVS tape, Tyco/US Surgical). **(D)** Microporous, multifilament mesh (GoreTex, Gore Medical).

structure is altered by irradiation of 10 kGy with considerable weakness (6).

Pore size is an important characteristic determining the ability of the host's immune system cells and microorganisms to penetrate the material. The pore sizes previously discussed refer to interfiber pore sizes. The multifilament meshes have in common that the intrafiber pore sizes are less than 10 μm. This factor is believed to be paramount in determining the risk of infection. These pores allow for entry of small microorganisms, but not larger polymorphonuclear leukocytes and macrophages. In addition, pores allow for ingrowth of fibroblasts and blood cells for collagen infiltration and angiogenesis.

A classification system for hernia repair meshes by Amid categorizes grafts according to pore size and filament characteristics of the mesh construction (Table 32.3) (7,8). This results in four types of synthetic graft materials. Relative to pelvic reconstructive surgery, only type I synthetic grafts are used with any frequency and are well tolerated. Other grafts are likely to be associated with increased reactivity, infection, and rejection.

More recently, polypropylene grafts have been modified to make them softer and more porous. The basic caveat here is use of a soft large-pore mesh for reconstructive surgery. Whether the soft and larger-pore meshes will improve outcomes is yet to be determined, but it makes theoretical sense. Recent reports regarding shrinkage of an implanted mesh over time may be related to the incorporated host collagen rather than the mesh itself but are

concerning. In the recent past, composite mesh materials have been developed by coating a synthetic mesh, such as polypropylene, with materials such as collagen. This combination would theoretically result in prompt restoration of pelvic support. However, many composite grafts have resulted in healing abnormalities, including infection and rejection, thus making the grafts inappropriate for use in pelvic reconstructive surgery. Nevertheless, new composite grafts will likely be marketed in hopes of improving manageability and outcomes.

Biologic Grafts

Historically, biologic grafts were initially used in reconstructive surgery. More recently, the availability of biologic grafts has increased in hopes of providing surgeons with a biologic material with prompt availability and ease of procurement. Biologic grafts are autologous (from the patient herself), allografts (from other human sources), or xenografts (from an animal source).

Autologous fascia lata slings represent the initial use of an autologous graft. Durability and success rates of this procedure were very good. However, the use of an autologous graft is associated with a need to harvest the graft and has associated donor-site complications, such as pain, seroma, and others. Autologous graft sites are typically fascia lata or abdominal wall fascia. Increased operative time and donor site complications have decreased the popularity of these grafts.

TABLE 32.3

Amid Classification of Biomaterials

Types	Filament	Pore Type	Pore Size	Example
Type I	Monofilament	Macroporous	>75 μm	Marlex (CR Bard) Prolene (Ethicon) Atrium (Atrium Medical)
Type II	Multifilament	Microporous	<10 μm	Gore-Tex (WL Gore)
Type III	Multifilament	Micromacroporous	<10–75 μm	Mersilene (Ethicon) Teflon (CR Bard)
Type IV	Monofilament	Submicroporous	<10 μm	Cellgard Silastic

Adapted from Cosson M. Amid classification of biomaterials. *Int Urogynecol J* 2003;14:169–178.

Allografts

Cadaveric source grafts were initially popular due to their availability from various tissue banks. However, as surgeons became more familiar with the variability in quality, limited availability, and possible risk of disease transmission, the use of allografts decreased significantly. As the demand for cadaveric grafts increased, the quality decreased. In addition, during the tissue preparation for implantation, chemical or radiation treatment of the graft may weaken its inherent structure, resulting in a reported increased failure rate, especially as related to suspensory procedures such as sacrocolpopexies (9). Chemical processing of allografts has resulted in more durable and higher-quality fascia lata. Tutoplast processed fascia lata (Mentor Corp., Santa Barbara, CA) has been used for slings as well as reinforcement of the anterior and posterior vaginal walls. Quality is more predictable, but its cost is higher. Yet another source of cadaveric graft material is derived from human dermis (Repliform Tissue Regeneration Matrix, LifeCell Corporation, Branchburg, NJ). It is a processed, acellular material that serves as a matrix for tissue ingrowth. Its use has also been applied to repair of anterior and posterior vaginal wall prolapse, as well as treatment of stress urinary incontinence (10).

Xenografts

Xenografts represent a growing area of graft utilization to augment prolapse repairs (Fig. 32.2).

Availability of animal source grafts is greater. Preparation for implantation represents the area of most significant controversy. Currently available sources include porcine and bovine products. Commonly used porcine products include small intestinal submucosa (SIS, Cook Biomedical, Bloomington, IN), dermal products (Intexen, American Medical Systems, Minnetonka, NY), among others. Other porcine dermal products include Pelvicol (Bard Urological, Covington, GA), which is treated by chemical cross-linking. Bovine products have included bovine pericardium (Veritas, Synovis Surgical Innovations, Minneapolis, MN).

It is unknown whether the animal source of a xenograft makes a significant difference in its implanted behavior. However, there are basic differences in how the material is prepared for implantation. Initially, materials were cross-linked chemically in order to stabilize molecular bonds and prevent degradation after implantation. This resulted in a material that became encapsulated and not integrated into host tissues (Fig. 32.3). Encapsulated materials may shrink and harden, resulting in alteration of vaginal wall anatomy. More recently, the trend has been toward utilization of non–cross-linked materials, which are incorporated into host tissue by neovascularization and collagen ingrowth (Fig. 32.4). These tissues thus become part of the host tissue as "neofascia" within a number of months. There is an ongoing debate regarding the importance of a biologic graft's longevity. The non–cross-linked material may be degraded by host enzymes, including col-

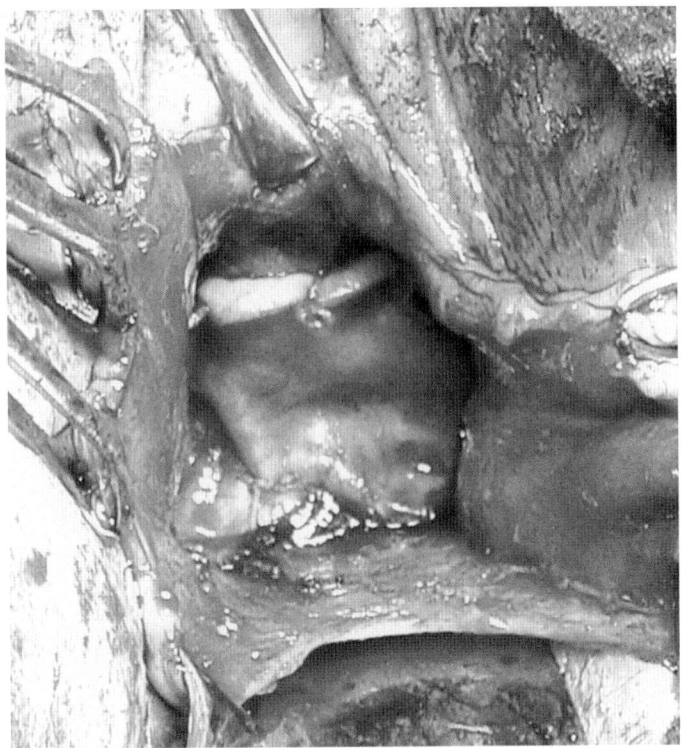

FIGURE 32.2 • Biologic bovine pericardium "collagen matrix" graft reinforcing a cystocele repair.

lagenases, prior to neovascularization and collagen ingrowth, resulting in weakening of the repair. Identification of those patients apt to rapid breakdown of an implanted biologic graft may become an important selection criterion in the future.

Besides issues relative to rate of degradation of an implanted biologic graft, other concerns relate to the likelihood of disease transmission (i.e., prions or viruses) or immune reactions due to persistence of animal antigens. To date, there has been no evidence of acute or latent disease transmission with the use of xenografts for vaginal surgery. Most grafts are completely acellular and thus should have no significant antigenicity. SIS has

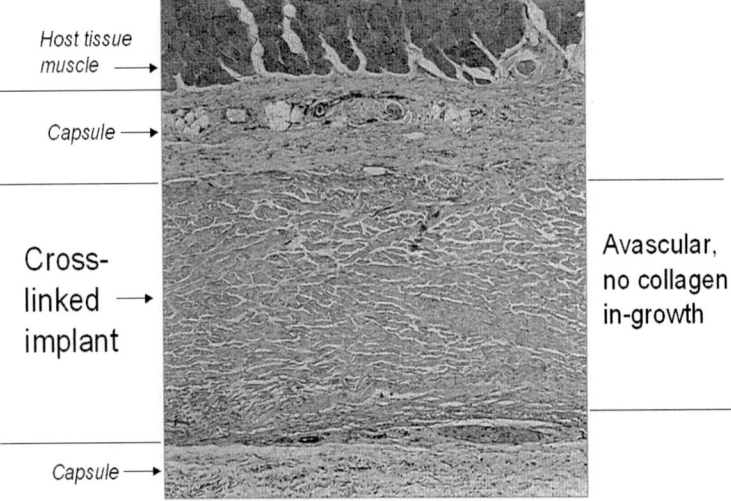

FIGURE 32.3 • Cross-linked graft may encapsulate and not be incorporated into host tissue.

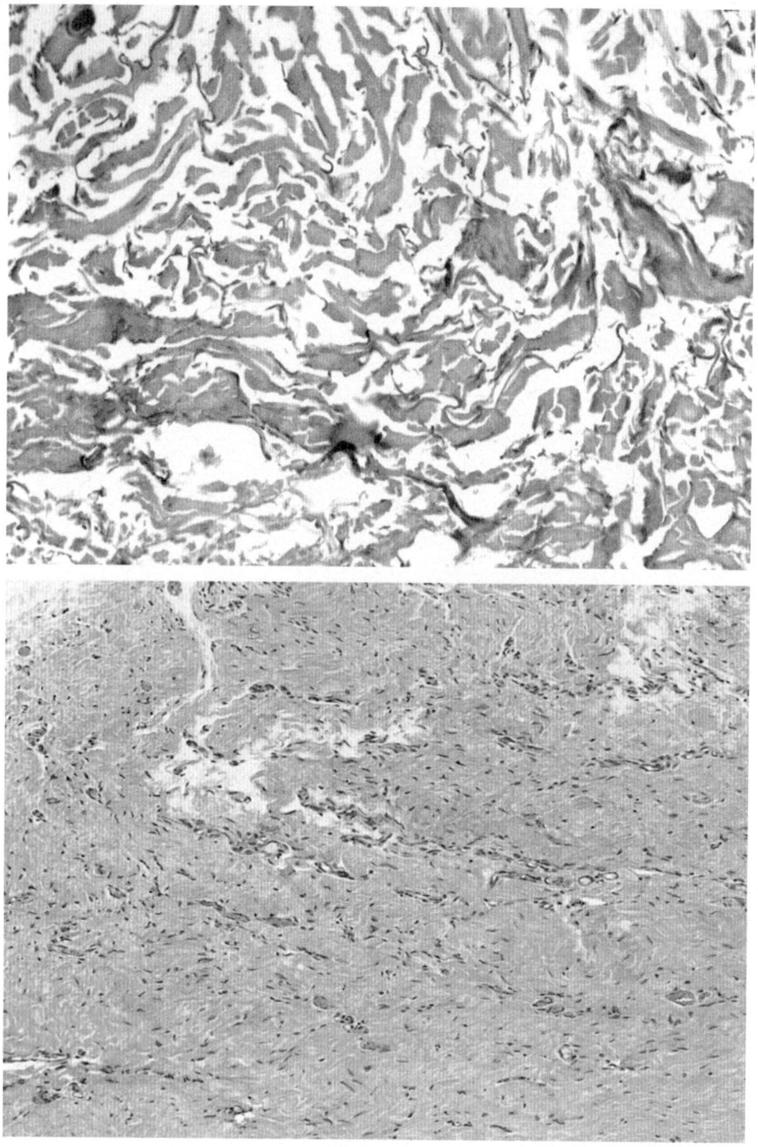

FIGURE 32.4 ● Non–cross-linked graft allows prompt neovascularization and collagen ingrowth.

been shown to have some cellular remnants, but the chemical preparatory treatment is designed to lend the graft nonimmunogenic.

The basic premise for the usage of a xenograft relates to the fact that an implanted biologic graft is a "collagen matrix," which will result in "neofascia" formation by collagen deposition into the biologic graft as it is broken down (see Fig. 32.4). This concept is well accepted in other areas of reconstructive surgery, including neurosurgery and orthopaedics. Whether this concept will improve pelvic reconstructive surgery outcomes remains to be seen.

Complications of Graft Use

Infection is one of the most concerning complications of mesh use in surgery. Macrophages and neutrophils are unable to gain access into the small pores of types II and III materials, which may be susceptible to bacterial invasion. These pores measure less than 10 μm in at least one dimension, allowing bacterial entry and proliferation. Complete removal of the graft is recommended for these types if infection develops. Type I grafts allow for host cell penetration and thus do not require removal if infected. Despite the widespread belief that pore size influences the host's ability to respond to infection, newer data refute this theory. Macrophages have been identified within small interstices of multifilament polypropylene mesh material, suggesting that pore size alone is not the sole determinant of infection rates (11).

Appearance of mesh through the surface of the tissue in which it has been implanted has been described using various terms: erosion, extrusion, exposure, or rejection. In the absence of specific definitions, a preferred term may be "healing abnormality." A consensus on classification terms was recently proposed based on a clinical roundtable including basic scientists and experienced pelvic surgeons (12). It was suggested that a general term such as "healing abnormality" be utilized rather than a specific term, which suggests a mechanism for abnormal healing. The proposed classification included four factors:

1. Time relative to implantation
2. Presence of inflammatory/granulation tissue
3. Location of abnormality relative to a suture line
4. Viscera involved

This can then lead to classification of a healing abnormality as simple or complex (Table 32.4). This simplified classification requires validation but should allow surgeons to better describe the healing abnormality and provide information to patients regarding its management. A simple healing abnormality will commonly respond to local estrogen administration and excision of exposed mesh segments in the office (Fig. 32.5). This conservative therapy will resolve symptoms in approximately 50% of involved patients. The other 50% of patients may require an outpatient operating room procedure to excise the exposed area, undermine the adjacent vaginal epithelium, and reclose the epithelium over the defect. In either case, the prognosis for healing is excellent and there is no need to consider removal of the implanted graft. A complex healing abnormality will likely require removal of the graft or a portion of it.

An inflammatory process may or may not be involved in a healing abnormality. Possible etiologies include infection, tissue atrophy, or lack of fibrin deposition in the expected area of scar formation. The latter theory has been studied by Junge, who evaluated collagen formation in recurrent hernia patients. Explanted meshes were analyzed in both a quantitative and qualitative manner. Decreased type I/III collagen ratios were found in explanted tissue, suggesting that differences in scar tissue composition may contribute to increased risk of hernia recurrence (13).

In light of these complications, some have made recommendations to optimize graft usage, as noted in Table 32.5 (14). Preimplantation soaking of an implant in an antibiotic solution is commonly used by urologic surgeons but has not been demonstrated to decrease healing abnormality rates in vaginal surgery. Optimizing tissue quality with local estrogen therapy and minimizing vaginal epithelial trimming during wound closure likely represent the two main areas where surgeons can have a positive impact on healing.

Clinical Applications

The use of grafts in pelvic reconstructive surgery is likely here to stay. The rate of graft use adoption has markedly exceeded the rate of increasing knowledge regarding graft biology. Surgeons should thus become familiar with the biology of a graft prior to implantation.

Currently, there are only a few areas where usage of a graft is clearly indicated. These include performance of a suburethral sling procedure, as well as sacrocolpopexy. No significant evidence is currently available demonstrating the superiority of a grafted versus nongrafted repair of the anterior or posterior vaginal walls. However, the rather high recurrence rate of genital prolapse has lead to increased graft utilization. Soft polypropylene mesh is the preferred graft material for sacro-

TABLE 32.4

Proposed Classification of Graft-Related Healing Abnormalities

	Simple	Complex
Timing relative to implantation	<12 weeks	>12 weeks
Site relative to suture line	At suture line	Other than at suture line
Presence of inflammatory tissue	None	Granulation
Affected viscera	Vagina	Bladder, rectum, or other

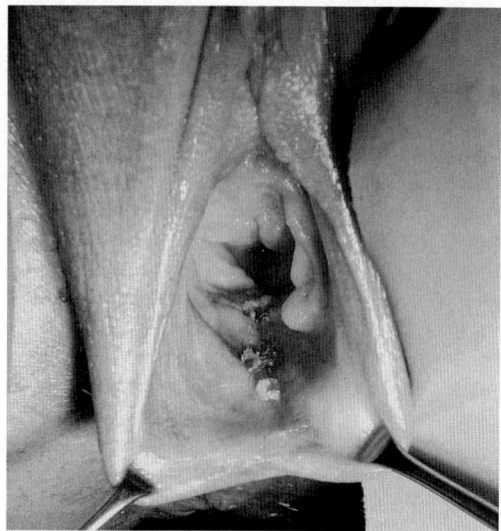

FIGURE 32.5 ● Simple healing abnormality after implantation of a type I polypropylene graft. This responded to local estrogen cream and trimming of visible mesh.

sary (slings and sacrocolpopexy). The choice of a synthetic versus biologic material is less clear when the graft is utilized in an area not under significant strain, where neofascia development is the goal (anterior or posterior vaginal walls).

TISSUE ADHESIVES

Biologically active adhesives may soon make suture use seem archaic. Cyanoacrylates have been successfully used for external skin closure (Dermabond). Once moisture is encountered, the liquid polymerizes into an impermeable solid form. It can be removed with acetone-containing compounds. To promote adequate wound healing, the patient should avoid water immersion in the immediate period after its application. The solidified compound sloughs off in approximately 1 to 2 weeks. Its efficacy is affected by excessive movement; thus, its use on joints is not advised. It is a question of time until a bonding agent able to be used internally becomes available.

CONCLUSIONS

Surgeons should select their reconstructive tools with care. Suture choices have become more limited due to clinical experience and reported outcomes. The same cannot be said about grafts due to the large variety of grafts available and limited data on outcomes and complications. Surgeons should thus keep themselves informed regarding new data on outcomes related to graft usage, both in the basic sciences as well as in the clinical

colpopexy as well as suburethral slings. This is reaching standard of care acceptance based on recent comparative studies (15). Biologic grafts may be theoretically superior for repair of the anterior or posterior vaginal walls due to the decreased likelihood of healing abnormalities. However, longevity is still an issue. Thus, synthetic graft materials are likely indicated at a site where tissue is under strain and neoligament formation is neces-

---

TABLE 32.5

Ten Suggestions for Using Artificial Graft Material

1 Minimize the choice of material when poor tissue quality, impaired wound healing, or susceptibility to infection is present.
2 Minimize local contamination.
3 Minimize the length of incisions that overlap with the graft.
4 Minimize the use of "flap" or "U-shaped" incisions.
5 Minimize the degree of dissection.
6 Minimize bleeding.
7 Minimize the amount of material used for the repair.
8 Minimize the intraoperative exposure time of the material.
9 Minimize tension.
10 Be familiar with the historical use and techniques involved with the choice of material.

Adapted from Niknejad K, Plzak LS III, Staskin DR, et al. Autologous and synthetic urethral slings for female incontinence. *Urol Clin North Am* 2002;29(3):597–611.

realm. Overall, patients appear to benefit from graft utilization, despite the lack of available objective outcome data at the current time. Future developments in tissue adhesives, genetic engineering, and understanding of the biologic behavior of implants will certainly soon have an impact on our utilization of surgical tools such as grafts.

REFERENCES

1. Luijendijk RW, Hop WC, van den Tol MP, et al. A comparison of suture repair with mesh repair for incisional hernia. *N Engl J Med* 2000;343(6):392–398.
2. Sanz LE. Sutures: a primer on structure and function. *Contemp Ob Gyn* 1990;35(32):99–106.
3. Fenner DE. New surgical mesh. *Clin Obstet Gynecol* 2000;43(3):650–658.
4. Julian TM. The efficacy of Marlex mesh in the repair of severe, recurrent vaginal prolapse of the anterior midvaginal wall. *Am J Obstet Gynecol* 1996;175(6): 1472–1475.
5. Baessler K, Hewson AD, Tunn R, et al. Severe mesh complications following intravaginal slingplasty. *Obstet Gynecol* 2005;106:713–716.
6. Brun JL, Bordenave L, Lefebvre F, et al. Physical and biologic characteristics of the main biomaterials used in pelvic surgery. *Biomed Mater Eng* 1992;2:203–225.
7. Cosson M, Debodinance P, Boukerrou M, et al. Mechanical properties of synthetic implants used in the repair of prolapse and urinary incontinence in women: which is the ideal material? *Int Urogynecol J* 2003; 14(3):169–178.
8. Amid P. Classification of biomaterials and their relative complications in an abdominal wall hernia surgery. *Hernia* 1997;1:15–21.
9. Fitzgerald MP, Mollenhauer J, Bitterman P, et al. Functional failure of fascia lata allografts. *Am J Obstet Gynecol* 1999;181:1339–1346.
10. Crivellaro S, Smith JJ, Kocjancic E, et al. Transvaginal sling using acellular human dermal allograft: safety and efficacy in 253 patients. *J Urol* 2004;172:1374–1378.
11. Rodeheaver G. IUGA Grafts Roundtable. *Int Urogynecol J* 2006;17(Supp 1):51–55.
12. Davila GW, Drutz H, Deprest J. Summary: IUGA Grafts Roundtable. *Int Urogynecol J* 2006;17(3).
13. Junge K, Klinge U, Rosch R, et al. Decreased collagen type I/III ratio in patients with recurring hernia after implantation of alloplastic prostheses. *Langenbecks Arch Surg* 2004;389(1):17–22.
14. Niknejad K, Plzak LS III, Staskin DR, et al. Autologous and synthetic urethral slings for female incontinence. *Urol Clin North Am* 2002;29(3):597–611.
15. Culligan PJ, Blackwell L, Goldsmith LJ, et al. A randomized controlled trial comparing fascia lata and synthetic mesh for sacral colpopexy. *Obstet Gynecol* 2005;106(1):29–37.

SECTION V

Appendices

I

Urogynecology and the Internet

Joseph M. Montella and Steven E. Swift

The Internet and the World Wide Web have changed the practice of medicine dramatically. Information that was once available to a select few in the field of medicine is now available to anyone with access to a computer and questions to be answered. Physicians are now more inclined to see patients who come prepared with information (at times inaccurate) and address these issues. The purpose of this appendix is to guide the reader to websites containing information pertinent to the field of urogynecology and female pelvic floor medicine. The following list of websites is by no means exhaustive because the World Wide Web is fluid, and there are bound to be several more sites related to the field by the time of publication of this text. The reader can use one of the variety of search engines on the web (e.g., Yahoo, Excite, Alta Vista) to explore the various physician- and patient-oriented websites. Also, each site has links to other sites that may be useful to the reader. Keep in mind that there are many sites with erroneous information, and it is incumbent on the physician to sort out the facts for the patients and correct any misconceptions.

GOVERNMENT SITES

- *www.nlm.nih.gov:* The United States National Library of Medicine provides an excellent resource for Medline, research funding opportunities, and library services.
- *www.niddk.nih.gov:* The link to the National Institute of Diabetes, Digestive, and Kidney Diseases provides a resource in government funding for research into urinary incontinence and pelvic floor disorders.
- *clinicaltrials.gov:* The U.S. National Institutes of Health, through its National Library of Medicine, has developed ClinicalTrials.gov to provide patients, family members, and members of the public with current information about clinical research studies.
- *www.niddk.nih.gov/health/kidney/nkudic.html:* The National Kidney and Urologic Diseases Information Clearinghouse (NKUDIC) is an information dissemination service established in 1987 to increase knowledge and understanding about diseases of the kidneys and urologic system among people with these conditions and their families, health care professionals, and the general public.
- *www.nichd.nih.gov:* The National Institute of Child Health and Development (NICHD) administers a multidisciplinary program of research, research training, and public information, nationally and within its own facilities, on reproductive biology and population issues; on prenatal development as well as maternal, child, and family health; and on medical rehabilitation. The Institute supports and conducts basic, clinical, and epidemiologic research in the reproductive sciences.
- *www.ahcpr.gov:* The Agency for Healthcare Research and Quality (formerly the Agency for Healthcare Policy and Research) offers information on government programs and grants.
- *www.hcfa.gov:* The website of the Health Care Financing Administration (HCFA), the federal agency that administers Medicare, Medicaid, and the State Children's Health Insurance Program (SCHIP), includes information on reimbursement, statistics, and publications.

PROFESSIONAL SOCIETIES

- *www.augs.org:* The American Urogynecologic Society, founded in 1979, is dedicated to research and education in urogynecology and to improved care for women with lower urinary tract disorders. This site provides both physician and patient education materials, research funding opportunities, links to government and congressional websites, and information on postgraduate fellowship training programs in urogynecology.

- *www.acog.org:* The American College of Obstetrics and Gynecology provides resources for physicians and patients as well as information on postgraduate courses in urogynecology.
- *www.auanet.org:* The American Urologic Association provides a wide range of services, including publications, the Annual Meeting, continuing medical education, and health policy advocacy.
- *www.continent.org:* The primary mission of the International Continence Society is to study the storage and voiding function of the lower urinary tract, its diagnosis, and the management of lower urinary tract dysfunction and to encourage research into pathophysiology, diagnostic techniques, and treatment.
- *www.iuga.org:* The International Urogynecological Association is an international organization committed to promoting and exchanging knowledge regarding the care of women with urinary and pelvic floor dysfunction.
- *sgsonline.org:* The goal of the Society of Gynecologic Surgeons is to promote the acquisition of knowledge and the improvement of skills in gynecologic surgery, to enhance the understanding of gynecology and gynecologic surgery through basic and clinical research, and to be a source of public and professional information.
- *www.iciq.net:* The International Consultation on Incontinence has a website with a modular quality-of-life questionnaire for all aspects of pelvic organ dysfunction. This site is being developed to serve as a online repository for a quality-of-life questionnaire with modules covering everything from nocturia to sexual dysfunction. The goal is to make this available to researchers investigating the impact of disease and treatment on the various aspects of pelvic floor dysfunction.
- *www.nafc.org:* The National Association for Continence (NAFC), formerly Help for Incontinent People (HIP), is a not-for-profit or-

ganization established in 1982 dedicated to improving the quality of life of people with incontinence. NAFC's purpose is to be the leading source of education, advocacy, and support to the public and to health professionals about the causes, prevention, diagnosis, treatments, and management solutions for incontinence.

- *www.simonfoundation.org:* The work of the Simon Foundation includes aid to patients with incontinence, aid to the families of those patients, creating public awareness, reviewing relevant legislation, and encouraging the medical profession's interest in incontinence and pelvic floor dysfunction.

MEMBERSHIP AND PATIENT-ORIENTED SITES

- *www.obgynlinx.com:* ObGynLinx.com is designed to keep obstetrics and gynecology professionals up to date with the latest medical developments by aggregating the top obstetrics and gynecology articles from hundreds of premier medical journals and categorizing the information into 14 subspecialties, including urogynecology.
- *womenshealth.medscape.com:* Medscape offers access to abstracts from conferences in all medical specialties, including gynecology, and offers continuing medical education (CME) credits as well as access to journal articles.
- *www.centerwatch.com:* This CenterWatch site is a comprehensive guide to clinical trials underway in every region of the United States, listed by disease or condition as well as research centers and additional resources specifically for each disease entity.
- *www.obgyn.net:* OBGYN.net includes such features as current clinical news, original articles, CME, cases of the month, an events locator and other interactive tools, professional forums in English and Spanish, and free procedure videos viewable online.
- *www.mybladder.com:* MyBladder is an online community dedicated to encouraging people with bladder control problems to seek help while promoting an understanding of bladder control problems and awareness of the latest treatment options.

II

Quality-of-Life Tools

Steven E. Swift

The following table is a short description of the various quality-of-life (QOL) tools for assessing urinary incontinence and pelvic organ prolapse. While it is extensive it may not be complete, as new tools are constantly being developed. The commonly used tools are the King's Health Questionnaire, IIQ, UDI, PFDI, and PDIQ. The King's Health Questionnaire and scoring sheet follow the list below. The others can be found in their entirety in Chapter 3.

TABLE 1

Description of Condition-Specific Health-Related Quality-of-Life and Symptom Severity Instruments

Name of Instrument	Target Population/Condition	Items, *n*	Subscales
Health-Related Quality-of-Life Tools for Urinary Incontinence			
CONTILIFE: a quality-of-life questionnaire for urinary incontinence (1)	Stress urinary incontinence	28	Daily activities, effort activities, self-image, emotional consequences, sexuality, well-being, global score
Incontinence Impact Questionnaire (2)	Urinary incontinence	30	Physical activity, travel, social, emotional
Incontinence Impact Questionnaire-Revised (3)	Urinary incontinence	30	Physical activity, travel, social, emotional, embarrassment
Incontinence Impact Questionnaire-Short Form (4)	Urinary incontinence	7	Not applicable
Incontinence Quality-of-life Questionnaire (5)	Urinary incontinence	22	Avoidance and limiting behaviors, psychosocial, social embarrassment
Incontinence Stress (6)	Urinary incontinence	20	Depressive, aesthetic/somatic, social
Overactive Bladder Questionnaire (7)	Continent and incontinent overactive bladder	33	Symptom bother, coping, concern, social interaction, sleep
Quality-of-life Questionnaire for Urinary Urge Incontinence (8)	Urge urinary incontinence	24	Activities, emotional, impact self-image, sleep, well-being

(continued)

TABLE 1 *(Continued)*

Name of Instrument	Target Population/Condition	Items, *n*	Subscales
Health-Related Quality-of-Life Tools for Urinary Incontinence			
Symptom Impact Index for Stress Incontinence in Women (9)	Stress urinary incontinence	3	Not applicable
Urge Impact Scale (10)	Urinary incontinence	24	Psychological burden, perception of personal control, self-concept
Urge Incontinence Impact Questionnaire (11)	Mixed urinary incontinence, urge urinary incontinence	32	Travel, activities, physical activities, feelings, relationships, sexual function, nighttime bladder control
Urinary Incontinence Handicap Inventory (12)	Elderly women, UI caused be detrusor activity	17	Not applicable
Urinary Incontinence Severity Score (13)	Urinary incontinence	10	Not applicable
York Incontinence Perceptions Scale (14)	Urinary incontinence	8	Not applicable
Symptom Severity Questionnaires for Urinary Incontinence			
Sandvik Incontinence Severity Index (15)	Urinary incontinence	2	Not Applicable
Urogenital Distress Inventory (2)	Urinary incontinence	19	Irritative symptoms, obstructive/ discomfort symptoms, stress symptoms
Urogenital Distress Inventory-short form (4)	Urinary incontinence	6	Irritative symptoms, obstructive/discomfort symptoms, stress symptoms
International Consultation on Incontinence Questionnaire (16)	Urinary incontinence, nocturia, naginal symptoms, bowel symptoms, neurogenic bladder, overactive bladder	Series of 16 modules	Irritative symptoms, obstructive symptoms, sexual symptoms, nocturia, stress and urge incontinence symptoms, fecal symptoms of incontinence and constipation.
Questionnaires That Cover Both Symptom Severity and Health-Related Quality-of-Life for Urinary Incontinence			
King's Health Questionnaire (17)	Urinary incontinence	21	Role limitations, physical limitations, social limitations, personal limitations, emotional problems, sleep/energy disturbance, severity (coping) measures, symptom severity, incontinence impact (single item), general health perception (single item)

(continued)

TABLE 1 *(Continued)*

Name of Instrument	Target Population/Condition	Items, *n*	Subscales
Health-Related Quality-of-Life Questionnaires for Pelvic Organ Prolapse			
Pelvic Floor Disorder Impact Questionnaire (18)	Pelvic organ prolapse	46	3 subsets; one each for urinary, prolapse, and colorectal-anal. Each covers travel, social, emotional, and physical activity.
Pelvic Floor Disorder Impact Questionnaire-short form (19)	Pelvic organ prolapse	7	Not applicable
Symptom Severity Questionnaires for Pelvic Organ Prolapse			
Pelvic Floor Distress Inventory (17)	Pelvic organ prolapse	93	3 subsets; one each for urinary symptoms (obstructive, irritative, stress incontinence), prolapse (general, anterior, posterior) symptoms, and colorectal-anal symptoms (obstructive, incontinence, pain/irritation, rectal prolapse)
Pelvic Floor Distress Inventory-short form (18)	Pelvic organ prolapse	20	Not applicable
Questionnaires That Cover Both Symptom Severity and Health-Related Quality-of-Life for Pelvic Organ Prolapse			
Prolapse Quality-of-Life Questionnaire (20)	Pelvic organ prolapse	38	Role limitations, physical/social limitations, personal relationships, emotions, sleep/energy, coping measures. Symptom severity for urinary, prolapse, and anal rectal symptoms.
Sexual Function Questionnaires for Prolapse and Urinary Incontinence			
Pelvic Organ Prolapse and Incontinence Sexual Function Questionnaire (21)	Pelvic organ prolapse and/or urinary incontinence	31	Behavioral/emotive, physical, partner-related
Epidemiology Questionnaires for Pelvic Organ Prolapse, Urinary Incontinence, and Fecal Incontinence			
Epidemiology of prolapse and incontinence questionnaire (22)	Pelvic organ prolapse, overactive bladder, stress urinary incontinence, and fecal incontinence	49	Pelvic organ prolapse, stress urinary incontinence, overactive bladder, fecal incontinence, and impact on quality of life for each.

KING'S HEALTH QUESTIONNAIRE
1998
Version 8

Name _____

Age _____ years

Today's date _____/_____/_____

This questionnaire asks about any problems you <u>may</u> have with your bladder or with incontinence of urine.

How would you describe your health at present?   Please tick one answer

Very good   ◯

Good   ◯

Fair   ◯   ⬛ 5

Poor   ◯

Very poor   ◯

How much do you think your bladder affects your life?   Please tick one answer

Not at all   ◯

A little   ◯   ⬛ 4

Moderately   ◯

A lot   ◯

Please write down <u>if</u> you have any of the following symptoms and mark how much these affect you.

	None	A little	Moderately	A lot	
Going to the toilet to pass urine very often	◯	◯	◯	◯	☐
Getting up at night to pass urine	◯	◯	◯	◯	☐
Urgency: A strong desire to pass urine					☐
Urge incontinence; urinary leakage associated with a strong desire to pass urine	◯	◯	◯	◯	☐
Stress incontinence: leaking urine with coughing, sneezing, etc.	◯	◯	◯	◯	☐
Wetting the bed at night	◯	◯	◯	◯	☐
Leaking urine with sexual intercourse	◯	◯	◯	◯	☐
Frequent urine infection	◯	◯	◯	◯	☐
Any other problems? Please specify.	◯	◯	◯	◯	☐
_____					☐
					☐
					☐

Office use   ☐   ☐ + ☐ + ☐

Below are some daily activities that can be affected by your bladder problem.
How much does your bladder problem affect you?
We would like you to answer every question. <u>Simply tick the circle that applies to you.</u>

ROLE LIMITATIONS	Not at all	Slightly	Moderately	A lot
To what extent does your bladder affect your household tasks (e.g., cleaning, shopping, etc.)?	○	○	○	○
Does your bladder affect your job or your normal daily activities outside the home?	○	○	○	○

PHYSICAL/SOCIAL LIMITATIONS	Not at all	Slightly	Moderately	A lot
Does your bladder affect your physical activities (e.g., going for a walk, etc.)?	○	○	○	○
Does your bladder affect your ability to travel?	○	○	○	○
Does your bladder limit your social life?	○	○	○	○
Does your bladder limit your ability to see/visit friends?	○	○	○	○

PERSONAL RELATIONSHIPS	Not Applicable	Not at all	Slightly	Moderately	A lot
Does your bladder affect your relationship with your partner?	○	○	○	○	○
Does your bladder affect your sex life?	○	○	○	○	○
Does your bladder affect your family life?	○	○	○	○	○

EMOTIONS	Not at all	Slightly	Moderately	A lot
Does your bladder make you feel depressed?	○	○	○	○
Does your bladder make you feel anxious or nervous?	○	○	○	○
Does your bladder make you feel bad about yourself?	○	○	○	○

SLEEP/ENERGY	Never	Sometimes	Often	All the time
Does your bladder affect your sleep?	○	○	○	○
Do you feel worn out/tired?	○	○	○	○

<u>Do you do any of the following?</u>
If so, how much?

	Never	Sometimes	Often	All the time
Use pads or incontinence pants to keep dry?	○	○	○	○
Be careful how much fluid you drink?	○	○	○	○
Change your underclothes when they get wet?	○	○	○	○
Worry that you smell?	○	○	○	○

THANK YOU, NOW PLEASE CHECK THAT YOU HAVE ANSWERED ALL THE QUESTIONS   ○

Office use   ☐ ☐ ☐   ☐ ☐   ☐ ☐ ☐ ☐

TO CALCULATE SCORE

1. *General Health Perceptions*
   Score = ([Score to GHPA – 1]/4) × 100
2. *Incontinence Impact*
   Score = ([Score to GHPB – 1]/3) × 100
3. *Role Limitations*
   Score = ([(Scores to RLA + RLB) – 2]/6) × 100
4. *Physical Limitations*
   Score = ([(Score to PLA + PLB) – 2]/6) × 100
5. *Social Limitations*
   Score = ([(Score to PLC + PLD + PRC) – 3] /9) × 100 **
   ** if score to PRC1 ≤ if 0 then . . .—2) /6) × 100
6. *Personal Relationships*
   Score = ([(Score to PRA + PRB) –2] /6) × 100 ***
   *** if score to PRA + PRB ≥ 2,
   if PRA + PRB = 1; . . . –1) /3) × 100
   if PRA + PRB = 0; . . . treat as missing value (not applicable)
7. *Emotions*
   Score = ([(Score to EMA + EMB + EMC) – 3] /9)× 100
8. *Sleep/Energy*
   Score = ([(Score to SEA + SEB) – 2] /6) × 100
9. *Severity Measures*
   Score = ([(Score to SMA + SMB + SMC + SMD) – 4] /12) × 100

GHPA:	question 1 page 1
GHPB:	question 2 page 1
RLA:	question 1 page 3
RLB:	question 2 page 3
PLA:	question 3 page 3
PLB:	question 4 page 3
PLC:	question 5 page 3
PLD:	question 6 page 3
PRA:	question 7 page 3
PRB:	question 8 page 3
PRC:	question 9 page 3
EMA:	question 1 page 4
EMB:	question 2 page 4
EMC:	question 3 page 4
SEA:	question 4 page 4
SEB:	question 5 page 4
SMA:	question 6 page 4
SMB:	question 7 page 4
SMC:	question 8 page 4
SMD:	question 9 page 4

The questions about urinary, bowel, and sexual symptoms do not have a score.

REFERENCES

1. Amarenco G, Arnould B, Carita P, et al. European psychometric validation of the CONTILIFE: a quality-of-life questionnaire for urinary incontinence. *Eur Urol* 2003;43:391–404.
2. Shumaker SA, Wyman JK, Uebersax JS, et al. Health-related quality-of-life measures for women with urinary incontinence: the Incontinence Impact Questionnaire and the Urogenital Distress Inventory. Continence Program in Women (CPW) Research Group. *Qual Life Res* 1994;3:291–306.
3. van der Vaart CH, de Leeuw JR, Roovers JP, et al. The effect of urinary incontinence and overactive bladder symptoms on quality of life in young women. *BJU Int* 2002;90:544–549.
4. Uebersax JS, Wyman JF, Shumaker SA, et al. Short forms to assess life quality and symptom distress for urinary incontinence in women: the Incontinence Impact Questionnaire and the Urogenital Distress Inventory. *Neurourol Urodyn* 1995;14:131–139.
5. Wagner TH, Patrick DL, Bavendam TG, et al. Quality of life of persons with urinary incontinence: development of a new measure, *Urology* 1996;47:67–71.
6. Yu LC, Kaltreider DL, Hu T, et al. The ISQ-P tool: measuring stress associated with incontinence. *J Gerontol Nurs* 1989;15:9–15.
7. Coyne K, Revicki D, Hunt T, et al. Psychometric validation of an overactive bladder symptoms and health-related quality-of-life questionnaire: the OAB-q. *Qual Life Res* 2002;11:563–574.
8. Marquis P, Amarenco G, Sapede C, et al. Development and validation of a disease-specific quality-of-life questionnaire for urinary urge incontinency. *Qual Life Res* 1995;4:458–459.
9. Black N, Griffiths J, Pope C. Development of a symptom severity index and a symptoms impact index for stress incontinence in women. *Neurourol Urodyn* 1996; 15:630–640.
10. DuBeau CE, Kiely DK, Resnick NM. Quality-of-life impact of urge incontinence in older persons: a new measure and conceptual structure. *J Am Geriatr Soc* 1999;47:989–994.
11. Lubeck DP, Prebil LA, Peeples P, et al. A health-related qualify-of-life measure for use in patients with urge urinary incontinence: a validation study. *Qual Life Res* 1999;8:337–344.
12. Rai GS, Kiniors M, Wientjes H. Urinary incontinence handicap inventory. *Arch Gerontol Geriatr* 1994;19:7–10.
13. Stach-Lempinen B,. Kujansuu E, Laippale P, et al. Visual analogue scale, urinary incontinence severity score, and 15 D-psychometric testing of three different health-related quality-of-life instruments for urinary incontinent women. *Scand J Urol Nephrol* 2001;35:476–483.
14. Lee PS, Reid DW, Saltmarche A, et al. Measuring the psychosocial impact of urinary incontinence: the York Incontinence Perceptions Scale (YIPS). *J Am Geriatr Soc* 1995;43:1275–1278.
15. Sandvik H, Hunskaar S, Seim A, et al. Validation of a severity index in female urinary incontinence and its implementation in an epidemiological survey. *J Epidemiol Comm Health* 1993;47:497–499.
16. Published online with all accompanying articles regarding validation of the individual modules at www.iciq.net.
17. Kelleher CJ, Cardozo LD, Khullar V, et al. A new questionnaire to assess the quality of life of urinary incontinent women. *Br J Obstet Gynaecol* 1997;104:1374–1379.

18. Barber MD, Kuchibhatia MN, Pieper CF, et al. Psychometric evaluation of 2 comprehensive condition-specific quality-of-life instruments for women with pelvic floor disorders. *Am J Obstet Gynecol* 2001;185:1388–1395.

19. Barber MD, Walters MD, Bump RC. Short forms of two condition-specific quality of life questionnaires for women with pelvic floor disorders (PFDI-20 & PFIQ-7). *Am J Obstet Gynecol* 2005;193:102–113.

20. Digesu GA, Khullar V, Cardozo L, et al. P-QOL: a validated questionnaire to assess the symptoms and quality of life of women with urogenital prolapse. *Int Urogynecol J* 2005;16:176–181.

21. Rogers R, Kammerer-Doak D, Villarreal A, et al. A new instrument to measure sexual function in women with urinary incontinence and pelvic organ prolapse. *Am J Obstet Gynecol* 2001;184:552–558.

22. Lukacz ES, Lawrence JM, Buckwalter JG, et al. Epidemiology of prolapse and incontinence questionnaire: validation of a new epidemiologic survey. *Int Urogynecol J* 2005;16:272–284.

Index